HEALTHCARE TECHNOLOGIES SERIES 1

Nanobiosensors for Personalized and Onsite Biomedical Diagnosis

Nanobiosensors for Personalized and Onsite Biomedical Diagnosis

Edited by Pranjal Chandra

The Institution of Engineering and Technology

Published by The Institution of Engineering and Technology, London, United Kingdom

The Institution of Engineering and Technology is registered as a Charity in England & Wales (no. 211014) and Scotland (no. SC038698).

First published 2016

The Institution of Engineering and Technology
Michael Faraday House
Six Hills Way, Stevenage
Herts, SG1 2AY, United Kingdom

www.theiet.org

British Library Cataloguing in Publication Data
A catalogue record for this product is available from the British Library

ISBN 978-1-84919-950-6 (hardback)
ISBN 978-1-84919-951-3 (PDF)

Typeset in India by MPS Limited
Printed in the UK by CPI Group (UK) Ltd, Croydon

This book is affectionately dedicated to
my loving daughter "Pranya",
wife "Ananya",
mother "Neelam",
and
father "Prof. Ramesh Chandra Srivastava".

Contents

About the Author **xix**

1 Gold nanoparticle-based electrochemical biosensors for biomedical diagnosis applications **1**
1.1 Introduction 1
1.2 Synthesis of AuNPs 3
1.2.1 Electrodeposition of AuNPs 3
1.2.2 Chemical synthesis of AuNPs 4
1.3 Functions of AuNPs in electrochemical biosensors 4
1.3.1 Improvement of electron transfer efficiency 5
1.3.2 Immobilization of biological recognition element 7
1.3.3 Signal generation and amplification 8
1.4 Conclusions and outlook 14
Acknowledgments 15
References 15

2 Development and application of microbiosensors for *in-vivo* diagnostics **21**
2.1 Introduction 21
2.2 *In-vivo* enzymatic biosensors 22
2.2.1 Commercialized continuous glucose monitoring systems (CGMS) 22
2.2.2 *In-vivo* enzymatic biosensor systems in development 24
2.3 Development of non-enzymatic *in-vivo* biosensors 29
2.4 Conclusion 30
References 30

3 Electrochemical biosensors: fabrication and applications in biodiagnostics **37**
3.1 Principle of electrochemical biosensor 37
3.1.1 Voltammetry 37
3.1.2 Potentiometry 38
3.1.3 Surface charge using field-effect transistors (FETs) 38
3.1.4 Conductometry 39
3.2 Electrochemical nucleic acid sensors 39
3.2.1 Detection of Genotoxicants/Pesticide 40
3.2.2 Detection of hybridisation can be done by different strategies 40

3.3 Electrochemical enzymatic sensor 42
3.3.1 Direct detection of analytes 42
3.3.2 Indirect detection of analytes via inhibition of enzyme activity 43
3.4 Electrochemical immunosensors 43
3.4.1 An indirect immunosensor 43
3.4.2 The direct immunosensor 44
3.5 Electrochemical whole cells based sensors 44
3.5.1 Based on the cellular activity of the cell 45
3.5.2 Based on cellular barrier behavior 45
3.6 Electrochemical aptasensors 45
3.7 Widely used materials in the construction of electrochemical biosensors 45
3.7.1 Conducting polymers 45
3.7.2 Carbon nanomaterial in electrochemical biosensors 47
3.7.3 Nanoparticles 48
3.8 Practical applications of the electrochemical biosensors 49
3.8.1 Biosensors of healthcare 49
3.8.2 Biosensors for environmental monitoring 50
3.8.3 Biosensors in food industry 51
3.8.4 Biosensors for cancer 52
3.8.5 Biosensors for pathogens 52
Acknowledgement 53
References 53

4 Microchip-based separation and detection methods for chemically and biologically valuable analytes 55
4.1 Introduction 55
4.2 Separation and detection methods for chemically and biologically valuable analytes 57
4.2.1 Separation and extraction of DNA 57
4.2.2 Separation of proteins 58
4.2.3 Separation of small biological analytes 62
4.2.4 Miscellaneous separation 64
4.3 Challenges and future outlook 67
4.4 Conclusion 67
Acknowledgment 68
References 68

5 Biosensors of *in vitro* detection of cancer and bacterial cells 73
5.1 Introduction 73
5.2 Biosensors of *in vitro* detection of cancer cells 75
5.2.1 Aptamers for detection of cancer cells 75
5.3 Biosensors of *in vitro* detection of bacterial cells 79
5.3.1 Electrochemical and optical nanobiosensors for bacterial cells detection 79

5.3.2 Microfluidics for bacterial cells detection 81
5.3.3 Paper-based nanobiosensors for bacterial cell detection 82
5.3.4 Lab-on-a-chip and chip-plate based nanobiosensors for bacterial cells detection 83
5.3.5 Perspectives of nanobiosensors in bacterial cells detection 83
5.4 Conclusion and final remarks 84
References 85

6 Biacore – a surface plasmon resonance-based technology 95
6.1 Introduction 95
6.2 Biacore technology 97
6.3 Principle in biacore system 97
6.4 Biacore sensing surfaces 99
6.5 Non-fouling on Biacore sensing surfaces 101
6.6 Biomolecular recognition in biacore system 102
6.7 Kinetic analyses 103
6.8 Refunctioning and regeneration of chip surfaces 103
6.9 Recommendations for controlled experiments 105
6.10 Conclusions 105
References 105

7 Implantable microbiosensors: towards *in vivo* monitoring 109
7.1 Introduction 109
7.2 Microbiosensor technologies 111
7.3 Analyte-specific biosensors 115
7.4 New materials for improving the *in vivo* stability of implantable microbiosensors 122
7.5 Conclusion and future prospects 129
Acknowledgement 130
References 130

8 Nanomaterials based biosensors: a smart approach towards on-site clinical diagnosis 139
8.1 Introduction 139
8.2 Conventional techniques for clinical diagnosis 141
8.3 Nanomaterials for clinical diagnosis 141
8.3.1 Metal nanoparticles 144
8.3.2 Quantum dots 145
8.3.3 Magnetic nanoparticles 146
8.3.4 Carbon nanostructures 148
8.3.5 Nanostructured conducting polymers 149
8.3.6 Nanostructured metal oxide 151
8.4 Challenges and future prospects 158
8.5 Conclusions 158
Acknowledgments 159
References 159

9 Optical waveguide-based biosensor for label-free monitoring of living cells **165**
Abstract 165
9.1 Label-free optical biosensors in cell adhesion research 165
9.2 The Epic BenchTop optical biosensor 167
9.3 Cell adhesion on tailored surfaces 169
9.4 The dependence of cell adhesion kinetics on the surface density of integrin ligands, as measured with the Epic BT biosensor 170
9.5 Outlook 175
Acknowledgment 175
References 175

10 Optical biosensors for the detection of food borne pathogens **181**
10.1 Introduction 181
10.2 Current technologies for pathogen detection 182
10.3 Enzyme-linked immunosorbent assay (ELISA) 182
10.4 Polymerase chain reaction (PCR) 183
10.5 Biosensors 183
10.5.1 Overview 183
10.5.2 Biorecognition techniques 184
10.5.3 Antibodies 184
10.5.4 Enzymes 184
10.5.5 Nucleic acids 184
10.6 Transduction techniques 185
10.6.1 Electrochemical 185
10.6.2 Piezoelectric 185
10.7 Sample preparation 185
10.8 Optical biosensors 186
10.8.1 Surface plasmon resonance (SPR) 186
10.9 Fluorescence 188
10.9.1 Auto-fluorescent protein (AFP) 189
10.9.2 Bioluminescence resonance energy transfer 189
10.9.3 Quantum dots 189
10.10 Surface enhanced Raman spectroscopy (SERS) 195
10.11 Other methods 199
10.11.1 Interferometry 199
10.11.2 Optical fibre 199
10.11.3 Carbon nanotubes 200
10.12 Conclusions and future prospects 202
Acknowledgements 204
References 204

11 Generation and optimisation of antibodies for biosensor applications **209**
11.1 Antibody generation for use in biosensors 209

11.2 Polyclonal antibody generation 211
11.2.1 Process of adaptive immune response 211
11.2.2 Hosts for polyclonal antibody production 212
11.2.3 Purification of polyclonal antibodies 214
11.3 Monoclonal antibody generation 215
11.3.1 Hybridoma cell production 215
11.3.2 Purification of monoclonal antibodies 216
11.3.3 Recombinant antibody generation 216
11.3.4 Generation of recombinant antibodies 217
11.3.5 Selection of recombinant antibodies through phage display 217
11.3.6 DiCAST, a novel technology of direct clone analysis and selection 219
11.3.7 Selection of recombinant antibodies using Biacore 4000 220
11.3.8 Expression of soluble recombinant antibodies 220
11.3.9 Purification of recombinant antibodies 221
11.4 Antibody optimisation for biosensor applications 221
11.4.1 Optimisation of antibody specificity, sensitivity and affinity for biosensors through genetic modification 221
11.4.2 Optimisation of antibody stability for biosensor applications 223
11.4.3 Optimisation of antibody immobilisation strategies for biosensors 224
11.5 Summary 225
Acknowledgements 225
References 225

12 Smartphone-based *in vitro* diagnostic technologies for personalized healthcare monitoring and management 231
12.1 Introduction 231
12.2 Signal detection in SP-based *in vitro* diagnostics 232
12.2.1 Colorimetric, fluorescent and luminescent detection 232
12.2.2 SPR detection 233
12.2.3 Lateral flow assays 236
12.2.4 Microscopy 236
12.2.5 Electrochemical detection 236
12.2.6 Cytometry 239
12.3 Applications of smartphone-based *in vitro* diagnostics 241
12.3.1 Detection of biomolecules, metabolites and biomarkers 241
12.3.2 Detection of microorganisms 242
12.3.3 Detection of other analytes 246
12.3.4 Other bio-analytical applications 246
12.4 Conclusions, challenges and future trends 246
References 247

13 Lateral flow biosensors **253**
13.1 Introduction 253
13.2 The mechanism of lateral flow immunoassay 253
13.3 Types of LFIA 255
13.3.1 Noncompetitive immunoassay 255
13.3.2 Competitive immunoassay 255
13.4 LFIA components 255
13.4.1 Antibodies 257
13.4.2 Membrane 258
13.4.3 Tracers 260
13.4.4 Pads 261
13.5 Important parameters for LFIA 262
13.5.1 Biomolecule immobilization 262
13.5.2 Biomolecule coverage on the tracer 264
13.5.3 Buffer and pH 264
13.6 Applications of lateral flow biosensors 264
13.7 Major hurdles facing the lateral flow biosensors 265
13.8 Future perspectives of lateral flow biosensors for personalized and onsite medicine 266
13.9 Conclusion 267
References 268

14 MicroRNAs and their applications in diagnosis for osteoarthritis **277**
14.1 Introduction 277
14.2 Potential miRNAs as early diagnostic biomarkers for OA 278
14.2.1 miR-146 279
14.2.2 miR-140 280
14.2.3 miR-22 280
14.2.4 miR-27b 281
14.3 MiRNAs biomarker detection technologies 282
14.4 Nano-biomaterials for molecular beacon-based miRNA detection 284
14.5 Conclusions 286
References 287

15 Electrochemical capacitive biosensors for point-of-care diagnostics: principles and applications **293**
15.1 Introduction 293
15.1.1 Electrochemistry and biosensors 293
15.1.2 Potentiometric, amperometric and impedimetric biosensors 298
15.2 Types of capacitance and capacitive phenomena 301
15.2.1 Electrostatic or geometrical capacitance 302
15.2.2 Double-layer capacitance 302
15.2.3 Dipolar capacitance of molecular layers 304
15.2.4 Electrochemical capacitance 306

15.3 Capacitive biosensors 309
15.4 Summarization and perspectives 313
References 314

16 AC electrokinetics-based capacitive biosensor as a platform technology for on-site detection of biospecific interactions 317
16.1 Introduction 317
16.2 Mechanisms 319
16.2.1 Capacitive detection of biomolecular binding on electrode surface 319
16.2.2 Direct detection of interfacial capacitance 320
16.2.3 ACEK enhancement of affinity sensing 321
16.3 Devices and methods 324
16.3.1 Interdigitated microelectrode sensors 324
16.3.2 Sample preparation and electrode functionalization 324
16.3.3 Measurement procedure 326
16.4 Experiments 326
16.4.1 Capacitive sensing for rapid analysis of surface quality control 326
16.4.2 Capacitance changes due to protein binding and detachment 327
16.4.3 Sensitive and quantitative detection 328
16.4.4 Effect of AC frequency 329
16.4.5 Effect of electrode designs 332
16.4.6 Selectivity in complex fluids 334
16.5 Conclusions 336
Acknowledgments 338
References 338

17 Fibre optical technology for monitoring and diagnostic applications 341
17.1 Introduction 341
17.1.1 Fibre optic technology 342
17.1.2 Bioreceptors 345
17.2 Immobilization 346
17.2.1 Adsorption 346
17.2.2 Microencapsulation 346
17.2.3 Entrapment 347
17.2.4 Cross-linking 347
17.2.5 Covalent bonding 347
17.3 Sensing schemes 347
17.3.1 Absorbance 348
17.3.2 Fluorescent 349
17.4 Surface plasmon resonance (SPR) 350
17.5 Advantageous and disadvantageous of optical fibre biosensors 350

17.6 Clinical and diagnostic applications 351
17.7 Biosensors for diabetes applications 352
17.7.1 Glucose as diabetes biomarker 352
17.7.2 Biosensors for glucose measuring 352
17.8 Biosensors for cardiovascular diseases applications 353
17.8.1 Cardiovascular disease biomarkers 353
17.8.2 Biosensors in cardiovascular disease 353
17.9 Biosensors for cancer applications 354
17.9.1 Cancer biomarkers 354
17.9.2 Biosensors in cancer disease 355
17.10 Conclusions 355
References 356

18 Nanobiosensors for the detection of circulating tumor cells 363
18.1 Introduction 363
18.2 Nanostructured interfaces designed for CTC detection 364
18.2.1 From micro to nano 364
18.2.2 From artificial to biomimetic 366
18.2.3 From traditional to smart 368
18.3 Purification and isolation strategy based on nanostructured interfaces 371
18.4 Conclusions and prospects 373
Acknowledgments 373
References 374

19 Design investigations for robust and continuous online heartbeat monitoring using wearable vs. Doppler-based non-contact vital signs biosensors 379
19.1 Wearable ECG sensors 379
19.1.1 Components of the wearable ECG sensor system 381
19.2 Implantable cardioverter defibrillator (ICD) 384
19.2.1 Components of the ICD system 385
19.3 Biosignal instrumentation amplifier (INA) 387
19.3.1 Biosignal Instrumentation Amplifier (INA) 389
19.3.2 INA design consideration 390
19.3.3 Fully differential folded-cascode based chopper stabilized INA 391
19.3.4 State-of-the-art performance comparison 398
19.4 Doppler-based non-contact vital signs (NCVS) sensor 398
19.4.1 Doppler radar principle for NCVS Sensor 400
19.4.2 Quadrature receiver and arc-tangent demodulation for NCVS sensors 401
19.4.3 Direct-conversion receiver and range correlation in NCVS sensors 403

19.4.4 Antenna characterization for NCVS sensor – directivity and radiation patterns 405
19.4.5 NCVS system evaluated with several antennas 406
19.4.6 Experimental results and analysis 411
19.5 Summary of heart beat sensing techniques 415
References 416

20 Lab on a chip for point-of-care analysis of drugs in body fluids 421
20.1 Introduction 421
20.2 Point-of-collection testing (POCT) 422
20.3 Lab-on-chip system for POCT 423
20.3.1 Materials and fabrication 423
20.3.2 Detection 425
20.3.3 POCT drug analysis in body fluids with lab-on-chip systems 428
20.4 Conclusions and future directions 438
References 439

21 Hydrogel-based biosensors: fundamentals and applications 443
21.1 Introduction 443
21.2 General properties of hydrogel 444
21.2.1 Equilibrium swelling 444
21.2.2 Swelling kinetics 446
21.2.3 Pore size/porosity of the gels 447
21.3 Immobilization of biomolecules and applications as biosensors 448
21.3.1 Physical deposition and cross-linking 449
21.3.2 Entrapment 449
21.3.3 Covalent immobilization 450
21.3.4 Electrostatic immobilization 452
21.3.5 Affinity-based immobilization 453
21.4 Multi-analyte detecting system 453
21.5 Summary 455
References 455

22 Applications of graphene microelectrodes in clinical analysis 459
22.1 Biosensors based on nanostructured materials 459
22.2 Graphene nanomaterials used in electrochemical biosensors fabrication 460
22.3 Miniaturized graphene electrochemical biosensors for health monitoring 461
22.3.1 Enzymatic biosensors 461
22.3.2 Immunosensors 465
22.3.3 DNA sensors 467

22.4 Conclusions and future prospects 468
Acknowledgments 469
References 469

23 Sensing of nucleic acids and cancer cells using nanostructure-SPR integrated with microfluidic chip 473
23.1 Introduction 473
23.2 Conventional SPR 474
23.3 Localized surface plasmon resonance (LSPR) 474
23.4 Nanostructure array SPR 476
23.5 Integration of SPR sensors with microfluidic chip 480
23.6 SPR sensors for multiplexing 480
23.7 SPR-based biosensors 482
23.7.1 SPR-based biosensors for detection of nucleic acids 483
23.7.2 SPR-based biosensors for detection of cancer cells 488
23.8 Conclusion 491
References 492

24 Surface plasmon resonance based miniaturized biosensors for medical applications 499
24.1 Introduction 499
24.2 Principle of SPR-sensors work 500
24.3 Types of SPR-sensors 502
24.3.1 SPR-sensors with prismatic coupling devices (couplers) 502
24.3.2 SPR-sensors with waveguide coupling devices 504
24.3.3 SPR-sensors with diffraction gratings 504
24.3.4 Localized SPR (LSPR) 504
24.4 Analytical parameters of SPR-sensors 505
24.5 Sensor surface functionalization 506
24.5.1 Covalent binding 506
24.5.2 Non-covalent binding 507
24.6 SPR-analysis formats 507
24.7 Mass-produced SPR-sensors 509
24.8 SPR-sensors for non-laboratory diagnostics 509
24.8.1 Commercial portable SPR-sensors 509
24.8.2 Recent works in portable SPR-sensors development 513
24.9 Conclusion 515
Acknowledgments 516
References 516

25 Methods for monitoring oxidative stress using conventional and advanced nanodiagnostics methods 521
25.1 Introduction 521
25.1.1 Oxidants 521
25.1.2 Antioxidants 522

25.2 Conventional methods for monitoring oxidative stress 523
25.2.1 Determination of total antioxidant activity 523
25.2.2 Method for monitoring lipid peroxidation 524
25.2.3 Measurement of redox status – reduced glutathione (GSH)/oxidized glutathione (GSSG) ratio 524
25.3 Measurement of oxidative status using various oxidative stress biomarkers 525
25.3.1 Determination of acetylcholinesterase activity 525
25.3.2 Determination of membrane sulfhydryl (–SH) group 526
25.3.3 Determination of protein carbonyl content 527
25.3.4 Determination of red blood cell osmotic fragility 529
25.4 Advanced nanodiagnostic methods for monitoring oxidative stress 529
25.4.1 Gold nanoparticle based assay for biomarker of oxidative stress 530
25.4.2 Detection of glutathione using biosensor 530
25.4.3 Detection of 3-nitro-L-tyrosine (3NT) using solid phase extraction (SPE) sorbent material 531
25.4.4 Microsensor arrays 533
25.4.5 Detection of 8-hydroxy-2'-deoxyguanosine (8OHdG) using immunosensor 533
25.5 Conclusion and the future 533
Acknowledgment 534
List of abbreviations 534
References 534

26 Metallic nanobiosensors for biological analysis and medical diagnostics 537
26.1 Introduction 537
26.2 Sensing principles 540
26.2.1 Sensing based on absorption of metal NPs 540
26.2.2 Sensing based on light scattering of metal NPs 544
26.2.3 Sensing based on interaction between metal NPs and fluorophore/reporter 547
26.2.4 Sensing based on intrinsic luminescent properties of metal NCs 550
26.2.5 Summary/outlook 554
26.3 Development of paper-based POC diagnostic devices 554
26.3.1 Dipstick assays 555
26.3.2 Lateral flow assays 555
26.3.3 Microfluidic paper analytical devices 556
26.3.4 Summary/outlook 557
26.4 Future perspectives 558
26.4.1 Commercialization potentials 558
26.4.2 Future challenges 558
References 559

27 Carbon nanomaterial based biosensors for onsite biomedical diagnosis **567**
27.1 Introduction 567
27.2 Basic instruction about carbon nanomaterials (CNMs) 567
27.3 CNMs-based biosensor and its applications 569
27.3.1 In vitro application of CNMs biosensor 569
27.3.2 In vivo application of CNMs-based biosensor 574
27.4 Conclusions 577
References 579

28 Nanoparticle-based sensing of oligonucleotides and proteins **583**
28.1 Introduction 583
28.2 Sensing of oligonucleotides 584
28.3 Sensing of protein 586
28.4 Conclusion 590
References 591

Index **593**

About the Author

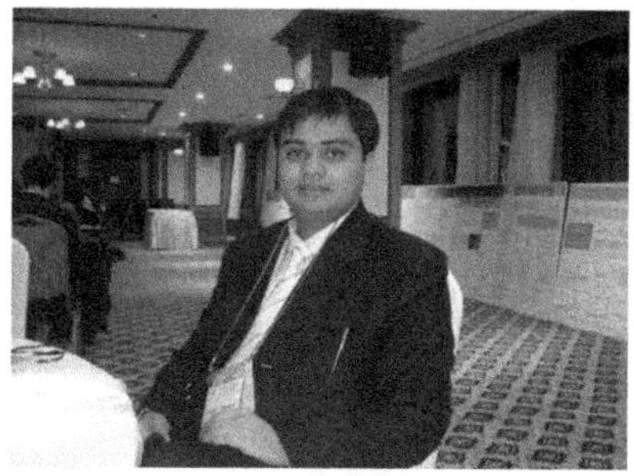

Dr. Pranjal Chandra is currently working as Assistant Professor and Principal Investigator in Department of Biosciences and Bioengineering at the Indian Institute of Technology Guwahati (IITG), Guwahati, India. He earned his PhD from the Institute of Biophysio Sensor Technology, Pusan National University, South Korea and did postdoctoral research at Technion – Israel Institute of Technology, Israel. His research group is working towards the development of cheap diagnostic methods based on nanobiosensors, microfluidic systems, paper based sensors for biomedical diagnostics and environmental monitoring. He is recipient of several awards and fellowships including the Ramanujan Fellowship awarded by Government of India. Dr. Chandra is editorial board member of various journals including *World Journal of Methodology, USA*.

About the Author

Chapter 1

Gold nanoparticle-based electrochemical biosensors for biomedical diagnosis applications

Ye Zhu[1]

1.1 Introduction

Detection of disease biomarkers based on specific binding interaction between the recognizer biomolecules and the target molecules is of significance for clinical diagnosis. Transduction of the binding event into a measurable signal is the essential task of such kind of detection. More than four decades ago, Clark and Lyons pointed out the significance in designing of biosensors as economical and fast tools for clinical studies [1]. Biosensors are analytical devices incorporating a biological recognition element with a physicochemical transducer [2]. When the biological recognition element binds with its specific target, the corresponding biological reaction can be monitored by the transducer and can be transduced into a detectable signal. The most common physicochemical transducers used for biosensors are classified to be electrochemical, optical, thermometric, piezoelectric etc. [2]. Among all them, biosensors based on electrochemical transducer have attracted considerable interest. For instance, electrochemical immunosensor, which is developed based on the antibody/antigen specific immune reaction, is a representative group of affinity biosensors for clinical diagnosis [3]. This kind of biosensors can transduce the specific binding between the antibody recognizer and the antigen target into detectable electrochemical signals, which might be amperometric, potentiometric, impedimetric or conductometric [1]. The schematic presentation of an electrochemical immunosensor is illustrated in Figure 1.1. Because of the high sensitivity, fast analytical time, inherent simplicity, miniaturization, low cost and power requirement, electrochemical biosensors have emerged as promising approach for clinical diagnosis and attracted considerable attention [4]. Especially, as the concept of 'point-of-care testing' has attracted growing attention, electrochemical biosensors have been widely explored as attractive and promising candidates for the

[1]School of Chemistry and Chemical Engineering, Shandong University, Jinan 250100, China

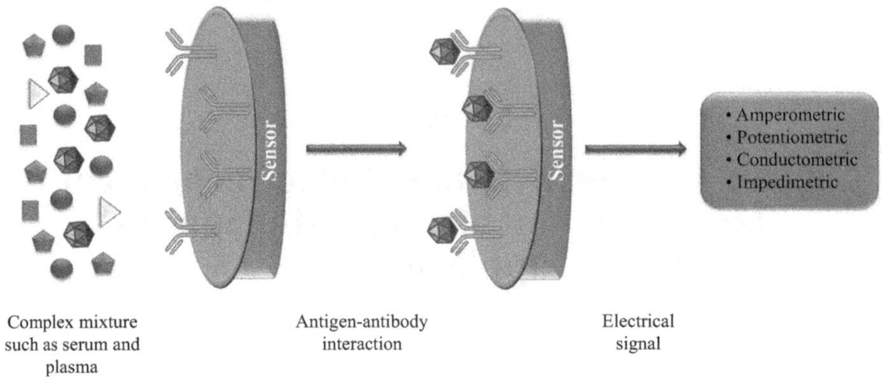

Figure 1.1 Schematic representation of electrochemical immunosensor [1]

development of portable systems and onsite monitoring devices for point-of-care medical diagnosis [5,6].

Owing to the rapid progress of interdisciplinary research, the development of electrochemical biosensors has been highly promoted by other advanced technologies and materials. Nanotechnology is the fast expanding area of research focusing on the development of novel diagnostic strategies [7]. Nanotechnology generates various nanomaterials (at 1–100 nm scale) with unique large surface area-to-volume ratio and size- and morphology-tunable electronic, conductive and catalytic properties [8]. The use of nanomaterials provides the electrochemical biosensors with high surface area for the immobilization of biological recognizers and thus facilitating better access of analytes to these recognizers, signal amplification, and label-free-real-time detection. Therefore, introduction of nanomaterials into fabrication of electrochemical biosensors leads to ultrasensitive detection of ultralow levels of disease biomarkers [7].

Among various nanomaterials, such as metal nanoparticles, carbon nanotubes, graphene, quantum dots, magnetic beads, and various nanocomposites, noble metal nanoparticles like gold nanoparticles (AuNPs) are the perfect raw materials for robust, rapid clinical diagnostics. The minute quantities required make AuNPs inexpensive, whilst their stability, sensitivity, and reproducibility as well as high-quality supplies give manufacture guarantee due to which AuNPs are already commercially available [9,10]. Furthermore, AuNPs possess excellent conductivity, biocompatibility, and catalytic properties [11,12]. They can be easily functionalized with selected chemical groups or combined with other materials to yield original nanohybrids and nanocomposite with new and improved characteristics [8,13]. These unique properties make AuNPs the ultimate nanoscale materials for diagnostic purposes. They have been widely employed for fabrication of electrochemical biosensors with high performance for various biomedical diagnoses.

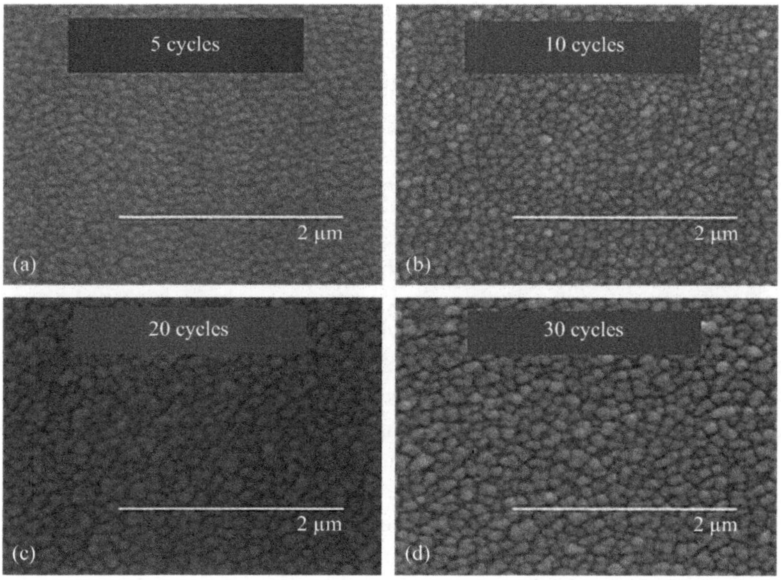

Figure 1.2 SEM images of AuNPs electrodeposited on ITO surface for (a) 5 cycles, (b) 10 cycles, (c) 20 cycles, and (d) 30 cycles of CV [19]

1.2 Synthesis of AuNPs

The synthesis approaches of AuNPs for electrochemical biosensors applications mainly include direct electrodeposition onto electrode surface and chemical reduction synthesis.

1.2.1 Electrodeposition of AuNPs

Electrodeposition of AuNPs onto electrode surface is a simple and effective modification approach, which can be achieved through several electrochemical techniques. AuNPs can be electrochemically deposited onto the pretreated electrode in $HAuCl_4$ solution by linear sweeping the potential from +1.4 V to +0.5 V (vs. Ag/AgCl) [14], cycling the potential between +0.1 V and +1.6 V [15], or applying a constant potential of −0.2 V [16–18]. Usually, the deposited AuNPs onto the electrode surface exhibit a size between 20 nm and 100 nm, which increases with the increasing potential scanning cycles or deposition time. Cheng *et al.* found that the size of deposited AuNPs was also significantly affected by the applied potential and supporting electrolyte concentration (as shown in Figure 1.2) [19]. Previous studies have demonstrated that AuNPs can effectively improve the electrode conductivity and extend the electroactive area of the working electrode [15–18]. In addition, AuNPs possess excellent biocompatibility and abundant surface chemical properties, and thus can easily interact with biomolecules. Due to the advantages of large active surface, biocompatibility, high conductivity, and convenience for immobilization of biomolecules, the deposition of AuNPs onto the electrode surface has been considered an outstanding technique to improve the sensitivity of the electrochemical sensors [15].

1.2.2 Chemical synthesis of AuNPs

AuNPs colloid solution can be prepared via chemically reducing gold ions by several reducing regents, such as sodium borohydride and sodium citrate. However, the high surface energy of AuNPs makes them extremely reactive and aggregation happens easily in the AuNPs system without protection or passivation of their surfaces. To avoid the aggregation and precipitation, chemically synthesized AuNPs are usually prepared in the presence of a stabilizer which binds to their surface to impart high stability and rich linking chemistry and provides the desired charge and solubility properties [20]. The most common synthesis route for AuNPs in aqueous phase is Turkevich method, which employs sodium citrate as both reductant and stabilizer [21,22]. In that method, sodium citrate is added into boiling $HAuCl_4$ solution, resulting in the formation of AuNPs companied by a color change of the solution. The AuNPs size varies with the gold-to-reductant ratio, concentration of reducing agent, and seed-mediated growth [21,22]. The diameters of AuNPs used for electrochemical biosensors are usually controlled in the range of 10–20 nm, which facilitates the further modification [23–25].

Except for typical Turkevich method, chemical synthesis of AuNPs by using sodium borohydride as the reductant was developed, which can be conducted at room temperature [26]. Recently, Alocilja developed a green alkaline based AuNPs synthesis procedure using a linear oligosaccharide (dextrin) as a coating agent. This procedure can produce AuNPs under alkaline conditions (pH 9) at room temperature, opening the possibility for explorations of biomolecule (DNA) functionalization during synthesis [27,28].

Compared with the electrodeposited AuNPs, chemical synthesized AuNPs can paly more roles in an electrochemical biosensor due to facile modification with biomolecules. As illustrated in Figure 1.3, proteins like antibody can interact with AuNPs through electrostatic interaction, hydrophobic interaction, and covalent conjugation [29], offering stable primary antibody immobilization or secondary antibody-AuNP bioconjugate for signal amplification. The strong affinity of AuNPs toward thiol-modified molecules through covalent Au-S bonds provides more possibility to design novel electrochemical biosensors for clinical diagnosis.

1.3 Functions of AuNPs in electrochemical biosensors

According to the roles of AuNPs playing in electrochemical biosensors, they can improve the analytical performance mainly in three aspects, (i) improvement of electron transfer efficiency, (ii) immobilization of biological recognition elements, and (iii) signal generation and amplification.

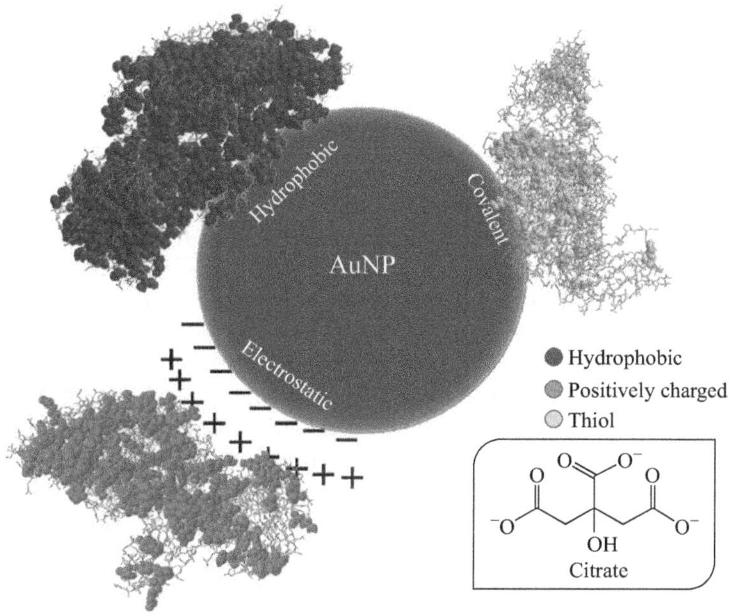

Figure 1.3 Schematic representations of the different modes of interaction involved in conjugation of antibodies to AuNPs [29]

1.3.1 Improvement of electron transfer efficiency

For an electrochemical biosensor, the electrode is a very important element which is applied as the platform for biological recognizer immobilization, the place where the biological reaction occurs, and the transducer to convert the biological or chemical information into measurable electronic signals. Therefore, effective modification of an electrode is crucial for the development of a satisfying electrochemical biosensor [30]. Common electrodes used in electrochemical sensors include glassy carbon electrode, metal electrode, screen printed electrode, indium tin oxide coated glass electrode, and so on. Most of them possess low conductivity and limited active area, which decelerates the electron transfer rate and limits the sensitivity of the electrochemical sensors. To solve these problems, using highly conductive and electroactive nanomaterial incorporated electrodes as signal transducers is a trend in recent electrochemical biosensor development. As the nanomaterial that can be easily synthesized and exhibits excellent conductivity, electrochemical activity, and high surface area-to-volume ratio, AuNPs are well suitable for the modification of electrode surface and can tremendously improve the sensitivity of the electrochemical sensors to detect biomarkers at ultralow level [7].

The electrodes are usually modified with AuNPs in different ways. The simplest way is to directly electrodeposit an AuNP layer onto the electrode surface. Electrochemical impedance spectra have demonstrated that the AuNP-deposited electrode exhibits lower impedance values than bare electrodes, and even bare gold electrode [15,16]. Cyclic voltammetric studies in $[Fe\ (CN)_6]^{3-/4-}$ solution have suggested that the electroactive area of the working electrode can be effectively extended by the deposited AuNPs [15,17,18]. By means of this simple and effective electrode modification method, a large number of electrochemical biosensors have been fabricated for biomedical diagnosis purpose. For instance, Shim's group reported a series of AuNP-deposited electrochemical biosensors for the detection of coenzymes, cancer biomarkers, and cancer cells [31–33]. Furthermore, they successfully developed a highly sensitive and stable AuNP-deposited microelectrode for in vivo detection of glutathione disulfide and oxidative stress monitoring [34]. Cheng *et al.* reported AuNP-modified indium tin oxide coated glassy electrode as a DNA sensor for impedimetric detection of a specific point mutation in apolipoprotein E gene, which was related to the progression of Alzheimer's disease [19]. Liu *et al.* fabricated an electrochemical DNA biosensor that was modified with graphene and AuNPs for the detection of mycobacterium tuberculosis [18]. All the above literatures demonstrated that electrodeposited AuNPs can effectively increase the conductivity and the electroactive area of the electrode and thus improve the sensitivity of the sensors.

Compared with the electrodeposited AuNPs, the modification of the electrodes with chemical synthesized AuNPs is diversified. Fakanya *et al.* fabricated screen-printed electrodes with gold colloid ink to detect inflammation biomarker C-reactive protein in serum samples. The developed electrode exhibited better performance than other control electrodes [35]. Wang and Li reported ultrasensitive electrochemical immunosensors for detection of cancer biomarkers based on AuNP-modified electrode [23,24]. AuNPs were attached onto the electrode through the chemical interaction with self-assembled 1, 6-hexanedithiol. Compared with the bare gold electrode, the AuNP-modified electrodes not only act as an effective conduction pathway for the electron transfer, but also provide more active sites for electron transfer and the adsorption of biomolecules. Furthermore, the AuNP-modified electrodes exhibited better uniformity, ensuring the reproducibility of the fabricated sensors [23].

To yield the advantages of various materials, nanocomposites composed of chemical synthesized AuNPs and other materials are often utilized to achieve multifunctionalized electrodes. Electrochemical immunosensors for detection of β-glucans and cancer biomarkers were constructed based on chitosan/AuNP nanocomposite, where the AuNPs can accelerate the electron transfer and lead to high detection sensitivity [36,37]. AuNPs can also be incorporated with polymer to form composite films and applied for different biosensor applications [38]. Shim's group synthesized AuNP-encapsulated conducting polymer layer through electropolymerization of self-assembled precursor monomer-encapsulated AuNP solution. The biosensors fabricated based on this kind of layer displayed enhanced performance in terms of higher conductivity, stability, and sensitivity as compared to their previous reports where AuNPs were electrodeposited onto the sensor surface before conducting polymer was attached [30,39,40]. Wang's group synthesized nanocomposite materials by in situ growth of AuNPs on the surface of multi-walled carbon nanotubes-COOH/graphene. The obtained materials exhibited enhanced fast electron transfer and excellent biocompatibility. The related biosensor showed prominently sensitivity for the detection of Bilirubin [41].

1.3.2 Immobilization of biological recognition element

For the biosensors, the stable immobilization of the biological recognizers onto the electrode is extraordinarily important and pivotal [14]. Because of the superior biocompatibility, high surface area-to-volume ratio, and abundant surface chemical properties, AuNPs are ideal immobilization platform for a lot of biomolecules. Since AuNPs have strongly affinity with functional groups such as CN, SH, and NH_2 [42], immobilization of biological recognition elements based on their interaction with AuNPs has attracted enormous interest. Zhuo *et al.* reported a sensitive electrochemical biosensor for progastrin releasing-peptide tumor marker, which used AuNP-functionalized graphene sheets nanocomposite film as the biosensor platform for immobilization of primary antibodies. The used nanocomposite film could increase the surface area for capturing more antibodies and could provide a favorable microenvironment for biomolecule and effectively keep their activities [43]. Because of strong interaction between AuNPs and SH group through covalent Au-S bond, electrodeposited AuNPs layer has been considered an outstanding platform for convenient immobilization of thiol-modified biomolecule [15]. A number of electrochemical biosensors, which employed electrodeposited AuNPs layer for the immobilization of thiol-modified DNA recognizers, were fabricated for the detection of engrailed-2 cancer biomarker, protein kinase A activity, and *Escherichia coli* [15–17]. Furthermore, tetrahedron-structured DNA probes were strongly anchored at electrodeposited AuNPs surface through the modified three thiol groups at vertices, leaving a free-standing probe at the top. This construction provided a well-ordered platform to meet the requirements of interacting with more target molecules, such as dihydronicotinamide adenine dinucleotide and microRNA [44,45]. Core/shell structured Fe_3O_4/Au magnetic nanoparticles were synthesized and used to load DNA aptamers as recognition element for detection of thrombin [46].

To improve the stability and efficiency for immobilization of recognition element, AuNPs can also be incorporated into nanocomposites, which can strongly increase the efficient surface of the electrode for loading more recognizer molecules. Horseradish peroxidase enzymes were immobilized onto the natural polyhydroxyalkanoate-AuNPs composite which was coated on an indium tin oxide glass plate for the analysis of artemisinin [38]. Shim's group synthesized AuNP-encapsulated conducting polymer composite through self-assemble and electrodeposition. The reactive functional groups (e.g. carboxylic acid groups or amine groups) on the conducting polymers were completely facing outward for covalent attachment of biorecognition element (antibody or aptamer) as shown in Figure 1.4 [30,39,40].

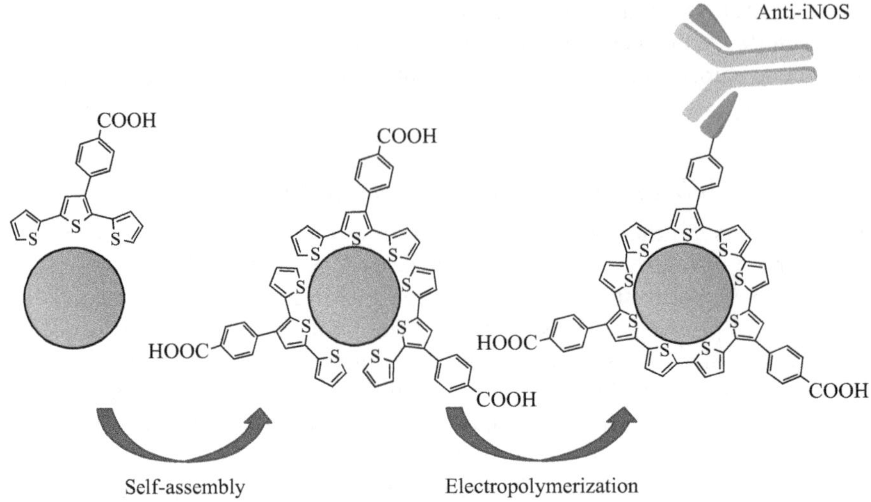

Figure 1.4 Self-assembly scheme of the TTBA monomer layer and electropolymerization of TTBA on AuNPs [39]

1.3.3 Signal generation and amplification

1.3.3.1 Signal generation

Except for modification of electrode surface in terms of promotion of electron transfer and immobilization of recognition element, AuNPs, which possess unique tunable physicochemical properties as well as good biological compatibility, conducting capability, and high surface area-to-volume ratio, are ideal candidates for electronic signal transduction of biological recognition events in electrochemical biosensors [47]. Biosensors employing AuNPs as tags or electrochemical labels have been developed. The AuNPs tags are linked with the recognition elements (such as antibody or DNA) to form bioconjugate. The detection process is based on the binding event between the target molecule and the specific recognizer that is conjugated to AuNP. Then, the electrochemical signal reflecting the specific binding event can be obtained by oxidizing the conjugated AuNPs in 1 M hydrochloride acid solution at a constant potential of 1.25 V, followed by the measurement of the dissolved $AuCl_4^-$ with voltammetry. Protein and DNA associated with various diseases were detected using such kind of AuNP tags [48,49]. Eksi *et al.* synthesized silver/gold core/shell bimetal nanoparticles, which were further conjugated with the antibodies specific to *Escherichia coli*. As a result, *Escherichia coli* were successfully detected by measuring the dissolved Au^{3+} ions [50].

1.3.3.2 Nanocarrier for signal amplification

To achieve ultrasensitive detection of biomolecules, new concept based on coupling the biocatalytic amplification of catalyst tags with additional amplification units and processes are highly desirable [51,52]. Nanomaterial-based bioamplification strategies using nanomaterial as a host for signal-generating labels have been developed for enormous signal enhancement [53–55]. As described above, the unique properties in terms of superior biocompatibility, high surface area-to-volume ratio, and abundant surface chemical properties make AuNPs the ultimate nanoscale materials to serve as a carrier for multi-amplification of detection signals. Actually, since the first report described a colloidal gold-antibody conjugate that served as an immunochemical marker [56], the use of AuNP-based biospecific conjugates in various fields of biology and medicine became very active [11]. There has been a wealth of works dealing with the application of functionalized AuNPs as carriers for signal amplification. Based on the strong interaction between AuNPs and the amine groups and cysteine residues contained in proteins [38], AuNPs are often used as the carriers for various proteins, such as antibody and enzymes. For instance, secondary antibody-AuNP bioconjugate was used instead of single secondary antibody for detection of hepatitis B surface antigen. The presence of AuNPs increased the immobilized amount of secondary antibody, and thus enhanced the sensitivity of the immunoassay [57,58]. A multi-nanomaterial electrochemical biosensor combining graphene, magnetic beads, and enzyme-labeled antibody-AuNP bioconjugate was developed for detection of carcinoembryonic antigen. The sensitivity of the sensor was enhanced by modifying the AuNPs with horseradish peroxidase and the detection antibody, to form the bioconjugate [59]. Zhuo *et al.* developed a novel electrochemical immunosensor using ferrocene and glucose oxidase multifunctionalized Au/TiO_2 nanocomposite as a trace label. Because of the large surface area and good biocompatibility of Au/TiO_2 nanocomposite, the high load amount of ferrocene and glucose oxidase were immobilized on the nano-Au/TiO_2 surface with good biological activity, resulting in the improvement of the intensity of the signal and ultrasensitive detection of small cell lung cancer biomarkers (as illustrated in Figure 1.5) [43].

Because of the strong interaction between AuNPs and thiol-modified DNA through Au-S bonds, a number of novel and effective signal amplification strategies combining AuNPs and DNA techniques were designed. For instance, Pu's group synthesized DNA-AuNP-polyaniline nanocomposite as a tracer label, which exhibited good biocompatibility and excellent electrochemical activity to amplify the electrochemical signal generated from $Fe(CN)_6^{4-/3-}$ indicator. This nanocomposite provided a simple preparation process for a signal-on DNA biosensor and resulted in high sensitivity for the detection of Mycobacterium tuberculosis over a broad linear range [18]. An electrochemical biosensor based on AuNP-DNA conjugate was developed for hybridization detection of specific K-ras gene that was highly associated with colorectal cancer. The AuNPs offered excellent electrochemical signal transduction and effective signal amplification by forming network-like thiocyanuric acid/AuNPs [49]. Wang's group developed a multiple signal amplification strategy for ultrasensitive detection of epithelial tumor biomarker mucin 1 protein based on hairpin oligonucleotide-functionalized AuNPs amplification coupled with enzyme-linkage reaction [60]. Zheng and coworkers synthesized graphene oxide-thionine-Au@SiO_2 functional nanocomposite which was used as a carrier for loading a large amount of signal DNA aptamer and hemin/G-quadruplex complex. Furthermore, the hemin/G-quadruplex complex could act as a bioelectrocatalytic peroxidase-mimicking DNAzyme for signal

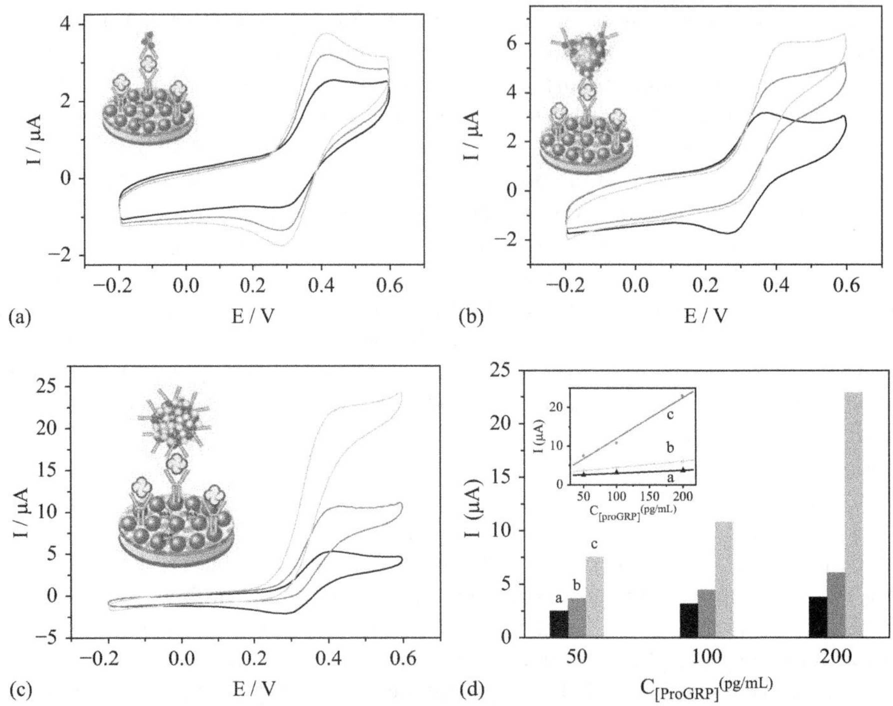

Figure 1.5 The CVs after the sandwich immunoreaction of the resulted immunosensor with variously labeled probes. (a) Fc-Ab_2, (b) GOD/Fc-Ab_2/nano-TiO_2 and (c) GOD/Fc-Ab_2/nano-Au/TiO_2. All of them were detected in the presence of 1.8 mM glucose in working buffer at 50 mV/s. (d) showed the voltammetric responses vs. ProGRP concentration for the three labeled probes [43]

amplification and thus greatly improved the sensitivity of the biosensors for *Escherichia coli* O157:H7 eaeA gene [17]. To further generate the detectable signal with a high signal-to-noise ratio, 'supersandwich mode' was constructed based on signal units composed of DNA-functionalized AuNP-based hybridization chain reaction, which could introduce the superior signal enhancement [37,45]. As illustrated in Figure 1.6, the AuNP-carried signal unit offered a large amount of loading sites for reporting molecules and thus resulted ultrasensitive detection of cancer biomarkers at trace level.

1.3.3.3 Nanocatalyst for signal amplification

As a nanometer-sized noble metal, AuNPs possess excellent electrocatalytic activities toward some small molecules like glucose, hydrogen peroxide, dopamine, and catechol, which significantly differ from their bulk counterparts. The high surface area-to-volume ratio and active sites of AuNPs constitute part of the

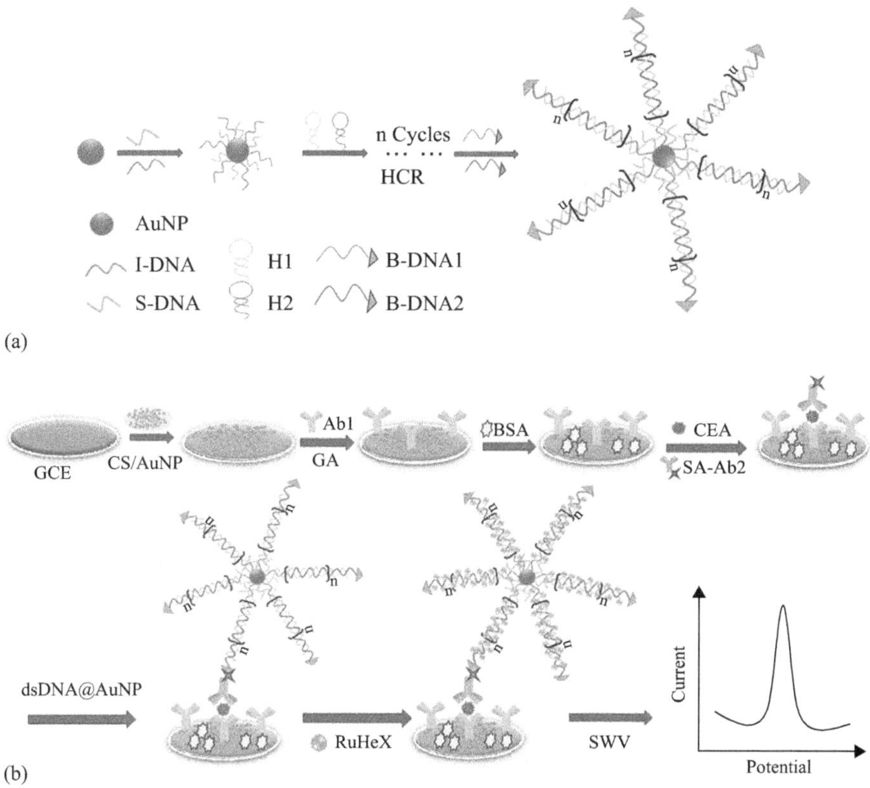

Figure 1.6 Schematic diagram of (a) the preparation of dsDNA@AuNP tag and (b) the immunosensor fabrication and electrochemical immunoassay procedure [37]

driving force in developing nanosized electrocatalysts [20]. Based on this unique electrocatalytic activity as well as biocompatibility, a large number of electrochemical sensors for clinical diagnosis have been widely developed [20,61]. Recently, Yuan' group reported a novel cholesterol biosensor based on AuNP-catalyzed luminol electrogenerated chemiluminescence. Owing to the catalytic activity of AuNPs toward luminol-H_2O_2 system, the detection sensitivity was significantly improved. The electrogenerated chemiluminescence method based on AuNPs is simple, sensitive, and low-cost, ensuring a promising alternative approach for cholesterol detection [62]. The electrocatalytic activity of AuNP tags toward hydrogen evolution reaction was carefully investigated by Merkoci and coworkers. They confirmed that AuNP tags could effectively catalytically reduce protons to hydrogen at an adequate potential in acidic medium, based on which a novel electrocatalytic device was developed for specific identification of tumor cells [63]. Furthermore, taking the advantage of this electrocatalytic activity of AuNP tags toward hydrogen evolution reaction, they exploited a magneto sandwich immunoassay based on porous magnetic microsphere platforms and AuNP-secondary antibody tags. The detectable signal was generated by AuNP tags and further enhanced by the high active area that was offered by the porous magnetic microsphere, resulting in successful detection of Alzheimer's disease biomarkers in real clinical samples [64].

Recently, functional materials composed of two or more components have attracted increasing interest, because the unique properties of each component can be combined for multiple purposes, or the new properties can be achieved due to the synergistic effect [20,65]. Based on this point, AuNPs, as one of the most common nanomaterials applied for biosensing, have been widely explored for combination with other components like metals, nanomaterials, polymers, and biomolecules. For instance, Liu *et al.* described a new label-free strategy based on catalytic signal amplification with single-wall carbon nanotubes wrapped with Au-Rh hollow nanospheres. The combination of Rh and Au provided the materials with biological macromolecule binding features and superior electrocatalytic activity toward hydrogen peroxide, resulting the potential application in monitoring human immunodeficiency virus curative effects through the detection of nuclear paraspeckle assembly transcript 1 [25]. Wei's group developed a novel and sensitive electrochemical immunosensor for ultrasensitive detection of pancreatic cancer biomarker carbohydrate antigen 199 by using Au@Cu_xO yolk-shell nanostructures as labels for signal amplification. The Au@Cu_xO nanostructures, consisting of AuNP yolk and porous Cu_xO shell, exhibited high electrocatalytic activity toward the reduction of hydrogen peroxide as analytical signal [66]. A simple and sensitive electrochemical strategy was designed using heme-AuNPs. The anchored heme-AuNPs showed strong electrocatalytic O_2 reduction, which were used for analysis of Alzheimer's disease biomarkers [67]. Polypyrrole nanofibers-supported AuNPs heterogeneous composite materials were synthesized in situ via hydrogen bonding interactions, which exhibited a high electrocatalytic activity toward glucose oxidation. Based on the synthesized hybrids, a nonenzymatic glucose sensor was developed and could be applied for routine analysis of glucose in clinical diagnosis [68]. Zheng *et al.* prepared core-shell structured Au@CdS nanoparticles with charge selective stabilizer, where a single AuNP core was coated with CdS quantum dots via an in situ self-assembly method. Because of the electrostatic interaction between negatively charged Au@CdS core-shell nanoparticle and positively charged dopamine analyte, the proposed hybrid materials exhibited selective electrocatalytic activity toward dopamine and were employed to fabricate a charge selective electrochemical sensor with good sensitivity and selectivity for dopamine detection in the presence of ascorbic acid and uric acid, as illustrated in Figure 1.7 [65].

Since Mirkin *et al.* demonstrated that AuNPs could in situ catalyze the deposition of silver and this phenomenon could be employed to enhance the sensitivity of a DNA hybridization assay [69,70], silver enhancement has been widely exploited for clinical diagnosis. The principle of silver enhancement is that in the presence of AuNPs catalyst, large amounts of silver ions can be chemically reduced by reductant like hydroquinone and deposit onto the surface of AuNPs catalyst.

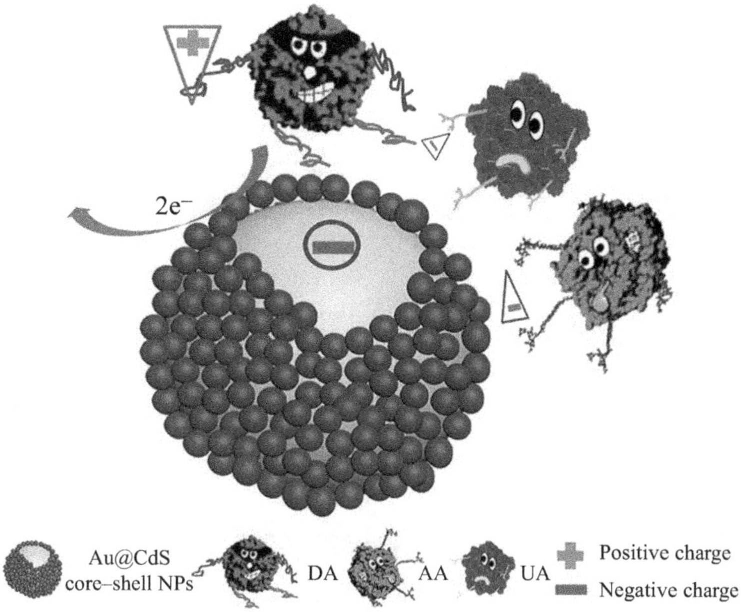

Figure 1.7 Schematic illustration of the reaction mechanism of the Au@CdS core–shell structure with DA in the presence of UA and AA [65]

As a result, small AuNPs labels can lead to a mass of big silver particles and thus the detectable signal can be significantly enhanced. Using AuNP-streptavidin conjugate as a catalyst for silver precipitation in the presence of silver ions and hydroquinone, Lin *et al.* developed a sensitive electro-microchip DNA-biosensor for bacteria detection [71]. Ju's group designed a multiple signal amplification strategy by using microbead-carried AuNPs as tracing tag to label signal antibody and AuNPs-induced silver deposition for anodic stropping analysis. This strategy was successfully employed for ultrasensitive immunosensing of cancer biomarkers with a very low detection limit, indicating potential application in clinical diagnosis [72]. In spite of efficient enhancement of detectable signal, the traditional silver enhancement method suffered from the unspecific deposition of silver resulted from the direct mixture of silver ions and reductant in the enhancer solution, which might compromise the detection sensitivity and accuracy [73]. To solve this problem, Merkoci's group proposed electroreduction silver ions with the catalytic effect of AuNPs and further optimized the silver electrodeposition potential to achieve the silver deposition only on the surface of the AuNPs and not on the electrode surface. This novel detection mode allowed the immunoassay with an enhanced sensitivity for further application in clinical analysis [73]. In addition, the hydrazine-AuNP-aptamer bioconjugate, where hydrazine served as the reductant instead of hydroquinone and was directly attached onto AuNPs catalyst to avoid the nonspecific silver deposition on the sensor surface, was designed by Zhu *et al.* and applied to reduce silver ions for

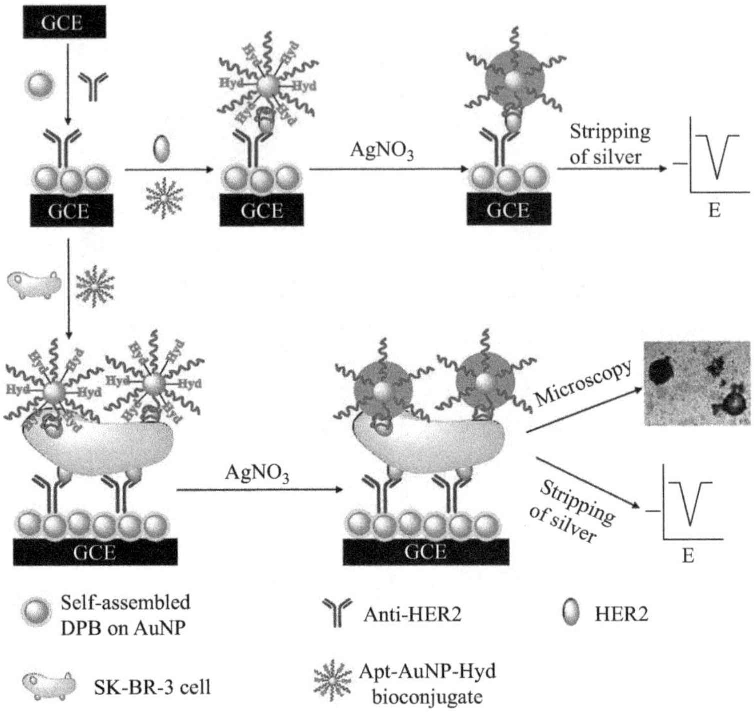

Figure 1.8 Schematic representation of the immunosensor for detection of HER2 protein and HER2-overexpresing SK-BR-3 breast cancer cells [40]

signal amplification selectively. As shown in Figure 1.8, the electrochemical sensor developed with this hydrazine-AuNP-aptamer bioconjugate was successfully applied to detect cancer biomarkers and breast cancer cells with ultrahigh sensitivity [40].

1.4 Conclusions and outlook

Due to the unique properties in terms of excellent conductivity, high surface area-to-volume ratio, abundant surface chemical properties, and superior electrocatalytic activity, AuNPs are considered to be promising nanomaterial for diagnostic purpose and biomedical applications. A large number of electrochemical biosensors based on AuNPs have been developed to detect various disease-related analytes like small molecules, DNA, proteins, and cells. The efficient functions of AuNPs in the biosensors are summarized in three aspects: (i) improvement of electron transfer efficiency, (iii) immobilization of biological recognition element, and (ii) signal generation and amplification. As a nanomaterial allowing abundant modification, AuNPs enable various novel and facile designs for electrochemical biosensors with high sensitivity and reliability. In particularly, the nanocomposites composed of AuNPs and other materials provide the biosensor with multiple functional platforms. The combination of AuNPs with DNA amplification techniques offers possibility of cascade signal amplification.

In spite of great progress that has been achieved in the development of AuNPs-based electrochemical biosensors for clinical diagnosis, challenges remain. Development of a single electrochemical biosensor for simultaneous detection of multiple biomarkers in a small sample volume will be of significance for practical disease diagnosis. Development of portable devices based on AuNPs will significantly promote the point-of-care medical diagnosis. With continuous efforts on exploring the properties and applications of AuNPs, we believe that AuNPs will play more important roles in the electrochemical biosensors to achieve various biomedical diagnostic purposes.

Acknowledgments

This work was supported by the National Science Foundation of China (21305077) and Research Award Fund for Outstanding Middle-aged and Young Scientist of Shandong Province (BS2013SW031). The author would like to thank her coworkers for their motivated contributions.

References

[1] Bahadir E.B., Sezginturk M.K. 'Applications of electrochemical immunosensors for early clinical diagnostics'. *Talanta*. 2015;**132**:162–174.

[2] Turner A.P.F., Karube I., Wilson G.S. *Biosensors: Fundamentals and Applications*. New York: Oxford University Press; 1987.

[3] Skladal P. 'Advances in electrochemical immunosensors'. *Electroanalysis*. 1997;**9**(10):737–745.

[4] Wilson G.S., Hu Y.B. 'Enzyme based biosensors for in vivo measurements'. *Chemical Reviews*. 2000; **100**(7):2693–2704.

[5] Drummond T.G., Hill M.G., Barton J.K. 'Electrochemical DNA sensors'. *Nature Biotechnology*. 2003;**21**:1192–1199.

[6] Wang J. 'Portable electrochemical systems'. *Trends in Analytical Chemistry*. 2002;**21**(4):226–232.

[7] Devi R.V., Doble M., Verma R.S. 'Nanomaterials for early detection of cancer biomarker with special emphasis on gold nanoparticles in immunoassays/sensors'. *Biosensors and Bioelectronics*. 2015;**68**:688–698.

[8] Pingarron J.M., Villalonga R. 'Advanced materials in electroanalysis'. *Electroanalysis*. 2015; **27**(9):2018.

[9] Kumar A., Boruah B.M., Liang X.J. 'Gold nanoparticles promising nanomaterials for the diagnosis of cancer and HIV/AIDS'. *Journal of Nanomaterials*. 2011; **2011**:202187.

[10] Howes P.D., Rana S., Stevens M.M. 'Plasmonic nanomaterials for biodiagnostics'. *Chemical Society Reviews*. 2014;**43**:3835–3853.

[11] Dykman L., Khlebtsov N. 'Gold nanoparticles in biomedical applications: recent advances and perspectives'. *Chemical Society Reviews.* 2012;**41**:2256–2282.

[12] Raju G.S.R., Benton L., Pavitra E., Yu J.S. 'Multifunctional nanoparticles: recent progress in cancer therapeutics'. *Chemical Communications.* 2015;**51**:13248–13259.

[13] Zhu X.Q., Li J., He H.P., Huang M., Zhang X.H., Wang S.F. 'Application of nanomaterials in the bioanalytical detection of disease-related genes'. *Biosensors and Bioelectronics.* 2015;**74**:113–133.

[14] Zhu Y., Son J.I., Shim Y.B. 'Amplification strategy based on gold nanoparticle-decorated carbon nanotubes for neomycin immunosensors'. *Biosensors and Bioelectronics.* 2010;**26**:1002–1008.

[15] Lee S., Jo H., Her J., Lee H.Y., Ban C. 'Ultrasensitive electrochemical detection of engrailed-2 based on homeodomain-specific DNA probe recognition for the diagnosis of prostate cancer'. *Biosensors and Bioelectronics.* 2015;**66**:32–38.

[16] Yin H.S., Wang M., Li B.C., Yang Z.Q., Zhou Y.L., Ai S.Y. 'A sensitive electrochemical biosensor for detection of protein kinase A activity and inhibitors based on Phos-tag and enzymatic signal amplification'. *Biosensors and Bioelectronics.* 2015;**63**:26–32.

[17] Li Y., Deng J., Fang L.C., *et al.* 'A novel electrochemical DNA biosensor based on HRP-mimicking hemin/G-quadruplex wrapped GOx nanocomposites as tag for detection of *Escherichia coli* O157:H7'. *Biosensors and Bioelectronics.* 2015; **63**:1–6.

[18] Liu C., Jiang D.N., Xiang G.M., Liu L.L., Liu F., Pu X.Y. 'An electrochemical DNA biosensor for the detection of Mycobacterium tuberculosis, based on signal amplification of graphene and a gold nanoparticle-polyaniline nanocomposite'. *Analyst.* 2014;**139**:5460–5465.

[19] Cheng X.R., Hau B.Y.H., Tatsuro E., Kagan K. 'Au nanoparticle-modified DNA sensor based on simultaneous electrochemical impedance spectroscopy and localized surface plasmon resonance'. *Biosensors and Bioelectronics.* 2014;**53**:513–518.

[20] Guo S., Wang E. 'Synthesis and electrochemical applications of gold nanoparticles'. *Analytica Chimica Acta.* 2007;**598**:181–192.

[21] Frens G. 'Controlleld nucleation for the regulation of the particle size in monodisperse gold suspensions'. *Nature Physical Science.*1973;**241**:20–22.

[22] Kimling J., Maier M., Okenve B., Kotaidis V., Ballot H., Plech A. 'Turkevich method for gold nanoparticle synthesis revisited'. *Journal of Physical Chemistry B.* 2006;**110**:15700–15707.

[23] Zhou J., Du L.P., Zou L., Zou Y.C., Hu N., Wang P. 'An ultrasensitive electrochemical immunosensor for carcinoembryonic antigen detection based on staphylococcal protein A-Au nanoparticle modified gold electrode'. *Sensors and Actuators B: Chemical.* 2014;**197**:220–227.

[24] Zheng D.Y., Zhu X.J., Ding X.R., Zhu X.L., Yin Y.M., Li G.X. 'Sensitive detection of CD147/EMMPRIN and its expression on cancer cells with electrochemical technique'. *Talanta*. 2013;**105**:187–191.

[25] Liu F., Xiang G.M., Zhang L.Q., *et al.* 'A novel label free long non-coding RNA electrochemical biosensor based on green L-cysteine electrodeposition and Au-Rh hollow nanospheres as tags'. *RSC ADVANCES*. 2015;**5**; 51990–51999.

[26] Jana N.R., Gearheart L., Murphy C.J. 'Seeding growth for size control of 5–40 nm diameter gold nanoparticles'. *Langmuir*. 2001;**17**:6782–6786.

[27] Anderson M.J., Torres-Chavolla E., Castro B.A., Alocilja E.C. 'One step alkaline synthesis of biocompatible gold nanoparticles using dextrin as capping agent'. *Journal of Nanoparticle Research*. 2011;**13**:2843–2851.

[28] Torres-Chavolla E., Alocilja E.C. 'Nanoparticle based DNA biosensor for tuberculosis detection using thermophilic helicase-dependent isothermal amplification'. *Biosensors and Bioelectronics*. 2011;**26**:4614–4618.

[29] Ilkhani H., Sarparast M., Noori A., Bathaie S.Z., Mousavi F. 'Electrochemical aptamer/antibody based sandwich immunosensor for the detection of EGFR, a cancer biomarker, using gold nanoparticles as a signaling probe'. *Biosensors and Bioelectronics*. 2015;**74**:491–497.

[30] Zhu Y., Chandra P., Song K.M., Ban C., Shim Y.B. 'Label-free detection of kanamycin based on the aptamer-functionalized conducting polymer/gold nanocomposite'. *Biosensors and Bioelectronics*. 2012;**36**:29–34.

[31] Lee K.S., Won M.S., Noh H.B., Shim Y.B. 'Triggering the redox reaction of cytochrome c on a biomimetic layer and elimination of interferences for NADH detection'. *Biomaterials*. 2010;**31**:7827–7835.

[32] Kim D.M., Noh H.B., Park D.S., Ryu S.H., Koo J.S., Shim Y.B. 'Immunosensors for detection of Annexin II and MUC5AC for early diagnosis of lung cancer'. *Biosensors and Bioelectronics*. 2009;**25**:456–462.

[33] Chandra P., Noh H.-B., Shim Y.-B. 'Cancer cell detection based on the interaction between an anticancer drug and cell membrane components'. *Chemical Communications*. 2013;**49**:1900–1902.

[34] Noh H.-B., Chandra P., Moon J.O., Shim Y.-B. 'In vivo detection of glutathione disulfide and oxidative stress monitoring using a biosensor'. *Biomaterials*. 2012;**33**:2600–2607.

[35] Wellington M.F., Ibtisam E.T. 'Detection of the inflammation biomarker C-reactive protein in serum samples: towards an optimal biosensor formula'. *Biosensors*. 2014;**4**:340–357.

[36] Liu D., Luo P., Sun W.W., Zhang L.P., Wang Z. 'Detection of b-glucans using an amperometric biosensor based on high-affinity interaction between Dectin-1 and β-glucans'. *Analytical Biochemistry*. 2010;**404**:14–20.

[37] Ge Y.Q., Wu J., Ju H.X., Wu S. 'Ultrasensitive enzyme-free electrochemical immunosensor based on hybridization chain reaction triggered double strand DNA@Au nanoparticle tag'. *Talanta*. 2014;**120**:218–223.

[38] Pinkee P., Keisham R., Bolin K.K., Raju K. 'Natural polyhydroxyalkanoate-gold nanocomposite based biosensor for detection of antimalarial drug artemisinin'. *Materials Science and Engineering C*. 2014;**37**:314–320.

[39] Koh W.C.A., Chandra P., Kim D.-M., Shim Y.-B. 'Electropolymerized self-assembled layer on gold nanoparticles: detection of inducible nitric oxide synthase in neuronal cell culture'. *Analytical Chemistry*. 2011; **83**: 6177–6183.

[40] Zhu Y., Chandra P., Shim Y. 'Ultrasensitive and selective electrochemical diagnosis of breast cancer based on a hydrazine–Au nanoparticle–aptamer bioconjugate'. *Analytical Chemistry*. 2013;**85**:1058–1064.

[41] Feng Q.L., Du Y.L., Zhang C., *et al*. 'Synthesis of the multi-walled carbon nanotubes-COOH/graphene/gold nanoparticles nanocomposite for simple determination of Bilirubin in human blood serum'. *Sensors and Actuators B: Chemical*. 2013;**185**:337–344.

[42] Grabar K.C., Freeman R.G., Hommer M.B., Natan M.J. 'Preparation and characterization of Au colloid monolayers'. *Analytical Chemistry*. 1995;**67**:735–743.

[43] Zhuo Y., Chai Y.Q., Yuan R., Mao L., Yuan Y.L., Han J. 'Glucose oxidase and ferrocene labels immobilized at Au/TiO_2 nanocomposites with high load amount and activity for sensitive immunoelectrochemical measurement of ProGRP biomarker'. *Biosensors and Bioelectronics*. 2011;**26**:3838–3844.

[44] Li Z.L., Su W.Q., Liu S.P., Ding X.T. 'An electrochemical biosensor based on DNA tetrahedron/graphene composite film for highly sensitive detection of NADH'. *Biosensors and Bioelectronics*. 2015;**69**:287–293.

[45] Liu L.Z., Song C., Zhang Z., *et al*. 'Ultrasensitive electrochemical detection of microRNA-21 combining layered nanostructure of oxidized single-walled carbon nanotubes and nanodiamonds by hybridization chain reaction'. *Biosensors and Bioelectronics*. 2015;**70**:351–357.

[46] Zhao J., Liu M.L., Zhang Y.Y., Li H.T., Lin Y.H., Yao S.Z. 'Apoferritin protein nanoparticles dually labeled with aptamer and horseradish peroxidase as a sensing probe for thrombin detection'. *Analytica Chimica Acta*. 2013;**759**:53–60.

[47] Guo S.J., Wang E.K. 'Synthesis and electrochemical applications of gold nanoparticles'. *Analytica Chimica Acta*. 2007;**598**:181–192.

[48] Omidfar K., Dehdast A., Zarei H., Sourkohi B.K., Larijani B. 'Development of urinary albumin immunosensor based on colloidal AuNP and PVA'. *Biosensors and Bioelectronics*. 2011;**26**:4177–4183.

[49] Wang X.Y., Shu G.F., Gao C.C., Yang Y., Xu Q., Tang M. 'Electrochemical biosensor based on functional composite nanofibers for detection of K-ras gene via multiple signal amplification strategy'. *Analytical Biochemistry*. 2014;**466**:51–58.

[50] Eksi H., Güzel R., Güven B., Boyaci I.H. Solak A.O. 'Fabrication of an electrochemical *E. coli* biosensor in biowells using bimetallic nanoparticle-labelled antibodies'. *Electroanalysis*. 2015;**27**(2):343–352.

[51] Wang J., Liu G., Jan M.R. 'Ultrasensitive electrical biosensing of proteins and DNA: carbon-nanotube derived amplification of the recognition and transduction events'. *Journal of America Chemistry Society*. 2004; **126**:3010–3011.

[52] Ding L., Bond A.M., Zhai J., Zhang J. 'Utilization of nanoparticle labels for signal amplification in ultrasensitive electrochemical affinity biosensors: a review'. *Analytica Chimica Acta*. 2013;**797**:1–12.

[53] Wang J. 'Nanomaterial-based amplified transduction of biomolecular interactions'. *Small*. 2005;**1**:1036–1043.

[54] Yu X., Munge B., Patel V., *et al.* 'Carbon nanotube amplification strategies for highly sensitive immunosensing of cancer biomarkers in serum and tissue'. *Journal of America Chemistry Society*. 2006;**128**:11199–11205.

[55] Mani V., Chikkaveeraiah B.V., Patel V., Gutkind J.S., Rusling J.F. 'Ultrasensitive immunosensor for cancer biomarker proteins using gold nanoparticle film electrodes and multienzyme-particle amplification'. *Journal of American Chemical Society*. 2009;**3**:585–594.

[56] Faulk W.P., Taylor G.M. 'An immunocolloid method for the electron microscope'. *Immunochemistry*. 1971;**8**:1081–1083.

[57] Ding C.F., Li H., Hu K.C., Lin J.M. 'Electrochemical immunoassay of hepatitis B surface antigen by the amplification of gold nanoparticles based on the nanoporous gold electrode'. *Talanta*. 2010;**80**:1385–1391.

[58] Alipour E., Ghourchian H., Boutorabi S.M. 'Gold nanoparticle based capacitive immunosensor for detection of hepatitis B surface antigen'. *Analytical Methods*. 2013;**5**:4448–4453.

[59] Jin B., Wang P., Mao H.J., *et al.* 'Multi-nanomaterial electrochemical biosensor based on label-free graphene for detecting cancer biomarkers'. *Biosensors and Bioelectronics*. 2014;**55**:464–469.

[60] Hu R., Wen W., Wang Q.L., *et al.* 'Novel electrochemical aptamer biosensor based on an enzyme-gold nanoparticle dual label for the ultrasensitive detection of epithelial tumour marker MUC1'. *Biosensors and Bioelectronics*. 2014;**53**:384–389.

[61] Merkoci A. 'Nanoparticles based electroanalysis in diagnostics applications'. *Electroanalysis*. 2013;**25**(1):15–27.

[62] Zhang M.H., Yuan R., Chai Y.Q., *et al.* 'A biosensor for cholesterol based on gold nanoparticles-catalyzed luminol electrogenerated chemiluminescence'. *Biosensors and Bioelectronics*. 2012;**32**;288–292.

[63] Escosura-Muniz A., Sanchez-Espinel C., Dıaz-Freitas B., Gonzalez-Fernandez A., Costa M.M., Merkoci A. 'Rapid identification and quantification of tumor cells using an electrocatalytic method based on gold nanoparticles'. *Analytical Chemistry*. 2009;**8**(24):10268–10274.

[64] Escosura-Muñiz A., Plichta Z., Horák D., Merkoçi A. 'Alzheimer′s disease biomarkers detection in human samples by efficient capturing through porous magnetic microspheres and labelling with electrocatalytic gold nanoparticles.' *Biosensors and Bioelectronics*. 2015;**67**:162–169.

[65] Zhang W.X., Zheng J.Z., Tan C.H., *et al.* 'Designed self-assembled hybrid Au@CdS core–shell nanoparticles with negative charge and their application as highly selective biosensors'. *Journal of Materials Chemistry B*. 2015;**3**:217–224.

[66] Guo A., Li Y., Cao W., *et al.* 'An electrochemical immunosensor for ultrasensitive detection of carbohydrate antigen 199 based on Au@CuxOS yolk–shell nanostructures with porous shells as labels'. *Biosensors and Bioelectronics*. 2015;**63**:39–46.

[67] Liu L., Zhao F., Ma F., Zhang L., Yang S., Xia N. 'Electrochemical detection of β-amyloid peptides on electrode covered with N-terminus-specific antibody based on electrocatalytic O_2 reduction by Aβ(1–16)-heme-modified gold nanoparticles'. *Biosensors and Bioelectronics*. 2013;**49**:231–235.

[68] Li C., Su Y., Lv X., *et al.* 'Controllable anchoring of gold nanoparticles to polypyrrole nanofibers by hydrogen bonding and their application in nonenzymatic glucose sensors'. *Biosensors and Bioelectronics*. 2012; **38**(1):402–406.

[69] Taton T.A., Mirkin C.A., Letsinger R.L. 'Scanometric DNA array detection with nanoparticle probes'. *Science*. 2000;**289**(8):1757–1760.

[70] Park S-J, Taton T.A., Mirkin C.A. 'Array-based electrical detection of DNA with nanoparticle probes'. *Science*. 2002;**295**(22):1503–1506.

[71] Yeh C.H., Chang Y.H., Chang T.C., Lin H. p., Lin Y.C. 'Electro-microchip DNA-biosensor for bacteria detection'. *Analyst*. 2010;**135**;2717–2722.

[72] Lin D., Wu J., Wang M., Yuan F., Ju H. 'Triple signal amplification of graphene film, polybead carried gold nanoparticles as tracing tag and silver deposition for ultrasensitive electrochemical immunosensing'. *Analytical Chemistry*. 2012;**84**:3662–3668.

[73] Escosura-Muniz A., Costa M.M., Merkoci A. 'Controlling the electrochemical deposition of silver onto gold nanoparticles: reducing interferences and increasing the sensitivity of magnetoimmuno assays'. *Biosensors and Bioelectronics*. 2009;**24**:2475–2482.

Chapter 2

Development and application of microbiosensors for *in-vivo* diagnostics

Lawrence Kulinsky[1]

2.1 Introduction

Biosensors are devices consisting of biological recognition element (such as enzymes, antibodies, receptors, or nucleic acids) and a transducer that produces a recordable output (electrical, chemical, mechanical, optical, or thermal) as a result of biorecognition event [1]. Typically, samples (such as blood or saliva) are taken from patients and placed for analysis into an *in-vitro* biosensor. Ease of sample collection – from finger prick drawing of blood for lateral flow strips used in ubiquitous self-administered electrochemical portable blood glucose measurement system [2] to biosensor integrated into contact lens able to continuous in-situ monitoring of glucose level in tears [3, 4], to portable and wearable systems for collection and analysis of analytes in breath, sweat, and tears [5] – makes *in-vitro* or *ex-vivo* testing increasingly easy, convenient, and reliable [6]. In some case, however, biosensors must be implanted *in-vivo* to collect real-time dynamic data of changing physiological state such as changing level of certain neurotransmitters in the brain as a result of external stimuli [7], or to monitor dynamically changing glucose level in diabetic patients where avoiding rapid transition from hyperglycemia to hypoglycemia is necessary to prevent hypoglycemic shock [8] and biosensors can be paired with the insulin pump for controlled release of insulin to maintain normoglycemia [9]; finally, continuous measurements of specific molecular indicators such as level of glucose and lactate are vitally important in cases of trauma-induced hemorrhages [10].

Enzymatic as well as non-enzymatic implantable microbiosensors are discussed with emphasis on biosensor longevity, sensitivity, and selectivity. These *in-vivo* biosensor systems have different levels of maturity: while most of the surveyed *in-vivo* biosensor systems are tested on animal models, some of the most mature *in-vivo* biosensors, such enzymatic amperometric biosensor platforms developed for diabetic patients, are undergoing clinical trials and several systems have been commercialized. This review focuses on the advances in development of

[1]Mechanical and Aerospace Engineering Department, University of California, Irvine

in-vivo microbiosensors in last five years. Many of the *in-vivo* microsensors that sometimes are loosely termed "biosensors," but that don't contain biological recognition elements. For example, *in-vivo* real-time detection of nitric oxide [11], non-enzymatic electrochemical sensors using direct oxidation of glucose on the electrode surface that don't have biological recognition elements (such as enzymes, proteins, oligonucleotides) [12], or boronic acid derivatives based fluorescence glucose sensors [13] fall outside this survey.

2.2 *In-vivo* enzymatic biosensors

Most of the *in-vivo* biosensors use enzymes as their biological recognition elements [14]. These biomolecules often belong to a class of enzymes called oxidoreductases that includes oxidases and dehydrogenases [15]. In amperometric enzymatic biosensors enzymes assist in converting the reactant of interest into a product (for example, glucose oxidase converts into gluconic acid) with liberation of electroactive substance (such as hydrogen peroxide). In the first generation of enzymatic blood glucose biosensors oxygen is used as the electron acceptor. To combat interference from other redox species, in the second generation of the enzymatic blood glucose biosensors mediators (also called artificial electron acceptors) shuttle electrons between the redox site of the enzyme and the surface of the working electrode. The most recent, third generation of enzymatic biosensors, have direct electron transfer between the redox center of the enzyme and the electrode [16].

2.2.1 Commercialized continuous glucose monitoring systems (CGMS)

Present state-of-the-art commercialized *in-vivo* biosensing technology is used in continuous glucose monitoring [17, 18]. Food and Drug Administration (FDA) in US has approved continuous glucose monitoring biosensor systems from several companies, including FreeStyle Navigator II (Abbott) [19], G4 Platinum (DexCom) [20], and Enlite (Medtronic) [21] (Figure 2.1). Needle-like biosensors are inserted subcutaneously and connected to non-implanted transmitters that contain power source and could transmit signal wirelessly to handheld device displaying the glucose concentration. Because these sensors measure glucose concentration not in blood, but in the interstitial fluid, periodic (approximately every 12 h) calibrations using finger stick-based blood glucose meters are required to establish a correlation between glucose level in subcutaneous tissues and blood glucose level of the patient [22]. Some errors in the measurements can be associated with discrepancies and time lag between glucose concentration changes in blood and subcutaneous tissue [23].

All the listed commercial continuous glucose monitoring systems (CGMS) use glucose oxidase (GOx) enzyme to catalytically oxidize glucose [24]. The Dexcom and Medtronic biosensors that don't use artificial mediators utilize oxygen (dissolved in interstitial fluid) as electron acceptor, while Freestyle enzymatic electrode uses osmium complex as a mediator to transfer charges from the redox center of the

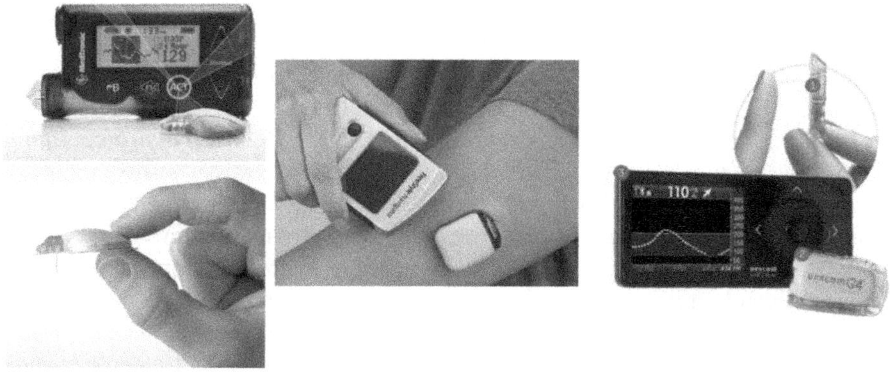

Figure 2.1 Commercial continuous glucose monitoring systems: (left) MiniMed 530G Insulin Pump (top) and Enlite Biosensor (bottom) (MiniMed); (center) Freestyle Navigator II (Abbott); (right) G4 Platinum (Dexcom) with (1) biosensor (2) transmitter and (3) receiver

enzyme to the electrode [25]. Presence of the mediator allows for shifting of the oxidation potential down and thus avoiding interference from various substances such as uric acid or acetaminophen and improving selectivity of the sensor.

The current level generated in *in-vivo* amperometric biosensors is proportional to the concentration of glucose in the subcutaneous fluid and it depends on several parameters, including the geometry of the microelectrode. For example, for needle-type enzymatic electrode [26] (utilized in DexCom biosensor system), the current profile is given by the modified Cottrel's equation (2.1):

$$i(t) = \frac{nFAD_{app}C^*}{r_e}\left[\frac{2exp(-0.05\pi^{0.5}\tau^{0.5})}{\pi^{0.5}\tau^{0.5}} + \frac{1}{ln(5.2945 + 0.7493\tau^{0.5})}\right];$$

$$\tau = \frac{4D_{app}t}{r_e^2} \tag{2.1}$$

where C^* is the bulk concentration of the glucose, A is the area of the microelectrode, n is the number of electrons transferred in a redox reaction, D_{app} is the diffusion coefficient of the electroactive species, F is the Faraday constant, and r_e is the radius of the needle electrode. Current profiles are available for the implantable enzymatic electrodes of various geometries [27].

In cases when no mediators are used and biosensors depend on stable oxygen concentration in fluid, a selective membrane (for example, from polyurethane [28, 29]) above the enzymatic layer allows to slow down the diffusion of the glucose, while smaller oxygen molecules are not slowed significantly by the membrane, providing a stable level of oxygen at the electrode surface albeit at a price of somewhat slower detection [30]. Permselective membranes could also block the passage to the sensor surface of endogenous species such as ascorbic acid or dopamine that are interfering with amperometric detection [31].

Lifetime of the implanted biosensor can be significantly reduced by the foreign body response and biofouling (attachment of cells to the implant) [32]. Foreign body response results in inflammation that typically proceeds in stages: *acute inflammatory phase* that follows implantation and lasts several days (where plasma proteins and macrophages move toward the implant), followed by *chronic inflammation* (during which intensive vascularization proceeds in tissues surrounding an implant and fibroblasts and vascular endothelial cells are proliferated), eventually leading to formation of collagenous fibrous capsule around the device, preventing normal operation of biosensor [33]. Biocompatible hydrophilic outer membranes can significantly reduce biofouling and foreign body response associated with insertion and implantation of the sensors. The success of the commercial *in-vivo* biosensors critically depend on selection and optimization of the proper outer polymer layer. For example, the biosensor of the Freestyle Navigator CGM system with functionalized vinyl pyridine-styrene copolymer layer coating implanted in the rabbit muscle did not exhibit encapsulation for more than a year [25]. Also, the smaller the implanted device, the less is the extent of the inflammatory response, so miniaturization of the biosensors is important [18].

Typically commercial *in-vivo* subcutaneous amperometric biosensors need to be replaced every 5 to 7 days [34]. Special applicators facilitate the insertion of these needle-type biosensors by the users into their abdominal area or to the back of the arm. Studies have shown that *in-vivo* CGMS's performance is comparable to that of microdialysis system where subcutaneous fluid is sampled via catheter, but the glucose measurement is performed with enzymatic assays *in-vitro* [35]. CGMS are continuously evolving and the current generation of these systems has improved longevity and accuracy as compared with previous generation of CGMS devices [36, 37]. Comparison of performance between Freestyle Navigator, G4 Platinum, and Enlite CGM systems has revealed that the accuracy of these systems measured as aggregate mean absolute relative difference (MARD) between sensors' measurements were $12.3 \pm 12.1\%$, $10.8 \pm 9.9\%$, and $17.9 \pm 15.8\%$, respectively [38].

Implanted continuous monitoring glucose microbiosensors can be paired with insulin (and potentially glucagon) pump for closed-loop drug delivery system, so-called artificial pancreas [26, 39–42]. Despite widespread application of CGMS and insulin pump combos (such as, Medtronic's MiniMed 530G insulin pump coupled with Enlite sensor), today there is no fully automated insulin administration and various degrees of user input are required to initiate administration of insulin bolus [43]. Challenges that are still remaining include dynamic nature of differences of glucose levels in blood and in subcutaneous adipose tissues, but accuracy, reliability, and longevity of CGMS still remain major areas for improvement [17, 39].

2.2.2 *In-vivo enzymatic biosensor systems in development*

In-vivo electrochemistry allows for real-time determination of physiological concentration of many biological molecules and compounds. Monitoring of glucose (critical not only for maintaining normoglycemia in diabetic patients but also for understanding of energy utilization in the brain), lactate (important for trauma management and for estimating the extent of oxygen deprivation after myocardial infarction), glutamate (one of the most important neurotransmitters in mammalian nervous system responsible for signaling and thus such neural functions as cognition, learning, and memory), dopamine (regulation of this neurotransmitter is affected during such neurological disorders as Huntington's and Parkinson's diseases) and other biomolecules can be performed by a new generation of enzymatic biosensors [44]. Rapid advancement in this area is connected to new developments in materials science, including implementation of new materials and of nanotechnology [45–48].

One research group immobilized glucose oxidase (GOx) together with Neutral Red (NR) electrochemical mediators on a flexible carbon fiber (FCF) 1 micron in diameter to obtain the second-generation biosensor. Bare 1 micron diameter CFC was used as a counter-electrode and both, the working and the counter-electrode were fixed within a flexible polypropylene 0.5 mm internal diameter flexible catheter. The system was tested *in-vitro* and then implanted into the thoracic region of a living rat (*Rattus novergicus*) [49]. The *in-vivo* detection of glucose was performed at normal (30 mg/dL) and elevated (200 mg/dL) levels.

Graphene is a very attractive material for biosensor electrodes due to its excellent electromechanical properties, especially extremely high surface area and charge-carrier mobility [50]. Recently, a joint group of researchers from Sweden and Pakistan reported on development and testing of third-generation graphene-based miniature biosensor for intracellular glucose measurements [51]. Glass capillary with the tip size of 0.7 μm was coated with graphene and dipped into GOx mix at room temperature and dried, resulting in the deposition of graphene-GOx conjugate. This microelectrode with corresponding Ag/AgCl reference microelectrode were used in potentiometric two electrode setup to measure glucose level in a single cell from a human subcutaneous adipose tissue sample. In potentiometry the potential difference is measured between the indicator electrode and the reference electrode at zero current. Graphene sheets are located in close vicinity to redox centers of the enzymes enabling a direct electron transfer resulting in an enhanced sensitivity of ~64 mV/decade with good linearity in the measurement range of 10 μM–1 mM of glucose. The biosensor also demonstrated superior selectivity: adding up to 500 μM of ascorbic acid or uric acid (reactants that typically cause strong interference in enzymatic biosensors) to 1000 μM of glucose generates only a weak transient signal. The biosensor measurements of 60 ± 10 mM glucose concentration corresponded well with nuclear magnetic resonance spectroscopy measurements of 70 mM in human muscle tissue.

A group of researchers from Clarkson University (USA) constructed glutamate oxidase (GmOx) biosensor designed to work well in conditions of hypoxia (oxygen deprivation) often associated with neurodegenerative diseases [52]. Oxidoreductase enzymes don't work reliably under low oxygen conditions since lack of oxygen (and not of the analyte of interest) becomes the limiting factor in biosensor measurement. To address this problem the chitosan immobilization matrix of the biosensor besides GmOx includes a composite of ceria and titania nanoparticles on the surface of the platinum microelectrode. The oxygen stored in cerium-oxide-rich nanoparticles can be released upon the reaction with hydrogen peroxide that is generated at the enzyme in contact with glutamate. This release process is catalyzed by the presence of titania nanoparticles. Amperometric detection was performed at a potential of 0.6 vs Ag/AgCl reference electrode in oxygenated and deoxygenated conditions. The sensitivities reported for these conditions were 793 pA/μM and 395 pA/μM and the corresponding limits of detection were 0.594 μM and 0.493 μM for oxygenated and deoxygenated conditions, respectively. Recordings were conducted also in cerebrospinal fluid. Preliminary *in-vivo* studies in Sprague-Dawley rats demonstrated the promise of this technology for real-time detection of glutamate.

The same research group used platinum-ceria nanoparticles (reported as having higher biocatalytic activity than pure ceria) immobilized together with lactate oxidase (Lox) enzyme on the surface of the platinum microelectrode [52]. The biosensor had a detection limit under hypoxic conditions of 100 pM. The biosensor also demonstrated high selectivity against the physiological levels of ascorbic acid due to the employment of o-phenylenediamine (o-PD) permselective layer deposited on the platinum electrode surface. *In-vivo* amperometric measurements (using applied potential of 0.55 V vs Ag/AgCl reference electrode) were successfully performed on the brain tissue of anesthetized rats.

In some cases a simultaneous *in-vivo* reading of several analytes is required. This capability is urgently required for managing trauma and its complications such as hemorrhage (abnormal blood flow) that is one of the leading causes of death following accidents and war injuries [53]. To efficiently monitor trauma, in addition to measurement of physical vital signs (heart rate, temperature, etc.), collecting data on physiologically relevant biochemical markers is critical. For example, glucose level indicates severity of injury or shock and lactate levels are indicative of hypoxia.

Researchers from Clemson University (USA) have developed an implantable integrated lactate and glucose biosensor to influence patient outcomes following trauma-induced hemorrhage [10]. The microchip contains the amperometric setup with microdisc electrode array of separately immobilized lactate oxidase and glucose oxidase enzymes. The biosensors exhibited linear dynamic ranges of 1.0–7.0 mM for lactate and 0.10–13.0 mM for glucose. Preliminary *in-vivo* studies were performed in a Sprague-Dawley rat hemorrhage model where wireless transmitting dual potentiostat was used to control the implanted biosensor chip.

The same group reported on further study of the implantable dual glucose and lactate biosensor with special emphasis on the techniques for enzyme immobilization [54]. If prior work used electroactive hydrogels for enzyme immobilization, in this study researchers demonstrated superiority of the entrapment with polypyrrole electropolymerization that included 1-ethyl-3-[3-dimethylaminopropyl] carbodiimide (EDC), N-hydroxysulfosuccinimide (Sulfo-NHS), and monomerization agent 4-(3-pyrrolyl)butyric acid and sulfonization/dopanization reagent 4-sulfobenzoic acid. *In-vivo* measurements in Sprague-Dawley model demonstrated that after 4 h there was a significant deterioration in sensitivity, response time, and detection limits due to biofouling.

One of the most active application areas for *in-vivo* biosensing in recent years has been the brain research. Many microbiosensors have been developed and tested to measure the levels of neurochemicals in the extracellular fluid to understand the molecular basis of brain functions for energy utilization and signal transmission [55]. One of the alternative to *in-vivo* biosensing measurement is the use of implanted microdialysis catheter for sampling of the intracellular fluid coupled with *in-vitro* biosensing. For example, research team of the Chinese Academy of Sciences has developed an efficient second-generation biosensor for measurement of the glucose levels in the brain. The synthesis process for assembly of all biosensing elements (enzyme glucose dehydrogenase, GDH; cofactor NAD+; mediator methylene green) are encapsulated into a nanoparticle and these biochemically active nanoparticles, together with single-walled nanotubes, form three-dimensional nanocomposite on a glassy carbon substrate. In the *In-vivo* study, the glucose levels of the samples taken from the striatum of guinea pigs were determined to be 0.31 ± 0.03 mM.

The same group later reported on the development of microdialysis cannula-coupled biosensor flow cell for online measurement of hypoxanthine [56]. The study demonstrated that biosensor fabricated utilizing xanthine oxidase enzyme (XOD) immobilized with low-potential mediator thionine absorbed onto nanotubes exhibits good selectivity against such interfering compounds as uric acid or ascorbic acid. Online measurements of brain microdialysates were performed on adult male Sprague-Dawley rats.

It is possible to combine advantages of microdialysis sampling approach (such as minimization of biofouling since biosensors in these setups are located outside the body) and portability and afforded mobility of implantable biosensors by using microfabrication (including soft lithography) to create an encapsulated enzymatic microreactor (EMR) coupled to microdialysis catheter [57]. The microfluidic chip was molded from polydimethylsiloxane (PDMS) and included fluidic channel with integrated micromixer allowing efficient mixing of glucose oxidase solution with microdialysis sample in nanoliter volumes. The EMR also included thin film platinum electrode and Ag/AgCl reference wire electrode. The researchers successfully demonstrated a short-term (4 h) application of the system for *in-vivo* continuous glucose monitoring on male Wistar rats.

Implantable biosensors are an attractive alternative to microdialysis approach since it's easier to miniaturize the biochip and make an implantable system. A number of research groups have developed and validated implantable micro-biosensors for monitoring various neurochemicals in brain extracellular fluid including D-serine [58], choline [59], glucose [60], glutamate [61], dopamine [62], lactate [63], and pyruvate [64], among others.

For enzymatic biosensors interferences from exogenous and endogenous electroactive substances present a serious issue that is usually dealt with in three ways: using mediators, co-immobilizing additional types of enzymes, and using permselective membranes. Utilization of mediators often allows for shifting an oxidation potential of the analyte of interest below that of interfering substances. For example, researchers have created bioelectrode with active surface being a three-dimensional matrix of multiwall carbon nanotubes (MWNTs), polyaniline, Glucose Oxidase, and Prussian Blue (mediator) [60]. The glucose biosensor exhibited negligible interference from such substances as sodium ascorbate, dopamine, 3,4-dihydroxyphenylacetic acid (DOPAC), and uric acid (UA). Another study reported using co-immobilized ascorbate oxidase enzyme to dramatically reduce interference from ascorbic acid for amperometric detection of glutamate [65]. Finally, utilization of permselective membranes at electrode surfaces presents a widely employed strategy for reduction of access of the interfering compounds to an electrode surface. Popular choices for the membranes are either self-assembled layers such as Nafion or electrodeposited polymer films such as poly(phenylenylenediamine) (PPD) and overoxidized polypyrrole (OPPy); usually the higher selectivity comes at a price of somewhat lower sensitivity [31]. One research group evaluated variety of permselective membranes including Nafion, OPPy, PPD, Overoxidized Polyaniline (OPANi), and Polypyrrole-poly(2-naphthol) in effectiveness at reducing interference for amperometric detection of glutamate [66]. Poly(m-PD) and Nafion-poly(m-PD) demonstrated the best selectivity in *in-vitro* and *in-vivo* experiments.

It is possible to use microfabrication to create biosensor probe. In one study a lithography was used on silicon wafer to mask it and etch out a 150 micron wide, 120 micron thick probe [67]. Platinum metal pads and traces were patterned on the surface of the probe and then PPy was electrodeposited, Nafion was coated, and L-glutamate oxidase layers were cross-linked with bovine serum albumin (BSA) and glutaraldehyde to create the biosensing layers on the surface of the electrode. *In-vivo* studies in male Sprague-Dawley rats followed. This experimental procedure utilized an Ag/AgCl wire reference electrode for amperometric measurements, however it is not the best choice of *in-vivo* reference electrode for a long-term study due to instability due to dissolution or delamination of AgCl film. The same research group microfabricated glutamate biosensor probe with electrochemically deposited iridium oxide reference electrode [68].

Microfabrication affords ease of fabrication of the microelectrode array on a single biosensor probe and thus multiple enzymes can be immobilized on a probe and various analytes can be measured simultaneously. For example, microfabricated silicon microprobe with platinum electrode array immobilized with choline oxidase and L-glutamate oxidase via cross linking with BSA and glutaraldehyde and subsequently covered by the electropolymerized PPD layer to improve selectivity of the sensor [69]. The biosensor exhibited limits of detection below 0.5 μM and sensitivity of 132 ± 20 μA $mM^{-1}cm^{-2}$ for choline and 95 ± 20 μA $mM^{-1}cm^{-2}$ for L-glutamate. The biosensor was successfully tested *in-vivo* in male Lister hooded rats. It is possible to implement a multi-analyte enzymatic biosensor by immobilizing enzymes on separate wire electrodes and collecting these electrodes into a bundle for implantation. This was a strategy implemented by a research group that fabricated multiplex biosensor device for simultaneous measurement of lactate, glucose, and pyruvate levels in the brain [64]. *In-vivo* testing confirming viability of the device was performed in male Wistar rats.

In order to realize implantable biosensor systems miniaturized biosensors required to be integrated with a wireless potentiostat and transceiver and incorporate a small footprint power supply [70, 71]. Several examples of integrated implantable biosensor platforms were demonstrated in recent years. One group has developed an implantable needle-type biosensor designed to continuously measure uric acid concentration in the interstitial fluids of the birds during various activities, including in flight [72]. The total system weighs just 6.5 g and consists of a biosensor (based on uricase enzyme immobilized on platinum-iridium wire and connected in two-electrode setup with Ag/AgCl reference paste electrode), microcontroller, read-out circuitry, and high capacity lithium polymer battery. *In-vivo* feasibility study included implantation of the biosensor system on the back of pigeons and collecting data during trials of flight and rest periods. Another group has developed a miniaturized wireless biosensor system to measure whole cholesterol concentration and tested the system *in-vivo* in fish [73]. The needle-type biosensor had an immobilized cholesterol oxidase and ferrocene mediator fixated in chitosan matrix on top of platinum-iridium wire electrode coated with Nafion. Reference Ag/AgCl wire was wrapped around the electrode wire. The integrated system included 3 V micro battery and wireless potentiostat weighing around 6 g. The biosensor was implanted into fish eyeball interstitial sclera fluid and successfully collected cholesterol data for 48 h.

2.3 Development of non-enzymatic *in-vivo* biosensors

Among significant present limitations of presently used enzymatic *in-vivo* biosensors are their relatively short lifetime (5–7 days for commercialized CGMS), attendant requirement for frequent implantation, and need for daily calibration and non-enzymatic biosensors might offer a viable *in-vivo* monitoring alternative since their life-time is not limited by enzyme stability and degradation [74]. Most of the recently developed non-enzymatic *in-vivo* biosensors belong to optical sensors based on ligand–receptor interactions [75].

The earliest type of the optical (fluorescence) receptor-based biosensors utilized glucose-binding protein concanavalin A (Con A) where glucose detection is enacted through fluorescent resonant energy transfer (FRET) between fluorescein isothiocyanate-bound dextran and tetramethylrhodamineisothiocyanate-bound Con A [76]. In this biosensor glucose competes with fluorescently labeled dextran to binding site of Con A. Once dextran binds to Con A, the fluorescence is quenched. Thus florescence intensity is proportional to glucose concentration. Researchers were able to implement this FRET-based detection in 2 mm diameter poly(ethylene glycol) (PEG) hydrogel microspheres [77]. Recent *in-vivo* studies included implanting optical fiber with Con A and fluorophore-conjugated betacyclodextrin subcutaneously into anesthetized canines for several hours and glucose with concentration up to 300 mg/dL was measured with good correspondence to plasma glucose reference [78]. It is possible to synthesize quantum dots conjugated to Con A to implement “smart tattoo” biosensor (microcapsules or nanocapsules implanted under a dermis) [74]. One group, for example, synthesized CdTe quantum dots (QD) conjugated with Con A for detection of lipopolysaccharide [79]. Recent review describes advances in utilizing novel materials such as graphene for carbohydrates monitoring, including with FRET-based detection [80].

Con A does not have a great specificity among carbohydrates (for example, it has stronger affinity to fructose than to glucose), therefore, glucose-binding proteins (GBPs) such as periplasmic binding protein (PBP) based on *E. coli* and that can be genetically engineered present a viable option to fluorescent detection of glucose with higher specificity [75]. Researchers have been working toward development of *in-vivo* biosensors based on glucose/galactose binding proteins [81] and some one group using genetically engineered GBP has demonstrated glucose sensing in whole porcine blood [82]. However, this is still a young research field without significant studies of continuous monitoring in animal models.

2.4 Conclusion

Progress in *in-vivo* microbiosensors in the last five years has been reviewed. Despite a significant progress made in *in-vivo* biosensing recently, there are still some significant challenges that need to be overcome in many disciplines related to selectivity, sensitivity, biocompatibility, longevity, and reliability of *in-vivo* biosensors and additional advances are needed in miniaturized controls and telemetry and power supplies before *in-vivo* microbiosensors will find wide adoption [5, 83, 84].

References

[1] Turner AP. Biosensors: sense and sensibility. *Chemical Society Reviews* 2013,**42**:3184–3196.

[2] Yetisen AK, Akram MS, Lowe CR. Paper-based microfluidic point-of-care diagnostic devices. *Lab on a Chip* 2013,**13**:2210–2251.

[3] Chu MX, Miyajima K, Takahashi D, *et al.* Soft contact lens biosensor for in situ monitoring of tear glucose as non-invasive blood sugar assessment. *Talanta* 2011,**83**:960–965.

[4] Kudo H, Arakawa T, Mitsubayashi K. Status of soft contact lens biosensor development for tear sugar monitoring: a review. *Electronics and Communications in Japan* 2014,**97**:52–56.

[5] Matzeu G, Florea L, Diamond D. Advances in wearable chemical sensor design for monitoring biological fluids. *Sensors and Actuators B: Chemical* 2015,**211**:403–418.

[6] Corrie S, Coffey J, Islam J, Markey K, Kendall M. Blood, sweat, and tears: developing clinically relevant protein biosensors for integrated body fluid analysis. *Analyst* 2015,**140**:4350–4364.

[7] Tsai T-C, Guo C-X, Han H-Z, *et al.* Microelectrodes with gold nanoparticles and self-assembled monolayers for in vivo recording of striatal dopamine. *Analyst* 2012,**137**:2813–2820.

[8] Koschwanez HE, Reichert WM. In vitro, in vivo and post explantation testing of glucose-detecting biosensors: current methods and recommendations. *Biomaterials* 2007,**28**:3687–3703.

[9] Kulinsky L, Madou MJ. BioMEMS for Drug Delivery. In: *MEMS for biomedical applications.* Edited by Bhansali S, Vasudev A, Woodhead Publishing; Cambridge, UK; 2012.

[10] Guiseppi-Elie A. An implantable biochip to influence patient outcomes following trauma-induced hemorrhage. *Analytical and Bioanalytical Chemistry* 2011,**399**:403–419.

[11] Keum DH, Jung HS, Wang T, *et al.* Microneedle biosensor for real-time electrical detection of nitric oxide for in situ cancer diagnosis during endomicroscopy. *Advanced Healthcare Materials* 2015,**4**:1153–1158.

[12] Toghill KE, Compton RG. Electrochemical non-enzymatic glucose sensors: a perspective and an evaluation. *International Journal of Electrochemical Science* 2010,**5**:1246–1301.

[13] Heo YJ, Shibata H, Okitsu T, Kawanishi T, Takeuchi S. Long-term in vivo glucose monitoring using fluorescent hydrogel fibers. *Proceedings of the National Academy of Sciences* 2011,**108**:13399–13403.

[14] Wilson GS, Gifford R. Biosensors for real-time in vivo measurements. *Biosensors and Bioelectronics* 2005,**20**:2388–2403.

[15] Wilson GS, Hu Y. Enzyme-based biosensors for in vivo measurements. *Chemical Reviews* 2000,**100**:2693–2704.

[16] Ferri S, Kojima K, Sode K. Review of glucose oxidases and glucose dehydrogenases: a bird's eye view of glucose sensing enzymes. *Journal of Diabetes Science and Technology* 2011,**5**:1068–1076.

[17] Vashist SK. Continuous glucose monitoring systems: a review. *Diagnostics* 2013,**3**:385–412.

[18] Vaddiraju S, Burgess DJ, Tomazos I, Jain FC, Papadimitrakopoulos F. Technologies for continuous glucose monitoring: current problems and future promises. *Journal of Diabetes Science and Technology* 2010,**4**:1540–1562.

[19] McGarraugh G, Brazg R, Weinstein R. FreeStyle Navigator continuous glucose monitoring system with TRUstart algorithm, a 1-hour warm-up time. *Journal of Diabetes Science and Technology* 2011,**5**:99–106.

[20] Garcia A, Rack-Gomer AL, Bhavaraju NC, *et al.* Dexcom G4AP: an advanced continuous glucose monitor for the artificial pancreas. *Journal of Diabetes Science and Technology* 2013,**7**:1436–1445.

[21] Adolfsson P, Örnhagen H, Eriksson BM, Cooper K, Jendle J. Continuous glucose monitoring—a study of the enlite sensor during hypo-and hyperbaric conditions. *Diabetes Technology & Therapeutics* 2012,**14**:527–532.

[22] Iscoe KE, Davey RJ, Fournier PA. Do different glucose levels at calibration influence accuracy of continuous glucose monitoring readings in vitro? *Journal of Diabetes Science and Technology* 2012,**6**:477–478.

[23] Basu A, Dube S, Slama M, *et al.* Time lag of glucose from intravascular to interstitial compartment in humans. *Diabetes* 2013,**62**:4083–4087.

[24] Yoo E-H, Lee S-Y. Glucose biosensors: an overview of use in clinical practice. *Sensors* 2010,**10**:4558–4576.

[25] McGarraugh G. The chemistry of commercial continuous glucose monitors. *Diabetes Technology & Therapeutics* 2009,**11**:S-17–S-24.

[26] Shichiri M, Yamasaki Y, Kawamori R, Hakui N, Abe H. Wearable artificial endocrine pancreas with needle-type glucose sensor. *The Lancet* 1982, **320**:1129–1131.

[27] Kotanen CN, Moussy FG, Carrara S, Guiseppi-Elie A. Implantable enzyme amperometric biosensors. *Biosensors and Bioelectronics* 2012,**35**: 14–26.

[28] Tapsak MA, Rhodes RK, Shults MC, McClure JD. Techniques to improve polyurethane membranes for implantable glucose sensors. Patent US 20030217966, Nov 27, 2003.

[29] Van Antwerp WP. Polyurethane/polyurea compositions containing silicone for biosensor membranes. Patent WO 1996030431, Oct 3, 1996.

[30] Wang J. In vivo glucose monitoring: towards 'Sense and Act' feedback-loop individualized medical systems. *Talanta* 2008,**75**:636–641.

[31] Cordeiro C, de Vries M, Cremers T, Westerink B. The role of surface availability in membrane-induced selectivity for amperometric enzyme-based biosensors. *Sensors and Actuators B: Chemical* 2016,**223**:679–688.

[32] Gifford R, Kehoe JJ, Barnes SL, Kornilayev BA, Alterman MA, Wilson GS. Protein interactions with subcutaneously implanted biosensors. *Biomaterials* 2006,**27**:2587–2598.

[33] Onuki Y, Bhardwaj U, Papadimitrakopoulos F, Burgess DJ. A review of the biocompatibility of implantable devices: current challenges to overcome foreign body response. *Journal of Diabetes Science and Technology* 2008,**2**:1003–1015.

[34] Mortellaro M, DeHennis A. Performance characterization of an abiotic and fluorescent-based continuous glucose monitoring system in patients with type 1 diabetes. *Biosensors and Bioelectronics* 2014,**61**:227–231.

[35] Mader J, Weinhandl H, Köhler G, *et al.* Assessment of different techniques for subcutaneous glucose monitoring in Type 1 diabetic patients during 'real-life' glucose excursions. *Diabetic Medicine* 2010,**27**:332–338.

[36] Christiansen M, Bailey T, Watkins E, *et al.* A new-generation continuous glucose monitoring system: improved accuracy and reliability compared with a previous-generation system. *Diabetes Technology & Therapeutics* 2013,**15**:881–888.

[37] Calhoun P, Lum J, Beck RW, Kollman C. Performance comparison of the Medtronic Sof-Sensor and Enlite glucose sensors in inpatient studies of individuals with type 1 diabetes. *Diabetes Technology & Therapeutics* 2013,**15**:758–761.

[38] Damiano ER, McKeon K, El-Khatib FH, Zheng H, Nathan DM, Russell SJ. A comparative effectiveness analysis of three continuous glucose monitors the Navigator, G4 Platinum, and Enlite. *Journal of Diabetes Science and Technology* 2014, **8**:699–708.

[39] Ang KH, Tamborlane WV, Weinzimer SA. Combining glucose monitoring and insulin delivery into a single device: current progress and ongoing challenges of the artificial pancreas. *Expert Opinion on Drug Delivery* 2015,**12**:1579–1582.

[40] Alvarez-Lorenzo C, Concheiro A. Smart drug delivery systems: from fundamentals to the clinic. *Chemical Communications* 2014,**50**:7743–7765.

[41] Brambilla D, Luciani P, Leroux J-C. Breakthrough discoveries in drug delivery technologies: the next 30years. *Journal of Controlled Release* 2014,**190**:9–14.
[42] Park K. Controlled drug delivery systems: past forward and future back. *Journal of Controlled Release* 2014,**190**:3–8.
[43] Kumareswaran K, Evans ML, Hovorka R. Closed-loop insulin delivery: towards improved diabetes care. *Discovery Medicine* 2012,**13**:159–170.
[44] Wilson GS, Johnson MA. In-vivo electrochemistry: what can we learn about living systems? *Chemical Reviews* 2008,**108**:2462–2481.
[45] Scognamiglio V. Nanotechnology in glucose monitoring: advances and challenges in the last 10 years. *Biosensors and Bioelectronics* 2013,**47**:12–25.
[46] Zhang L, Wang J, Tian Y. Electrochemical in-vivo sensors using nanomaterials made from carbon species, noble metals, or semiconductors. *Microchimica Acta* 2014,**181**:1471–1484.
[47] Satvekar R, Tiwale B, Pawar S. Emerging trends in medical diagnosis: a thrust on nanotechnology. *Medicinal Chemistry* 2014,**4**:407–416.
[48] Rahman MM, Ahammad AJS, Jin J-H, Ahn SJ, Lee J-J. A comprehensive review of glucose biosensors based on nanostructured metal-oxides. *Sensors* 2010,**10**:4855–4886.
[49] Iost RM, Sales FC, Martins MV, Almeida MC, Crespilho FN. Glucose biochip based on flexible carbon fiber electrodes: in vivo diabetes evaluation in rats. *ChemElectroChem* 2015,**2**:518–521.
[50] Kuila T, Bose S, Khanra P, Mishra AK, Kim NH, Lee JH. Recent advances in graphene-based biosensors. *Biosensors and Bioelectronics* 2011,**26**: 4637–4648.
[51] ul Hasan K, Asif MH, Hassan MU, *et al.* A miniature graphene-based biosensor for intracellular glucose measurements. *Electrochimica Acta* 2015,**174**:574–580.
[52] Sardesai NP, Ganesana M, Karimi A, Leiter JC, Andreescu S. Platinum-doped ceria based biosensor for in vitro and in vivo monitoring of lactate during hypoxia. *Analytical Chemistry* 2015,**87**:2996–3003.
[53] Kotanen CN, Guiseppi-Elie A. Monitoring systems and quantitative measurement of biomolecules for the management of Trauma. *Biomedical Microdevices* 2013,**15**:561–577.
[54] Kotanen CN, Karunwi O, Guiseppi-Elie A. Biofabrication using pyrrole electropolymerization for the immobilization of glucose oxidase and lactate oxidase on implanted microfabricated biotransducers. *Bioengineering* 2014,**1**:85–110.
[55] Zhang M, Yu P, Mao L. Rational design of surface/interface chemistry for quantitative in vivo monitoring of brain chemistry. *Accounts of Chemical Research* 2012,**45**:533–543.
[56] Mao L, Zhang Z, Hao J, Xiao T, Yu P. Online electrochemical systems for continuous neurochemical measurements with low-potential mediator-based electrochemical biosensors as selective detectors. *Analyst* 2015,**140**:5039–5047.

[57] Moon B-U, de Vries MG, Cordeiro CA, Westerink BH, Verpoorte E. Microdialysis-coupled enzymatic microreactor for in vivo glucose monitoring in rats. *Analytical Chemistry* 2013,**85**:10949–10955.

[58] Zain ZM, O'Neill RD, Lowry JP, *et al.* Development of an implantable d-serine biosensor for in vivo monitoring using mammalian d-amino acid oxidase on a poly (o-phenylenediamine) and Nafion-modified platinum–iridium disk electrode. *Biosensors and Bioelectronics* 2010,**25**:1454–1459.

[59] Baker KL, Bolger FB, Lowry JP. A microelectrochemical biosensor for real-time in vivo monitoring of brain extracellular choline. *Analyst* 2015,**140**: 3738–3745.

[60] Li R, Guo D, Ye J, Zhang M. Stabilization of Prussian blue with polyaniline and carbon nanotubes in neutral media for in vivo determination of glucose in rat brains. *Analyst* 2015,**140**:3746–3752.

[61] Hamdan SK. In vivo electrochemical biosensor for brain glutamate detection: a mini review. *The Malaysian Journal of Medical Sciences: MJMS* 2014,**21**:12–26.

[62] Njagi J, Chernov MM, Leiter J, Andreescu S. Amperometric detection of dopamine in vivo with an enzyme based carbon fiber microbiosensor. *Analytical Chemistry* 2010,**82**:989–996.

[63] Schuvailo O, Soldatkin O, Lefebvre A, Cespuglio R, Soldatkin A. Highly selective microbiosensors for in vivo measurement of glucose, lactate and glutamate. *Analytica Chimica Acta* 2006,**573**:110–116.

[64] Cordeiro C, de Vries M, Ngabi W, Oomen P, Cremers T, Westerink B. In vivo continuous and simultaneous monitoring of brain energy substrates with a multiplex amperometric enzyme-based biosensor device. *Biosensors and Bioelectronics* 2015,**67**:677–686.

[65] Rahman MA, Kwon N-H, Won M-S, Choe ES, Shim Y-B. Functionalized conducting polymer as an enzyme-immobilizing substrate: an amperometric glutamate microbiosensor for in vivo measurements. *Analytical Chemistry* 2005,**77**:4854–4860.

[66] Wahono N, Qin S, Oomen P, Cremers T, de Vries M, Westerink B. Evaluation of permselective membranes for optimization of intracerebral amperometric glutamate biosensors. *Biosensors and Bioelectronics* 2012,**33**:260–266.

[67] Wassum KM, Tolosa VM, Tseng TC, Balleine BW, Monbouquette HG, Maidment NT. Transient extracellular glutamate events in the basolateral amygdala track reward-seeking actions. *The Journal of Neuroscience* 2012,**32**:2734–2746.

[68] Tolosa VM, Wassum KM, Maidment NT, Monbouquette HG. Electrochemically deposited iridium oxide reference electrode integrated with an electroenzymatic glutamate sensor on a multi-electrode arraymicroprobe. *Biosensors and Bioelectronics* 2013,**42**:256–260.

[69] Frey O, Holtzman T, McNamara R, *et al.* Enzyme-based choline and l-glutamate biosensor electrodes on silicon microprobe arrays. *Biosensors and Bioelectronics* 2010,**26**:477–484.

[70] Farina D, Alvau MD, Puggioni G, *et al.* Implantable (Bio) sensors as new tools for wireless monitoring of brain neurochemistry in real time. *World* 2014,**3**:1–17.

[71] Carrara S, Ghoreishizadeh S, Olivo J, *et al.* Fully integrated biochip platforms for advanced healthcare. *Sensors* 2012,**12**:11013–11060.

[72] Gumus A, Lee S, Ahsan SS, *et al.* Lab-on-a-bird: biophysical monitoring of flying birds. *PloS One* 2015,1–10.

[73] Takase M, Murata M, Hibi K, Huifeng R, Endo H. Development of mediator-type biosensor to wirelessly monitor whole cholesterol concentration in fish. *Fish Physiology and Biochemistry* 2014,**40**:385–394.

[74] Heo YJ, Takeuchi S. Towards smart tattoos: implantable biosensors for continuous glucose monitoring. *Advanced Healthcare Materials* 2013,**2**:43–56.

[75] Borisov SM, Wolfbeis OS. Optical biosensors. *Chemical Reviews* 2008,**108**:423–461.

[76] Meadows D, Schultz JS. Fiber-optic biosensors based on fluorescence energy transfer. *Talanta* 1988,**35**:145–150.

[77] Russell RJ, Pishko MV, Gefrides CC, McShane MJ, Cote GL. A fluorescence-based glucose biosensor using concanavalin A and dextran encapsulated in a poly (ethylene glycol) hydrogel. *Analytical Chemistry* 1999,**71**:3126–3132.

[78] Liao K-C, Chang S-C, Chiu C-Y, Chou Y-H. Acute response in vivo of a fiber-optic sensor for continuous glucose monitoring from canine studies on point accuracy. *Sensors* 2010,**10**:7789–7802.

[79] Ebrahim S, Reda M, Hussien A, Zayed D. CdTe quantum dots as a novel biosensor for serratia marcescens and lipopolysaccharide. *Spectrochimica Acta Part A: Molecular and Biomolecular Spectroscopy* 2015,**150**:212–219.

[80] Wang Y, Qu K, Tang L, *et al.* Nanomaterials in carbohydrate biosensors. *TrAC Trends in Analytical Chemistry* 2014,**58**:54–70.

[81] Pickup JC, Khan F, Zhi Z-L, Coulter J, Birch DJ. Fluorescence intensity- and lifetime-based glucose sensing using glucose/galactose-binding protein. *Journal of Diabetes Science and Technology* 2013,**7**:62–71.

[82] Siegrist J, Kazarian T, Ensor C, *et al.* Continuous glucose sensor using novel genetically engineered binding polypeptides towards in vivo applications. *Sensors and Actuators B: Chemical* 2010,**149**:51–58.

[83] Kricka LJ, Polsky TG, Park JY, Fortina P. The future of laboratory medicine—a 2014 perspective. *Clinica Chimica Acta* 2015,**438**:284–303.

[84] Hasan A, Nurunnabi M, Morshed M, *et al.* Recent advances in application of biosensors in tissue engineering. *BioMed Research International* 2014,**1**:1–18.

Chapter 3

Electrochemical biosensors: fabrication and applications in biodiagnostics

Nirmal Prabhakar[1] and Himkusha Thakur[1]

3.1 Principle of electrochemical biosensor

Based on their operating principle, the electrochemical biosensors can employ potentiometric, amperometric and impedimetric transducers depending on which aspects of the cell need to be measured. It involves the measurement of the potential and/or current in an electrochemical cell containing the target analyte and converting the chemical information into a measurable amperometric signal. Electrochemical sensing usually requires a reference electrode, a counter electrode and a working electrode/sensing electrode. The reference electrode, commonly made from Ag/AgCl, is kept at a distance from the reaction site in order to maintain a known and stable potential. The working electrode serves as the transduction element in the biochemical reaction, while the counter electrode establishes a connection to the electrolytic solution so that a current can be applied to the working electrode (Figure 3.1).

3.1.1 Voltammetry

Voltammetry is an electro-analytical method that can analyse a target by applying a constant or varying time-dependent potential to an electrochemical cell and measuring the resulting change in the current as a function of that potential. It can provide quantitative and qualitative information about the species involved in the oxidation or reduction reaction. Using different voltammetric techniques as Amperometry, Cyclic voltammetry, Differential pulse voltammetry, and Square wave voltammetry, different voltammograms are obtained (amperometry does not result in voltammogram). These voltammograms are analysed to know the concentration of the analyte as biocatalytic reaction rates are often chosen to be first order dependent on the bulk analyte concentration and such steady-state currents are usually proportional to the bulk analyte concentration.

[1]Department of Biochemistry, Punjab University, Chandigarh 160014, India

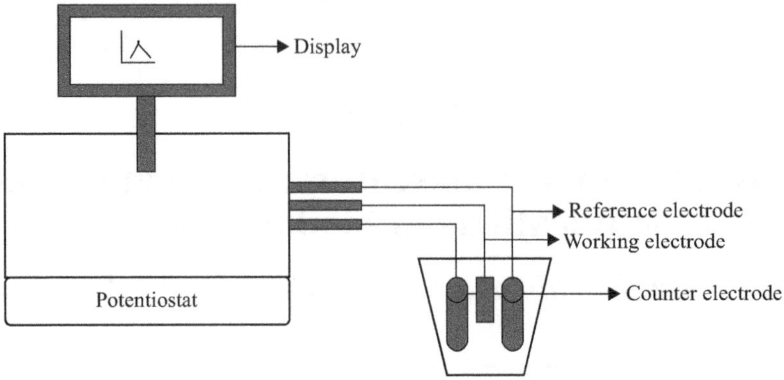

Figure 3.1 Diagram of potentiostat used in electrochemical studies

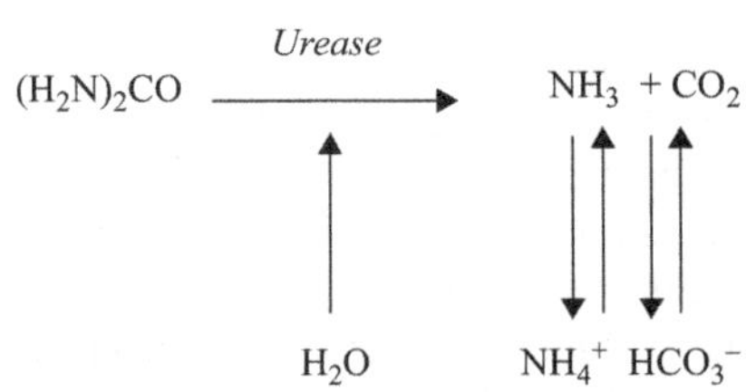

Figure 3.2 Principle of potentiometric urea biosensor

3.1.2 Potentiometry

Potentiometry passively measures the potential of a solution between two electrodes, affecting the solution very little in the process. The potential is then related to the concentration of one or more analytes. The transducer may be an ion-selective electrode (ISE) which is an electrochemical sensor based on thin films or selective membranes as recognition elements.

The potentiometric sensor has the characteristic that are different from voltammetric sensors as the measured species (such as H^+, NH_4^+) is not consumed and the output of the biosensor is in voltage and proportional to natural log of concentration. Taking an example of potentiometric urea biosensor, urea biorecognition is based on highly effective and selective hydrolysis of this compound catalysed by urease (Figure 3.2). These products alkalise the microenvironment at the surface of pH-sensor causing a decrease in its potential. So, potentiometric devices measure the accumulation of a charge potential at the working electrode.

3.1.3 Surface charge using field-effect transistors (FETs)

An important variation of the systems used to determine ion concentrations are the ion-sensitive field-effect transistors (ISFETs). An ISFET is composed of an ion-selective membrane applied directly to the insulated gate of the FET. When such

ISFETs are coupled with a biocatalytic layer, they become biosensors, and are usually called either enzyme field-effect transistors (ENFETs) or immunological field-effect transistors (IMFETs). The ISFET principle is based on a local potential generated by surface ions from a solution. This potential modulates the current flow across a silicon semiconductor. The transistor gate surface in ISFET is covered by a selective membrane; for pH detection such as silicon nitride (Si_3N_4), alumina (Al_2O_3), zirconium oxide (ZrO_2) and tantalum oxide (Ta_2O_5).

3.1.4 Conductometry

The conductometric biosensors are based on the fact that almost all enzymatic reactions involve either consumption or production of charged species and, therefore, lead to a global change in the ionic composition of the tested sample. Biosensors based on the conductometric principle present a number of advantages: (a) thin-film electrodes are suitable for miniaturisation and large scale production using inexpensive technology, (b) they do not require any reference electrode, (c) transducers are not light sensitive, (d) the driving voltage can be sufficiently low to decrease significantly the power consumption, (e) large spectrum of compounds of different nature can be determined on the basis of various reactions and mechanisms.

The inverse value of conductance is called resistance and hence for this reason such systems have also been named as impedimetric sensors. Electrochemical Impedimetric Spectroscopy (EIS) measures the response of an electrochemical system to an applied potential as a function of the frequency resulting in an impedance spectra known as Nyquist plot. The conductometric devices can be used to study biomolecular reactions on the sensing electrode that produce changes in the concentration of charged species in a solution. Another approach is to directly monitor the changes in conductance of an electrode as a result of the immobilisation of biomolecules as enzymes or complementary antibody-antigen pairs, etc. onto the electrode surface.

Based on the varied biomolecules being used for the fabrication of electrochemical biosensors, different detection strategies can be discussed that are very frequently employed in the electrochemical transduction.

3.2 Electrochemical nucleic acid sensors

Nucleic acids (NA) are perhaps the most widely used biomolecules in the field of biosensors due to their tremendous promise for obtaining sequence-specific information in a faster, simpler, and cheaper manner. NA biosensors have two major applications: sensing of genotoxicants (pesticide/toxicants, etc.) and detection of hybridisation to identify wide range of targets. ***Nucleic acid based electrochemical biosensors can be further categorised on the basis of detection strategy involved***. For example, most of the genotoxicants are detected based upon the electroactivity of NAs only, i.e., with or without the use of any mediator or a label. While the specific hybridisation reactions that are conducted to detect the presence of a particular target (e.g. pathogen or a biomarker of a disease) use the redox mediators, covalent bound labels or enzymes coupled to NA.

3.2.1 Detection of Genotoxicants/Pesticide

Guanine Oxidation is used for the detection of Genotoxicants/Pesticides, with or without reagent. The reagent-less techniques use no additional chemical reagents such as indicators or redox mediators to generate an analytical signal. In damaged DNA, the chemical nature of individual nucleotide is changed and this change is recorded by the biosensor. Most of the label-free NA biosensors employ guanine base (of the immobilised DNA) as a source of analytical signal to be interpreted, although all the NA bases have been reported to be electrochemically oxidisable, this is because guanine has low oxidising potential in comparison to other bases and any modification in the guanine is often accompanied by a loss of the guanine peak. The guanine oxidation current can be measured with or without an aid of reagent. The other strategy is to measure the current mediated by a reagent as metal complex (e.g. Ruthenium complex) in a solution. The advantage of this approach is to bring the far situated guanines to the close vicinity of the electrode surface for direct electro oxidation.

3.2.2 Detection of hybridisation can be done by different strategies

3.2.2.1 Monitoring guanine oxidation

The change in the guanine oxidation peak current has application in detection of not only in genotoxicants but for hybridisation also. Single stranded DNA (probe specific to some gene) that is used as probe has exposed nitrogenous bases especially guanine for oxidation. While in the case of dsDNA (hybridised form), there will be less availability of the guanine leading to falling of guanine oxidation current. The lowering of guanine oxidation current is thus the indication of the presence of complementary DNA-specific organism.

3.2.2.2 Redox mediators

These are small size compounds that enable the reversible exchange of electrons with the electrode and preferentially bind either to ssDNA or dsDNA. The most used electron mediators are ferrocene (Fc), $K_3Fe[(CN)]_6^{3-/4-}$, $Ru(bpy)_3^{3+/2+}$, $Os(bpy)_3^{3+/2+}$ and phenothiazine dye methylene blue (MB). NA biosensor for the detection of pathogen can be developed by immobilisation of oligonucleotide complementary to the one specific to pathogen. When the target DNA (test sample) containing a specific sequence matches that of the immobilised oligonucleotide probe DNA because of complementarity, a hybrid duplex DNA is formed at the electrode surface. Such hybridisation event is detected via the decreased current signal of an electroactive indicator such as MB gets intercalated in between the DNA duplex and can show very minimised MB peak current (Figure 3.3).

3.2.2.3 Electrochemically detectable label (or tracer)

is the other detection strategy, a label being attached to the NA that considerably improves the specificity and hence the detection, as the labelled DNA can be easily distinguished from the unlabelled one. These labels could be the electroactive groups, some of the widely used such labels include Fc tethered to the ends of

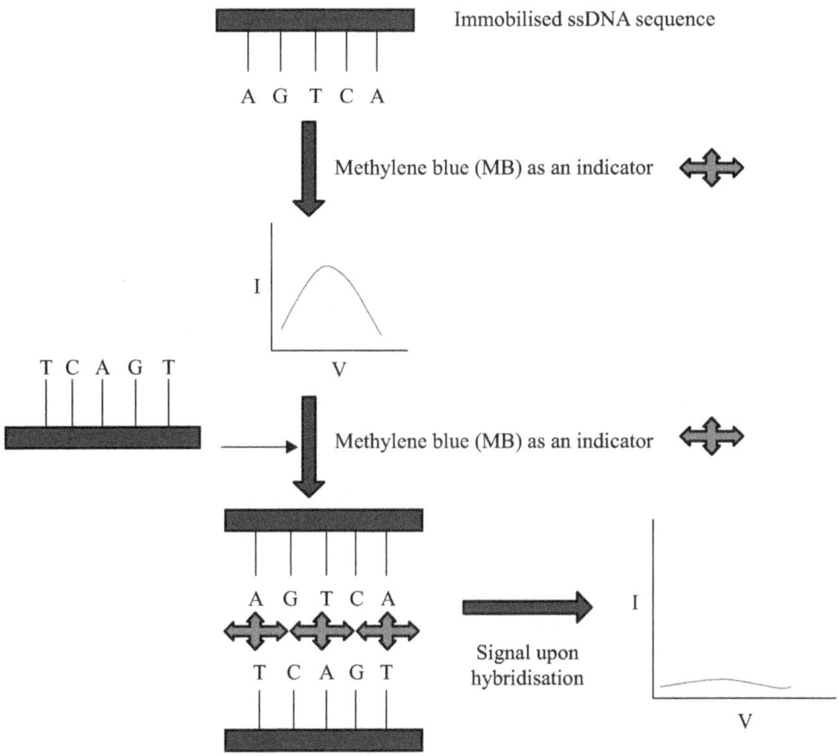

Figure 3.3 Electrochemical DNA biosensor for detection of hybridization using MB as an electroactive indicator

synthetic ODNs. When the complementary Fc labelled target DNA hybridised with the capture probe immobilised on the matrix, the Fc moiety comes closer to the electrode and a significant anodic current peak is observed because of the oxidation of the Fc. But if there is a mismatch, the binding to the capture probe becomes much weaker. As a result, fewer Fc molecules will be present in the vicinity of the electrode and much diminished or may be negligible anodic peak will be observed. Thus upon recognising the complementary sequence, voltammogram will show a well-defined anodic current peak, hence confirming hybridisation.

3.2.2.4 Enzymes as an aid to the electrochemical detection

have been put forward lately in terms of sandwich assays. The Fc labelling is frequently coupled with an enzyme-based electrochemical detection. The two enzymes that are largely used in such sandwich assays are alkaline phosphatase and horse radish peroxidase. For example, a biotinylated target probe is used to hybridise with its complementary capture probe (the modification like biotinylation can be either on capture probe being immobilised on the matrix or on the target probe, depending upon the design of strategy being used). Avidin-Alkaline Phosphatase (ALP) conjugate is bound to another DNA sequence complementary to the target probe.

Because of the biotin–avidin interactions, this avidin-ALP conjugate binds to the biotinylated target probe. When the substrate is added, it is catalysed by ALP to form an electroactive product. This compound after oxidation releases electrons that take part in the redox cycle of ferrocene (Fc^+ to Fc) (ferrocene present on the matrix) and thus producing the analytical signal. This signal is enhanced in the presence of the hybridisation as comparison to the mismatch sequence.

3.2.2.5 The electrochemical molecular beacons

attracted great attention as a tool for the solution of DNA hybridisation analysis. They are composed of an oligonucleotide forming a hairpin-like stem-loop structure, with a label. The sequence of the oligonucleotide with Fc as a label is chosen to form readily the stem-loop structure at the electrode surface. Within this structure Fc is located close to the electrode surface, producing a distinguished cyclic voltammetric redox pair in the absence of the complementary DNA. These voltammetric signals were due to electron tunnelling between Fc and the electrode. Hybridisation of target with the oligonucleotide results in the formation of a rigid rod like duplex DNA, and the Fc label is moved away from the electrode surface. This change in the Fc distance from the electrode surface results in a decreased or absence of the Fc electrochemical signal.

3.3 Electrochemical enzymatic sensor

Enzymes are first biomolecules used in the development of biosensors because of their high catalytic activity and selectivity toward substrates. Redox enzymes catalyse oxidation or reduction reactions with direct electron transfer making them highly suitable for electrochemical sensors that provide continuous real-time monitoring of the target biomolecules. The relatively simple layout consists of a bio-recognition layer of enzymes attached to a working electrode, and a transducer as shown in a Figure 3.4.

The enzyme-based biosensors can be divided into two main categories depending upon the detection principles.

3.3.1 Direct detection of analytes

Many metabolites like glucose, cholesterol, amino acids, uric acid, lactate, etc. are detected using this direct strategy and involves more or less same principle, i.e., the

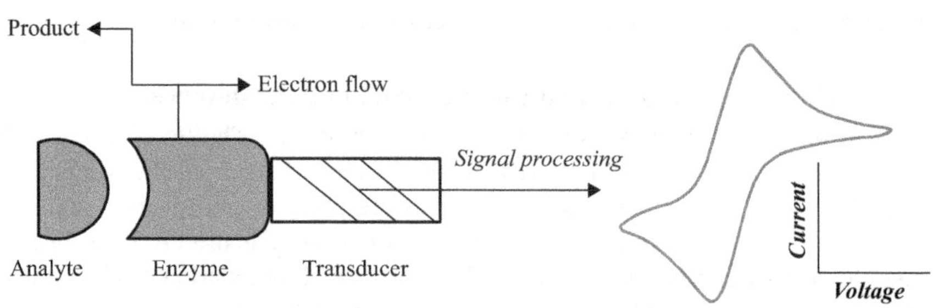

Figure 3.4 Illustration showing an enzymatic biosensor

substrate to be determined diffuses into the enzyme layer where the enzymatic reaction occurs, i.e., S + R - - - - P + R′ (in presence of enzyme), producing a product (P or R′) or consuming a coreactant (R) which can be measured electrochemically.

Enzyme-based electrochemical biosensor for the detection of cholesterol using cholesterol oxidase (ChOx) has been fabricated widely. Cholesterol, in the presence of ChOx, generates cholestenone and hydrogen peroxide, which further breaks down to oxygen and protons, releasing electrons. These produced electrons are responsible for the change in current peak that is directly proportional to the concentration of cholesterol. Increased concentration corresponds to the increased current because of the enhanced release of the electrons.

3.3.2 Indirect detection of analytes via inhibition of enzyme activity

It is based upon the inhibition assays to determine the concentration of the inhibitor in the assayed sample by measuring the percent of inhibition of the biocatalyst immobilised on the biosensor. This strategy is generally employed for the detection of food and environmental contaminants, primarily among them pesticides, herbicides and heavy metals. Organophosphate (OP) and carbamate insecticides are considered to be the most potent cholinesterase inhibitors for the commonly existing pollutants. Acetylcholinesterase (AChE)-based electrochemical sensors for the detection of pesticides (OP) present a perfect example of inhibition-based enzymatic biosensors. In AchE-based sensors, acetylthiolcholine is taken as substrate and thiocholine being produced can be monitored using electrochemical methods. The enzyme activity is indirectly proportional to the pesticide concentration.

$$\text{Acetylthiocholine} + H_2O \longrightarrow \text{Thiocholine} + \text{Acetic acid}$$

$$2\ \text{Thiocholine} \longrightarrow \text{Dithio-bis-choline} + 2H^+ + 2e^-$$

A well-defined current peak can be observed in the absence of pesticide, while the presence will replace the substrate in the enzymatic reaction to occupy the active sites of the enzymes, thus inhibiting the enzymatic activity. This results in much diminished current peak when analysed in the presence of the substrate.

3.4 Electrochemical immunosensors

An immunosensor is a device comprising of an antigen or antibody species coupled to a signal transducer, which detects the binding of complementary species.

3.4.1 An indirect immunosensor

An indirect immunosensor uses a separate labelled species that is detected after binding by, e.g., fluorescence or luminescence (i.e. a heterogeneous immunoassay). A direct device detects the binding by a change in potential difference, current, mass, heat properties (i.e. a homogenous immunoassay).

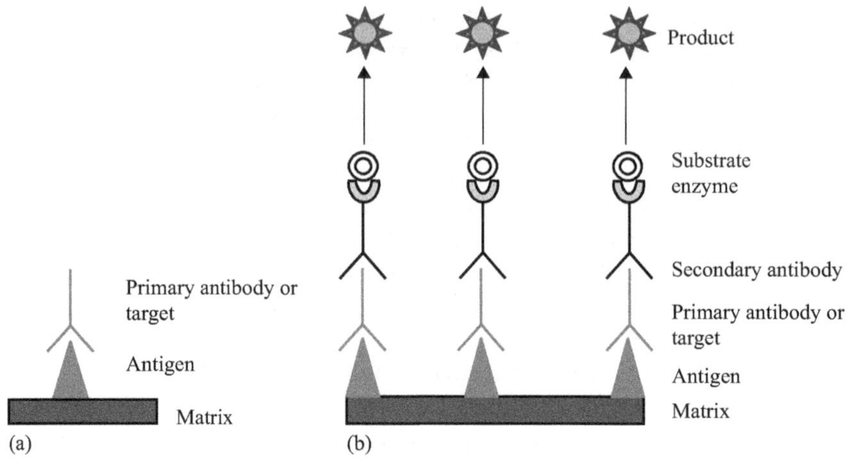

Figure 3.5 Illustration showing (a) direct and (b) indirect immunosensor

The indirect immunosensor involves the sandwich assay where the primary antibody Ab1 (immobilised on a suitable matrix) captures the target microbe. This is labelled using the secondary antibody-enzyme conjugate (Ab2-Enz), and the added enzyme substrate is converted to electrochemically active product measurable at the electrode (Figure 3.5).

3.4.2 The direct immunosensor

The direct immunosensor measures the change in the current or impedance because of the captured microbe that is blocking access of a suitable redox probe to the electrode. This is measured either using voltammetry or electrochemical impedance spectroscopy. Electrochemical immunosensors have been fabricated for wide range of targets including biomarkers involved in tumour detection, pathogens, or detection of different diseases.

3.5 Electrochemical whole cells based sensors

Whole cells, as the biological recognition elements in biosensors, can identify the physiological events and provide the analytical information as a living cell is considered to be an electrochemical dynamic system. Using whole cells as biomolecule gives advantages over others especially when compared with enzyme, as whole cells are less expensive and more stable during the production process. Different types of cells can be incorporated into electrochemical biosensor, including microorganisms, mammalian cells and recombinant cells in the immobilisation format of single cell, cell layer and cell network.

The cell based electrochemical biosensors mainly involve the monitoring of cellular activity/function and cellular barrier behaviour.

3.5.1 Based on the cellular activity of the cell

The cellular activity of a cell is the metabolism which depends on the intracellular and extracellular environment, leading to the changes of pH, oxygen and ion concentrations. This change can be observed in the form of electrochemical signal. The detection of cellular metabolites can give direct evidence of the activation of specific receptors and thus decoding the associated disease. In one of the whole cells based cholinesterase biosensor used for pesticide detection, the whole cells of *Arthrobacter globiformis* containing choline oxidase were fixed on a probe. Generated current was proportional to bacteria respiration [1].

The biggest advantage of using this type is the high stability of the response and long life-time of the sensor at ambient temperature, due to the conservation of the enzyme in its natural micro-environment inside the immobilised cells.

3.5.2 Based on cellular barrier behaviour

The cells are known to have excellent insulating properties and this property is exploited by biosensor based on cellular barrier behaviour, as it can affect the local ionic environment at the electrode interface (e.g. inhibition of flow of electrons), that can lead to change of resistance or current. The increased magnitude of electron-transfer resistance is related to the number of immobilised cells. Thus electrochemical techniques can be used to analyse the biological status of cells, including cellular viability, morphology, cell number, and adhesion, proliferation and apoptosis of cells.

3.6 Electrochemical aptasensors

Aptamers are artificial DNA or RNA oligonucleotides selected in vitro that are small in size, chemically stable, cost effective, which have the ability to bind to various target analytes as proteins (enzymes, prions, antibodies, growth factors, gene regulatory factors, cell adhesion molecules and lectins), pathogenic bacteria, viruses, pesticides, toxins, heavy metals, etc. with strong affinities and specificities and even exceeding than antibodies. Systematic Evolution of Ligands by Exponential Enrichment (SELEX) is the most accepted technique to generate the aptamer sequences that specifically bind to a target ligand or ligands (Figure 3.6).

The same immobilisation as well as detection strategies are employed here as well except that instead of hybridisation there is a formation of three-D complex and the change in the current is the indication of formation of aptamer-analyte complex.

3.7 Widely used materials in the construction of electrochemical biosensors

3.7.1 Conducting polymers

The biggest reason of using conducting polymers is their most notable property of inherent electrical conductivity, which is closely connected to the charge transfer

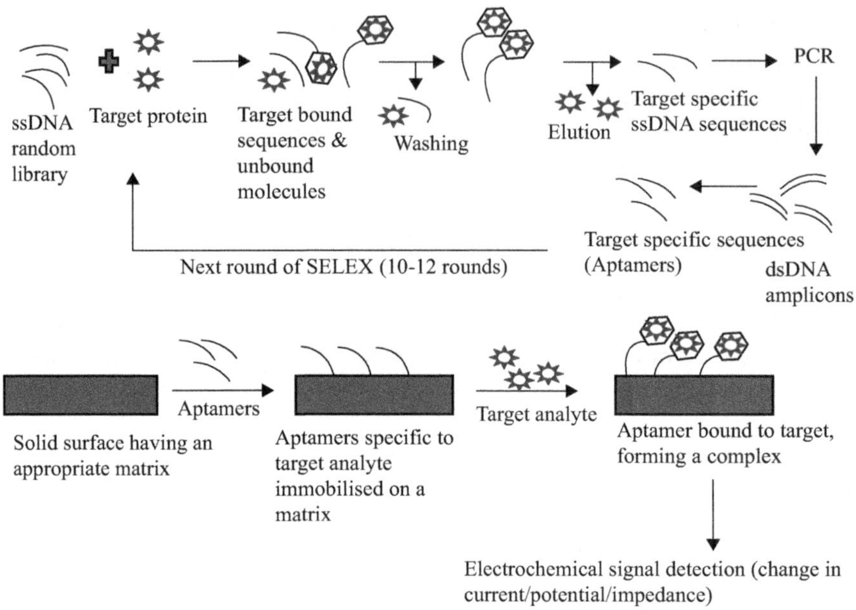

Figure 3.6 Schematic diagram of SELEX procedure

rate and electrochemical redox efficiency. Conducting polymers contain π-electron backbone responsible for their electrical conductivity, low energy optical transitions, low ionisation potential and high electron affinity. These extended π-conjugated systems of the conducting polymers have single and double bonds alternating along the polymer chain. Due to their chemical and structural diversity, these are considered as better candidates as immobilisation matrices in construction of electrochemical biosensors. Conducting polymers also share the strengths of polymers over other materials, including low-temperature synthesis and processing, large-area manufacture, flexibility and cost effectiveness.

Though they are conductive in nature but still have lower level of conductivity compared to metal, and poor solubility that can be improved through doping with a suitable dopant or modifying the polymer with some functional groups or making polymer composite/hybrid.

The preparation of polymers from their monomers can be done by using chemical or even biochemical methods or electropolymerically, to form polymeric particles of different and controlled size. Electrochemical polymerisation can control the thickness and morphology of deposited layer by application of well-defined potential and current. Some of the conducting polymers that are used frequently are Polypyrrole, Polyaniline, Thiophene based polymers, etc.

Polypyrrole has number of properties as redox activity, ability to form nanowires with room temperature conductivity (10^{-4} to 10^{-2} S cm^{-1}), ion-exchange and ion discrimination capacities, electrochromic effect depending on electrochemical polymerisation conditions and charge/discharge processes, strong absorptive properties toward gases, proteins, DNA, catalytic activity, corrosion protection properties, its biocompatibility, capability to transduce energy arising from interaction of analyte and analyte-recognising-site into electrical signals that are easily monitored.

Polyaniline is one of the most important conducting polymers. Polyaniline (PANI) has very good electrochemical activity and chemical stability and has been widely used in the DNA biosensor. Compared with a gold nanoparticle (GNP)- or carbon nanotube-based biosensor, the conducting PANI-based biosensor has some advantages: low-temperature synthesis, tunable conductivity and no need for purification or catalytic deposition processing. Unfortunately, PANI is usually less favourable as the element in biosensor construction because of its relative lower conductivity than the carbon nanotube as well as their non-oriented nanofibre morphology, leading to low detection sensitivity. The thermal stability of PANI is superior to other polymers. The processability and conductivity of PANI are also fairly good. From economic point of view, PANI is significantly superior to others because the aniline monomer is less expensive than other monomers.

Thiophene based polymers are one of the more extensively studied and like other conducting polymers are π-conjugated systems. Among thiophenes, poly (3,4-ethylendioxythiophene) (PEDOT) is widely used in the fabrication of biosensors and exhibits relatively high electrical conductivity and also is very stable even during the electrochemical changes. Poly(thiophene) and its derivatives, such as PEDOT are known to be the most stable conducting polymers currently available. This polymer can be simply obtained by anodic oxidation of the relevant monomer but shows high insolubility, that is overcome by the addition of dopants like Lithium Perchlorate (LP) or poly(styrenesulfonate) (PSS). These PEDOT:PSS or PEDOT:LP dispersions consist of a conducting PEDOT polycation and a counter anion, having a higher molecular weight than the previous one acts as a stabiliser keeping the PEDOT chain dispersed in the aqueous medium and also maintain the electron neutrality. PEDOT has been quite useful for making nanomaterial composites mainly due to its excellent stability and the possibility to prepare the corresponding PEDOT polymer hybrid matrices [2].

3.7.2 Carbon nanomaterial in electrochemical biosensors

Carbon nanotubes are built from sp^2 carbon units and are seamless structure with hexagonal honeycomb lattices with closed topology and tubular structure. There are two distinct structural families in carbon nanotubes, multi-wall carbon nanotubes (MWCNTs) and single-wall carbon nanotubes (SWCNTs). Carbon nanotubes have unique mechanical properties, electronic properties in combination with chemical stability. For sensing applications, carbon nanotubes have some advantages: small size with larger surface; high sensitivity, fast response and good reversibility at room temperature as a gas molecule sensor; enhanced electron transfer. CNTs also support an easy biomolecule immobilisation with retention of activity in biosensors and by providing the different functional groups such as carboxylic moieties for covalent linking of CNT to biorecognition elements (or other materials) [3].

On the other side, Graphene has also attracted strong scientific and technological interest in recent years because of its unique physicochemical properties: high surface area, excellent thermal conductivity and electric conductivity, and strong mechanical strength. Graphene-based electrodes have shown superior performance in terms of electrocatalytic activity [4] than carbon nanotubes-based ones. In comparison with carbon nanotubes, graphene exhibits potential advantages of low cost, high surface area, ease of processing and less toxicity. Graphene exhibits excellent electron transfer promoting ability and excellent catalytic behaviour toward small biomolecules such as H_2O_2, NADH, which makes graphene extremely attractive for enzyme-based biosensors.

3.7.3 Nanoparticles

The nanoparticles with unique properties have found broad application in many kinds of analytical methods. Owing to their small size (normally in the range of 1–100 nm), nanoparticles exhibit unique chemical, physical and electronic properties that are different from those of bulk materials. The basic functions of nanoparticles can be mainly classified as: (1) immobilisation of biomolecules (due to their large specific surface area and high surface free energy); (2) catalysis of electrochemical reactions (high surface energy); (3) enhancement of electron transfer (conductivity and tiny dimensions); (4) labelling biomolecules (small size and property of being modified) and (5) acting as reactant (chemical activity).

Nanoparticles are largely used in enzymatic biosensors as enzymes usually lack direct electrical communication with electrodes due to deeply seated active centres of enzymes surrounded by thick insulating protein shells.

Nanoparticles can be broadly classified into five categories including Fullerenes, Carbon nanotubes, Metal and Metal Oxide nanoparticles, Quantum dots and Polymeric Nanoparticles.

Metal nanoparticles have generally excellent conductivity and catalytic properties, which make them suitable for acting as 'electronic wires' to enhance the electron transfer between redox centres in proteins and electrode surfaces, and as catalysts to increase electrochemical reactions. Nanoparticles possess a drawback of aggregation that reduces their high surface area-to-volume ratio and subsequently effectiveness, but by appropriately dispersing metal and metal oxide nanoparticles into synthetic and naturally occurring polymers, many of the shortcomings can be overcome without compromising the parent properties of the nanoparticles.

The distinctive properties of GNPs have played an important role in increased interest over the last few years toward their coupling with biomolecules directly or indirectly. The GNPs provide a biomolecule friendly stable surface for their immobilisation that maintain their biological activities. Also, GNPs allow direct electron transfer between redox proteins and bulk electrode materials, which allows electrochemical sensing to be performed without the need for electron-transfer mediators. Like other nanoparticles, GNPs exhibit high surface-to-volume ratio and improved electron conducting property. GNP-modified matrices can be prepared in three ways: (1) by binding GNPs with functional groups of self-assembled monolayers (SAM), (2) by direct deposition of nanoparticles on a transducer, (3) by incorporating GNPs into the electrode by mixing them with the other components in the composite electrode matrix, e.g., preparing hybrids like PEDOT-GNPs.

3.8 Practical applications of the electrochemical biosensors

3.8.1 Biosensors of healthcare

For the determination of substances in biological fluids such as blood, serum and urine, etc., or to determine a certain biomarker of a disease, biochemical laboratories need much more reliable, cost effective as well as fast methods and biosensors can fulfil that demand.

3.8.1.1 Glucose

Blood glucose monitoring is a way of testing the concentration of glucose in the blood and is of utmost importance in the care of diabetes mellitus. There are various types of invasive and non-invasive glucometres and non-invasive have gained quite a popularity because of absence of drawing blood by puncturing the skin. NovioSense has developed a technique to measure different metabolites in basal tear fluid, based on a non-invasive sensor that is not visible when worn by subjects. The developed miniature electrochemical sensor is capable of detecting these metabolites and their respective concentrations, via an enzymatic reaction using an electrochemical cell.

The company Integrity Applications has worked upon generation of another non-invasive device for detection of glucose and has moved toward clinical trials potential regulatory approval in the U.S. This GlucoTrack uses an ear lobe clip-on similar to pulse oximetres to spot glucose levels through the skin. The sensor uses three different technologies to estimate blood glucose and sends its readings to a smartphone-like device that displays the numbers and keeps track of previous tests. Currently there are very few examples of point of care testing sensors that are available over the counters.

3.8.1.2 Cholesterol

Cholesterol biosensors based on electrochemical transduction hold an important place in the diagnostics due to high-rate of clinical disorders, such as heart disease, coronary artery disease, cerebral thrombosis, etc. (caused by the anomalous levels of cholesterol in blood). Umar *et al.* have developed a highly sensitive cholesterol amperometric biosensor based on the immobilisation of cholesterol oxidase (ChOx) onto the ZnO nanoparticles that has shown detection limit of 0.37 nM with a response time of less than 5 seconds [5]. From the commercialisation point of view, Oxford Biosensors have developed a portable hand-held device (Multisense^{TM}) for cholesterol detection. The project to develop smart integrated miniaturised sensors

(SIMS) is being led by Professor Tony Killard at University of the West of England, Bristol for the detection of cholesterol.

3.8.1.3 Urea

Urea is a nitrogen compound widely used, such as fertiliser in agriculture and as a nitrogen source for animal feeding stuff additive. The determination of urea is of great importance in areas such as clinical analysis, food industry, cosmetics and environmental assessment. In the environmental area, the large amount of urea in wastewater and water bodies can encourage the eutrophication process. Determination of blood urea nitrogen is an important routine test widely used in clinical laboratories. Urease enzyme has been widely used by researchers to develop a biosensor [6].

3.8.1.4 Celiac disease (Anti-gliadin antibody as biomarker) sensor

Celiac disease is an autoimmune disorder that can occur in genetically predisposed people where the ingestion of gluten leads to damage in the small intestine. When people with celiac disease eat gluten (a protein found in wheat, rye and barley), their body mounts an immune response that attacks the small intestine. The diagnosis of Celiac disease requires to test for levels of antibodies like Immunoglobulin A anti-tissue transglutaminase or high levels of another antibody, anti-gliadin antibody may also be detected. However, anti-gliadin antibody levels are useful in monitoring response to treatment, because they will usually begin to fall within several months of successful treatment of celiac disease. An immunosensor has been developed for the detection of autoantibodies directed against wheat gliadin, involved in celiac disease [7].

3.8.1.5 Oxidative stress

Hydrogen peroxide (H_2O_2), along with the hydroxyl radical (OH) and superoxide anion (O_2^-), belongs to a group of molecules known as reactive oxygen species (ROS). The sensing of the level of these ROS as H_2O_2 can be of great help in diagnosing the associated diseases. One such type of biosensor had a fast response of less than 2 s with a good LOD [8]. Other than the direct detection of ROS, several biomarkers of oxidative stress as glutathione (GSH), 3-nitrotyrosine (NT), homocysteine (Hcys) and cysteine (Cys) can be identified.

3.8.2 Biosensors for environmental monitoring

Environmental monitoring is critical to know whether the quality of our environment is getting better or worse. Environmental monitoring helps to create a baseline for the impact of pollutants like harmful gases, heavy metals, toxins, pesticides, genotoxicants, etc. in the air, land and water.

3.8.2.1 Pesticides

Due to the large amounts of pesticides commonly used in agriculture/horticulture, their impact on health, early and accurate pesticide analysis is important. Electrochemical biosensor for the detection of pesticides has been discussed in Section 3.3.2 too.

3.8.2.2 Heavy metals

Heavy metals can be toxic to living organisms and these can make important alterations to the biochemical cycles of life. The main threats to human health from heavy metals are associated with exposure to lead, cadmium, mercury and arsenic. Adam *et al.* developed a new heavy metal biosensor based on interaction of heavy metal ions (Cd^{2+} and Zn^{2+}) with phytochelatin. The authors have used the sensor to determine heavy metals in a biological sample – human urine and platinum in a pharmaceutical drug [9]. Lead (Pb), another harmful heavy metal, can come from automobile exhausts, old paints, mining wastes, incinerator ash or water from lead pipes and is known to cause damage to the nervous system. Kaur *et al.* developed a potentiometric biosensor based on urease inhibition by Pb (II) ions for its estimation in milk samples [10].

3.8.2.3 Toxic gases

Many electrochemical biosensors have been prepared for the detection of toxic gases as carbon monoxide. When a chemically reactive gas passes through the diffusion barrier it is either oxidised (accepts oxygen and/or gives up electrons) or reduced (gives up oxygen and/or accepts electrons), depending upon the gas. The resulting potential difference between the two electrodes causes a current to flow and is proportional to the concentration of the gas. One of an example is the detection of formaldehyde (a colourless, flammable, strong-smelling chemical that is commonly used as an industrial fungicide, germicide and disinfectant). Lin *et al.* have developed a formaldehyde sensor using TiO_2 nanotube arrays with detection limit is estimated to be around 0.04 ppm [11].

3.8.2.4 Genotoxicants

The detection of genotoxicants that could be present in water, food, soil and plant samples, or the presence of analytes (carcinogens, drugs, mutagenic pollutants, etc.) have been widely done by using DNA biosensors. These targets have binding affinities for the structure of DNA. Binding of small molecules to DNA and their subsequent effect is generally studied with electrochemical signal of guanine and has been discussed in detail under Section 3.2.1.

3.8.3 Biosensors in food industry

Acrylamide is formed when certain carbohydrate-rich foods are fried, baked or roasted at temperatures above 120 °C and is of concern as a possible carcinogen. Stobiecka *et al.* have designed a voltammetric biosensor for the detection of acrylamide with LOD of 1.2×10^{-10} M [12].

Another harmful substance found in commonly consumed item is benzene. Presence of benzene in soft drinks has been reported and is of concern for human health due to the carcinogenic nature of benzene. A biosensor was formed with biological sensing element (*Pseudomonas putida* F1), which could detect the presence of benzene [13]. Various types of sensors for detection of heavy metals like lead in the food sample have been reported as discussed in Section 3.8.2.2.

To detect the polyphenols in the tea using tyrosinase has been an interesting use of biosensors. Major quality attributes such as colour and astringency are directly linked with polyphenol contents. The voltage response due to the catalytic activity of tyrosinase on tea PP is measured as a method of quality assessment.

Short chain fatty acids are liberated by lipolysis that are responsible for rancid flavours found in milk and can be used to evaluate the freshness of milk by monitoring the oxygen consumption of the bacteria (*Arthrobacter nicotianae*) [14].

3.8.4 Biosensors for cancer

Early diagnosis of cancer is important because when abnormal tissue or cancer is found early, it may be easier to treat. Biomarkers are therefore invaluable tools for cancer detection, diagnosis, patient prognosis and treatment selection. There is a wide range of cancer biomarkers that can help to detect cancer at the early or late stages of cancer. Biosensors are highly sensitive methods for measuring cancer diagnosis markers present at ultra-low levels during early stages of the disease. An immunosensor was designed for detection of human epidermal growth factor receptor 2 (HER2) using a differential pulse voltammetry (DPV) method. Anti-HER2 antibodies attached to a suitable matrix and under optimal conditions, the immunosensor was responsive to HER2 concentrations over a wide range with a satisfactory detection limit as low as 0.995 pg/ mL and a favourable sensitivity. The reliability of the method in clinical analysis was proved by successful quantisation of HER2 levels in serum samples obtained from patients [15].

Many researchers have worked upon the detection of Telomerase activity using electrochemical measurements. Telomerase is considered as important biomarker for cancer cells and it is responsible for the immortality of cells and uncontrolled growth of cancer cells.

3.8.5 Biosensors for pathogens

Pathogen detection is of utmost importance because of health and safety concern. The main disadvantages of conventional pathogen detection methods are the multistep procedure and long-time requirements. A rapid, portable and accurate diagnostic technique can be provided by a biosensor and thus prevention from the outbreak of any epidemic.

Campylobacter jejuni (a food pathogen) is a gram-negative bacteria that can lead to the development of Guillian-Barre Syndrome (GBS), a disorder of the peripheral nervous system often leading to partial paralysis. Ivnitski *et al.* developed a new ion-channel biosensor based on supported bilayer lipid membrane for direct and fast detection of *Campylobacter* species. The biosensor showed good sensitivity and selectivity to *Campylobacter* species [16].

Salmonella is a bacterium that can cause fever, diarrhoea and abdominal cramps if salmonella-infected food is taken. Ma *et al.* have developed an aptasensor that showed a detection limit as low as 3 cfu/mL and this novel method is specific and fast, and it has the potential for real sample detection [17].

Sexually transmitted diseases (STDs) are a public health problem, and their prevalence is rising even in developed nations, in the era of HIV/AIDS. A sequence-specific electrochemical STD sensor based on self-assembled monolayer specific to detection of Gonorrhoea, an STD, has been fabricated by Singh *et al.* [18].

An electrochemical biosensor for the detection of short DNA sequences related to the human immunodeficiency virus type 1 (HIV-1) has been developed by Wang *et al.* [19].

Nakamura *et al.* used an electrode system consisting of a basal-plane pyrolytic graphite (BPG) electrode and a porous nitrocellulose detection of bacteria in urine. *Escherichia coli* is the most common causative agent of urinary tract infection (UTI). With this system $5\times10^2 \pm 5\times10^5$ cells/mL was measured in urine samples [20].

Acknowledgement

Authors acknowledge the insightful discussions with labmates that helped in framing this chapter.

References

[1] Stoytcheva M., Zlatev R., Valdez B., Magnin J.P., Velkova Z. 'Electrochemical sensor based on *Arthrobacter globiformis* for cholinesterase activity determination'. *Biosens. Bioelectron.* 2006, vol. 22, pp. 1–9.

[2] Istambouliea G., Sikorab T., Jubeteb E., Ochotecob E., Marty J.L., Noguer T. 'Screen-printed poly(3,4-ethylenedioxythiophene) (PEDOT): a new electrochemical mediator for acetylcholinesterase-based biosensors'. Talanta. 2010, vol. 82, pp. 957–961.

[3] Sergei A. Usanov, Archakov A., Shumyantseva V., *et al.* 'Cholesterol amperometric biosensor based on cytochrome P450scc'. *Biosens. Bioelectron.* 2004, vol. 19, pp. 971–976.

[4] Y. Wang, Y.M. Li, L.H. Tang, J. Lu, J.H. Li. 'Application of graphene-modified electrode for selective detection of dopamine'. *Electrochem.Commun.* 2009, vol. 11, pp. 889–892.

[5] Umar A., Rahman M.M., Vaseem M., Hahn Y.B. 'Ultra-sensitive cholesterol biosensor based on low-temperature grown ZnO nanoparticles'. *Electrochem. Commun.* 2009, vol. 11, pp. 118–121.

[6] Ali S.U., Ibupoto Z.H., Salman S., Nur O., Willander M., Danielsson B. 'Selective determination of urea using urease immobilized on ZnO nanowires'. *Sens. Actuators. B.* 2011, vol. 160, pp. 637–643.

[7] Balkenhohl T., Lisdat F. 'An impedimetric immunosensor for the detection of autoantibodies directed against gliadins'. *Analyst.* 2007, vol. 132, pp. 314–322.

[8] Bian X., Lu X., Jin E., Kong L., Zhang W., Wang C. 'Fabrication of Pt/polypyrrole hybrid hollow microspheres and their application in electrochemical biosensing towards hydrogen peroxide'. *Talanta.* 2010, vol. 81, pp. 813–818.

[9] Adam V., Zehnalek J., Petrlova J., *et al.* 'Phytochelatin modified electrode surface as a sensitive heavy-metal ion biosensor'. *Sensors.* 2005, vol. 5, pp. 70–84.

[10] Kaur H., Kumar S., Verma N. 'Enzyme-based colorimetric and potentiometric biosensor for detecting Pb (II) Ions in Milk'. *Braz. Arch. Biol. Technol.* 2014, vol. 57, pp. 613–619.

[11] Lin S., Li X. 'A selective room temperature formaldehyde gas sensor using TiO_2 nanotube arrays'. *Sens. Actuators, B.* 2011, vol. 156, pp. 505–509.

[12] Stobiecka A., Radecka H., Radecki J. 'Novel voltammetric biosensor for determining acrylamide in food samples'. *Biosens. Bioelectron.* 2007, vol. 22, pp. 2165–2170.

[13] Rasinger J.D., Marrazza G., Briganti F., Scozzafava A., Mascini M., Turner A.P.F. 'Evaluation of an FIA operated amperometric bacterial biosensor, based on Pseudomonas Putida F1 for the detection of benzene, toluene, ethylbenzene, and xylenes (BTEX). *Anal. Lett.* 2007, vol. 38, pp. 1531–1547.

[14] Vo-Dinh T., Cullum B. 'Biosensors and biochips: advances in biological and medical diagnostics'. *Fresenius J. Anal. Chem.* 2000, vol. 366, pp. 540–551.

[15] Emami M., Shamsipur M., Saber R., Irajirad R. 'An electrochemical immunosensor for detection of a breast cancer biomarker based on antiHER2–iron oxide nanoparticle bioconjugates'. *Analyst.* 2014, vol. 139, pp. 2858–2866.

[16] Ivnitski D., Wilkins E., Tien H.T., Ottova A. 'Electrochemical biosensor based on supported planar lipid bilayers for fast detection of pathogenic bacteria'. *Electrochem. Commun.* 2000, vol. 2, pp. 457–460.

[17] Ma X., Jiang Y., Jia F., Yu Y., Chen J., Wang Z. 'An aptamer-based electrochemical biosensor for the detection of Salmonella'. *J. Microbiol. Methods.* 2014, vol. 98, pp. 94–98.

[18] Singh R., Sumana G., Verma R., *et al.* 'DNA biosensor for detection of Neisseria gonorrhoeae causing sexually transmitted disease'. *J. Biotechnol.* 2010, vol. 150, pp. 357–365.

[19] Wang J., Cai X., Rivas G., Shiraishi H., Farias P.A.M., Dontha N. 'DNA electrochemical biosensor for the detection of short DNA sequences related to the human immunodeficiency virus'. *Anal. Chem.* 1996, vol. 68, pp. 2629–2634.

[20] Nakamura N., Shigematsu A., Matsunaga T. 'Electrochemical detection of viable bacteria in urine and antibiotic selection'. *Biosens. Bioelectron.* 1991, vol. 6, pp. 575–580.

Chapter 4

Microchip-based separation and detection methods for chemically and biologically valuable analytes

Shabi Abbas Zaidi[1], Akbar Nawab[2] and Bishnu P. Joshi[3]

4.1 Introduction

Electrophoresis is an outstanding and multifaceted technique to detect various complex biological samples such as nucleic acids, proteins, and oligonucleotides. It relies on the generation of some detectable signals due to migration behavior of charged species existing in any sample under the influence of applied electric field. Owing to the versatility of the principle of electrophoresis, it has been successfully adapted in advanced capillary electrophoresis (CE) technique which is considered a more sophisticated separation technique over gel electrophoresis (GE) and High Performance Liquid Chromatography (HPLC). Here, varying micropore sizes of capillaries are usually employed to perform separation of various charged particles of different sizes. These separations are facilitated by the application of high voltages, generating electro-osmotic (EOF) and electrophoretic flow of buffer solutions and ionic species, respectively, within the capillary. Some of the commendable features of CE are summarized below [1].

1. Capable to provide efficient and fast separation.
2. One capillary can be regularly used several times just by changing the experimental conditions and electrolytes without diminishing its efficiency.
3. Due to micropore size of capillary, minute amount of sample (only tens of nL) and electrolytes are required, making it environmentally friendly and ideal for the analysis of harmful and costly samples.
4. It is a cheap alternative to LC as capillaries of CE cost a tenth of the price of a LC column.
5. Portable, making it suitable for point-of-care analysis.

[1]Department of Chemistry, Kwangwoon University, Seoul 139-701, Korea
[2]Department of Anatomy and Cell Biology, College of Medicine, University of Florida, Gainesville, Florida 32610, USA
[3]Department of Internal Medicine, Division of Gastroenterology, University of Michigan Health System, Ann Arbor, Michigan 48109, USA

Recently, the phenomenal advancement on microelectronics/nanoelectronics has opened up vast horizons for miniaturization. This trend is widely used in chemical laboratories in processing various experimental fields. One of the remarkable achievements is scaling down the entire biological or chemical analysis onto a microfluidic chip or channel refereed as "Lab-on-a-chip" or a "microchip" (i.e., micro total analysis system, μTAS). It shows amazing characteristics including increased analysis speed, fewer samples and reagent consumption, higher throughput, reduced instrument size and therefore increased portability, environmental compatibility, and cost effectiveness [2]. The fabrication design of a microchip is very simple, consisting of the few fundamental elements including a sample injection zone, an electrophoresis separation channel, and a system for the detection of the migrating analytes as shown in Figure 4.1.

The need for more efficient injection zone, separation of various complex samples with different size and charges, and their detection methods have paved the ways to tailor the fundamental parts of a microchip in different ways. The chip-based separations become somewhat more complicated, given a more complex network of connected channels and much smaller reservoir dimensions which are more susceptible to the effects of evaporation, buffer depletion, and Laplace pressures arising from surface tension [3].

Several detection methods such as absorbance, mass spectrometry, refractive index, laser induced fluorescence (LIF), electrochemical, and other detection methods have been coupled with microchip CE. However, the most popular detection method used so far with microchips has been LIF. Since LIF can introduce undesired complexity for the analysis of biological samples due to derivatization, electrochemical detections are considered the well-suited methods for

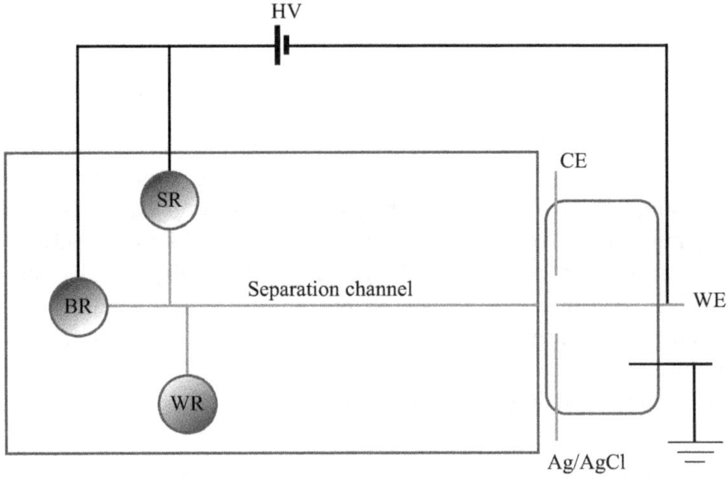

Figure 4.1 Schematic of a simple T-cross microchip. SR, sample reservoir; BR, buffer reservoir; WR, waste reservoir; WE, working electrode; and CE, counter electrode

detection of separated species [2]. We recommend some good reviews for readers which could provide more basic and fundamental insights about microchip systems [3, 4–7].

In this work, we discuss the utilization of microchip-based separation systems for chemically and biologically valuable analytes. We have described the details of many substantial articles explaining the design of microchips, and utilities for their preparation, so that readers might understand the principles behind such devices and relevant detection strategies. The current challenges and future outlook have been discussed in detail in order to provide a clear understanding about the fundamentals of sensor design and performance that have the real possibility of upgrading the field. We have categorized this work into many sections based on their applications for the convenience.

4.2 Separation and detection methods for chemically and biologically valuable analytes

4.2.1 Separation and extraction of DNA

The study of DNA (deoxyribose nucleic acid) and its interaction with protein is considered very crucial for their role in many cellular functions [8]. Hence, besides qualitative detection, the quantitative determination of them is necessary [9, 10].

Xu *et al.* separated specific double-stranded DNA (ds-DNA) fragments by selecting a series of mixed poly(ethylene oxide) (PEO) matrices in a commercially available polymethylmethacrylate (PMMA) microchip system. Among many matrices, PEO with an intermediate MW of 4×10^5 is found to be a dominant factor for separating small DNA fragment pairs (e.g., 82 and 88 bp), while PEO with a high MW of 8×10^6 plays an important role in separating intermediate and large fragments (e.g., 271 and 281 bp, 506 and 517 bp, 7 and 10 kbp). High-concentration PEO mixtures exhibited better resolution for short fragments, while dilute PEO mixtures show better resolution for long fragments. Wide DNA fragments from 20 bp to 40 kbp were successfully separated within 4 min [11].

Kim *et al.* utilized a conventional glass double-T microchip for DNA fragment analysis based on on-line pre-concentration base stacking (BS) technique with a microchip capillary gel electrophoretic (MCGE) separation step in a poly(vinylpyrrolidone) (PVP) sieving matrix. Since the BS occurs simultaneously with the electrokinetic injection of $OH-$ and DNA sample, the stacking is initiated at the low-conductivity zone of the microchip channel, which resulted in an increased focusing of different sizes of DNA fragment samples. Compared to a conventional MCGE separation with a normal electrokinetic injection, the peak heights of 50–2650-base pair (bp) DNA fragments on the MCGE-BS separation were increased 3.9–8.0-fold [12].

Duarte *et al.* fabricated a polyester-toner (PeT) microfluidic device with channel depth up to ~270 μm by a novel technique where a CO_2 laser is used to create the microchannel in polyester sheets containing a uniform layer of printed toner, and multilayer devices can easily be constructed consequently. Using PeT microchips, more than 65% DNA can be recovered from 0.60 μL of blood, concentrated and compatible with downstream microchip-based PCR amplification using dynamic solid phase extraction (dSPE). In addition, the PCR process is capable to amplify a 520 bp fragment of λ-phage DNA, making this technique a potential candidate for genetic analysis without being expensive and involving complexity [13].

Duarte *et al.* employed the similar PeT channel for DNA separations of 100 and 1000 bp with polymer solutions (0.5% m/v hydroxyethylcellulose or hydroxypropylcellulose). The system provided high plate numbers within 4 min for 1000 bp fragments [14]. Cao *et al.* utilized thiol-modified DNA-binding AuNPs (gold nanoparticles) as a tag. The target DNA was sandwiched between Au NPs and probe DNA labeled with horseradish peroxidase (HRP) for DNA separation. The tagging helps to create electrophoretic mobility between free probe and probe-target complex, resulting into the separation of a 27-mer DNA fragments with different sequences with high speed and resolution [15].

A mathematical model was developed for a microchip with simultaneous optimization of separation length (L) and electric field strength (E), taking into account the various factors affecting the separation including sample injection, detector, diffusion, and Joule heating for high speed separation of DNA [16]. In order to separate DNA-protein complex using electrophoretic mobility shift assay (EMSA) on PMMA-based microchip, a complex of human nuclear factor-kB (rhNF-kB) and its consensus ds-oligonucleotide fluorescently labeled with Cy5, was separated within 200 s [8].

Two powerful techniques including Droplet-based microfluidics and slip chip methods were combined to make a microchip-CE (MCE) platform fabricated by PMMA sheets for the separation of 30 sub-nL sample droplets containing fluorescent dyes or DNA fragments. This method exhibited high theoretical plates compared to the other microchip-based DNA separations [17].

Ghanim and Abdullah developed a disposable DNA biosensor poly (dimethylsiloxane) (PDMS) microchip with electrochemical detection using printed circuit board (PCB) substrate made of copper. The results demonstrate that DNA fragments ranging from 250 to 10000 bp can be separated easily at 18 V/cm, proving its utility [18].

4.2.2 Separation of proteins

Proteomics is a vital branch of biology where various biological problems related to proteins, their identification in cells, tissues, or body fluids are studied. The separation and detection of proteins in complex biological matrices is a daunting task. Microchip electrophoresis (MCE) has been proved futile in this area, resulting into many critical and valuable reports in this particular area [19, 20].

Nagata *et al.* employed a polyethylene glycol (PEG)-coated PMMA plastic microchip for high-speed separation of proteins of molecular weight 21.5–116.0 kDa within 8 s using a SDS-linear polyacrylamide solution [21]. Lu *et al.* showed that different electrophoretic mobilities of surfactant denatured proteins help to separate α-lactalbumin, ovalbumin, conalbumin), and β-galactosidase using MCE in free solution with LIF detection. The free solution mobilities were not correlated with the molecular weights of the proteins [22].

Shadpour described a 2D separation of proteins using a PMMA microchip. First, the Alexa Fluor 633 conjugated proteins, ranging in size from 38 to 110 kDa were separated in the first dimension based on size using SDSμ-CGE followed by the second dimension consisted of a fast MEKC separation, which sorted proteins based on differences in their interactions with SDS surfactants poised well above their critical micelle concentration. The geometrical layout of the chips is shown in Figure 4.2. The proteins were detected with LIF within 12 min [23].

Kustos *et al.* studied protein profile of a Candida albicans strain on commercial microchip with LIF detection inducing the changes in protein by different anti-fungal agents. The microchip performed well in protein profiling of 40-kDa protein and up regulation of a 60-kDa protein compared to CE which separated only 19-kDa peak, and up-regulation of a 60-kDa protein [24].

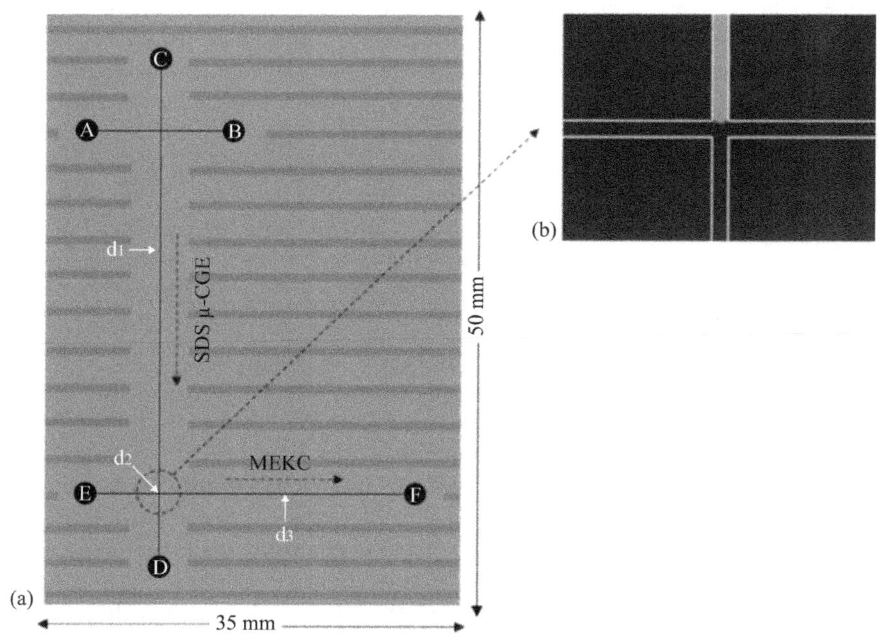

Figure 4.2 (a) Geometrical layout of the PMMA microelectrophoresis chip used for 1D and 2D separations. Solution reservoirs: (A) sample, (B) sample waste, (C) SDS μ-CGE buffer, (D) SDS μ-CGE buffer waste, (E) MEKC buffer, and (F) MEKC buffer waste.
(b) Fluorescence image of the sieving matrix/MEKC interface at the intersection of the SDS μ-CGE and MEKC dimensions. The fluorescence was generated by seeding the sieving matrix with fluorescein. Reproduced with permission from ACS from Reference 24

A simple PDMS microchip with gold and copper integrated microelectrodes was fabricated for the separation of protein mixture of Cy3-extravidin and Cy3-IgG. One water-soluble ionic liquid (IL), 1-butyl-3-methylimidazolium dodecanesulfonate (BAS) which works as IL and surfactant was employed as a running buffer provided high separation at physiological pH compared to other supporting electrolytes or surfactants. Moreover, the BAS buffer also eliminated the protein adsorption on PDMS channel [25].

Okada *et al.* separated Lysozyme, trypsin inhibitor, and carbonic anhydrase proteins on a conventional poly(methylmethacrylate) (PMMA) microchip making sodium dodecyl sulfate-protein complexes (SDS-PC) using linear-poly(acrylamide) (L-PA) of molecular weights between 600 and 1000 KDa with fluorescent detection method. In order to remove protein adsorption, channel walls of PMMA microchip were modified with methylcellulose [26].

For a size-based separation of proteins from 18 to 116 kDa (β-Lactoglobulin, Carbonic anhydrase, Ovalbumin, BSA, and β-Galactosidase), Root *et al.* developed an acid-labile surfactant (ALS) as a replacement for SDS in a poly-(N-hydroxyethylacrylamide) polymer-coated glass microchip with fluorescence detector. Despite no significant differences in migration times and peaks broadening between ALS and SDS, ALS can provide significant advantages in terms of integrating protein separation modalities, as well as the front-end separation with spectrometry compared to SDS [27].

Cong and coworkers successfully demonstrated the step-wise gradient of voltage on the separation of proteins extracted from *Escherichia coli* by isoelectric focusing in a 50% v/v c-MAPS and polyacrylamide coated microchip. The step-wise increase in electric field with the strength up to 1500 V/cm exhibited superior resolution of proteins compared to the fixed electric field strength of 750 V/cm [28]. Wang *et al.* exploited online isotachophoresis concentrations for the separation of bovine serum albumin (BSA) and its immunoassay in a simple microchip GE with mAb in a T-cross PMMA microchip with an inverted fluorescence microscope to view the protein separations. The study showed 2000-fold concentration of BSA immune complex due to isotachophoresis [29].

In order to delineate protein adsorption on microchip wall, porous liquid crystalline lipid-based nanoparticles (LCNPs) were used for the separation of green fluorescent protein (GFP) in cyclic olefin polymer coated microchip with integrated fiber grooves for LIF detection. The LCNPs were made by lipids of soy phosphatidylcholine, glycerol dioleate and polysorbate 80, and oleic acid with geometric diameter of 50–100 nm [30].

Zhang *et al.* demonstrated the surface grafting strategy for Alkyne-PEG by “Click” chemistry in T-cross PDMS microchips with to enhance separation performance for both amino acids and proteins. Comparison of protein separation using PDMS microchips before and after surface modification suggested greatly improved electrophoretic performance of the PEG-functionalized PDMS microchips [31]. Zheng *et al.* investigated the rapid separation of high-density lipoprotein (HDL) labeled with NBD C6-ceramide by MCE with LIF. This method offered efficient separation of the subclasses HDL2 and HDL3 of HDL in 4 min [32].

To quantify the glycomic-profile changes as disease biomarkers, Novotny group reported a highly reproducible combination of a glycomic sample preparation/ solid-phase derivatization of glycoprotein-derived N-linked glycans with their subsequent microchip-based separation and mass-spectrometric (MS) measurements. This method was subsequently and successfully applied on 30 human blood serum samples (15 cancer-free and 15 Stage IV breast cancers) to search for potential N-linked glycan biomarkers [33].

An ion-permeable membrane, consisting of acrylamide, N,N-methylene-bisacrylamide and 2-(acrylamido)-2-methylpropanesulfonate was photo-polymerized in PMMA microchip for on-chip concentration of anionic proteins α-fetoprotein (AFP) and heat shock protein 90 (HSP90) which were excluded from the porous membrane based on both size and charge by Nge and coworkers. The schematic of microchip design is shown in Figure 4.3. This method provided a 410-fold

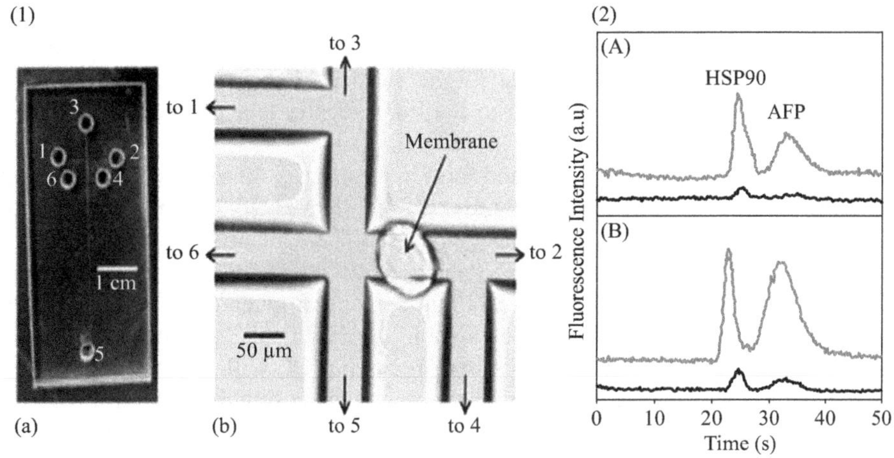

Figure 4.3 *(1) Photograph of a microchip and zoom view of a pre-concentration membrane. (a) Photograph of the microchip for sample pre-concentration. Reservoir labels are 1, sample; 2, sample waste; and 3–6, buffer. The channel connected to reservoir 4 helped to empty the monomer solution from the channel leading to reservoir 2 after polymerization of the gel. The channel leading to reservoir 6 provides cross-T injection, while the channel connected to reservoir 1 provides offset-T injection. (b) Photomicrograph of microchannel intersection region showing position of the polymerized membrane, indicated by the black arrow. (2) Pre-concentration and μ-CE of cancer-related proteins. Mixture of HSP90 and AFP; (A) 10 nM and (B) 20 nM. Pre-concentration time; 1 min. The bottom traces represent μ-CE without pre-concentration, while the top traces denote pre-concentration followed by separation. Reproduced with permission from John Wiley & Sons from Reference 35*

pre-concentration factor for fluorescent labeled cancer proteins followed by separation in 1 min [34].

Xu *et al.* separated and enriched acetylated proteins and peptides using a microchip coupled to MALDI-MS in order to acquire information on the acetylation sites. Prior to separation, silanol-covered surface of PDMS microchip was coated with poly (diallyldimethylammonium chloride). This method was successful to separate and enrich the 72.5 fmolμL^{-1} of acetylated BSA and 72.5 fmolμL^{-1} of tryptic BSA-Ac and subsequently identified with MALDI-MS technique [35].

4.2.3 Separation of small biological analytes

Various types of biogenic monoamines and their metabolites were separated and detected by employing electrophoretic separation on microchip using a combined enzyme-catalyzed system consisting of nicotinamide adenine dinucleotide coenzyme in its reduced form (NADH) on the amperometric electrode [36]. Lunte group demonstrated the use of rapid CO_2 laser ablation (3 s) for the patterning of CE microchannels in PDMS. This patterning minimized the EOF and nonspecific adsorption of hydrophobic analytes to the surface. The PDMS microchip was applied for separation and detection of the fluorescently labeled neurotransmitters aspartate and glutamate [37].

Ding and Garcia separated and detected phenol, 4,6-dinitro-o-cresol and pentachlorophenol, on a simple T-cross PDMS fabricated CE microchip with pulsed amperometric detection using gold wire. The separation of analytes were achieved within 3 min with Limit of detection (LOD) of 2.8 fmol, 1.1 fmol, and 1.6 fmol forphenol, 4,6-dinitro-o-cresol and pentachlorophenol, respectively [38]. Four toxic alkaloids, colchicine, thiocolchicine, colchicoside, and thiocolchicoside were separated on a conventional T-cross microchip-CE with UV detector by Lu *et al.* Compared to simple CE method, the microchip resulted in five times sensitivity enhancements with LODs ranging from 2 to 6 mg L^{-1} depending upon the specific alkaloid and the dimension of the optical cell [39].

Alvarez *et al.* demonstrated the separation of *p*-aminophenol and l-ascorbic acid using a cyclic olefin copolymer modified PMMA chip. Different working electrode alignment such as in-channel or end-channel has been tested in conjunction with several materials including gold, platinum, or carbon for sensitive detection [40]. Duarn and coworkers utilized a polycarbonate (PC)-CE microchip to separate the potassium, sodium and lithium ions in a 20 mM MES/His buffer within a minute at 28.5 kV/m with a contactless conductivity detector. The LODs for the ions were 100 μM [41].

Pumera *et al.* studied two different types of modifications in microchips where a negatively charged *N*-(trimethoxysilylpropyl) ethylenediamine triacetic-acid (TETT)-based sol and a methyltrimethoxysilane (MTMOS)-based sol were used as pseudo stationary phases in running buffer to separate and observe the selectivity between nitroaromatic explosives and environmental pollutants, aminophenols, respectively, in the electrophoresis separations. There were no concentration limitations of these sol additives unlike micellar additives that require a minimum surfactant concentration ($\geq$CMC) [42].

Piccin *et al.* proposed an effective microchip protocol based on electrophoretic-separation and electrochemical detection with glassy carbon electrode for nitrate explosive: ethylene glycol dinitrate, pentaerythritol tetranitrate, propylene glycol dinitrate, and glyceryl trinitrate. Under optimized conditions, the compounds were separated within 120 s with excellent LOD and response time compared to other reports on the separation techniques of nitrate ester explosives [43].

Pozo-Ayuso *et al.* proposed a novel dual-channel MCE on glass substrates for the first time with electrochemical detection. In this design, the possibility of carrying out two simultaneous measurements for the separation of dopamine, *p*-aminophenol, and hydroquinone was studied successfully where the form of injection was of paramount importance in such a way that the simple introduction of an electrode in reservoir A (without applying any voltage) was necessary for obtaining signals which were similar in both channels, with slight differences attributed to electrode distance from the channel outlet and alignment. The design of the proposed plan and the simultaneous separation are shown in Figure 4.4 [44].

Gustafsson *et al.* described the fabrication of silicon-based microchip for electrochromatographic separations where UV-transparent waveguides for detection and integrated couplers for optical fibers on the chip were combined. The microchip was covalently coated with hydrophobic octylsilanes for reverse phase separation of acetophenone, valerophenone, and hexanophenone within 2 min [45].

In our work, a method for simultaneous detection of anticancer drugs was developed by integrating the pre-concentration and separation steps in a microfluidic device on an amperometric biosensor made by ds-DNA and cardiolipin modified screen printed electrodes at the end of separation channel. The pre-concentration was performed by combining two techniques of field amplified sample stacking (FASS) and field amplified sample injection (FASI) which improved concentration of anticancer drugs ~1093 times. The schematic diagram of the microfluidic device and the biosensor fabrication are shown in Figure 4.5. This method exhibited very low detection limits of four drugs between 1.2 and 5.5 fM [46].

Kumar *et al.* performed separation of hydrazine, methylhydrazine, and 1,1-dimethylhydrazine in ~30 s based on a commercial PMMA microchip consisting of two-cross channels with contactless conductivity detection with LODs of 11.9, 35.5, and 337.8 ng/mL, respectively [47].

A microchip CE system hyphenated with a microwave-induced plasma optical emission spectrometry (MIP-OES) was used for copper species. The separation channel was interfaced to MIP-OES through an extremely low flow demountable direct injection high efficiency nebulizer (D-DIHEN) directly at the liquid exit of the chip. This method allowed analyzing sample volumes of 25 nL with baseline separation of copper species (Cu(II) and $Cu(EDTA)^{2}$) within 90 s [48]. Chand *et al*, separated cysteine and homocysteine using a PDMA microchip with on-chip microfabricated gold microelectrodes. For separation, 1.5% (w/v) agarose gel was coated inside the channel to effectively separate the analytes as agarose gel creates a drag force due to its sieving action. Cysteine and homocysteine were detected in 92 s and 104 s, respectively [49]. Ye *et al.* developed a method where double T-MCE was used to separate free and HRP-labeled cortisol

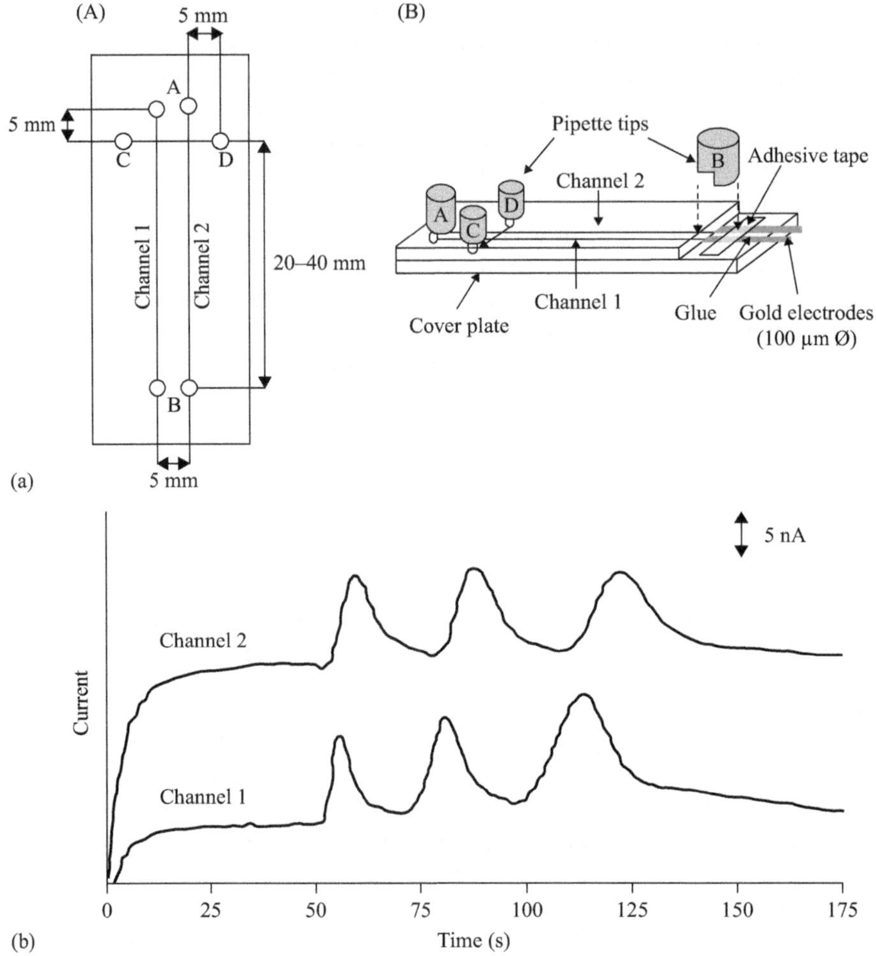

Figure 4.4 *(a) Dual-channel microchip designs (A) including reservoirs and electrochemical detector (B). (b) Simultaneous electropherograms for a sample mixture of 100 μM DA, pAP and HQ (each) using a dual-channel microchip. Conditions: Running buffer, 25 mM MES–His pH 5.95; Vinj = +500 V for 5 s; Vsep = +750 V; Ed = +1.2 V (vs Ag/AgCl). Reproduced with permission from Elsevier from Reference 45*

(immunoreaction) with chemiluminescence (CL) detection. The separation was accomplished within 60 s providing a linear range between 9 and 900 nM and LOD of 4.2 nM [50].

4.2.4 Miscellaneous separation

Ninonuevo *et al*. developed a nanoliquid chromatography-mass spectrometry (nano LC-MS) method for the separation of oligosaccharides (i.e., mixtures of alditols

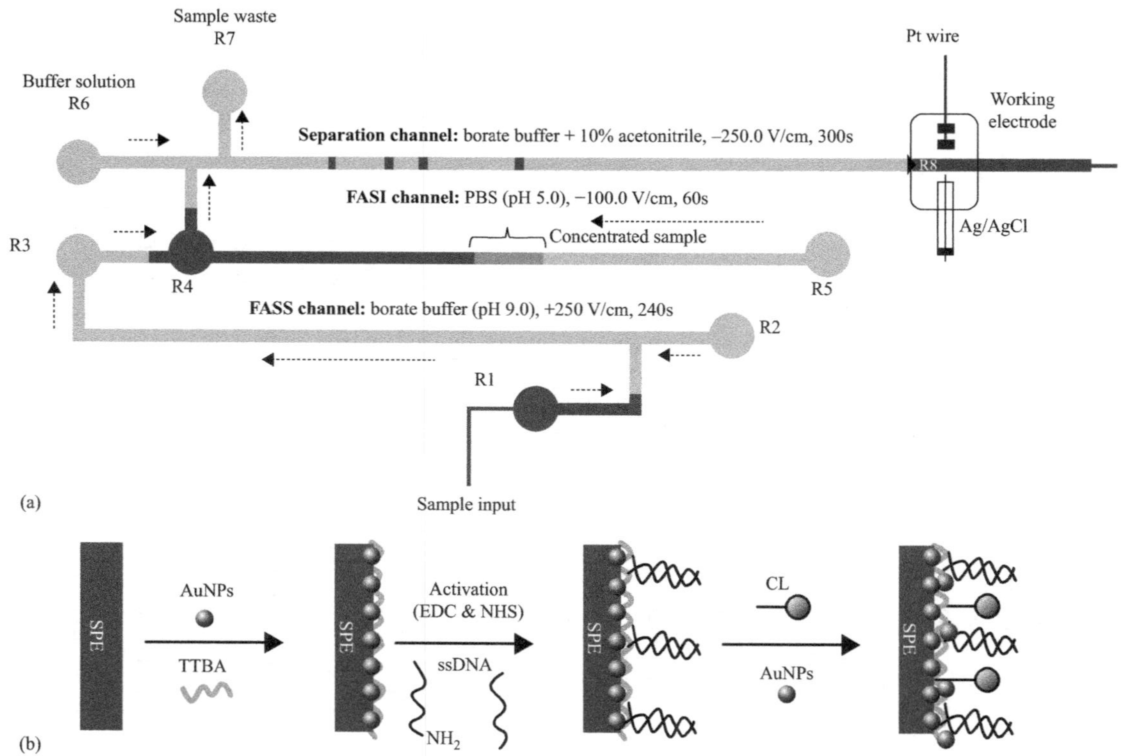

Figure 4.5 *(a) Schematic diagram of the microfluidic device. (b) Schematic representation of the biosensor fabrication (TTBA, 5,2':5',2''-terthiophene-3'-carboxylic acid and CL, cardiolipin). Reproduced with permission from Elsevier from Reference 47*

from mucins and human milk oligosaccharides employing graphitized carbon chromatography (GCC) on microchip [51]. The microchip was employed for the chiral separation of tryptophan enantiomers on protein-stationary phase immobilized in a PMMA microchip with LIF detection. In the stationary phase, BSA conjugated with the shortened carboxylic single-walled carbon nanotubes (SWCNTs) was employed as the chiral selector. This method separated tryptophan enantiomers in 70 s with a resolution factor of 1.35 [52].

Soper group demonstrated a method for low abundant point mutations in genomic DNA using a combination of an allele-specific ligase detection reaction (LDR) with free-solution conjugate electrophoresis (FSCE) to generate and analyze the genetic products. The separation was performed and compared in a commercial capillary array electrophoresis (CAE) system and a PMMA microchip with only a Tris-based running buffer containing additives to suppress the EOF. The results showed that PMMA microchip took just 85 s as compared to 11 min in CAE method for the separation of LDR-dt conjugates [53].

Oblak and coworkers exploited the fact that the concentration of reduced form of glutathione (GSH) levels in the RBCs obtained from patients suffering from type 2 diabetes is lower in comparison to those RBCs obtained from healthy controls. Hence, they demonstrated a simple quantification method to observe this fact in either a six- or twelve-channel microchip PDMA as well as simultaneous determination of the antioxidant without prior separation. The control and samples of RBCs were run in parallel channels in microchip. The results suggest that GSH concentrations in the RBC may be useful in screening for resistance to C-peptide *in vivo* [54].

Rhazi *et al.*, separated and quantified glutenin subunits in a commercial microchip CE-SDS system which seems very complicated where integration of the sample loading, staining, separation, destaining, and detection were carried out in a single chip. This approach provides response in just 45 s [55]. Aota *et al.* proposed cell-free plasma separation from 200 μL of human whole blood *via* axial migration of blood cells and cross-flow filtration of blood cells and vessels in a octadecyltrichlorosilane coated microchip simultaneously. In addition, axial migration process helps to prevent clogging and hemolysis. With this method, 65% of the plasma from 200 μL of whole blood was successfully separated in 25 min [56].

Wu *et al.* enriched and separated sialylated human milk oligosaccharides (SHMOs) isomers using nanoLC-Chip/QTOF MS using microchip packed with porous graphitized carbon (PGC) with good precision [57]. Due to the importance of Haptoglobin phenotyping (Hp) in various major diseases, the separation and detection of it were performed on SDS treated glass microchip with LIF detection by Huang *et al.* It could differentiate Hp 1-1 and Hp 2-2 in 150 s compared to normal CE which needs 400 s [58].

Recently, the molecular imprinted polymer-Fe_3O_4@polynorepinephrine NPs-based PDMS MCE system was used for the separation of L-tryptophan, L-valine, L-threonine, Gly-L-Phe, and *S*-ofloxacin or *S*-binaphthol [59]. In another report, a microchip consisting two microchannels including a Y-type double-helix reaction microchannel and a parallel separation channel was employed for efficient mixing and chemical reactions followed by its utilization in the separation. Five aldehydes were derivatized and could be driven through separation microchannels by just siphoning for good separation [60]. Lucca *et al.* developed a novel graphene-modified electrode to be used as amperometric sensor in a T-cross microchip device for the separation of an anionic mixture containing iodide and ascorbate [61].

4.3 Challenges and future outlook

Despite many advantages, there are many challenges in microchip-CE systems. First, the fabrication of microchip is a multistep process. Polymer microchips need tedious preparation, however, it is easy as compared to the fabrication of glass microchips which demands more effort and careful handling. Furthermore, the generation of background signals from microchip is another issue which can be delineated by exploiting different types of raw materials for plastic microchip fabrication. For good separation performance, the design of microchip also needs attention in order to minimize the dispersion and stagnant flow of sample and buffer cause turbulence in the analysis. Thus, the microchip with cylindrical design or some other alternatives are used. Various kinds of detectors and coupling of different mass spectrometric systems are also somewhat problematic, nevertheless, many good solutions have been proposed for them.

Since CE has made its niche in the LC dominant area, the next task should be to open the ways where the raised challenges are reduced as much as possible. Furthermore, after its successful commercialization due to its portability and rapid operation, more commercial products and transfer of the knowledge generated from LC to microchip CE systems to provide more robust and reliable, portable analytical systems are needed. Moreover, the most challenging part is to search and work on the general processes which could be utilized universally.

4.4 Conclusion

Based on the above-mentioned discussion, it can be concluded that in the last decade or so, microchip-based separations have grown tremendously, showing potential in various kinds of separations. It is worth noticing that microchip-CE has been exploited a lot in the separation, enrichment, quantification of proteins, DNA, and small analytes. Furthermore, it was noted that the type of detection method was also of paramount importance before analyzing the samples. One of the other outstanding aspects of microchip-CE system is its fast response time where no other techniques can compete with it. Most of the separation and detection of analytes were carried out within few minutes unless a complex approach for the integration of channels for simultaneous procedures was employed. However, in those analyses too, the total analysis time was quite lower in comparison to other techniques where many processes are carried out one after other such as sample pretreatment, loading, separation, and detection. In addition, the automation of these systems has also been realized, reducing the efforts during analysis. The other excellent features of microchip-CE is its environmental friendly approach as very little amount of samples and running buffers are required for analysis. Finally, various pre-concentration strategies can be applied easily in microchip-CE in order to analyze the sample despite its low volume in a complex mixture.

Acknowledgment

Shabi Abbas Zaidi is thankful to Kwangwoon University for funding in 2016.

References

[1] Breadmore M.C. "Capillary and microchip electrophoresis: challenging the common conceptions." *Journal of Chromatography A.* 2012; **1221**: 42–55.
[2] Liu Y., Vickers J.A., Henry C.S. "Simple and sensitive electrode design for microchip electrophoresis/electrochemistry." *Analytical Chemistry.* 2004; **76**: 1513–1517.
[3] Crabtree H.J., Cheong E.C.S., Tilroe D.A., Backhouse C.J. "Microchip injection and separation anomalies due to pressure effects." *Analytical Chemistry.* 2001; **73**: 4079–4086.
[4] Stefan Nagl S., Schulze P., Ludwig M., Belder D. "Progress in microchip enantioseparations." *Electrophoresis.* 2009; **30**: 2765–2772.
[5] Lin S., Lin T.Y., Fuh M.R. "Recent developments in microfluidic chip-based separation devices coupled to MS for bioanalysis." *Bioanalysis.* 2013; **5(20)**: 2567–2580.
[6] Breadmore M.C., Tubaon R.M., Shallan A.I., *et al.* "Advances in enhancing the sensitivity of electrophoresis and electrochromatography in capillaries and microchips." *Electrophoresis.* 2015; **36**: 36–61.
[7] Qian W., Zhang Y., Chen W., "Capturing cancer: emerging microfluidic technologies for the capture and characterization of circulating tumor cells." *Small.* 2015; **11**: 3850–3872.
[8] Inoue S., Kaji N., Kataoka M., *et al.* "Rapid qualitative evaluation of DNA transcription factor NF-jB by microchip electrophoretic mobility shift assay in mammalian cells." *Electrophoresis.* 2011; **32**: 3241–3247.
[9] Sinville R., Soper S.A., "High resolution DNA separations using microchip electrophoresis." *Journal of Separation Science.* 2007; **30**: 1714–1728.
[10] Lin Y., Huang M.F., Chang H.T., "Nanomaterials and chip-based nanostructures for capillary electrophoretic separations of DNA." *Electrophoresis.* 2005; **26**: 320–330.
[11] Xu F., Jabasini M., Baba Y., "Screening of mixed poly (ethylene oxide) solutions for microchip separation of double-stranded DNA using an orthogonal design approach." *Electrophoresis.* 2005; **26**: 3013–3020.

[12] Kim D.K., Kang S.H. "On-channel base stacking in microchip capillary gel electrophoresis for high-sensitivity DNA fragment analyses." *Journal of Chromatography A.* 2005; **1064**: 121–127.

[13] Duarte G.R.M., Price C.W., Augustine B.H., Carrilho E., Landers J.P. "Dynamic solid phase DNA extraction and PCR amplification in polyester-toner based microchip." *Analytical Chemistry.* 2011; **83**: 5182–5189.

[14] Duarte G.R.M., Coltro W.K.T., Borba J.C., Price C.W., Landers J.P., Carrilho E. "Disposable polyester–toner electrophoresis microchips for DNA analysis." *Analyst.* 2012; **137**: 2692–2698.

[15] Cao W., Chen L., Fu Y., Tan Z., Qu B. "A highly efficient and versatile microchip capillary electrophoresis method for DNA separation using gold nanoparticle as a tag." *Journal of Separation Science.* 2011; **34**: 939–946.

[16] Ni Y., Dou X., Cheng S., Zhu Y. "Design of separation length and electric field strength for high-speed DNA electrophoresis." *Electrophoresis.* 2011; **32**: 238–245.

[17] Hassan S., Morgan H., Zhang X., Niu X. "Droplet interfaced parallel and quantitative microfluidic-based separations." *Analytical Chemistry.* 2015; **87**: 3895–3901.

[18] Ghanim M.H., Abdullah M.Z. "Design of disposable DNA biosensor microchip with amperometric detection featuring PCB substrate.' *BioChip Journal.* 2013; **7(1)**: 51–56.

[19] Suzuki S. "Highly sensitive methods using liquid chromatography and capillary electrophoresis for quantitative analysis of glycoprotein glycans." *Chromatography.* 2014; **35**: 1–22.

[20] García-Campana A.M., Taverna M., Fabre H. "LIF detection of peptides and proteins in CE." *Electrophoresis.* 2007; **28**: 208–232.

[21] Nagata H., Tabuchi M., Hirano K., Baba Y. "High-speed separation of proteins by microchip electrophoresis using a polyethylene glycol-coated plastic chip with a sodium dodecyl sulfate-linear polyacrylamide solution." *Electrophoresis.* 2005; **26**: 2687–2691.

[22] Lu C., Smith A.E., Craighead H.G. "Separation of denatured proteins in free solution on a microchip based on differential binding of alkyl sulfates with different carbon chain lengths." Chemical Communication. 2005; 183–185.

[23] Shadpour H., Soper S.A. "Two-dimensional electrophoretic separation of proteins using poly(methyl methacrylate) microchips." *Analytical Chemistry.* 2006; **78**: 3519–3527.

[24] Kustos I., Nyul A., Lóránd T., Kocsis B., Kilár F. "Effect of antifungal agents on protein composition of Candida albicans studied by capillary electrophoresis and chip technology." *Journal of Biochemical and Biophysical Methods.* 2006; **69**: 57–65.

[25] Xu Y., Li J., Wang E. "Microchip micellar electrokinetic chromatography based on one functionalized ionic liquid and its excellent performance on proteins separation." *Journal of Chromatography A.* 2008; **1207**: 175–180.

[26] Okada H., Kaji N., Tokeshi M., Baba Y. "Poly(methylmethacrylate) microchip electrophoresis of proteins using linear-poly(acrylamide) solutions as separation matrix." *Analytical Sciences.* 2008; **24**: 321–325.

[27] Root B.E., Zhang B., Barron A.E. "Size-based protein separations by microchip electrophoresis using an acid-labile surfactant as a replacement for SDS." *Electrophoresis.* 2009; **30**: 2117–2122.

[28] Cong Y., Liang Y., Zhang L., Zhang W., Zhang Y. "Improved protein separation by microchip isoelectric focusing with stepwise gradient of electric field strength." *Journal of Separation Science.* 2009; **32**: 462–465.

[29] Wang J., Zhang Y., Mohamadi M.R., Kaji N., Tokeshi M., Baba Y. "Exceeding 20000-fold concentration of protein by the on-line isotachophoresis concentration in poly(methyl methacrylate) microchip." *Electrophoresis.*2009; **30**: 3250–3256.

[30] Ohlsson P., Ordeig O., Nilsson C., Harwigsson I., Kutter J., Nilsson S. "Microchip electroseparation of proteins using lipid-based nanoparticles.". *Electrophoresis.* 2010; **31**: 3696–3702.

[31] Zhang Z., Feng X., Xu F., Liu X., Liu B.F. "'Click' chemistry-based surface modification of poly(dimethylsiloxane) for protein separation in a microfluidic chip." *Electrophoresis.* 2010; **31**: 3129–3136.

[32] Zheng H., Cong H., Wang H., Jin Q., Zhao J. "A microchip-based method for rapid separation of subclasses of high-density lipoprotein." *Chromatographia.* 2010; **71**: 1119–1124.

[33] Alley W.R., Madera M.J., Mechref Y., Novotny M.V. "Chip-based reversed-phase liquid chromatography-mass spectrometry of permethylated n-linked glycans: a potential methodology for cancer-biomarker discovery." *Analytical Chemistry.* 2010; **82**: 5095–5106.

[34] Nge P.N., Yang W., Pagaduan J.V., Woolley A.T. "Ion-permeable membrane for on-chip pre-concentration and separation of cancer marker proteins." *Electrophoresis.* 2011; **32**: 1133–1140.

[35] Xu L., Wang W., Zhang Z., Yang P., Fan H., Kong J. "Microchip-based strategy for enrichment of acetylated proteins." *Microchimica Acta.* 2013; **180**: 613–618.

[36] Kova M.V., Schwarz M.A. "Enzymatic sensitivity enhancement of biogenic monoamines on a chip." *Electrophoresis.* 2005; **26**: 2701–2707.

[37] Fogarty B.A., Heppert K.E., Cory T.J., Hulbutta K.R., Martind R.S., Lunte S.M. "Rapid fabrication of poly(dimethylsiloxane)-based microchip capillary electrophoresis devices using CO_2 laser ablation." *Analyst.* 2005; **130**: 924–930.

[38] Ding Y., Garcia C.D. "Pulsed amperometric detection with poly(dimethylsiloxane)-fabricated capillary electrophoresis microchips for the determination of EPA priority pollutants." *Analyst.* 2006; **131**: 208–214.

[39] Lua Q., Copper C.L., Collins G.E. "Ultraviolet absorbance detection of colchicine and related alkaloids on a capillary electrophoresis microchip." *Analytica Chimica Acta.* 2006; **572**: 205–211.

[40] Castano-Alvarez M., Fernandez-Abedul M.T., Costa-Garcıa A. "Amperometric detector designs for capillary electrophoresis microchips.". *Journal of Chromatography A.* 2006; **1109**: 291–299.

[41] Duran P., Zhu K.Y., Swallow A., Noui-Mehidi N., Leech P., Glenn F. Detection of inorganic ions on a capillary electrophoresis microchip using a conductivity technique, *Biomedical Applications of Micro- and Nanoengineering III*, edited by Dan V. Nicolau, Proc. of SPIE Vol. 2006; **6416**: 64160J.

[42] Pumera M., Wang J., Grushka E., Lev O. "Organically modified sols as pseudostationary phases for microchip electrophoresis." *Talanta.* 2007; **72**: 711–715.

[43] Piccin E., Dossi N., Cagan A., Carrilho E., Wang J. "Rapid and sensitive measurements of nitrate ester explosives using microchip electrophoresis with electrochemical detection." *Analyst.* 2009; **134**: 528–532.

[44] Pozo-Ayuso D.F., Castano-Alvarez M., Fernandez-la-Villa A., *et al.* "Fabrication and evaluation of single- and dual-channel (Π-design) microchip electrophoresis with electrochemical detection." *Journal of Chromatography A.* 2008; **1180**: 193–202.

[45] Gustafsson O., Mogensen K.B., Ohlsson P.D., Liu Y., Jacobson S.C., Kutter J.P. "An electrochromatography chip with integrated waveguides for UV absorbance detection." *Journal of Micromechanics and Microengineering.* 2008; **18**: 055021 (7pp).

[46] Chandra P., Zaidi S.A., Noh H.B., Shim Y.B. "Separation and simultaneous detection of anticancer drugs in a microfluidic device with an amperometric biosensor." *Biosensors and Bioelectronics.* 2011; **28**: 326–332.

[47] Kumar A., Burns J., Hoffmann W., Demattio H., Malik A.K., Matysik F. "Determination of hydrazines by chip electrophoresis with contactless conductivity detection." *Electrophoresis.* 2011; **32**: 920–925.

[48] Matusiewicz H., Slachcinski M. "Interfacing a microchip-based capillary electrophoresis system with a microwave induced plasma spectrometry for copper speciation." *Central European Journal of Chemistry.* 2011; **9**: 896–903.

[49] Chand R., Han D., Islam K., Yeon I.J., Ko S.S., Kim Y.S. "Microchip capillary electrophoresis based separation and detection of cysteine and homocysteine." *Advanced Materials Research.* 2013; **647**: 482–486.

[50] Ye F., Yang T., Huang Y., Li S., Zhao S. "Homogeneous immunoassay of cortisol based on microchip electrophoresis with chemiluminescence detection." *Analytical Methods.* 2013; **5**: 5657–5661.

[51] Ninonuevo M., An H., Yin H., *et al.* "Nanoliquid chromatography-mass spectrometry of oligosaccharides employing graphitized carbon chromatography on microchip with a high-accuracy mass analyzer." *Electrophoresis.* 2005; **26**: 3641–3649.

[52] Weng X., Bi H., Liu B., Kong J. "On-chip chiral separation based on bovine serum albumin-conjugated carbon nanotubes as stationary phase in a microchannel." *Electrophoresis.* 2006; **27**: 3129–3135.

[53] Sinville R., Coyne J., Meagher R.J., *et al.* "Ligase detection reaction for the analysis of point mutations using free solution conjugate electrophoresis in a polymer microfluidic device." *Electrophoresis.* 2008; **29(23)**: 4751–4760.

[54] Oblak T.D., Meyer J.A., Spence D.M. "A microfluidic technique for monitoring bloodstream analytes indicative of C-peptide resistance in type 2 diabetes." *Analyst.* 2009; **134**: 188–193.

[55] Rhazi L., Bodard A.L., Fathollahi B., Aussenac T. "High throughput microchip-based separation and quantitation of high-molecular-weight glutenin subunits." *Journal of Cereal Science.* 2009; **49**: 272–277.

[56] Aota A., Takahashi S., Mawatari K., Tanaka Y., Sugii Y., Kitamori T. "Microchip-based plasma separation from whole blood via axial migration of blood cells." *Analytical Sciences.* 2011; **27**: 1173–1178.

[57] Wu S., Grimm R., German J.B., Lebrilla C.B. "Annotation and structural analysis of sialylated human milk oligosaccharides." *Journal of Proteome Research.* 2011; **10**: 856–868.

[58] Huang B., Huang C., Liu P., Wang F., Na N., Ouyang J. "Fast haptoglobin phenotyping based on microchip electrophoresis." *Talanta.* 2011; **85**: 333–338.

[59] Chen J., Liang R., Wang X., Qiu J. "A norepinephrine coated magnetic molecularly imprinted polymer for simultaneous multiple chiral recognition." *Journal of Chromatography A.* 2015; **1409**: 268–276.

[60] Peng X., Zhao L., Guo J., *et al.* "Double-helix micro-channels on microfluidic chips for enhanced continuous on-chip derivatization followed by electrophoretic separation." *Biosensors and Bioelectronics.* 2015; **72**: 376–382.

[61] Lucca B.L., Lima F., Coltro W.K.T., Ferreira S.V. "Electrodeposition of reduced graphene oxide on a Pt electrode and its use as amperometric sensor in microchip electrophoresis." *Electrophoresis.* 2015; **36**: 1886–1893.

Chapter 5

Biosensors of *in vitro* detection of cancer and bacterial cells

Seda Nur Topkaya[1] *and Mostafa Azimzadeh*[2]

5.1 Introduction

Over the past decades, biosensor systems are of great importance because of their capability to solve a potentially large number of analytical problems and challenges in multiple disciplines. They allow imaging and quantitative measurement of specific biomolecules and reactions both *in vivo* and *in vitro* [1–3]. The increasing worldwide demand for biosensors has resulted in considerable developments for detection of analyte of interest at levels of sophistication not possible before. Biosensors have enabled for highly sensitive, specific, rapid, low-cost and easy to handle detection systems. More advantages of the biosensor applications are that they can be miniaturized (lab-on-a-chip (LOC) devices) and offer robust results compared with classical analytical techniques such as immunohistochemistry or ELISA [4, 5]. Among wide range of applications of biosensors, the most notable one is in the field of medicine, which can be conveniently divided into *in vitro* and *in vivo* detections. In addition, the field of biosensors may be further categorized as two broad types instrumentation: (1) high-throughput laboratory machines capable of fast and accurate measurement of complex biological interactions and components; (2) easy-to-use portable devices for use by non-experts for Point-of-Care Testing (POCT) purposes [6]. In both categorizations, three integrated components are necessary to fabricate an effective biosensor: (i) a recognition element to interact with a target analyte; (ii) a signal transducer to generate a measurable signal from an analyte-biomolecular layer interaction and (iii) an electronic system for output analysis. A recognition element should be implemented as the receptor molecule to identify specifically the analyte due to playing an important part in the success of the sensitivity and specificity of the sensor device. The most widely used sensing elements are the antibodies, enzymes and synthetic molecular recognition elements such as nanomaterials, molecular

[1]Department of Analytical Chemistry, Faculty of Pharmacy, Ege University, Izmir, Turkey
[2]Department of Life Science Engineering, Faculty of New Sciences and Technologies, University of Tehran, Tehran, Iran

imprinted polymers, aptamers, metal oxides and peptides. Other component of the biosensor is a transducer that converts recognition events into the electrical signals. Transducers can be classified as electrochemical (amperometric, potentiometric, conductimetric, impedance), optical (colorimetric, fluorescence, luminescence, interferometry), calorimetric (thermistor) and mass sensitive (piezoelectric, acoustic wave) transducers. Among them, electrochemical transducers are the most widely used in biosensors, however recently, optical and mass sensitive biosensors are becoming more popular and their use is expanding in practical applications. In Figure 5.1, the components of a biosensor for the detection of cancer and bacterial cells have been shown.

This chapter describes some representative examples of *in vitro* detection of cancer and bacterial cells within the scope of biosensor systems. In cancer cell detection, priority is given to aptamers-based biosensors and the detailed information about the detection of cancer cells with the help of aptamers is explained. In the case of bacterial cells detection, electrochemical and optical biosensors that produce an electronic or optical signal proportional to the specific interaction between the target and the recognition molecule immobilized on the biosensor is

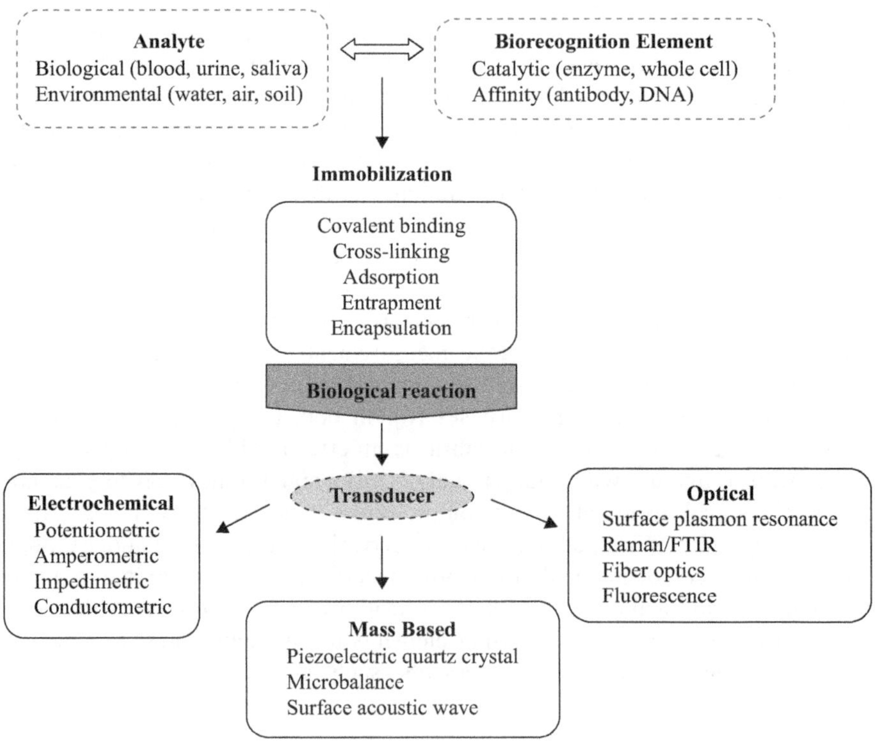

Figure 5.1 The components of the biosensor with various types of transducers for biosensing

elaborately exampled. In addition, microfluidics, LOC and paper-based detection systems for *in vitro* bacterial cells detection are emphasized in the chapter.

5.2 Biosensors of *in vitro* detection of cancer cells

Recent advancements in the field of biomedicine have opened the avenues for the significant achievements in cancer detection. Cancer is a highly complex disease and mainly characterized by (i) unlimited cell division and self-sufficient growth; (ii) invasion of nearby tissues and metastasis to distant organs; (iii) resistance to anti-growth signaling; (iv) apoptosis and (v) continuous angiogenesis [7]. Cancer mainly leads to changes in cell morphology/physiology and clinicians have diagnosed cancer is primarily based on the morphology of tumor cells or tissues for decades. Recently, biosensors for cancer cell detection is on rise to translate the knowledge of early-cancer detection strategies into clinically relevant methods that could be used as diagnostic and treatment purposes for cancer management to better understand the nature, properties and tendency to invasion of the cancer cells.

One of the most investigated biosensors, cell-based biosensors, combines living cells with the transducers, detects biochemical/electrochemical properties directly in real time and convert the changes into the measurable signals by transducers. In these applications, cell lines and primary cultured cells are mainly used as the cell sources. Compared to molecular-based biosensors, cell-based biosensors have superior properties as responding optimally to external stimuli in a physiologically related manner, having a broad spectrum of detection capabilities, long-term recording in a non-invasive way and providing highly sensitive and rapid analysis time for in situ monitoring [8]. Furthermore, cell-based biosensors present more extensive and complex functional data as signaling pathways than the immunochemical methods [9, 10]. Additionally, specific reaction between the actuators and cells can provide the intracellular and extracellular microenvironment condition, which can be applied in drug screening and testing [11, 12]. Despite the advantages over the conventional detection methods, cell-based biosensors suffer from poor efficacy outside of the laboratory since cells are extremely sensitive to changes in environmental conditions as pH, temperature, humidity and media composition and their limited portability for practical large-scale applications. However, advancements in nanotechnology and cell/tissue engineering approaches give a promising future for meeting these challenges.

5.2.1 Aptamers for detection of cancer cells

Aptamers are composed of short single-stranded DNA or RNA oligonucleotides that are capable of binding to target molecules through a specific three-dimensional structure with high affinity and selectivity and forming unique tertiary structures. Aptamers is composed of the Latin word *aptus* (meaning to fit) and the Greek suffix *mers* (meaning to particle).

They are produced with SELEX (Systematic Evolution of Ligands by Exponential Enrichment) [13, 14], which is an *in vitro* selection process, follows a series of steps:

i. Chemical synthesis of the oligonucleotides library having 10^{13}–10^{16} single-stranded nucleic acid molecules;
ii. Incubation of target molecules with an oligonucleotides library;
iii. Separation of oligonucleotides and target complexes from the unbound ones with different separation techniques;
iv. Amplification of the bound sequences (polymerase chain reaction (PCR) for DNA aptamer or by reverse transcriptase PCR for RNA aptamer);
v. Sequencing.

These steps are usually repeated 8–15 times before an enriched pool of nucleic acids with high binding affinity and specificity is obtained [15]. The drawbacks of the method are that the aptamer candidates identified through SELEX may bind to any epitopes on the protein surface during the incubation step that decreases the selectivity of the system and conformation of the isolated proteins might be changed during purification. Since its discovery in 1990, approximately 20 types of the original SELEX process have been developed to improve the conventional SELEX process [16].

Aptamers and aptamer-functionalized agents have been used extensively for targeted therapeutics, molecular diagnostics, *in vivo* imaging and biomarker discovery [17–20]. Aptamers have been also widely applied to cancer research for diagnosis due to having the potential to serve as molecular probes for specific recognition of oncoproteins, cancer cells, metabolites and biomarkers from complex mixtures [21–23]. Because of the complex environment of cancer cell surface, the aptamers selected by SELEX method may exhibit low or no affinity towards the targets. To overcome these challenges, a method named Cell-SELEX has been reported to isolate aptamers from living cells as targets, such as cancer cells [24, 25]. In Cell-SELEX, instead of using purified protein targets as it is done in SELEX, whole living cells are used as the targets, which generate cell-specific aptamers by employing the differences at the molecular level between any two-cell lines. Aptamers are selected for cell surface biomarkers, which are in their native structures and complexes. After typically 8–20 rounds of selection using positive (cancer cells) and negative targets (healthy cells or non-target cells), aptamers that distinguish cancer from healthy controls can be identified. In Cell-SELEX, prior data of the target proteins such as their structure, conformation and expression levels are not required [26]. One problem with the Cell-SELEX is that a high degree of non-specific background binding of oligonucleotides to cells causes slow convergence.

5.2.1.1 Applications of aptamers for *in vitro* cancer cells and biomarkers detection

Biomarkers is defined by the National Institutes of Health Biomarkers Definitions Working Group as "a characteristic that is objectively measured and evaluated as an indicator of normal biological processes, pathogenic processes, or pharmacologic responses to a therapeutic intervention" [27]. Biomarkers can be divided into three categories including: (1) diagnostic biomarkers, which help to early detection of a disease; (2) prognostic biomarkers, which allow to investigate the prognosis of tumors and (3) predictive biomarkers, which can be used to differentiate between various cancers and help in designing therapy plans for the patient [28]. Biomarkers can be specific cells, molecules, genes and gene products, enzymes or hormones. They indicate the changes in the expression of a certain protein that can be measured in tissues, body fluids or in the blood. As a result, each biomarker is an indicative of a particular disease process. In some cases, biomarkers may serve as potential drugs and prognostic targets. In the literature, there are many different cancer biomarkers, which can be categorized into the protein, hormone and oncogene-related cancer markers, embryonic and carbohydrate antigens and enzymatic tumor markers [29]. In particular, cell surface biomarkers provide crucial information for identifying cell types by acting as cell surface signatures. Affordable multiple biomarker detection methods, rapid sample processing times, minimal labor and small sample volumes are important parameters to be considered for biomarker analysis.

Aptamers can be coupled to various transduction platforms to demonstrate their applicability for cancer cells and biomarkers detection. In biosensor systems, when the component of the biosensor is an aptamer, it is defined as an aptasensors [30]. Within the field of biosensors, aptasensors can be generally classified according to their signal-transduction method. Generally, electrochemical, optical and mass-sensitive assays are the most popular platforms to detect cancer cells and biomarkers. Examples of aptasensors for cancer cells and biomarkers detection and their respective sensitivities are listed in Table 5.1.

As it is clearly seen from the Table 5.1, electrochemical detection of cancer cells/biomarkers with the aptamers are relatively dominant than the other detection systems. A living cell can be described as an electrochemical dynamic system so electrochemical biosensors have been widely used for cell type, concentration, viability, proliferation, apoptosis analysis due to allowing the continuous response for online control [48–50]. For instance, a recent study reported that TLS11a aptamers grafted on gold disk electrode could detect HepG2 cancer cells by specifically binding to the membrane surface of hepatocellular carcinoma cells using electrochemical impedance spectroscopy. They concluded that TLS11a aptamer has high affinity to human liver cancer cells when applied as the recognition layer in an electrochemical biosensor [51]. In another study, an electrochemical sensor is fabricated by directly conjugating two cell-specific aptamers, TLS1c and TLS11a, which specifically recognize MEAR cancer cells via the formation of amide bonds on the surface of a glassy carbon electrode. The detection sensitivity is higher than modified with a single type of aptamer alone, showing a very promising potential for rare cells-related clinical applications [52]. As an example of the direct cancer cell detection using aptasensors, an aptamer-conjugated Fluorescence Resonance Energy Transfer (FRET) silica nanoparticles assay was developed [53]. Through doping different ratio of different dyes into silica nanoparticles, different colored nanoparticles were obtained by a single wavelength excitation and then, FRET

Table 5.1 Aptasensors for cancer cells/biomarkers detection and their respective sensitivities

Transducer	Analytical method	Target cell/ biomarkers	Detection limit (cell mL^{-1})	Reference
Electrochemical	EIS and ASV	HL-60 Cell	1000	[31]
Electrochemical	EIS and CV	K562 Cell	1000	[32]
Electrochemical	DPV	HeLa Cell	10	[33]
Electrochemical	DPV	K562 Cell	14	[34]
Electrochemical	DPV	CCRF-CEM Cell	10	[35]
Electrochemical	SWSV	SK-BR-3 Cell	26	[36]
Electrochemical	CV	CEA Biomarker	0.2 ng/mL	[37]
Electrochemical	CV and EIS	EN2 Biomarker	5.62 fM	[38]
Optical	SERS	SK-BR-3 Cell	10	[39]
Optical	SPR	MCF-7 Cell	500	[40]
Optical	SPR	VEGF165 Biomarker	25 pg/mL	[41]
Optical	Fluorescence	SMMC-7721 Cell	1000	[42]
Optical	Colorimetry	HeLa Cell	100	[43]
Optical	LSPR and ECL	CEA Biomarker	1.52×10^{-6} ng/mL	[44]
Optical-Mass	SPR and QCM	tPSA Biomarker	0.39 ng/mL	[45]
Mass	SAW	MCF-7 Cell	32	[46]
Mass	QCM	CCRF-CEM Cell	1160	[47]

Abbreviations: EIS, Electrochemical Impedance Spectroscopy; ASV, Anodic Stripping Voltammetry; CV, Cyclic Voltammetry; DPV, Differential Pulse Voltammetry; SWSV, Square Wave Stripping Voltammetry; SERS, Surface Enhanced Raman Scattering; SPR, Surface Plasmon Resonance; LSPR, Localized Surface Plasmon Resonance; ECL, Enhanced Electrochemiluminescence; QCM, Quartz Crystal Microbalance; SAW, Surface Acoustic Wave; CEA, Carcinoembryonic antigen; EN, Engrailed-2 Protein; VEGF165, Vascular Endothelial Growth Factor-165; tPSA, total Prostate Specific Antigen.

nanoparticles were modified by aptamers specific for different cancer cell lines. FRET-Silica Nanoparticles aptamer conjugates successfully achieved to detect simultaneous detection of different cancer cells (T-cell leukemia and B-cell lymphoma).

Nanomaterials are also preferred for the aptamer-based cancer cells detections. For instance, researchers have developed a colorimetric assay for sensitive cancer cells detection using aptamers conjugated with gold nanoparticles. The aptamers-gold nanoparticles conjugates on the target cell surface resulted in a significant color change because the gold nanoparticles were in close proximity that allowed their surface plasmon resonances to overlap, while the non-target cells did not display any change in color. The detection limit based on simple absorbance measurements was 90 cells. Thousand target cells were readily detected by the naked eye [54]. In both transducer types, label free and labeled methods could be used depend on a detection strategy. Labels such as redox species, enzymes, nanoparticles and nanomaterials have been extensively used for recognition process. Alternatively, labeled target molecules or secondary capture agents (in the case of a sandwich-type assay) are often used in aptasensors. Labels are generally attached to terminal groups of aptamers via covalent interactions. The position of the interaction is significantly important due to not to interfering of the folding of the aptamer. The appropriate position of label prevents the loss of activity of the stability of the aptamer.

5.3 Biosensors of *in vitro* detection of bacterial cells

Infection diseases caused by bacteria have been producing serious health problems for human, animals and plants. Recent findings have confirmed that they could cause cancers [55–57], affect somatic cell reprogramming [58, 59] and B cells [60, 61]. Reliable and specific detection is a key issue to avoid harmful effects of bacteria and prevent their contagious [62, 63]. Several methods have been used for the bacteria determination, including the culture and colony counting method [64–66], PCR [67–69] and immunology-based methods [70, 71]. Along with the conventional detection methods, nanobiosensors, which take advantages of using nanomaterials within the biosensors systems, have gained great attention for bacterial cells detection from the environmental and biological samples due to providing high surface-to-volume ratio, surface activity, catalytic efficiency and adsorption ability [72, 73]. The large nanostructured surface areas enable attachment of large amount of captured bacterial cells and thus provide better and specific interaction between the targets and the transducers. Nanomaterials are composed of thousands of molecules or atoms that are aggregated into shapes such as rods, wires, tubes, pores, particles and arrays of these shapes. Nanomaterials could be classified as carbon nanotubes (CNTs), graphene, quantum dots (QDs), magnetic, gold, metal and silver nanoparticles. The remarkable sensitivity of nanomaterials-based biosensors also provides opportunities for detecting bacterial cells at concentrations very low down to even 1 CFU mL^{-1}. Limit of detection (LOD) of bacteria detection is reported in a standard bacteria-quantifying unit; Colony-Forming Unit per milliliter (CFU mL^{-1}).

In this section, we aim to review recent advances and innovations in the field of nanobiosensors for sensitive bacterial cells detection in three main categories including electrochemical/optical nanobiosensors, microfluidics and LOC systems.

5.3.1 Electrochemical and optical nanobiosensors for bacterial cells detection

Herein, we collect recently published electrochemical and optical nanobiosensors for bacterial cells detection (Table 5.2). In electrochemical and optical nanobiosensors, different types of bioreceptors are used such as antibody, aptamer, enzyme and oligonucleotides which immobilize on the surface of nanoparticles, electrodes and chips through chemical binding, electrostatic and hydrophobic interactions, trapping in a matrix or a capsule via a linker [74, 75]. Electrochemical

Table 5.2 Different assays and innovations in electrochemical- and optical-based nanobiosensors for bacterial cells detection

Transducer	Detection components technique, bioreceptors	Bacteria type	LOD (CFU mL^{-1})	Reference
Amperometric	Sandwich/Super paramagnetic Beads, Ab	*Escherichia coli*	457	[77]
Amperometric	Sandwich/Chitosan–MWCNTs–SiO_2, Ab	*Escherichia coli*	250	[78]
Amperometric	Nanocomposite, Ab, Enzyme, Pt	*Escherichia coli*	15	[79]
Voltammetric	Iron oxide@Au, CdS Biolabels, Ab	*Salmonella typhimurium*	13	[80]
Voltammetric	Bovine Serum Albumin-GO, AuNPs and Ab	*Shewanella oneidensis*	12	[81]
Voltammetric	Aptamer1-Magnetic Beads, Aptamer 2-AgNP	*Staphylococcus aureus*	1	[82]
Impidimetric	Bioimprinted, Chitosan-Graphene	Sulfate-reducing bacteria	7000	[83]
Impidimetric	Hyaluronic Acid-Alumina Membrane, Ab	*Escherichia coli*	10	[84]
Impidimetric	AuNP-Graphene, Streptavidin, Biotin-Ab	*Escherichia coli*	150	[85]
Conductometric	Ab-Coated Magnetic NP	*Escherichia coli*	1000	[86]
Colorimetric	Collecting on membrane in the vial, Ab	*Listeria monocytogenes*	120	[87]
Colorimetric	Electrostatic aggregation of Cysteine-NP	*Escherichia coli*	100	[88]
Fluorescent	Fluorescent-based Molecular Beacons	*Escherichia coli*	100	[89]
Fluorescent	Dual FRET Aptamers	*Vibrio parahaemolyticus*	25	[90]
Fluorescent	Aptamers nanoparticles	*Salmonella typhimurium*	50	[91]
Raman-based	Ab Immobilized on Nanoclusters	*Escherichia coli*	100	[92]
Raman-based	Two NP-Ab, Magnetic Trap	*Staphylococcus aureus*	1	[93]
SPR	Plasmonic ELISA array, Ab-NP	*Treponema pallidum*	1 pg/mL of Ab	[94]
SPR	ssDNA-NP aggregation	*Serratia marcescens*	5 pM DNA	[95]

Abbreviations: Ab, Antibody; NP, Nanoparticle; MWCNTs, Multi-Walled Carbon Nanotubes; Pt, Platin; FRET, Fluorescence Resonance Energy Transfer; SPR, Surface Plasmon Resonance.

nanobiosensors are taking advantages of electrochemical techniques together with remarkable futures of nanotechnology and extraordinary bio-selectivity of biosensors. Optical-based detection methods are widely used in bacterial detection because they are sensitive, fast, compact and resistance to electrical noise. In optical nanobiosensors different types of nanomaterials are being used as tag or label to enhance the sensitivity and readout signals [76].

5.3.2 Microfluidics for bacterial cells detection

Microfluidics is characterized by manipulation of fluids at the sub-millimeter length scale on a chip device that have been applied for many purposes as single cell analysis and culture, POCT, clinical and forensic analysis [96]. They can be integrated with different sample manipulation tasks such as lysis, extraction and amplification of bacteria samples before the detection process [97]. For the detection of various bacteria, microfluidics-based platforms offer many advantages including speed, cost, portability, high throughput automation, superior safety, improved efficiency and process parallelization [97, 98]. The components of a microfluidic device (force source, detector and transducer type, reservoir for sample, waste and outlet and collector), materials of the chip, patterns of the channels and the fluidics transport mechanism should be carefully selected for each specific application in order to achieve sensitive bacterial cells detection [98, 99]. Fluidic transport have been developed in two main methods; active and passive; passive forces such as capillary, gravity, surface tension and active forces such as centrifugal, micro pump, electric and/or electrophoretic forces [96, 99]. The detection part can be combined with different types of transducers ranging from electrical, electrochemical, optical and piezoelectric, etc. Among them, optical transducers such as colorimetric, fluorescent and Surface-Enhanced Raman Spectroscopy (SERS) are the most attractive and preferred in many types of microfluidic devices.

Different types of nanomaterials have been widely used in microfluidics systems. For instance, researchers developed a microfluidic dielectrophoresis device that used silica-coated SERS nanoprobes. In the study, the practical detection limit with a measurement time of 10 min was estimated to be 70 CFU mL^{-1} [100]. Another SERS-based microfluidic device used iron oxide–gold core–shell nanotag, while the vertically aligned carbon nanofibers were embedded on the silicon microfluidic chip. Dielectrophoresis achieved to capture and concentrate nanotag-labelled *Escherichia coli* on a little nanoelectrode. The detection limit was found as 210 CFU mL^{-1} in less than 1 min. Figure 5.2 presents a brief overview of this microfluidic dielectrophoresis device under a Raman microscope for bacteria detection [101].

As an example of utilization nanomaterials within the microfluidics, hybrid system composed of polydimethylsiloxane/paper/glass were developed with integrated aptamer-functionalized graphene oxide which could successfully detect *Lactobacillus acidophilus* with a detection limit of 11.0 CFU mL^{-1} in 10 min [102]. In another study, specific antibody modified QDs which are attaching to pathogenic *Salmonella* typhimurium was used. For selective detection of *Salmonella,* anti-Salmonella polyclonal antibodies were covalently immobilized onto the quantum dot surface. Then, super paramagnetic particles and a microfluidic chip were used to separate and concentrate the cells from the sample. The fluorescence signal from the quantum dot nanoparticles attached to *Salmonella* in the samples was measured with a portable fluorometer. This simple and portable device could detect down to 1000 CFU mL^{-1} *Salmonella* in food samples [103].

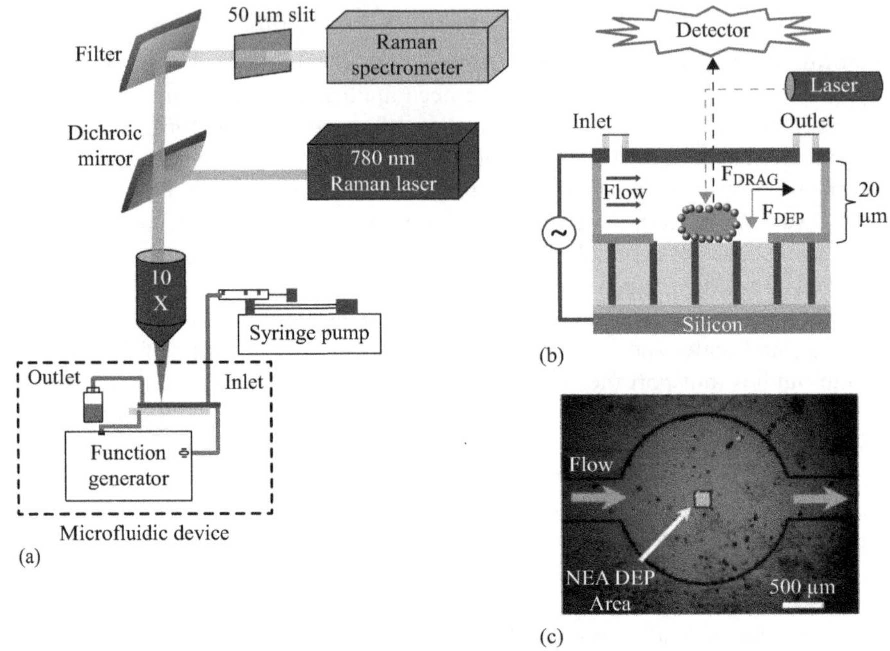

Figure 5.2 Schematic of the microfluidic dielectrophoresis device for SERS-based bacterial cells detection. Reprinted with permission from Reference 118

5.3.3 Paper-based nanobiosensors for bacterial cell detection

Paper- or membrane-based platforms are microfluidics/LOC devices that simply are made from paper matrices that could transmit sample fluids through it. [97, 104]. They are also called as Lateral Flow Assay (LFA) or Lateral Flow Immunochromatographic Assay (LFIA). They can be made of different materials such as cellulose, nitrocellulose, polycarbonate, or even office papers, with diverse shapes, thickness, structures and textures [97, 104]. Paper-based nanobiosensors mainly use gold nanoparticles which have been functionalized with aptamer [105], antibody [106] and DNA [107] for colorimetric detection of different bacterial cells. For instance, enzyme-functionalized gold nanoparticles in inkjet-printed enzymatic test strips in water sample was used to detect *E. coli* in less than 5 min with detection limit as 100 CFU mL^{-1} [108]. Recently, another researchers have succeeded to detect 100 CFU mL^{-1} *E. coli* in bottled water and milk by using photoluminescence quenching ability of graphene oxide and antibody modified QDs as a label [109].

5.3.4 Lab-on-a-chip and chip-plate based nanobiosensors for bacterial cells detection

LOC is a chip-based device that takes advantages of microfluidics and also integrates several automated laboratory functions onto a small miniaturized chip platform [104]. Since they can be integrated with different chemical and biological laboratory tasks, they are used for many different applications from single cell culture and examination, drug-cell interaction, cell and bacteria detection, tissue- and organ-on-a-chip, nanoparticles synthesis and toxicity tests [110]. Regarding their application in bacterial cells detection, many biosensors have been published in recent years because they can be a perfect medium for portable, ease-of-use, fast and real-time medical diagnostics. They also have high reproducibility due to standardization and automation of fabrication and working procedures [104]. The chip- or plate-based devices can be miniaturized in a small chip or plate, which can make a medium for attachment of nanoparticles and patterns, immobilizing bioreceptors and for the detection part. They are mainly based on some detector and transducers such as plasmonic-based [111, 112] electrochemical electrode embedded chips [113, 114] and electronics chips [115]. In Table 5.3, we collect the representative examples of microfluidics and LOC systems for sensitive bacterial cells detection.

Two distinctive LSPR-based methods have been developed based on AuNP which is functionalized with aptamer [111] and antibody [112], but in a voltammetric-based detection methods on electrode chips which have designed for DNA-based detection of *E. coli*, used ssDNA probe that attached to the chips surface applied 3D structures [116, 117]. In addition, the electronically based detection systems have been used for bacterial detection. For example, an *E. coli* detection system have been developed based on single walled carbon nanotubes (SWCNTs) and immobilized antibodies onto the junction sensor consists of gold tungsten microwires coated with polyethylenimine (PEI) and SWCNTs were aligned to form a cross-bar junction, functionalized with streptavidin and biotinylated antibodies. The system could detect 100 CFU mL^{-1} bacteria in less than 5 min by measuring changes in electrical current [118].

5.3.5 Perspectives of nanobiosensors in bacterial cells detection

As the bacterial infection is a main health problem and directly related to our health and quality of life, detection of them with the fast, simple, sensitive, specific and reliable methods have always been the main challenges. So far, tremendous accomplishments have been made in design and fabrication of different nanobiosensors that have been developed using cutting-edge techniques to enhance the sensitivity and selectivity of bacteria detection platforms. In the present section, we described general ideas and examined recent advances in this filed in different categories such as their transducer type, shape and structure of applied nanomaterials, target bacteria, limit of detection and brief overview of their detection mechanism. Due to important role of microfluidics and LOC methods in bacterial

Table 5.3 Selection of different methods in microfluidics and lab-on-a-chip nanobiosensors for bacterial cells detection

Method	Transducer/mechanism	Target bacteria	LOD (CFU mL^{-1})	Reference
Microfluidic	SERS/dielectrophoresis, Ab-NP-beads	*Salmonella choleraesuis Neisseria lactamica*	70	[100]
Microfluidic	SERS/dielectrophoretic, nanotag, chip	*Escherichia coli*	210	[101]
Microfluidic	Fluorescent/Ab-QD, magnet trap	*Salmonella typhimurium*	1000	[103]
Nanofluidic	Fluorescent/electrokinetic trap of bacteria	*Escherichia coli*	1000	[119]
Paper-based	Colorimetric/Ap-NP attachment	*Salmonella enteritidis*	10	[105]
Paper-based	Colorimetric/Ab-AuNP, enzyme activity	*Escherichia coli*	100	[106]
Paper-based	Colorimetric/ssDNA-NP attachment	*Listeria monocytogenes*	20	[107]
Paper-based	Photoluminescent/Ab-QD	*Escherichia coli*	100	[109]
Chip	LSPR/ Ap-AuNP coated silica NP-glass chip	3 pathogenic bacteria	30	[111]
Chip	LSPR/ Ab-NP, capture Ab, magnetic field	*Escherichia coli*	50	[112]
Chip	Voltammetric/ ssDNA-3D chip	*Escherichia coli*	150	[113]
Chip	Voltammetric/ssDNA-3D Nano electrodes	*Escherichia coli*	4	[114]
Chip-plate	Electronic/polyethylenimine, NP, Ab	*Escherichia coli*	100	[115]

Abbreviations: Ab, antibody; Ap, aptamer; NP, nanoparticle; QD, quantum dots.

cells detection, the focus of this section was on them. They are perfect for point-of-care detection of bacteria with embedding different laboratory task (sample preparation, separation and detection) into a small fluidics chip and enhancing its potential such as the time- and cost-effective, simple and contamination-free detection.

5.4 Conclusion and final remarks

The main goal of cancer and bacterial cells detection-based biosensor systems is that moving the knowledge to POCT as point-of-care applications has great clinical potential. There are several challenges in moving biosensors to POCT for cancer and bacterial cells detection such as development of sensitive biomarker assays within the multi-channel biosensors; advances in sample preparation and analyte enrichment; miniaturization and integration and advanced manufacturing techniques. Ultra-sensitive, highly specific, non-invasive and robust detection technologies for diagnosis, prognosis and prevention are required. It is urgently necessary to accelerate the translation of nanomedicine-based detection methods and devices to clinical care.

References

[1] Li L.L., Y.Q. Wang, L.J. Pan, Y. Shi, W. Cheng and Y. Shi, "A nanostructured conductive hydrogels-based biosensor platform for human metabolite detection." *Nano Letters.* 2015; **15**(2): pp. 1146–1151.

[2] Zhang, Y.L., P. Zuo, and B.C. Ye, "A low-cost and simple paper-based microfluidic device for simultaneous multiplex determination of different types of chemical contaminants in food." *Biosensors & Bioelectronics.* 2015; **68**: pp. 14–19.

[3] Yang, G., K.L. Kampstra, and M.R. Abidian, "High-performance conducting polymer nanofiber biosensors for detection of biomolecules." *Advanced Materials.* 2014; **26**(29): pp. 4954–4960.

[4] Campbell, K., A.C. Huet, C. Charlier, C. Higgins, P. Delahaut, and C.T. Elliott, "Comparison of ELISA and SPR biosensor technology for the detection of paralytic shellfish poisoning toxins." *Journal of Chromatography B: Analytical Technologies in Biomedical and Life Sciences.* 2009; **877**(32): pp. 4079–4089.

[5] Cork, J., R.M. Jones, and J. Sawyer, "Low cost, disposable biosensors allow detection of antibodies with results equivalent to ELISA in 15 min." *Journal of Immunological Methods.* 2013; **387**(1–2): pp. 140–146.

[6] Turner, A.P.F., "Biosensors: sense and sensibility." *Chemical Society Reviews.* 2013; **42**(8): pp. 3184–3196.

[7] Hanahan, D. and R.A. Weinberg, "The hallmarks of cancer." *Cell.* 2000; **100**(1): pp. 57–70.

[8] Liu, Q.J., C.S. Wu, H. Cai, N. Hu, J. Zhou, and P. Wang, "Cell-based biosensors and their application in biomedicine." *Chemical Reviews.* 2014; **114** (12): pp. 6423–6461.

[9] Daringer, N.M., R.M. Dudek, K.A. Schwarz, and J.N. Leonard, "Modular extracellular sensor architecture for engineering mammalian cell-based devices." *Acs Synthetic Biology.* 2014; **3**(12): pp. 892–902.

[10] Brauchle, E. and K. Schenke-Layland, "Raman spectroscopy in biomedicine – non-invasive in vitro analysis of cells and extracellular matrix components in tissues." *Biotechnology Journal.* 2013; **8**(3): pp. 288–297.

[11] Ramasamy, S., D. Bennet, and S. Kim, "Drug and bioactive molecule screening based on a bioelectrical impedance cell culture platform." *International Journal of Nanomedicine.* 2014; **9**: pp. 5789–5809.

[12] Weltin, A., K. Slotwinski, J. Kieninger, I. Moser, G. Jobst, and M. Wego, "Cell culture monitoring for drug screening and cancer research: a

transparent, microfluidic, multi-sensor microsystem." *Lab on a Chip.* 2014; **14**(1): pp. 138–146.

[13] Tuerk, C. and L. Gold, "Systematic evolution of ligands by exponential enrichment – RNA ligands to bacteriophage-T4 DNA-polymerase." *Science.* 1990; **249**(4968): pp. 505–510.

[14] Ellington, A.D. and J.W. Szostak, "In vitro selection of RNA molecules that bind specific ligands." *Nature.* 1990; **346**(6287): pp. 818–822.

[15] Stoltenburg, R., C. Reinemann, and B. Strehlitz, "SELEX-A (r)evolutionary method to generate high-affinity nucleic acid ligands." *Biomolecular Engineering.* 2007; **24**(4): pp. 381–403.

[16] Aquino-Jarquin, G. and J.D. Toscano-Garibay, "RNA aptamer evolution: two decades of SELEction." *International Journal of Molecular Sciences.* 2011; **12**(12): pp. 9155–9171.

[17] Reinemann, C. and B. Strehlitz, "Aptamer-modified nanoparticles and their use in cancer diagnostics and treatment." *Swiss Medical Weekly.* 2014; **144**: 1–12.

[18] Souada, M., B. Piro, S. Reisberg, G. Anquetin, V. Noel, and M.C. Pham, "Label-free electrochemical detection of prostate-specific antigen based on nucleic acid aptamer." *Biosensors & Bioelectronics.* 2015; **68**: pp. 49–54.

[19] Zhang, H.M., Y.L. Ma, Y. Xie, Y. An, Y.S. Huang, and Z. Zhu,"A controllable aptamer-based self-assembled DNA dendrimer for high affinity targeting, bioimaging and drug delivery." *Scientific Reports.* 2015; **5**, 1–8.

[20] Coles, D.J., B.E. Rolfe, N.R.B. Boase, R.N. Veedu, and K.J. Thurecht, "Aptamer-targeted hyperbranched polymers: towards greater specificity for tumours in vivo." *Chemical Communications.* 2013; **49**(37): pp. 3836–3838.

[21] Bamrungsap, S., T. Chen, M.I. Shukoor, Z. Chen, K. Sefah, Y. Chen, "Pattern recognition of cancer cells using aptamer-conjugated magnetic nanoparticles." *ACS Nano.* 2012; **6**(5): pp. 3974–3981.

[22] Zhao, B.J., P. Wu, H. Zhang, and C.X. Cai, "Designing activatable aptamer probes for simultaneous detection of multiple tumor-related proteins in living cancer cells." *Biosensors & Bioelectronics.* 2015; **68**: pp. 763–770.

[23] Xiang, D.X., S. Shigdar, G. Qiao, T. Wang, A.Z. Kouzani, S.F. Zhou, "Nucleic acid aptamer-guided cancer therapeutics and diagnostics: the next generation of cancer medicine." *Theranostics.* 2015; **5**(1): pp. 23–42.

[24] Shangguan, D., Y. Li, Z.W. Tang, Z.H.C. Cao, H.W. Chen, P. Mallikaratchy, "Aptamers evolved from live cells as effective molecular probes for cancer study." *Proceedings of the National Academy of Sciences of the United States of America.* 2006; **103**(32): pp. 11838–11843.

[25] Wang, Y.Y., Y. Luo, T. Bing, Z. Chen, M.H. Lu, N. Zhang, "DNA aptamer evolved by cell-SELEX for recognition of prostate cancer." *PLoS ONE.* 2014; **9**(6): 1–10.

[26] Phillips, J.A., D. Lopez-Colon, Z. Zhu, Y. Xu, and W.H. Tan, "Applications of aptamers in cancer cell biology." *Analytica Chimica Acta.* 2008; **621**(2): pp.101–108.

[27] Biomarkers Definitions Working, G., "Biomarkers and surrogate endpoints: preferred definitions and conceptual framework." *Clinical Pharmacology & Therapeutics.* 2001; **69**(3): pp. 89–95.

[28] Ray, S., P.J. Reddy, S. Choudhary, D. Raghu, and S. Srivastava, "Emerging nanoproteomics approaches for disease biomarker detection: a current perspective." *Journal of Proteomics.* 2011; **74**(12): pp. 2660–2681.

[29] Diamandis, E.P., "Cancer biomarkers: can we turn recent failures into success?" *Journal of National Cancer Institute.* 2010; **102**(19): pp. 1462–1467.

[30] O'Sullivan, C.K., "Aptasensors – the future of biosensing." *Analytical and Bioanalytical Chemistry.* 2002; **372**(1): pp. 44–48.

[31] Zhang, J.J., T.T. Zheng, F.F. Cheng, J.R. Zhang, and J.J. Zhu, "Toward the early evaluation of therapeutic effects: an electrochemical platform for ultrasensitive detection of apoptotic cells." *Analytical Chemistry.* 2011; **83** (20): pp. 7902–7909.

[32] Hao, C., L. Ding, X.J. Zhang, and H.X. Ju, "Biocompatible conductive architecture of carbon nanofiber-doped chitosan prepared with controllable electrodeposition for cytosensing." *Analytical Chemistry.* 2007; **79**(12): pp. 4442–4447.

[33] Wang, T.S., J.Y. Liu, X.X. Gu, D. Li, J. Wang, and E. Wang, "Label-free electrochemical aptasensor constructed by layer-by-layer technology for sensitive and selective detection of cancer cells." *Analytica Chimica Acta.* 2015; **882**: pp. 32–37.

[34] Lu, C.Y., J.J. Xu, Z.H. Wang, and H.Y. Chen, "A novel signal-amplified electrochemical aptasensor based on supersandwich G-quadruplex DNAzyme for highly sensitive cancer cell detection." *Electrochemistry Communications.* 2015; **52**: pp. 49–52.

[35] Chen, X.J., Y.Z. Wang, Y.Y. Zhang, Z.H. Chen, Y. Liu, Z.L. Li, "Sensitive electrochemical aptamer biosensor for dynamic cell surface N-glycan evaluation featuring multivalent recognition and signal amplification on a dendrimer-graphene electrode interface." *Analytical Chemistry.* 2014; **86**(9): pp. 4278–4286.

[36] Zhu, Y., P. Chandra, and Y.B. Shim, "Ultrasensitive and selective electrochemical diagnosis of breast cancer based on a hydrazine-Au nanoparticle-aptamer bioconjugate." *Analytical Chemistry.* 2013; **85**(2): pp. 1058–1064.

[37] Dai, Z., J. Chen, F. Yan, and H.X. Ju, "Electrochemical sensor for immunoassay of carcinoembryonic antigen based on thionine monolayer modified gold electrode." *Cancer Detection and Prevention.* 2005; **29**(3): pp. 233–240.

[38] Lee, S., H. Jo, J. Her, H.Y. Lee, and C. Ban, "Ultrasensitive electrochemical detection of engrailed-2 based on homeodomain-specific DNA probe recognition for the diagnosis of prostate cancer." *Biosensors & Bioelectronics.* 2015; **66**: pp. 32–38.

[39] Beqa, L., Z. Fan, A.K. Singh, D. Senapati, and P.C. Ray, "Gold nano-popcorn attached SWCNT hybrid nanomaterial for targeted diagnosis and

photothermal therapy of human breast cancer cells." *ACS Applied Materials & Interfaces*. 2011; **3**(9): pp. 3316–3324.

[40] Chen, H.X., Y.F. Hou, Z.H. Ye, H.Y. Wang, K. Koh, Z.M. Shen, "Label-free surface plasmon resonance cytosensor for breast cancer cell detection based on nano-conjugation of monodisperse magnetic nanoparticle and folic acid." *Sensors and Actuators B-Chemical.* 2014; **201**: pp. 433–438.

[41] Cho, H., E.C. Yeh, R. Sinha, T.A. Laurence, J.P. Bearinger, and L.P. Lee, "Single-step nanoplasmonic VEGF165 aptasensor for early cancer diagnosis." *ACS Nano.* 2012; **6**(9): pp. 7607–7614.

[42] Xie, Q., Y.Y. Tan, Q.P. Guo, K.M. Wang, B.Y. Yuan, J. Wan, "A fluorescent aptasensor for sensitive detection of human hepatocellular carcinoma SMMC-7721 cells based on graphene oxide." *Analytical Methods.* 2014; **6** (17): pp. 6809–6814.

[43] Chen, C.H., Y.F. Liu, Z.H. Zheng, G.H. Zhou, X.H. Ji, H.Z. Wang, "A new colorimetric platform for ultrasensitive detection of protein and cancer cells based on the assembly of nucleic acids and proteins." *Analytica Chimica Acta.* 2015; **880**: pp. 1–7.

[44] Wang, D.F., Y.Y. Li, Z.Y. Lin, B. Qiu, and L.H. Guo, "Surface-enhanced electrochemiluminescence of Ru@SiO_2 for ultrasensitive detection of carcinoembryonic antigen." *Analytical Chemistry.* 2015; **87**(12): pp. 5966–5972.

[45] Uludag, Y. and I.E. Tothill, "Cancer biomarker detection in serum samples using surface plasmon resonance and quartz crystal microbalance sensors with nanoparticle signal amplification." *Analytical Chemistry.* 2012; **84**(14): pp. 5898–5904.

[46] Chang, K., Y. Pi, W.P. Lu, F. Wang, F. Pan, F.K. Li, "Label-free and high-sensitive detection of human breast cancer cells by aptamer-based leaky surface acoustic wave biosensor array." *Biosensors & Bioelectronics.* 2014; **60**: pp. 318–324.

[47] Shan, W.Q., Y.L. Pan, H.T. Fang, M.L. Guo, Z. Nie, Y. Huang, "An aptamer-based quartz crystal microbalance biosensor for sensitive and selective detection of leukemia cells using silver-enhanced gold nanoparticle label." *Talanta.* 2014; **126**: pp. 130–135.

[48] Du, D., J. Cai, H.X. Ju, F. Yan, J. Chen, X.Q. Jiang, "Construction of a biomimetic zwitterionic interface for monitoring cell proliferation and apoptosis." *Langmuir.* 2005; **21**(18): pp. 8394–8399.

[49] Du, D., S.L. Liu, J. Chen, H.X. Ju, H.Z. Lian, J.X. Li, "Colloidal gold nanoparticle modified carbon paste interface for studies of tumor cell adhesion and viability." *Biomaterials.* 2005; **26**(33): pp. 6487–6495.

[50] Zhong, X., H.J. Bai, J.J. Xu, H.Y. Chen, and Y.H. Zhu, "A reusable interface constructed by 3-aminophenylboronic acid functionalized multiwalled carbon nanotubes for cell capture, release, and cytosensing." *Advanced Functional Materials.* 2010; **20**(6): pp. 992–999.

[51] Kashefi-Kheyrabadi, L., M.A. Mehrgardi, E. Wiechec, A.P.F. Turner, and A. Tiwari, "Ultrasensitive detection of human liver hepatocellular

carcinoma cells using a label-free aptasensor." *Analytical Chemistry.* 2014; **86**(10): pp. 4956–4960.

[52] Qu, L.M., J.H. Xu, X.F. Tan, Z. Liu, L.G. Xu, and R. Peng, "Dual-aptamer modification generates a unique interface for highly sensitive and specific electrochemical detection of tumor cells." *ACS Applied Materials & Interfaces.* 2014; **6**(10): pp. 7309–7315.

[53] Chen, X.L., M.C. Estevez, Z. Zhu, Y.F. Huang, Y. Chen, L. Wang, "Using aptamer-conjugated fluorescence resonance energy transfer nanoparticles for multiplexed cancer cell monitoring." *Analytical Chemistry.* 2009; **81**(16): pp. 7009–7014.

[54] Medley, C.D., J.E. Smith, Z. Tang, Y. Wu, S. Bamrungsap, and W.H. Tan, "Gold nanoparticle-based colorimetric assay for the direct detection of cancerous cells." *Analytical Chemistry.* 2008; **80**(4): pp. 1067–1072.

[55] Boccellato, F. and T.F. Meyer, "Bacteria moving into focus of human cancer." *Cell Host Microbe.* 2015; **17**(6): pp. 728–730.

[56] Viljoen, K.S., A. Dakshinamurthy, P. Goldberg, and J.M. Blackburn, "Quantitative profiling of colorectal cancer-associated bacteria reveals associations between Fusobacterium spp., enterotoxigenic bacteroides fragilis (ETBF) and clinicopathological features of colorectal cancer." *PLoS ONE.* 2015; **10**(3): 1–21.

[57] Chow, S.C., S.D. Gowing, J.J. Cools-Lartigue , C.B. Chen, J. Berube, H.W. Yoon, "Gram negative bacteria increase non-small cell lung cancer metastasis via toll-like receptor 4 activation and mitogen-activated protein kinase phosphorylation." *International Journal of Cancer.* 2015; **136**(6): pp. 1341–1350.

[58] Ito, N. and K. Ohta, "Reprogramming of human somatic cells by bacteria." *Development Growth and Differentiation.* 2015; **57**(4): pp. 305–312.

[59] Campisi, L., S.M. Soudja, J. Cazareth, D. Bassand, A. Lazzari, and F. Brau, "Splenic CD8 alpha(+) dendritic cells undergo rapid programming by cytosolic bacteria and inflammation to induce protective CD8(+) T-cell memory." *European Journal of Immunology.* 2011; **41**(6): pp. 1594–1605.

[60] Nothelfer, K., P.J. Sansonetti, and A. Phalipon, "Pathogen manipulation of B cells: the best defence is a good offence." *Nature Reviews Microbiology.* 2015; **13**(3): pp. 173–184.

[61] Jones, M.K., M. Watanabe, S. Zhu, C.L. Graves, L.R. Keyes, and K.R. Grau, "Enteric bacteria promote human and mouse norovirus infection of B cells." *Science.* 2014; **346**(6210): pp. 755–759.

[62] Arora, P., A. Sindhu, H. Kaur, N. Dilbaghi, and A. Chaudhury, "An overview of transducers as platform for the rapid detection of foodborne pathogens." *Applied Microbiology and Biotechnology.* 2013; **97**(5): pp. 1829–1840.

[63] Gubala, V., L.F. Harris, A.J. Ricco, M.X. Tan, and D.E. Williams, "Point of care diagnostics: status and future". *Analytical Chemistry.* 2012; **84**(2): pp. 487–515.

[64] Chen, C.Y., G.W. Nace, and P.L. Irwin, "A 6 $\times$ 6 drop plate method for simultaneous colony counting and MPN enumeration of Campylobacter

jejuni, Listeria monocytogenes, and Escherichia coli." *Journal of Microbiological Methods.* 2003; **55**(2): pp. 475–479.

[65] Fazal, N., R. Bartlett, D.A. Lammas, and D.S. Kumararatne, "A comparison of the different methods available for determining BCG-macrophage interactions invitro, including a new method of colony counting in broth." *FEMS Microbiology Immunology.* 1992; **105**(5–6): pp. 355–362.

[66] Hayama, K., N. Maruyama, and S. Abe, "Cell preparation method with trypsin digestion for counting of colony forming units in Candida albicans-infected mucosal tissues." *Medical Mycology.* 2012; **50**(8): pp. 858–862.

[67] Edouard, S., E. Prudent, P. Gautret, Z.A. Memish, and D. Raoult, "Cost-effective pooling of dna from nasopharyngeal swab samples for large-scale detection of bacteria by real-time PCR." *Journal of Clinical Microbiology.* 2015; **53**(3): pp. 1002–1004.

[68] Postollec, F., S. Bonilla, F. Baron, S. Jan, M. Gautier, and A.G. Mathot, "A multiparametric PCR-based tool for fast detection and identification of spore-forming bacteria in food." *International Journal of Food Microbiology.* 2010; **142**(1–2): pp. 78–88.

[69] Jiang, X.R., W.W. Jing, L.L. Zheng, S.X. Liu, W.J. Wu, and G.D. Sui, "A continuous-flow high-throughput microfluidic device for airborne bacteria PCR detection." *Lab on a Chip.* 2014; **14**(4): pp. 671–676.

[70] Gutierrez, J. and J. Liebana, "Immunological methods for the detection of structural components and metabolites of bacteria and fungi in blood." *Annales De Biologie Clinique.* 1993; **51**(2): pp. 83–90.

[71] Ferguson, C.M.J., N.A. Booth, and E.J. Allan, "An ELISA for the detection of Bacillus subtilis L-form bacteria confirms their symbiosis in strawberry." *Letters in Applied Microbiology.* 2000; **31**(5): pp. 390–394.

[72] Singh, R., M.D. Mukherjee, G. Sumana, R.K. Gupta, S. Sood, and B.D. Malhotra, "Biosensors for pathogen detection: a smart approach towards clinical diagnosis." *Sensors and Actuators B: Chemical.* 2014; **197**: pp. 385–404.

[73] Marín, S. and A. Merkoçi, "Nanomaterials based electrochemical sensing applications for safety and security." *Electroanalysis.* 2012; **24**(3): pp. 459–469.

[74] Perumal, V. and U. Hashim, "Advances in biosensors: principle, architecture and applications." *Journal of Applied Biomedicine.* 2014; **12**(1): pp. 1–15.

[75] Xu, S., "Electromechanical biosensors for pathogen detection." *Microchimica Acta.* 2012; **178**(3–4): pp. 245–260.

[76] Méjard, R., H.J. Griesser, and B. Thierry, "Optical biosensing for label-free cellular studies." *TrAC Trends in Analytical Chemistry.* 2014; **53**: pp. 178–186.

[77] Hassan, A.R., A. de la Escosura-Muniz, and A. Merkoci, "Highly sensitive and rapid determination of Escherichia coli O157:H7 in minced beef and water using electrocatalytic gold nanoparticle tags." *Biosensors and Bioelectronics.* 2015; **67**: pp. 511–515.

[78] Li, Y., P. Cheng, J. Gong, L. Fang, J. Deng, W. Liang, "Amperometric immunosensor for the detection of Escherichia coli O157:H7 in food specimens." *Analytical Biochemistry.* 2012; **421**(1): pp. 227–233.

[79] Li, Y., L. Fang, P. Cheng, J. Deng, L. Jiang, H. Huang, "An electrochemical immunosensor for sensitive detection of Escherichia coli O157:H7 using C60 based biocompatible platform and enzyme functionalized Pt nanochains tracing tag." *Biosensors and Bioelectronics.* 2013; **49**: pp. 485–491.

[80] Freitas, M., S. Viswanathan, H.P. Nouws, M.B. Oliveira, and C. Delerue-Matos, 'Iron oxide/gold core/shell nanomagnetic probes and CdS biolabels for amplified electrochemical immunosensing of Salmonella typhimurium." *Biosensors and Bioelectronics.* 2014; **51**: pp. 195–200.

[81] Wen, J., S. Zhou, and Y. Yuan, "Graphene oxide as nanogold carrier for ultrasensitive electrochemical immunoassay of Shewanella oneidensis with silver enhancement strategy." *Biosensors and Bioelectronics.* 2014; **52**: pp. 44–49.

[82] Abbaspour, A., F. Norouz-Sarvestani, A. Noori, and N. Soltani, "Aptamer-conjugated silver nanoparticles for electrochemical dual-aptamer-based sandwich detection of staphylococcus aureus." *Biosensors and Bioelectronics.* 2015; **68**: pp. 149–155.

[83] Qi, P., Y. Wan, and D. Zhang, "Impedimetric biosensor based on cell-mediated bioimprinted films for bacterial detection." *Biosensors and Bioelectronics.* 2013; **39**(1): pp. 282–288.

[84] Joung, C.K., H.N. Kim, M.C. Lim, T.J. Jeon, H.Y. Kim, and Y.R. Kim, "A nanoporous membrane-based impedimetric immunosensor for label-free detection of pathogenic bacteria in whole milk." *Biosensors and Bioelectronics.* 2013; **44**: pp. 210–215.

[85] Wang, Y., J. Ping, Z. Ye, J. Wu, and Y. Ying, "Impedimetric immunosensor based on gold nanoparticles modified graphene paper for label-free detection of Escherichia coli O157:H7." *Biosensors and Bioelectronics.* 2013; **49**: pp. 492–498.

[86] El Ichi, S., F. Leon, L. Vossier, H. Marchandin, A. Errachid, J. Coste, "Microconductometric immunosensor for label-free and sensitive detection of Gram-negative bacteria." *Biosensors and Bioelectronics.* 2014; **54**: pp. 378–384.

[87] Shim, W.-B., C.-W. Lee, M.-G. Kim, and D.-H. Chung, "An antibody–magnetic nanoparticle conjugate-based selective filtration method for the rapid colorimetric detection of Listeria monocytogenes." *Analytical Methods.* 2014; **6**(22): pp. 9129–9135.

[88] Raj, V., A.N. Vijayan, and K. Joseph, "Cysteine capped gold nanoparticles for naked eye detection of E. coli bacteria in UTI patients." *Sensing and Bio-Sensing Research.* 2015; **5**: pp. 33–36.

[89] Cao, J., C. Feng, Y. Liu, S. Wang, and F. Liu, "Highly sensitive and rapid bacteria detection using molecular beacon-Au nanoparticles hybrid nanoprobes." *Biosensors and Bioelectronics.* 2014; **57**: pp. 133–138.

[90] Duan, N., S. Wu, S. Dai, T. Miao, J. Chen, and Z. Wang, "Simultaneous detection of pathogenic bacteria using an aptamer based biosensor and dual fluorescence resonance energy transfer from quantum dots to carbon nanoparticles." *Microchimica Acta.* 2014; **182**(5–6): pp. 917–923.

[91] Wang, R., Y. Xu, T. Zhang, and Y. Jiang, "Rapid and sensitive detection of Salmonella typhimurium using aptamer-conjugated carbon dots as fluorescence probe." *Analytical Methods.* 2015; **7**(5): pp. 1701–1706.

[92] Najafi, R., S. Mukherjee, J. Hudson Jr., A. Sharma, and P. Banerjee, "Development of a rapid capture-cum-detection method for Escherichia coli O157 from apple juice comprising nano-immunomagnetic separation in tandem with surface enhanced Raman scattering." *International Journal of Food Microbiology.* 2014; **189**: pp. 89–97.

[93] Drake, P., P.-S. Jiang, H.-W. Chang, S.-C. Su, J. Tanha, L.-L. Tay, "Raman based detection of Staphylococcus aureus utilizing single domain antibody coated nanoparticle labels and magnetic trapping." *Analytical Methods.* 2013; **5**(16): p. 4152.

[94] Nie, X.M., R. Huang, C.X. Dong, L.J. Tang, R. Gui, and J.H. Jiang, "Plasmonic ELISA for the ultrasensitive detection of Treponema pallidum." *Biosensors and Bioelectronics.* 2014; **58**: pp. 314–319.

[95] Wang, X., Y. Li, J. Wang, Q. Wang, L. Xu, J. Du, "A broad-range method to detect genomic DNA of multiple pathogenic bacteria based on the aggregation strategy of gold nanorods." *Analyst.* 2012; **137**(18): pp. 4267–4273.

[96] Su, W., X. Gao, L. Jiang, and J. Qin, "Microfluidic platform towards point-of-care diagnostics in infectious diseases." *Journal of Chromatography A.* 2015; **1377**: pp. 13–26.

[97] Rivet, C., H. Lee, A. Hirsch, S. Hamilton, and H. Lu, "Microfluidics for medical diagnostics and biosensors." *Chemical Engineering Science.* 2011; **66**(7): pp. 1490–1507.

[98] Bridle, H., B. Miller, and M.P. Desmulliez, "Application of microfluidics in waterborne pathogen monitoring: a review." *Water Research.* 2014; **55**: pp. 256–271.

[99] Lee, H., L. Xu, D. Koh, N. Nyayapathi, and K.W. Oh, "Various on-chip sensors with microfluidics for biological applications." *Sensors (Basel).* 2014; **14**(9): pp. 17008–17036.

[100] Lin, H.Y., C.H. Huang, W.H. Hsieh, L.H. Liu, Y.C. Lin, C.C. Chu, "On-line SERS detection of single bacterium using novel SERS nanoprobes and a microfluidic dielectrophoresis device." *Small.* 2014; **10**(22): pp. 4700–4710.

[101] Madiyar, F.R., S. Bhana, L.Z. Swisher, C.T. Culbertson, X. Huang, and J. Li, "Integration of a nanostructured dielectrophoretic device and a surface-enhanced Raman probe for highly sensitive rapid bacteria detection." *Nanoscale.* 2015; **7**(8): pp. 3726–3736.

[102] Zuo, P., X. Li, D.C. Dominguez, and B.C. Ye, "A PDMS/paper/glass hybrid microfluidic biochip integrated with aptamer-functionalized graphene oxide nano-biosensors for one-step multiplexed pathogen detection." *Lab on a Chip.* 2013; **13**(19): pp. 3921–3928.

[103] Kim, G., J.H. Moon, C.Y. Moh, and J.G. Lim, "A microfluidic nano-biosensor for the detection of pathogenic Salmonella." *Biosensors and Bioelectronics.* 2015; **67**: pp. 243–247.

[104] Yoon, J.Y. and B. Kim, "Lab-on-a-chip pathogen sensors for food safety." *Sensors (Basel)*. 2012; **12**(8): pp. 10713–10741.

[105] Fang, Z., W. Wu, X. Lu, and L. Zeng, "Lateral flow biosensor for DNA extraction-free detection of Salmonella based on aptamer mediated strand displacement amplification." *Biosensors and Bioelectronics*. 2014; **56**: pp. 192–197.

[106] Cho, I.H., A. Bhunia, and J. Irudayaraj, "Rapid pathogen detection by lateral-flow immunochromatographic assay with gold nanoparticle-assisted enzyme signal amplification." *International Journal of Food Microbiology*. 2015; **206**: pp. 60–66.

[107] Liu, H., F. Zhan, F. Liu, M. Zhu, X. Zhou, and D. Xing, "Visual and sensitive detection of viable pathogenic bacteria by sensing of RNA markers in gold nanoparticles based paper platform." *Biosensors and Bioelectronics*. 2014; **62**: pp. 38–46.

[108] Creran, B., X. Li, B. Duncan, C.S. Kim, D.F. Moyano, and V.M. Rotello, "Detection of bacteria using inkjet-printed enzymatic test strips." *ACS Applied Material Interfaces*. 2014; **6**(22): pp. 19525–19530.

[109] Morales-Narvaez, E., T. Naghdi, E. Zor, and A. Merkoci, "Photoluminescent lateral-flow immunoassay revealed by graphene oxide: highly sensitive paper-based pathogen detection." *Analytical Chemistry*. 2015; **87** (16): pp. 8573–8577.

[110] Sackmann, E.K., A.L. Fulton, and D.J. Beebe, "The present and future role of microfluidics in biomedical research." *Nature*. 2014; **507**(7491): pp. 181–189.

[111] Yoo, S.M., D.K. Kim, and S.Y. Lee, "Aptamer-functionalized localized surface plasmon resonance sensor for the multiplexed detection of different bacterial species." *Talanta*. 2015; **132**: pp. 112–117.

[112] Wang, Y., W. Knoll, and J. Dostalek, "Bacterial pathogen surface plasmon resonance biosensor advanced by long range surface plasmons and magnetic nanoparticle assays." *Analytical Chemistry*. 2012; **84**(19): pp. 8345–8350.

[113] Yamashita, Y., T. Ikeda, M. Matsuda, D. Maji, T. Hoshino, and T. Mizushima, "Purification and characterization of HSP-inducers from Eupatorium lindleyanum." *Biochem Pharmacol*. 2012; **83**(7): pp. 909–922.

[114] Shahabadi, N., Z.M. Kalar, and A.V. Rayegani, "DNA interaction studies of an antiviral drug, ribavirin, using different instrumental methods." *DNA Cell Biology*. 2012; **31**(5): pp. 876–882.

[115] Klemm, K., M. Radic Stojkovic, G. Horvat, V. Tomisic, I. Piantanida , and C. Schmuck, "Interactions of multicationic bis(guanidiniocarbonylpyrrole) receptors with double-stranded nucleic acids: syntheses, binding studies, and atomic force microscopy imaging." *Chemistry*. 2012; **18**(5): pp. 1352–1363.

[116] Soleymani L., Z. Fang , and B. Lam, *et al*., "Hierarchical nanotextured microelectrodes overcome the molecular transport barrier to achieve rapid, direct bacterial detection." *ACS Nano*. 2011; **5**(4): pp. 3360–3366.

[117] Besant J.D., J. Das, E.H. Sargent, and E.O. Kelley, "Proximal bacterial lysis and detection in nanoliter wells using electrochemistry." *ACS Nano*,. 2013; **7**(9): pp. 8183–8189.

[118] Yamada K., C.-T. Kim, J.-H. Kim, J.-H. Chung, H.G. Lee, and S. Jun, "Single walled carbon nanotube-based junction biosensor for detection of Escherichia coli." 2014; *PLoS ONE*. **9**(9): e105767.

[119] Wang, Z., T. Han, T.-J. Jeon, S. Park, and S.M. Kim, "Rapid detection and quantification of bacteria using an integrated micro/nanofluidic device." *Sensors and Actuators B: Chemical*. 2013; **178**: pp. 683–688.

Chapter 6

Biacore – a surface plasmon resonance-based technology

Subash C.B. Gopinath[1,2,], Uda Hashim[1], M.K. Md Arshad[1] and Thangavel Lakshmipriya[1]*

6.1 Introduction

Surface Plasmon Resonance (SPR) is operating based on optical phenomenon, very commonly in use for the sensing applications [1]. The principle of SPR was first observed by Wood in the year 1902 and after different developments by researchers; in 1968 Kretschmann and Raether formulated the complete optical set-up. The first demonstration for biomolecular interactions using the SPR-principle was in 1983 by Lundstrom [2]. Unless otherwise stated, all SPR-based sensors are designed based on the configuration of Kretschmann [3]. After the above initiations, several SPR-based sensor systems have been generated with the choices for placement of the measurement chip, surface priming, composition of buffers, immobilization procedures and so on. These developments include a fiber optic SPR sensor with a wavelength interrogation and this sensor has a multimode optical fiber with locally exposed core and a thin gold film. The light reflected back to the fiber by a mirror at the end of the sensing area and a fiber optic coupler was used to separate the reflected light from incoming illumination [4]. Similarly, another fiber optic SPR sensor is reported; however, the fiber was illuminated by a monochromatic light through special optics to selectively excite fiber modes, and detect changes [5].

The development of mobile, compact and cost-effective sensing devices with potential for field applications were developed with miniaturized SPR sensors using the attenuated total reflection method as an alternative to laboratory SPR systems [6]. A conventional prism coupled with a rectangular thin glass substrate with an SPR active metal layer has been described [7, 8].

[1]Institute of Nano Electronic Engineering (INEE), Universiti Malaysia Perlis, 01000 Kangar, Perlis, Malaysia
[2]School of Bioprocess Engineering, Universiti Malaysia Perlis, 02600 Arau, Perlis, Malaysia
[*]Corresponding author

SPR-based Autolab Esprit is an instrument with double channel and auto-sampler. It has an optional electrochemical cuvette that facilitates to measure on a three-electrode system such as a fixed contact point to the gold layer of the sensor disk (gold is working as electrode), replaceable Ag/AgCl reference electrode and fixed platinum counter electrode. The cuvette designed for the Autolab SPR is pre-eminently suitable to obtain the signal at equilibrium. In this system, injection of the solution directly to the sensor surface is possible by means of automatic, semi-automatic or manually due to open configuration of this system. This system has also provided static incubation with unlimited time for monitoring the analysis such as cell-free protein synthesis. Thus, Autolab Esprit system is one of the SPR systems ideal for label-free monitoring the biomolecular interactions in real time [9].

SPR-based waveguide sensor has designed with Kretschmann configuration, in which modifications in the dielectric environment near the sensing surfaces with a high sensitivity by measuring changes in reflectivity. Reflected spectra are measured by rotating the resonator with respect to the laser and recording the reflected signal intensity as a function of the angle of incidence. Shifts in this resonance are resulting from the changes in the local refractive index as a result of the adsorption of biomolecules [10, 11]. Nevertheless, the overall principle and the considerations concerning the waveguide design are strikingly similar to an SPR device, with the only difference being the mode used for the measurements is not a surface mode but a waveguide mode [12]. In the waveguide sensor device any kind of solid material that reflects light and optically isolates the waveguide from the substrate can be used as the reflecting layer. Silver and gold are the typical materials for the reflecting layer, since the use of these metals provides a good sensitivity [13].

The self-assembled monolayer of gold colloids on the glass substrate was used widely in several SPR-sensors. Based on this, the localized surface plasmon resonance (LSPR)-based optical biosensor is also currently of considerable interest in the fabrication and optical characterization of gold nanoparticles on solid supports. The changes in the complex dielectric function in the vicinity of the interface between the metal and the media cause the variations of the local environments experienced by metal nanoparticles. The LSPR spectra can be obtained on UV–Vis absorption spectrometer and the resonance condition on the local dielectric environment enables a molecular sensing. The binding of analyte to the biosensor surface causes a change in the absorbance which was responsive to the concentration of biomolecules attached. This LSPR sensing yields similar results to the SPR technique as much simpler instrument [14]. Advances in SPR based techniques for bioanalysis were overviewed by Phillips and Cheng [15]. Recently, collections of publications appeared in the literature with various applications of SPR including studies on G-protein receptor signaling [16], incorporation of a transmembrane protein into liposomes [17], membrane binding of antimicrobial peptides [18], studies on glycol-conjugates [19] and high-throughput analyses [20].

6.2 Biacore technology

Even though there are vast developments in the past with SPR principles, biacore technology is one of the well-established SPR, founded in 1984 by a Sweden-based company and for the biomolecular interactions their system was launched in 1990 and further expansion was performed in 1995 by launching different instrumental set-ups namely, BIAlite, Biacore 1000 and Biacore 3000. Automated biacore system was introduced in 1999 towards several applications. Presently, a well-established biacore model T100 is available with higher sensitive advanced features and for high-throughput analysis [1].

Biacore technology is used to identify the biomolecules assisted with its appropriate partner. In addition to identifying biomolecules, this system is also in use for drug discovery, finding the binding strength, protein screening and inhibiting assay, also to generate the high-affinity ligand from the nucleic acid library. Various kind of sensing surface and surface modification are formulated with the biacore system. Through the surface modification, the reduction of signal-to-noise ratio and ultimate improvement in the limit of detection was achieved for the bimolecular interactions. Biacore technology is also allowed monitoring weak macromolecular interactions that are not possible by other sensors. In this chapter, we discuss about the overall biacore system and their special features and applications for the binding analyses of the biomolecules.

6.3 Principle in biacore system

Biacore system operates based on SPR principle and designed to check the biomolecular interaction. When polarized light hit the prism, results total internal reflection of monochromatic or electromagnetic waves [1]. The reflectivity measurements can be done for biomolecular recognition with the changes in the local index of refraction upon adsorption of the target molecule to the metal surface. The surface plasmons on the sensing plate have a penetration depth of a few hundred nanometers, leads to the variations in the signal obtained as spectral changes indicate that the biomolecular interactions occurred at the interface. In the simplest case of an SPR measurement, a probe or so-called ligand is immobilized on the sensor surface previous to the measurement and then the analyte (binding partner) pass on it. Depends on the ligand and the analyte binding the total internal reflection will be changed. These changes can be plotted in the sensogram (Figures 6.1 and 6.2) and these changes help to find the binding affinity, binding strength and the kinetics of the biomolecules (Figure 6.3). These changes are suited to measure the differences in binding with real time response. There are different tailor-made sensing surfaces available commercially in chips formats for different biomolecular analyses (Figure 6.4a–f).

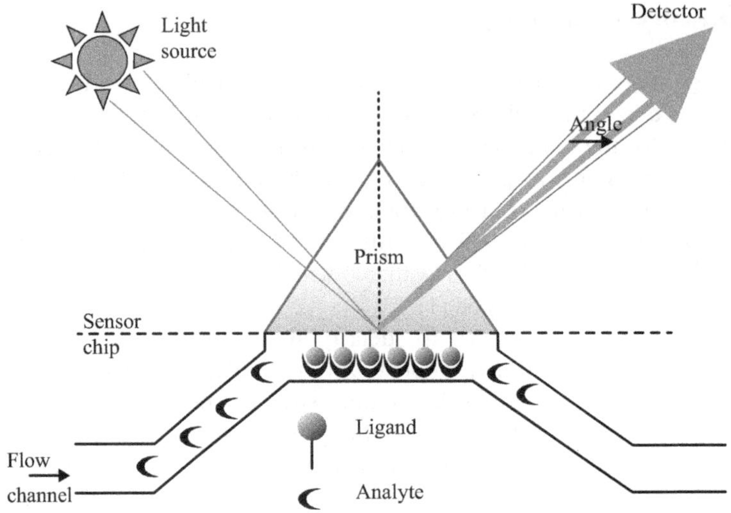

Figure 6.1 Set-up for biacore-based surface plasmon resonance. The angular changes will be detected by detector, to reflect the biomolecular interactions

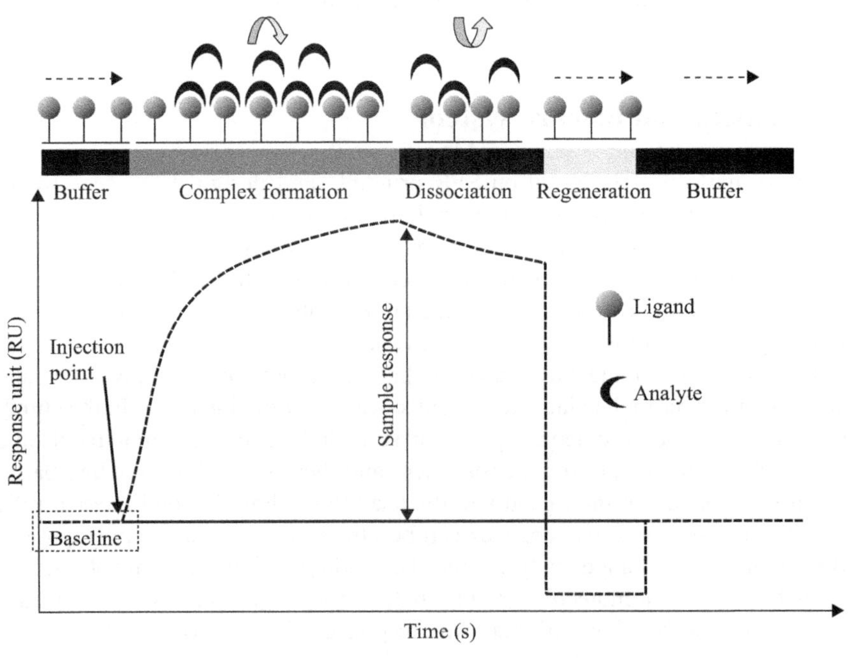

Figure 6.2 Association and dissociation process during biomolecular interactions on biacore. Injection point, responses and other processes are indicated

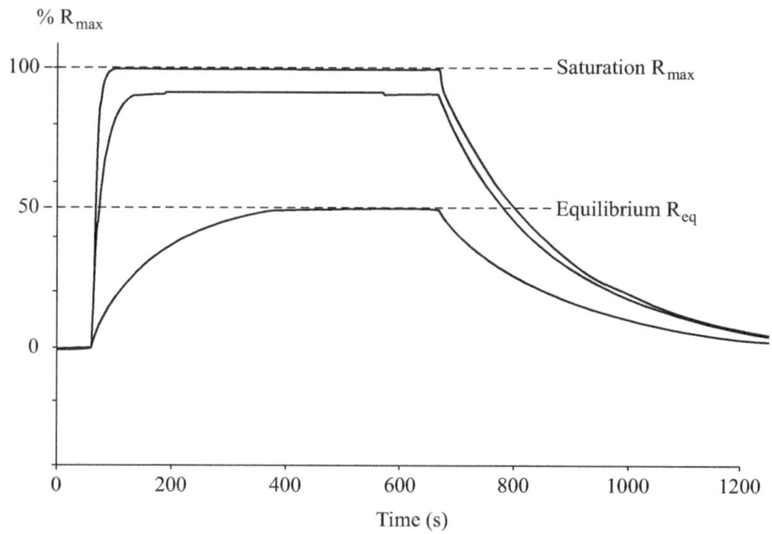

Figure 6.3 Kinetic analyses on biacore. Saturation (R_{max}) and equilibrium (R_{eq}) states are indicated

6.4 Biacore sensing surfaces

In biacore system generally gold coated glass chips are used to check and identify the biomolecules. These gold coated sensing surfaces from biacore are very stable under various conditions such as pH and organic solvents. On the gold surface, the appropriate chemical modifications have been made for the end-users. CM5 is the dextron coated gold chip and is used for wide range of biomolecular applications such as immobilization of antibody, peptide and oligonucleotides. CM4 chip is with lower carboxymethylation level than CM5 and is suitable to immobilize different molecules in terms of size compared to CM5. Similarly, CM3 chip has been coated with shorter dextron and used to immobilize the larger molecules on the sensing surface. Sensor chip has streptavidin immobilization with the dextron coated gold surface, is commonly used for the analyses of biotinylated ligands such as antibody and the oligonucleotides. Sensor chip L1 has the lipophilic modification on the dextron surface and it captures the liposomes. Sensor chip NTA is for the immobilization of the poly-histidine tagged ligands. Chip HPA is the flat hydrophilic surface to capture the lipid monolayers (Table 6.1; Figure 6.4a–f). Apart from the commercially available modified surface sensing chip, only plain gold is also very useful to researches to establish their own ideas and surface modification to improve their results. Many ways are followed to immobilize the ligand molecules on the gold surface such as through chemical linkers, or electrostatic attraction. For example, generally the COOH-terminated ligands on the sensing surface can capture the amine-ended molecules. On the other hand, molecules such as PEGylated ligand can immobilize on the Au surface via the electrostatic interaction.

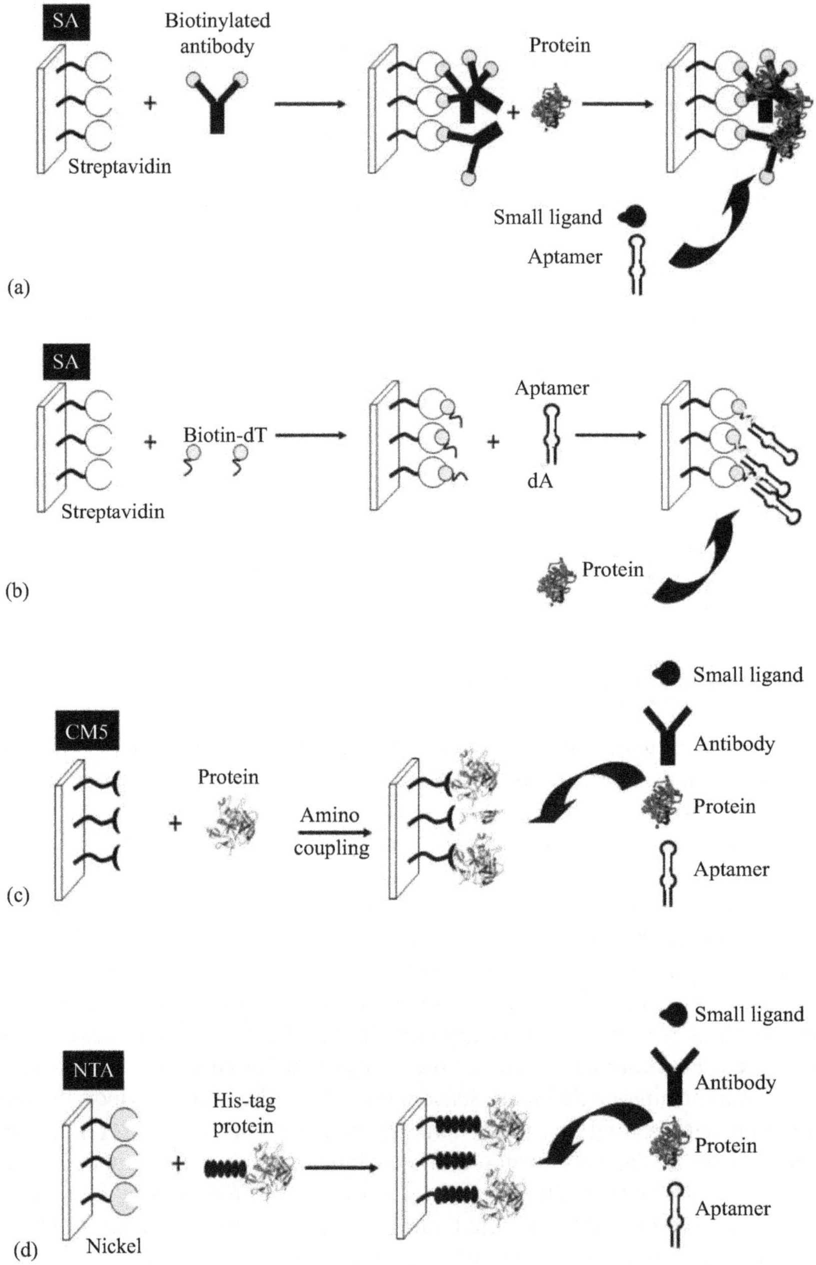

Figure 6.4 (*Continued*)

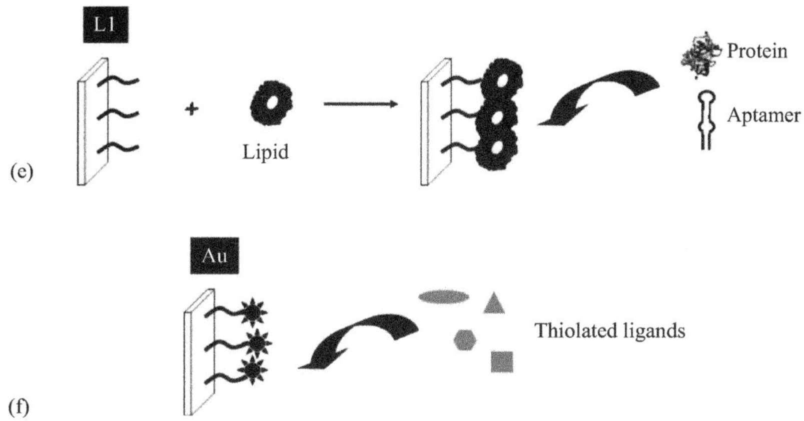

Figure 6.4 Different biomolecular interactions on biacore chips. Interactions of (a) antibody and antigen; further analyses on this surface with other biomolecules are indicated (b) aptamer and protein; (c) protein and biomolecules; (d) recombinant protein and biomolecules; (e) Lipid and biomolecules; (f) attachment of thiolated molecules on gold surface

Table 6.1 Commonly used Biacore chip-surfaces for bio-molecular interactions

Chip	**Surface**	**Ligands**	**Analytes**	**Figure**
SA	Carboxymethylated dextran	Pre-immobilized streptavidin	Biotinylated molecules	6.2a & b
CM3, CM4 & CM5	Carboxymethylated dextran	Ligands with $-NH_2$, $-SH$, $-CHO$, $-OH$ and $-COOH$	Suitable bio-molecules	6.2c
NTA	Carboxymethylated dextran	Pre-immobilized nitrilotriacetic acid	Histidine-tagged molecules	6.2d
L1 & HPA	Carboxymethylated dextran	Pre-immobilized with lipophilic groups	Liposomes, lipoglycans, Phospholipids	6.2e
Au	Gold	User-defined surface chemistries	Suitable bio-molecules	6.2f

6.5 Non-fouling on Biacore sensing surfaces

Even though successful modifications can be done on the sensing surface for bio-molecular interactions, non-fouling is one of the primary criteria in the sensing developments, which decides the quality of any given sensor. Blocking free areas on the sensing surface is important, because the sensitivity and limit of detection are highly improved with the suitable blocking materials. In the biacore sensing chip generally ethanolamine has been used as the blocking agent on carboxylated modified surfaces after attaches the probe. This blocking agent drastically reduce the bio-fouling in most cases. However, in some cases, example using serum samples, other suitable blocking agents must be used. Lakshmipriya *et al.*, [21] used Poly-ethylene glycol (PEG) as the blocking agent for the interactive analyses of human clotting factor IX and immunoglobulin-conjugated gold nanoparticles. They proved that the limit of detection was improved several fold with the assistance of PEG-based block polymers by the reduction in signal-to-noise ratio.

6.6 Biomolecular recognition in biacore system

Molecular identification, recognition and differentiation are the important applications in the fields such as medical, food and environmental. Especially, it is more important in the field of medical diagnosis to identify the diseases for early diagnosis. Biacore system fulfils these applications and effectively identified the diseases by the assistance of ligands such as antibody or aptamer or DNA or other molecules, which bind the appropriate analyte molecule [1, 22–29]. As shown in the Figure 6.4a–f, biacore system helps identifying the analyte molecule, which is in the solution state, against its suitable ligand molecule, which is previously immobilized on the sensing solid surfaces.

For example, Gopinath *et al.*, [27] have analyzed Aptamer–gD interactions using BIAcore T100 on a dextran-coated sensor chip. In this case, to determine the binding rate constants of the generated aptamers, with 24-mer poly(A) nucleotides at their 3′ ends, which could anneal to the complementary biotinylatedoligo (dT) [5′-Biotin-(T_{24})-3′] was used. For the analyses, initially, the biotinylatedoligo $(dT)_{24}$ was attached to the streptavidin by dissolving the oligo in binding buffer. The excess or unbound biotinylatedoligo was washed away with binding buffer at a flow rate of 20 μl/min for 10 min. To analyze the binding kinetics, 20 μl aptamer was injected (100 nM final concentration) at a flow rate of 2 μl/min for 10 min. This resulted in an increase of approximately 1200 RU upon aptamer binding to the complementary biotinylatedoligo. Single cycle kinetics were measured with five different concentrations of gD protein (10, 20, 40, 80 and 160 nM) by injecting the protein through both the experimental flow-cell (FC2) and the control flow-cell (FC1) with a flow rate of 30 μl/min and a total volume of 60 μl. The dissociation time was set for 2 min to obtain a smooth curve. Sensograms were corrected for non-specific binding by subtracting the aptamer attached curve (FC2) by the control curve (FC1), and the binding kinetics was evaluated. The sensor chip was then washed with a buffer solution, followed by the injection of a 10 mM NaOH solution to strip the aptamer from the biotinylated (dT) 24 before the next sample analysis.

6.7 Kinetic analyses

The most prominent benefit of direct detection using SPR biosensor technology is the determination of kinetics of (bio)molecular interactions. Biacore is associated with the evaluation biacore evaluation software, which fits with a 1:1 binding model. The interaction with the biomolecules can be calculated according to the equation $A + B = AB$ where A is the analyte and B is the ligand immobilized on the sensor surface. Reaction rate and equilibrium constants of interactions can be determined, e. g. the interaction $A + B = AB$ can be followed in real time with SPR technology. The association constant is the reaction rate of complex (AB) formation, giving the number of complexes formed per time at unit concentration of A and B. As soon as the complex AB is formed, its dissociation can commence. The dissociation rate constant describing this process expresses the number of AB complexes dissociating per unit time. The rate of association is used to measure from the forward reaction, and the dissociation rate can be measured from the reverse reaction.

The kd values depicting the ratio of the 'on' and 'off' rates of each aptamer were globally fitted for the five different concentrations using the Langmuir model assuming 1:1 ligand:analyte interaction. A good fit to the Langmuir model is used to decide based on the Chi^2 value. The Chi^2 is a statistical measure of closeness of experimental data to the theoretical mode used to determine the Kd, i.e. it describes how results agree with curve-fitting of the model used. Chi^2 values lower than the noise RU, indicate a good fit. The calculation can be done by injecting multiple concentrations of sample to be analyzed against the immobilized ligand (multiple cycle kinetics) and this process involves the repeated regeneration and attachment of analyte. However, in the recent version of Biacore T100 single cycle kinetics is possible by injecting consequent injection of multiple concentration of analyte against ligand without involving generation step. Gopinath *et al.* [26] have calculated both kd analyses and inhibition constant using in competition reactions. Similarly, Sekiya *et al.* [30] have also carried out the competition analysis with heparin for their RNA-aptamer and mouse prion protein interactions using biacore.

Exhaustive benchmark thermodynamic study using biacore technology was also achieved by several researchers as carried out by Navratilova *et al.* [31] Thermodynamics is a branch of physics that studies the effects of changes in temperature, pressure and volume on physical systems at the macroscopic scale by analyzing the collective motion of their particles using statistics. In short, heat means "energy in transit" and dynamics relates to "movement"; thus, in essence thermodynamics studies the movement of energy. Thermodynamics describes how systems respond to changes in their surroundings and it can be applied to a wide variety of topics in science and engineering.

6.8 Refunctioning and regeneration of chip surfaces

To generate the chip with no molecules, the attached surface molecules are generally regenerated with agents that have extreme ionic strength and pH. The

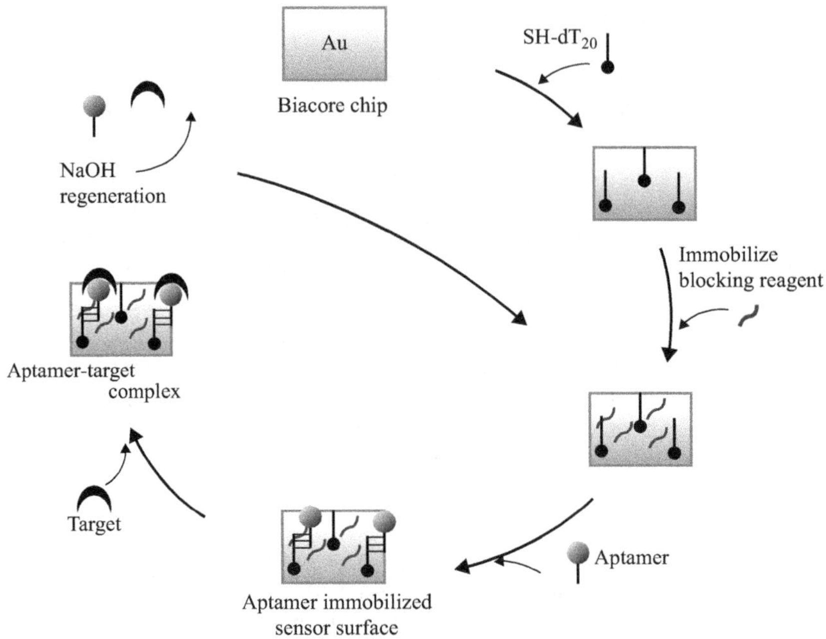

Figure 6.5 Regeneration process on biacore chip. Regeneration of aptamer is shown

following agents with extreme ionic strength are usually recommended by the manufacturer namely, Acetonitrile, DMSO, DTE, EDTA, Ethanol, Ethanolamine, Ethylene glycol, Formamide, Formic acid, Glycine pH 1.5–3.0, HCl, Imidazole, $MgCl_2$, NaOH, NaCl, SDS, Surfactant P20 and Urea. In Figure 6.5, the regeneration of aptamer attached on biotinylatedoligos by NaOH is shown. Regeneration of aptamer attachment is shown by the studies carried out by Gopinath *et al.* [22, 26] Chatelier *et al.* [32] have reconditioned and reused the biacore sensor research grade chips attached with covalently immobilized protein/peptide, by enzymatic and chemical treatment using Pronase E and Bromoacetic acid, respectively.

Even though, biacore chips are with choices of surfaces, these chips are relatively expensive. To reduce the cost by re-functionalizing the biacore chip's surface and to extend its lifetime especially for the application in resource-poor setting, Yuan *et al.*, [33] described a protocol to re-functionalize the biacore chips' surface for multiple times to analyze biomolecular interactions without interfering analysis from previously used surface or analytes. They have demonstrated how to strip-off the previously used biacore chips and re-functionalize the surface of the chip with streptavidin to measure biomolecular interactions, for example, RNA–protein interactions. Initially, a used biocore chip was collected and stripped-off all coated materials from the gold using piranha solution and re-functionalized the biacore chip as described earlier [33]. Their protocol permitted us to use safe and efficient regeneration of the commercial biacore chips. This is not only of great advantage to extend the lifetime of these chips but also makes them commercially more affordable, especially in a resource-poor setting. The time range for the entire protocol is ~1 day, including stripping off previously immobilized materials and re-functionalization of gold surface.

6.9 Recommendations for controlled experiments

With all the above conditions, to make the perfect analyses and genuine output in the biacore system, the following recommendations are usually considered.

1. Inclusion of surfactants in the flowing buffer will reduce the non-specific binding.
2. High-ionic strength will reduce the positive charged molecule interactions on especially net negative charged CM-series chips.
3. Use of salt like NaCl will reduce the non-specific electrostatic effects, drastically.
4. Performance of subtraction with background flow with flow-cell without ligand is highly recommended.
5. Chips can be re-used several times, better to keep them immersed in buffer solution when not in use.
6. Before starting the experiments, the baseline needs to be adjusted.
7. Filter and degas the buffers before use.
8. Optimization of pH to attach the ligand especially proteins.
9. Immobilization of high concentration of ligand to create maximum analyte binding.

6.10 Conclusions

With the above-mentioned set-ups, biaocre-based SPR technology has several appealing advantages which include reproducible results, stable baselines, low non-specific binding, high chemical stability, high sensitivity, regeneration and re-use, fast and convenient capture of biomolecules, surface stability in several conditions, series of binding steps can be performed compared with other analytical techniques, automatic sample handling, programmable for experimental performance without users' present, choice of ligand, label-free detection and real-time analysis. With these applications, biacore served for scientific community about two decades with several products by drastic improvements and expect for more advanced systems from to obtain comprehensive information.

References

[1] Gopinath, S.C.B. Biosensing applications of surface plasmon resonance-based Biacore technology. *Sens. Actuators B: Chem.* 2010; 150: 722–733.

[2] Tudos, A.J. and Schasfoort, R.B.M. Introduction to surface plasmon resonance. In. *Handbook of Surface Plasmon Resonance*. Schasfoort, R.B.M. and Tudos, A.J. (Eds.). Springer, United Kingdom, 2008; pp. 1–14.

[3] Kretschmann E. Die bestimmungoptischerkonstanten von metallendurchanregung von oberflachenplasmaschwingungen. *Z. Physik.* 1971; 241: 313–337.

[4] Jorgenson, R.C. and Yee, S.S. A fiber optic chemical sensor based on surface plasmon resonance. *Sens. Actuators B: Chem.* 1994; 12: 213–220.

[5] Ronot-Trioli, C., Trouillet, A., Veillas, C. and Gagnaire, H. Monochromatic excitation of surface plasmon resonance in an optical-fibre refractive-index sensor. *Sens. Actuators A Phys.* 1996; 54: 589–593.

[6] Vidal, M.M.B., Lopez, R., Aleggret, S., Alonso-Chamarro, J. and Garces, I. Determination of probable alcohol yield in musts by means of an SPR optical sensor. *J. Mateo. Sens. Actuators B*. 1993; 11: 455–459.

[7] Foster, M.W., Ferrel, D.J. and Lieberman, R.A. Surface plasmon resonance biosensor miniaturization. *Proc. SPIE.* 1994; 2293: 122–131.

[8] Homola, J., Yee, S.S. and Gauglitz, G. Surface plasmon resonance sensors: review. *Sens. Actuators B: Chem.* 1999; 54: 3–15.

[9] Kausaite, A., van Dijk, M., Castrop, J., *et al.* Surface plasmon resonance label-free monitoring of antibody antigen interactions in real time. *Biochem. Mol. Bio. Edu.* 2007; 35: 57–63.

[10] Gopinath, S.C.B., Awazu, K. and Fujimaki, M., *et al.* Influence of nanometric holes on the sensitivity of waveguide plasmon: a label-free nano-sensor to analyze RNA-aptamer ligand interactions. *Anal. Chem.* 2008; 80: 6602–6609.

[11] Gopinath, S.C.B., Awazu, K., Kumar, P.K.R. and Tominaga, J. Monitoring surface-assisted biomolecular assembly by means of evanescent-field-coupled waveguide-mode nanobiosensors. *Anal. Bioanal. Chem.* 2009; 394: 481–488.

[12] Fujimaki, M., Rockstuhl, C., Wang, X., *et al.* Biomolecular sensors utilizing waveguide modes excited by evanescent fields. *J. Microscopy.* 2008; 229: 320–326.

[13] Fujimaki, M., Rockstuhl, C., Wang, *et al.* Silica-based monolithic sensing plates for waveguide-mode sensors. *Optic. Exp.* 2008; 16: 6408–6416.

[14] Bi, N., Sun, Y., Tian, Y., *et al.* Analysis of immunoreaction with localized surface plasmon resonance biosensor. *Spectrochimica Acta Part A.* 2010; 75: 1163–1167.

[15] Phillips, K.S. and Cheng, Q. Recent advances in surface plasmon resonance based techniques for bioanalysis. *Anal. Bioanal. Chem.* 2007; 387: 1831–1840.

[16] Komolov, K.E. and Koch, K.W. Application of surface plasmon resonance spectroscopy to study G-protein coupled receptor signalling. *Methods Mol. Biol.* 2010; 627: 249–260.

[17] Granéli, A. Incorporation of a transmembrane protein into a supported 3D-matrix of liposomes for SPR studies. *Methods Mol. Biol.* 2010; 627: 237–248.

[18] Hall, K. and Aguilar, M.I. Surface plasmon resonance spectroscopy for studying the membrane binding of antimicrobial peptides. *Methods Mol. Biol.* 2010; 627: 213–223.

[19] Duverger, E. Lamerant-Fayel, N. Frison, N. Monsigny, M. Carbohydrate-lectin interactions assayed by SPR. *Methods Mol. Biol.* 2010; 627: 157–178.

[20] Takeda, H., Goshima, N. and Nomura, N. High-throughput kinase assay based on surface plasmon resonance,. *Methods Mol. Biol.* 2010; 627: 131–145.

[21] Lakshmipriya, T., Horiguchi, Y. and Nagasaki, Y. Co-immobilized poly (ethylene glycol)-block-polyamines promotes sensitivity and non-biofouling on gold sensor surface for detection of Factor IX in human plasma. *Analyst.* 2014; 139: 3977–3985.

[22] Gopinath, S.C.B., Balasundaresan, D., Akitomi, J. and Mizuno, H. An RNA aptamer that discriminates bovine factor IX from human factor IX. *J. Biochem.* 2006; 140: 667–676.

[23] Gopinath, S.C.B., Shikamoto, Y., Mizuno, H. and Kumar, P.K.R. A potent anti-coagulant RNA aptamer inhibits blood coagulation by blocking specifically an extrinsic clotting pathway. *Thromb. Haemos.* 2006; 95: 767–771.

[24] Gopinath, S.C.B., Sakamaki, Y., Kawasaki, K. and Kumar, P.K.R. An efficient RNA aptamer against human influenza B virus hemagglutinin. *J. Biochem.* 2006; 139: 837–846.

[25] Gopinath, S.C.B., Misono, T., Mizuno, T., Kawasaki, K. and Kumar, P.K.R. An RNA aptamer that distinguishes between closely related human influenza viruses and inhibits hemagglutinin-mediated membrane fusion. *J. Gen. Virol.* 2006; 87: 479–487.

[26] Gopinath, S.C.B., Shikamoto, Y., Mizuno, H. and Kumar, P.K.R. Snake venom-derived factor IX binding protein specifically blocks the Gla domain-mediated-membrane binding of human factors IX and X. *Biochem. J.* 2007; 405: 351–357.

[27] Gopinath, S.C.B., Hayashi, K. and Kumar, P.K.R. Aptamer that binds to the gD protein of herpes simplex virus-1 and efficiently inhibits viral entry. *J. Virol.* 2012; 86: 6732–6744.

[28] Gopinath, S.C.B. and Kumar, P.K.R. Biomolecular discrimination by Surface Plasmon Resonance. *Analyst.* 2014; 139: 2678–2682.

[29] Gopinath, S.C.B., Hayashi, K., Lee, J., *et al.* Analyses of compounds that interfere the herpes simplex virus-host receptor interactions using surface plasmon resonance. *Anal. Chem.* 2013; 85: 10455–10462.

[30] Sekiya, S., Noda, K., Nishikawa, F., Yokoyama, T., Kumar, P.K.R. and Nishikawa, S. Characterization and application of a novel RNA aptamer against the mouse prion protein. *J. Biochem.* 2006; 139: 383–390.

[31] Navratilova, I., Papalia, G.A., Rich, R.L., *et al.*, Biosensor-surface plasmon resonance: quantitative analysis of small molecule-nucleic acid interactions. *Methods.* 2007; 42: 150–161.

[32] Chatelier, R.C., Gengenback, T.R., Griesser, H.J., Brigham-Burke, M. and O'Shannessy, D.J. A general method to recondition and reuse Biacore sensor chips fouled with covalently immobilized protein/peptide. *Anal. Biochem.* 1995; 229: 112–118.

[33] Yuan, Y., Gopinath, S.C.B. and Kumar, P.K.R. Regeneration of commercial Biacore chips to analyze biomolecular interactions. *Opt. Engg.* 2011; 50: 034402–1–6.

Chapter 7

Implantable microbiosensors: towards *in vivo* monitoring

Chian Chee Hoe[1] and Zhiqiang Gao[1]

7.1 Introduction

The miniaturisation of biosensors – microbiosensors has definite advantages over conventional biosensors [1–5]. For example, minute amounts of sample are needed for successful tests; implantation of the microbiosensors is feasible and consequently enables *in vivo* monitoring in real-time. Also, various microbiosensors could be integrated to construct multifunctional microbiosensor assays [6]. For continuous real time *in vivo* measurements, other than small size, the microbiosensors should be useful for easy placement within a blood vessel (i.e. artery for blood gases/pH; vein for glucose/lactate) or under the skin in subcutaneous space (mainly for glucose) and exhibit long-term stability. They should not leach any toxic substances into the wearer and provide reliable results that are comparable with *in vitro* tests [1, 7–9], but a few processes can lead to wrong analytical results for implanted biosensors. Biofouling is one of these processes and it consists of the build-up of proteins, cells and other biological materials on the surface of the implanted biosensor. Proteins rapidly adsorb onto the surface of biosensor immediately after it is implanted. The adsorption of proteins to solid surfaces often changes the proteins' shape, which often leads to denaturation of the proteins and the formation of a gel-like layer of denatured proteins. This gel-like layer is responsible for a number of damaging processes referred to as membrane biofouling, fibrous encapsulation and membrane biodegradation, which ultimately result in biosensor failure *in vivo* [10]. The deposition of active cells on the surface of the implanted biosensor also severely affects oxygen concentration in the implantation site, thus leading to significant errors in the response of the implanted biosensor [11]. Discrepancies can also be observed when blood flow fluctuates in the blood vessel where the biosensor is implanted, or when the implanted biosensor contacts with the wall of the blood vessels where inherent metabolism of endothelial cells can affect the performance of the biosensor in the identical way as

[1]Department of Chemistry, National University of Singapore, Singapore 117543

adhered blood cells (wall effect) [12]. Furthermore, thrombus formation in patients can occur randomly since it depends on factors such as the inherent coagulation tendency of a particular patient and the velocity of blood flow within the lumen of the vessel in which the biosensor is implanted. The unpredictability of the performance of the implanted biosensor especially intravascular due to these biological factors makes the measurements unreliable, thus forestalling therapeutics aid. These issues are less common when implanting biosensors within much larger blood vessels, for example the pulmonary artery, where greater blood flow and the wider vessel diameter reduce the probability for these problems. Research into areas of biosensors indwelling in the vascular bed is less popular. These intravascular biosensors are less attractive mainly because they require surgery to implant and explant. It will be very troublesome if a biosensor malfunctions and has to be extracted. The invasive, complicated implantation procedure also limits the appeal of this location for implantation [13]. In contrast, microbiosensors implanted under the skin (subcutaneous measurements), like those developed for monitoring glucose levels, do not experience the same issues of platelet activation and thrombus formation. However such biosensors are subjected to their own problems such as biocompatibility issues, primarily from inflammatory responses that can affect their accuracy. Most of the biosensors implanted in the subcutaneous tissue are 0.05–5.0 mm in diameter. Implantation is usually done by using a guide cannula. The process of inserting the biosensors will cause some minor damage to the surrounding tissue like breaking of capillaries. Only 5 min is required for changes in blood glucose concentration to be reflected in the subcutaneous tissue [14] and there is minimal chance of life-threatening reactions, such as thrombosis with subcutaneously implanted biosensors [15]. There are a few sources of failure or lack of success of subcutaneously implanted biosensors. The first is again the passive loss of sensitivity resulting from uptake of relatively low molecular weight (<15 kDa) species such as lipids, protein fragments and a variety of small endogenous molecules on or into the biosensor. This process is relatively fast and has generally been referred to as the "run-in" time, which only lasts 2–4 h. Also, the biosensor membrane needs time to be hydrated and for the establishment of required mass transfer balance in the local environment before steady operation can be accomplished [16]. The second source of failure is the disturbance of oxygen and target analyte levels in the tissue surrounding the biosensor resulting from injury of tissue and the ensuing acute inflammatory response as mentioned earlier. Nonetheless, the duration of the acute inflammatory response, comprising several distinct processes, is relatively short. First, a blood clot, mainly made of fibrin, is formed to close the wound. Then, blood and tissue proteins such as cytokines and growth factors are released and leukocytes adhere to the endothelium of the blood vessels and permeate through the injured site, these are mostly neutrophils. Monocytes are finally mobilised to the injured site and these differentiate into macrophages. These phagocytic cells act to remove foreign materials like bacteria and dead cells to clean up the wound site. This acute inflammation response commonly causes biosensor instability over the first 48 h but can result in clean-up of the small amount of capillary blood that may have accumulated. A number of clinical trials have suggested that subcutaneously implanted biosensors can function accurately up to two weeks if they survive the initial days [17]. For long-term subcutaneous implantation, two other issues can ensure. There could be a total loss of enzymatic activity that will inevitably affect the response of the implanted biosensor. In addition, the capsule formation caused by the foreign body reaction may eventually block the access of the analyte and oxygen to the biosensor.

7.2 Microbiosensor technologies

Going by the different transducing devices used in implantable microbiosensors, implantable microbiosensors can be classified as electrochemical and optical. The latter presents the chance to continuously monitor different substances with fast response, low cost and high reliability [18–21]. On the other hand, due to the simplicity of producing an electrochemical microbiosensor and its ease of operation in the continuous mode, electrochemical transduction has been widely considered as the most suitable type of transduction for producing *in vivo* biosensors. Implantable electrochemical microbiosensors can be classified into three types based on the mechanisms that govern their operation; they are potentiometric, conductometric and voltammetric. The potentiometric biosensors rely on the measurement of the potential difference between two electrodes, one indicator electrode (the microbiosensor) and one reference electrode at equilibrium of the electrochemical cell. The potential of the indicator electrode varies with the activity or concentration of the analyte. That potential is measured with respect to the reference electrode. The change in the potential is directly related to the concentration in a logarithmic way. For example, Mataveli and colleagues constructed a potentiometric microbiosensor for the detection of adrenaline [22]. In their work, the biological recognition element employed for the biosensor is a polyphenol oxidase. The biosensor and the reference electrode were inserted in the jugular veins of the rats (Wistar). The concentration of adrenaline that they injected was calculated as 1.23 μM. After three injections with the same adrenaline concentration, the biosensor responses were 20.5, 9.47 and 4.87 mV, respectively. The calculated adrenaline concentrations, using the equation of matrix-matching calibration curve, were 8.63, 2.49 and 1.48 μM for the three consecutive injections, respectively. The different values obtained for the same quantity of adrenaline injected are most likely due to the metabolism of the rats. Generally, adrenaline is completely eliminated from the blood after 10 min of an intravenous injection. The reason the signal response decrease, according to them, is due to the interval between the injections was about 6 min and after the second injection the receptors were already activated and consequently the adrenaline metabolism rate has increased. Considering the complexity of the sample, the results are deem encouraging.

Applications of conductometric microbiosensors are limited due to the variable ionic background of clinical samples and the requirement to measure small conductivity changes under a high ionic strength. Nevertheless, one commercial system for the measurement of urea in serum, plasma and urine is a BUN analyser (Beckman–Coulter) [23]. In addition, Lee *et al.* reported a conductometric glucose microbiosensor using layer-by-layer assembled single-walled carbon nanotubes (SWNTs) and glucose oxidase (GOx) onto a planar substrate electrode [24]. Protons passing through the SWNT multilayer greatly affect the electronic conductance of the SWNTs. Based on the conductance change caused by protons, glucose concentration can be determined by the local pH changes caused by the oxidation of glucose catalysed by GOx. At a bias voltage of 0.6 V, the overall sensitivity and the resolution of the conductometric biosensor were 10.8 and 1.0 pM, respectively. This planar biosensor is beneficial since it can be utilised for continuous monitoring using the simplicity of the electronic detection and are low-cost due to the possibility of mass production. More importantly, it can be incorporated into implantable devices for possible *in vivo* applications.

Implantable amperometric microbiosensors continue as the dominant *in vivo* format for the detection, monitoring and reporting of bioanalytes. Amperometry is an electrochemical technique usually used in the commercial implantable microbiosensors. Amperometric microbiosensors are more sensitive and more suited for mass production than their potentiometric counterparts [25]. Consequently, a large number of implantable glucose microbiosensors, based on different designs, materials and membrane coatings have been developed over the past 30 years. The first demonstration of such biosensors for *in vivo* glucose monitoring was reported by Shichiri *et al.,* in 1982 [26]. His group developed a needle-type glucose biosensor which relied on a platinum anode held at +0.6 V (vs a silver electrode) to monitor the hydrogen peroxide produced enzymatically during the oxidation of glucose. The enzyme (GOx) was immobilised in a bovine serum albumin matrix with a cellulose-diacetate/heparin/polyurethane coating (Figure 7.1). The coating was used to widen the dynamic range of the biosensor. The majority of glucose biosensors used for *in vivo* applications are based on the GOx-catalysed oxidation of glucose by oxygen owing to concerns about potential leaching of mediators [27]. The needle-type glucose biosensor was tested in panrea-tectomised dogs and the implantable device produced excellent control of blood glucose for up to seven days.

Most of the biomolecules that can be detected and measured in the body (biomarkers) are not electroactive, glucose being the commonest example. The enzymes that are included in the biosensors can allow the binding of the electro-inactive species of interest and catalyse their oxidation or reduction to produce electroactive products for example hydrogen peroxide in the case of glucose. Based on the fabrication method, enzyme-based electrochemical biosensors can be categorised into first-generation, second-generation and third-generation biosensors [28, 29]. The first-generation glucose biosensors relay on the use of oxygen as substrate and they detect either oxygen or hydrogen peroxide produced. One advantage of this type of biosensors is that measuring of hydrogen peroxide formation is much simpler, specifically when the implantable biosensors are very small [30]. However, a predominant issue of the first-generation biosensors is their low selectivity since the amperometric measurement of hydrogen peroxide requires high operating potentials, thereby being susceptible to interferences from

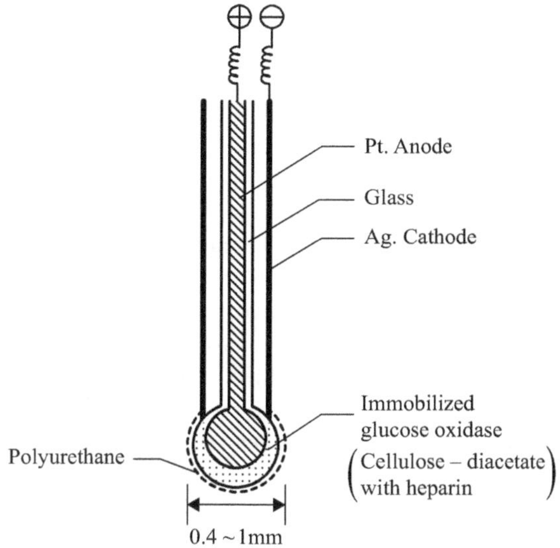

Figure 7.1 One of the first needle type glucose biosensors. Reproduced with permission from Reference 26

co-existing electroactive species [31]. From the late 1980s till now, extensive efforts were dedicated to eliminate the interference from co-existing electroactive species, such as uric acid, ascorbic acid, dopamine and certain drugs [32, 33]. Another problem lies in the fact that if the oxygen concentration is to be monitored, it is not easy to reproduce the results due to the variation in oxygen content in biological fluids, known as the 'oxygen deficit'.

The use of artificial redox mediators was introduced for the second-generation biosensors in order to fabricate biosensors which operate at moderate potentials. The improvements were realised by replacing oxygen with artificial electron acceptors, namely redox mediators. These redox mediators are able to ferry electrons from the enzyme to the surface of the substrate electrode [31]. Consequently, the mediators are reduced and they are re-oxidised electrochemically at the electrode, thus producing an amperometric signal and the oxidised form of the mediators are regenerated [34]. The enzymes that are to be used for the detection of the analyte of interest must be able to donate or accept electrons to or from the electrochemically active redox mediators. The redox mediators should also be rather specific for the electron transfer pathway between the biological recognition element and the electrode surface. There should not be a difference in potential of less than $\Delta E \sim 50$ mV between the different cofactors and the artificial redox mediators as this allow for the tuning of the desired operating potential. The redox mediators are required to be able to be immobilised on the electrode surface and/or the enzymes. Although hard to fulfil, especially in biological implanted systems, the redox mediators should not be toxic. The affinity of the enzymes for the specific redox mediators also has considerable impact on the performance of the biosensors.

One of the most fundamental disadvantages of using either the natural (first-generation) or an artificial (second-generation) free diffusing redox mediators in implantable biosensors design is the need for the availability of sufficient natural (e.g. oxygen) or artificial mediators to the active site of the enzymes and later at the electrode surface in order to achieve a detectable current signal. Furthermore, these artificial redox mediators must be securely fixed within the biosensors to prevent leakage as well as to provide biosensor stability [35]. It is important to note that not all redox mediators are biocompatible. Tetrathialfulvalene (TTF), ferricyanide, quinines, thionine, tetracyanoquinodimethane (TCNQ) and ferrocene were commonly used as the artificial redox mediators. Amongst them, ferrocene appears to be one of the most suitable redox mediators because it does not react with oxygen, stable in both the oxidised and reduced forms, independent of pH and react fast with enzymes [36].

The third-generation biosensors are reagentless and they operate on direct electron transfer between the enzyme and the electrode without the use of any redox mediators. These biosensors are basically still being researched on [31, 37]. The absence of the mediators provides the biosensors with superior selectivity in the sense that they could function in a potential window closer to the redox potential of the enzyme itself and therefore less susceptible to interfering species. This also signifies the removal of one additional reagent in the biosensors. For example, with their high surface area, excellent mechanical properties, excellent chemical stability and high electrical conductivity, graphene and carbon nanotubes (CNTs) are now extensively being exploited in the construction of third-generation micro- and nanobiosensors [38, 39]. Moreover, covalent functionalisation of graphene and CNTs further modulates their chemical and electronic properties of CNTs while offering the possibility of covalent conjugation to proteins [40] and allowing graphene and CNTs to behave both as an immobilisation matrix and as a redox mediator or electrocatalyst at the same time [41]. Conducting organic salts, such as TTF-TCNQ, are also known to mediate the redox reaction of flavoproteins, GOx for example, in addition to pyrrole-quinolinequinone enzymes (GDH-PQQ). However, for the continual development of the third-generation biosensors, we need to overcome the demanding challenge to the successful realisation of direct electron transfer between the enzyme and the electrode. Also, only a few enzymes including peroxidases have been shown to be able to directly exchange electrons with the electrode [42].

Several other approaches on the direct electron transfer of electrons from enzyme to the electrode have been developed in the past few years. For instance, Palmisano *et al.* reported a reagentless, third-generation glucose biosensor that is essentially oxygen- and interference-free. Such reagentless features are made possible through the synthesis of TTF-TCNQ onto an anti-interference layer of non-conducting over-oxidised poly(pyrrole) $(PPy)_{ox}$ film (Figure 7.2). The devised procedure has the potential to be adapted to mass-scale production and onward for *in vivo* experimentation. Based on a combination of adsorption and cross-linking of recently discovered cellobiose dehydrogenase from the ascomycete Corynascus thermophiles onto commercially available screen-printed electrodes, Zafar and

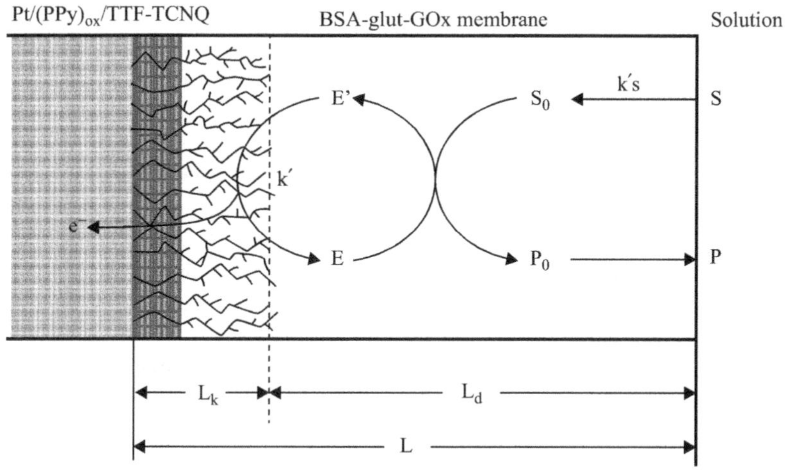

Figure 7.2 Schematic representation of processes involved in a Pt/(PPy)ox/TTF-TCNQ/BSA-glut-GOx enzyme electrode. S, P: substrate and product, respectively. E, E': oxidised and reduced form of the enzyme, respectively. Reproduced with permission from Reference 37

co-workers developed a third-generation glucose biosensor by simple modification of the screen-printed electrodes with CNTs [43]. Its low detection limit, a relatively wide dynamic range, high selectivity and stability bestow this third-generation glucose biosensor good potential to be applied for both *in vitro* and *in vivo* glucose monitoring. By making a nanoporous working electrode via the deposition of platinum nanoparticles, a needle-type implantable electrochemical glucose biosensor with great *in vivo* sensitivity was recently reported. Short-term *in vivo* tests showed that this biosensor can reproducibly track glycemic events despite the large background currents commonly encountered during animal testing. They were also focused on evaluating the long-term *in vivo* (one month) performance of this biosensor. With the variety of nanomaterials growing, their potential applicability in this third generation of electrochemical biosensors will also do the same.

7.3 Analyte-specific biosensors

Lactate (lactic acid, $pK_a = 3.86$) is an important biomarker/metabolite to sports and healthcare professionals because of its significance in several conditions including lactic acidosis, heart failure, severe infections, alcohol addiction, liver disease, ketoacidosis, severe dehydration, hemorrhage and shock [44]. Lactate levels provide data on anaerobic threshold which is very important for accommodating training programs in sports. For example, Spehar-Deleze *et al.* reported an implantable amperometric lactate microbiosensor for minimally invasive continuous *in vivo* monitoring. It was based on a small and easy to insert needle-typed system where a sensing platinum wire was inserted into a stainless steel tube that works as a linked counter and reference electrode [45]. An enzyme layer was introduced between two polymer membranes which allow high selectivity, a wide dynamic range and good biocompatibility. The biosensors had been fully evaluated *in vitro* and tested *in vivo* in rats. The measured values of tissue lactate obtained with their biosensor were compared with lactate levels measured in blood by the commercial LactatePro analyser. Although the collected concentrations were in the same range, no clear correlation between blood and tissue values was found. Cold sterilisation by gamma radiation, necessary for human studies, is currently being investigated. Their work will provide critical information on lactate levels in different physiological compartments and increase our understanding of physiological processes related to endurance sports [45].

Being the major excitatory neurotransmitter in the brain of mammals, Glutamate, an amino acid, plays an instrumental role in neurotransmission and neurotoxicity and is also involved in several neurological disorders such as epilepsy, Parkinson's disease and Alzheimer's disease. Qin *et al.* reported that the second-generation biosensors have relatively low reproducibility and low sensitivity [46]. Additionally, the design of the first-generation biosensors is more robust than the second generation that uses carbon fibres as substrate electrodes. As mentioned earlier, the detection of hydrogen peroxide requires a relatively high oxidation potential; this will cause other electroactive species like dopamine and ascorbic acid to be also oxidised. This is a big problem since the glutamate microbiosensor will eventually be used to monitor glutamate levels from extracellular fluid in brain areas rich in such potential interfering species. Several different approaches have been employed to overcome this problem but so far none of them are very effective [47, 48]. Wahono and colleagues reported on a needle-type glutamate microbiosensor (25 μm in diameter) constructed with a newly designed silica-based platinum electrode [49]. They first tested the membranes with the highest sensitivity for hydrogen peroxide *in vitro* and possessing the best selectivity against interferants. Then they assessed the performance of these membranes in short lasting (3–4 h) *in vivo* experiments. Later, it was observed that the biosensor protected by a poly(m-phenylenediamine) membrane deposited onto the platinum electrode has the best *in vitro* performance. Still, evaluation of these membranes after implantation showed poor selectivity against dopamine. Finally, they studied the ability of their biosensors to assess the effect of glutamate transport blocker DL-TBOA on modulating glutamate concentration in the prefrontal cortex of anaesthetised rats. The biosensors displayed a rapid 35-fold surge in extracellular glutamate after the introduction of DL-TBOA.

Dopamine is one of the most important catecholamines and is classified as a biological group of excitatory chemical neurotransmitters. It plays a critical role in the working of the central nervous, cardiovascular and hormonal systems. Low levels of dopamine in living bodies can result in several fatal diseases, such as Parkinson's and Alzheimer's diseases [50]. Quantification of dopamine is normally achieved using *in vivo* microdialysis to sample dopamine in the extracellular space followed by either electrochemical, coulometric or fluorescence detection of dopamine in the dialysate [51]. Unfortunately, microdialysis is rather time consuming and dopamine fluctuations can only be assessed on a time scale of tens of minutes to hours. Thus, dopamine quantification through *in vivo* microdialysis is not suitable for *in vivo* monitoring because dopamine levels are known to vary within fractions of seconds [52]. On the other hand, dopamine is electroactive which can be detected electrochemically with a microelectrode. However, direct electrochemical detection of dopamine suffers from limitations such as the need for background subtraction and electrode passivation. The oxidation potential for dopamine is between 0.3 and 0.6 V which is unfavourably high so that a number of electroactive substances, such as other catecholamine neurotransmitters, ascorbic acid and nitric oxide in the central nervous system, can also be oxidised, thus causing severe interference. Therefore, it is difficult to discriminate dopamine from those interfering substances [53]. Njagi *et al.* reported a tyrosinase-based implantable microbiosensor for dopamine [54]. It was demonstrated that the microbiosensor is relevant to make real-time *in vivo* monitoring of dopamine in the brain of anaesthetised rats. The microbiosensor is made up of a carbon fibre microelectrode coated with a biocatalytic layer containing tyrosinase planted in a chitosan biopolymer matrix and a mixture of cerium oxide/titanium oxide (CeO_2/TiO_2) (Figure 7.3). In the absence of CeO_2/TiO_2, very low oxidation currents of dopamine were obtained with the tyrosinase microbiosensor. Compared to the fast scan cyclic voltammetry commonly used for *in vivo* measurements of dopamine, the tyrosinase-based

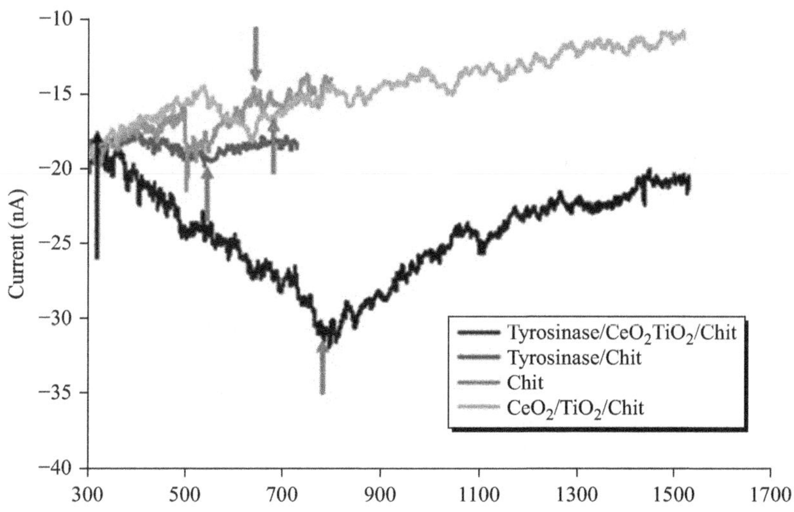

Figure 7.3 Amperometric responses of the tyrosinase-based microbiosensor in the absence and presence of the metal oxides and of the control electrode in the absence of enzyme to dopamine during electrical stimulation of the median forebrain bundle. The black arrow shows the onset of the electrical stimulation and the grey arrows indicate when stimulation was stopped. Reproduced with permission from Reference 54

biosensor offered several advantages like minimised electrode passivation due to the enzymatic/electrochemical cycling of the o-dopaquinone at the electrode surface, a relatively low operating potential and a low detection limit. The low operating potential effectively eliminated many common interferences found in brain fluids. Furthermore, this microbiosensor did not contain any other coating membranes and the materials used are biocompatible, making it an attractive candidate for uses in *in vivo* monitoring of dopamine.

Nitric oxide (NO) is an important signal transduction molecule involved in physiological functions such as blood pressure control, neurotransmission and constant monitoring of the immune system towards microorganisms, foreign tissue and diseases caused by altered cells, especially cancer cells. Excess amount of NO has been shown to cause some diseases [55]. NO is especially difficult to detect because of its low concentration, short half-time, low stability and high reactivity with reactive oxygen species present in biological systems [56]. NO is also naturally occurring metabolite released by nearly every type of cell in the body, including inflammatory cells. It is able to prevent platelet adhesion and thrombosis and also in wound healing [57]. Koh *et al.* recently reported the fabrication of a NO microbiosensor based on cytochrome c, a hemeprotein, immobilised onto nano-structured conducting polymer layers for *in vivo* monitoring of NO release stimulated by cocaine [58]. It was reported that Nafion coatings can effectively eliminate the interferences from oxygen, superoxide and hydrogen peroxide. The response time of this microbiosensor was less than 15 s. Thus, it is well suited to measure the extracellular fluctuation of NO in biological systems in real-time (Figure 7.4). Indeed, this microbiosensor was successfully implanted into the rat striatum and the basal NO concentration was determined to be 92 ± 5 nM. The microbiosensor efficiently detected the increased levels of extracellular NO in the striatum due to repeated injections of cocaine for seven days. In this aspect, the NO microbiosensor is an attractive platform to monitor extracellular NO levels in response to stimulant drug exposure.

Oxidative stress is caused by potent oxidising which are known as reactive oxygen species, such as hydrogen peroxide, superoxide anion, singlet oxygen and hydroxyl radical, and is associated with a number of diseases including inflammatory diseases, ischemic-reperfusion injury, atherosclerosis, cancer and aging [59]. Reactive oxygen species, on one hand, defend the body against viral or bacterial attack, but can, on the other hand, lead to oxidative damage of proteins, DNA and lipid peroxidation [60]. Real-time detection of reactive oxygen species is an analytical challenge because of its low concentration, high reactivity and short life-time. In addition, reactive oxygen species, once produced, are quickly attacked by other active biomolecules [61] and scavenged by superoxide dismutases (SODs) or antioxidants. Looking at one of the main reactive oxygen species superoxide anion, it would seems again that electrochemical method would offer a facile route to *in vivo* monitoring of unstable superoxide anion because of its high sensitivity. However first-generation biosensors could not differentiate the H_2O_2 generated from SOD-catalysed superoxide anion dismutation reaction from those that are present in biological tissues and thus may not be suitable for practical *in vivo* detection of

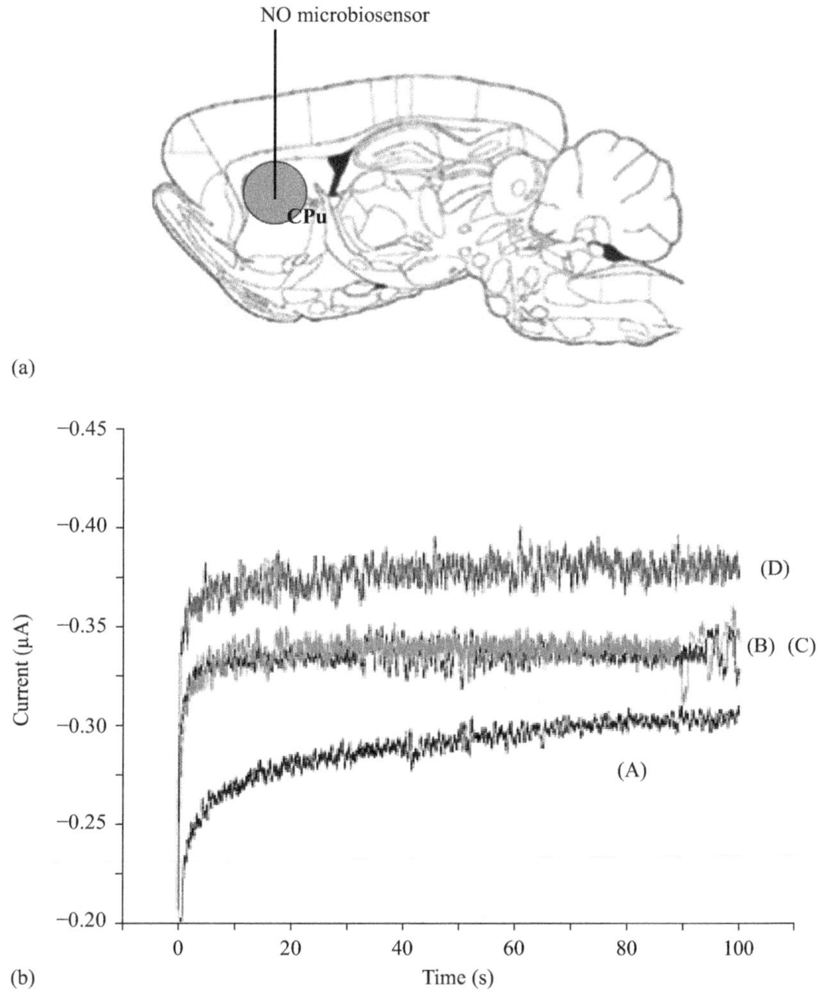

Figure 7.4 (a) Microbiosensor placement on a coronal section of rat brain. The microbiosensor was placed unilaterally into the centre of right dorsal striatum. CPu: caudate putamen (dorsal striatum). (b) In vivo amperometric responses recorded with a null (A) and cyt c/poly-TTCA microbiosensor in the saline (B), acute (C) or seven days repeated cocaine (D) injected rat dorsal striatum. Reproduced with permission from Reference 58

superoxide anion [62]. Ganesana *et al.* reported the use of cytochrome c (Cyt c) in the preparation of a miniaturised electrochemical biosensor for superoxide anion and experiments on real-time monitoring of the production and inactivation of superoxide anion by natural and engineered antioxidants in acutely prepared brain slices from mice [63]. Superoxide anion produced from the hippocampal region of the brain in

400-mm-thick sections were well within the range of detection of the electrode. When the slices were exposed to ischemic (decreased blood supply) conditions the superoxide anion production was increased by 200 per cent. In addition, measurements from the slices were stable over a 3–4-h period. Exogenous addition of SOD also lead to a decrease of the superoxide anion, this shows that the electrode is very specific in its sensing. This study demonstrated that electrochemical biosensors are promising for studying real-time dynamics of reactive oxygen species in a biological model.

It is now understandable that simultaneously monitoring several analytes continuously is vital. In one of the early studies, the correlation between ascorbate and glutamate was identified [64]. One area where monitoring of multiple analytes is useful is in neuroscience, where there is a growing interest in *in vivo* continuous and simultaneous monitoring of metabolism-related biomarkers, like glucose, lactate and pyruvate. Simultaneous monitoring of glucose and lactate has already been successfully described, even coupled to a telemetric device [65]. However, the device did not allow the necessary spatial resolution needed for monitoring in a discrete brain area. Cordeiro *et al.* developed a microbiosensor array for *in vivo* real-time simultaneous monitoring of the three major biomarkers in brain energy metabolism (Figure 7.5) [66]. The microbiosensor array was implanted in the medial prefrontal cortex of an anaesthetised adult male Wistar rat for *in vivo* evaluation. After an equilibration period, baseline brain levels of glucose (1.37 $\pm$ 0.2 mM), lactate (1.57 $\pm$ 0.4 mM) and pyruvate (0.37 $\pm$ 0.1 mM) were established.

The implantable microbiosensor array was able to measure the basal levels of glucose, lactate and pyruvate simultaneously. The high spatial resolution allowed them to monitor small and fast changes in brain of the target analytes that is not possible to be tracked by state-of-the-art *in vivo* brain monitoring techniques. Subsequently, the microbiosensor array recorded the responses of the animals when submitted to hyperglycemic (40 per cent glucose) and hypoglycemic (5 U/kg insulin).

In view of strong commercial interest, a few companies have been investigating such systems, but are only looking at monitoring the level of glucose in blood. These devices are termed as continuous glucose monitoring (CGM) systems. They have the ability of warning a diabetic patient (or medical care giver of a diabetes patient) of forthcoming hypoglycemic/hyperglycemic events [67]. The advantages of CGM in diabetic management are very clear to the diabetic population, as it lowers the HbA1c (glycated haemoglobin) level [68]. CGM devices are also expected to eventually accomplish the concept of an artificial pancreas, owing to the utilisation of constant feedback of analytical information from the glucose biosensor to activate an insulin delivery pump [69]. The earliest CGM device was developed by MiniMed in 2000, back then, data were only analysed after the monitoring process by the medical doctors [70]. Current CGM devices provide real-time display of data and the first real-time CGM device was released in 2005 by Guardian [71]. Currently, there are several FDA-approved CGM devices on the market.

In all CGM devices, instead of blood glucose, interstitial glucose is measured [72]. The access of the enzyme to interstitial glucose is limited by their design to guarantee that oxygen concentration (which is very low compared to glucose) is not

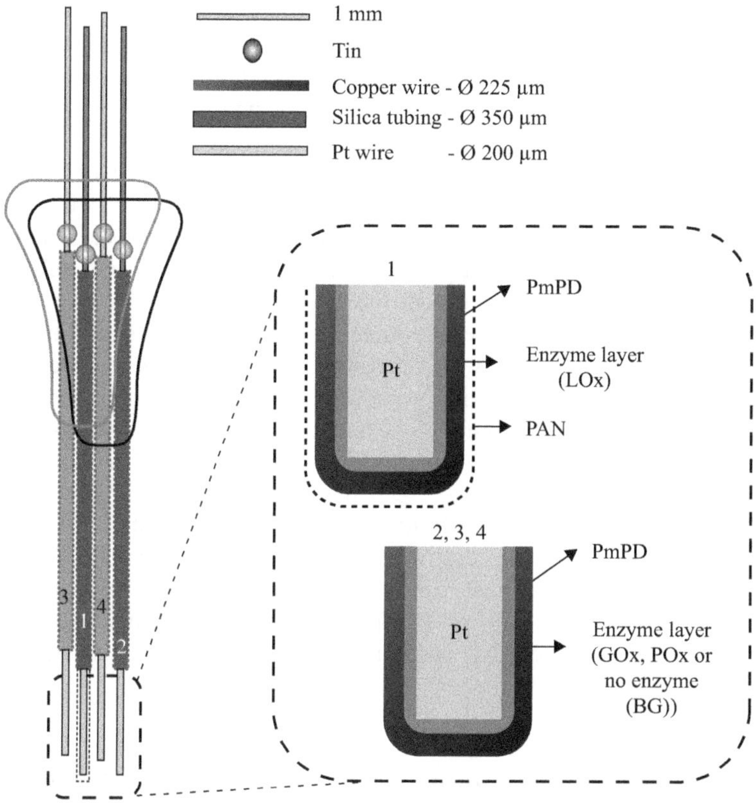

Figure 7.5 Schematic representation of the microbiosensor assembly: 1 – lactate biosensor; 2 – glucose biosensor, 3 – pyruvate biosensor, 4 – background biosensor. Reproduced with permission from Reference 66

rate limiting to the overall reaction rate [73]. The biosensor must be replaced every three days although some may last up to a week [31]. The main reason for the need to replace the biosensors so frequently is biofouling due to the reaction to the implanted biosensors. A reading is taken every 3–5 min which gives the sensing electrode, oxygen and glucose in the measured area chance to re-equilibrate. One might argued that this reading/signal from the biosensor to the transmitter is not truly continuous [74]. Upon receiving the signal, the transmitter will send a wireless signal to a portable processor which might be standalone. After which, the processor will calibrate this reading to true blood glucose obtained from external blood glucose metre. One must continue to perform finger stick blood sugar testing several times a day to ensure that the continuous monitor is correctly calibrated. Although using the same type of electrodes and enzyme, one of the big differences among the CGM devices is how inaccuracy problem is tackled. For example, either a polymer membrane is engaged to address the oxygen deficit problem or a barrier membrane is included to reduce the glucose flow, therefore reducing the production of hydrogen peroxide, which causes damage to the biosensor [75]. On the other hand, a highly efficient redox mediator such as osmium-based redox polymers can also substantially improve the accuracy because of its low operating potential and excellent mediating power [76, 77]. The effectiveness and safety of CGM devices is dependent on their accuracy and reliability. Edward *et al.* compared three CGM systems (FreeStyle Navigator from Abbott Diabetes Care, G4 Platinum from Dexcom and Enlite from Medtronic) in adult and paediatric subjects with type one diabetes under closed-loop blood-glucose control [78]. Twenty-four subjects with type one diabetes participated in one 48-h closed-loop blood glucose control experiment. Their blood sugar levels, measured from venous plasma obtained every 15 min, were paired in time with corresponding CGM glucose measurements obtained from the three CGMs that were worn at the same time by each subject. The Navigator and G4 Platinum (G4) had the best overall performance with an aggregate mean absolute relative difference (MARD) of all paired points of 12.3 ± 12.1 per cent and 10.8 ± 9.9 per cent, respectively. Both had lower MARDs of all paired points than Enlite (17.9 ± 15.8 per cent, $P < 0.005$). Very large errors (MARD > 50 per cent) were less frequent with the G4 (0.5 per cent) than with the Enlite (4.3 per cent, $P = 0.0001$). Their comprehensive head-to-head comparison of the commercial CGM systems revealed substantial discrepancies in their analytical performance. The Navigator and G4 were found to outperform the Enlite in these areas.

7.4 New materials for improving the *in vivo* stability of implantable microbiosensors

With the advent of microfabrication technology, mass production of microbiosensors to be implanted intravascularly or subcutaneously with required dimensions are now quite effortless done. For this consideration, the prevention of the extensive use of implantable microbiosensors in the clinical area is not due to miniaturisation, although it used to be a big challenge. The reason implantable biosensors are not so successful in clinical use lies largely in the shortage of reliable analytical efficiency of the implanted biosensors. In comparison to the outstanding stability and sensitivity of most biosensors' function *in vitro*, there is always a decrease in sensitivity after implantation, arising from a rapid decrease of *in vivo* signal followed by a total loss of the biosensor function within hours or days [79]. The biofouling of the biosensor and loss of enzyme activity due to the foreign body reaction after implantation are the major causes. More specifically, the performance problems appear to be from the biological responses of the host body instead of any actual changes to the responsiveness of the implanted biosensors. Biocompatibility is a key challenge for implantable biosensors and, although many attempts have been made to address this issue, it still remains challenging. The biocompatibility of implantable medical device has been defined as 'the ability of the device to carry out its intended function within flowing blood, with minimal interaction between device and blood that adversely affects device performance and without inducing uncontrolled activation of cellular or plasma protein cascades' [80]. Strictly speaking, an implanted device is biocompatible when its function is not affected by blood components and defence system of the host. In this section, we will have a close look at some of the new materials developed to address the biocompatibility issue. One of the usual ways would be to minimise protein adsorption and host response on the surface. The reduction of biofouling has chiefly been achieved by the construction of outer membranes or coatings that present themselves as a biocompatible interface, which protects the underlying enzyme and electrode from the immune system [81]. The use of this kind of coating/membranes is described as the passive strategy. Nafion, cellulose acetate, various hydrogels, polytetrafluoroethylene, polyvinyl chloride and many other polymeric materials have been explored, but their extent of effectiveness varies. Based on epoxy-enhanced polyurethane, which includes 30–40 per cent epoxy resin and 60–70 per cent polyurethane, Yu *et al.* developed an outer protective membrane for implantable biosensors [82]. This new membrane was designed to increase the *in vivo* durability and lifetime of implantable biosensors. This epoxy-polyurethane membrane was shown to be porous and is of excellent durability. It possessed long-term stability and lasting for four to eight months in solutions at room temperature for a biosensor with such a membrane. (Figure 7.6)

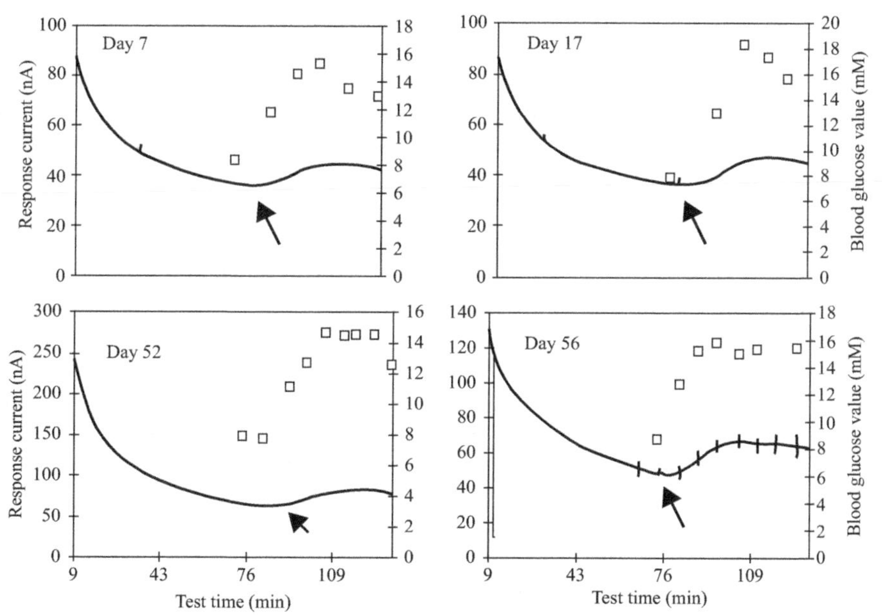

Figure 7.6 The response (solid line) of the implantable biosensor to glucose injections (indicated by arrows) at different days compared with blood glucose values (square box) measured by a glucose metre. Reproduced with permission from Reference 82

Large reduction of inflammatory response *in vivo* is also accomplished by surface modification to form hydrogels using hydrophilic polymers. The way they reduce biofouling is that these polymers are able to make the surface remarkably hydrophilic, so that proteins will have difficulty to go through the gel due to a tightly bound layer of water. Novel hydrogels were also developed by Yu and co-workers based on a co-polymer of hydroxyethyl methacrylate and 2,3-dihydroxypropyl methacrylate to protect implanted glucose biosensors from biofouling [83]. They also improved the porosity and mechanical properties of the hydrogels by using N-vinyl-2-pyrrolidinone and ethyleneglycol dimethacrylate. *In vivo* experiments involving rats which were subcutaneously implanted with eight such microbiosensors were tested per week over four weeks. The epoxy-polyurethane membrane has a low permeability and it act as an additional diffusion-limiting membrane between the hydrogel layer and the enzyme layer. All of the implanted biosensors continued to function for at least 21 days and three out of eight biosensors still functioned in day 28. Further analysis revealed that the fibrous capsules surrounding the hydrogel-coated biosensors were thinner than those without the hydrogel costings after 28 days of implantation.

Koschwanez *et al.* tested the hypothesis that porous poly-L-lactic acid coatings reduce fibrosis and also promote formation of blood micro-vessel in tissue adjacent to the implanted biosensor surface [84]. A three-week study of non-functional glucose biosensors involving subcutaneous rats showed the foreseen effect of porous coatings promoting the vessel formation and decreasing deposition of collagen. However, it is important to note that, whether the device has been placed intravascularly or sub-cutaneously will affect the foreign body response [85]. It was found that in contrast to subcutaneous, percutaneous functional biosensors with and without the porous coatings showed no significant difference in terms of histology or biosensor response. This could be due to the additional mechanical stresses introduced by percutaneous tethering may cancel the beneficial effects of the porous coatings. Ju *et al.* developed a porous collagen scaffold around implantable glucose biosensors for improving their biocompatibility [86]. Nordihydroguaiareticacid (NDGA)-treated collagen scaffolds were stable without physical deformation in the subcutaneous tissue of rats for four weeks. Compared to NDGA-cross-linked scaffolds, glutaraldehyde (GA)-treated collagen scaffolds were badly damaged following implantation, although both types of scaffolds (NDGA and GA-cross-linked) were stable *in vitro*. Moreover, the application of the highly porous NDGA-cross-linked scaffolds to implantable glucose biosensors did not significantly affect the function of the biosensors. The synthetic polymer, polyurethane, is known to possess the attractive mechanical properties for implantable biomedical device applications but is relatively inert. On the contrary, extracellular matrix derivatives which are natural bioactive materials lack mechanical properties that are longed for implantable devices. Mixed properties – bioactivity together with mechanical strength – can be attained by using electrospinning which can present a way to produce coaxial fibres with core-shell structure made by these different types of synthetic and natural materials [87]. In addition, compared to traditional membranes, the electrospun polyurethane membranes displayed advantages in having adjustable composition, structure and thickness. Furthermore, these membranes have been shown to have minimal effect on the functionality of the biosensors while maintaining a very low susceptibility to biofouling and fibrous encapsulation. Such membranes are expected to play an important role in engineering tissue responses to the implanted biosensors.

Instead of non-specific binding reduction using membranes, coatings and hydrogels, another approach can be used when specific functions inducing intended biological responses are introduced. The most obvious issues of this approach are suppressing the defence reactions near the implanted biosensor and improving new vascular tissues growth around the biosensor. One way is the application of the controlled release of drugs that prevent inflammation and inhibit fibrosis – active strategy, in addition to support growth of vascularised tissue so as to not severely impair delivery of analytes to the biosensor. This way, the drug release can provide advantages by reducing fundamental side effects and improving therapeutic responses. It has been shown that continuous local delivery of dexamethasone around the implanted biosensor can help to control inflammation [88]. Local drug delivery for implantable biosensors can be achieved through a coating made of hydrogel or microspheres embedded hydrogel composite [89]. However, dexamethasone release from hydrogel typically only lasts for two days. Microspheres or nanoparticles/hydrogel composites offer a much longer dexamethasone release time in comparison with hydrogels [90]. For example, Wang *et al.* developed a novel polymeric composite membrane consisting of poly(lactic-co-glycolic)acid (PLGA) microsphere dispersed in poly(vinyl alcohol) (PVA) hydrogels The polymeric composite membrane showed controlled release of dexamethasone-21 phosphate disodium. It is therefore can be used as a 'smart' drug eluting membrane for implantable microbiosensors to improve their biocompatibility [91]. The polymeric microspheres slowly released tissue-modifying drugs at the implantation site to control the inflammation and encapsulation of the implant, while the hydrogel allowed fast diffusion of analyte to the sensing elements. Both normal and diabetic rats were used in the study to investigate the effect of diabetes on tissue-biosensor interactions. A rigid coating around dummy biosensors was formed by the application of the PLGA/PVA hydrogel composite and it stayed all in one piece throughout a month. However, the diabetic rats exhibited lowered intensity and slowed onset of the foreign body response following implantation of drug free dummy biosensors in comparison to those of normal rats. The dummy biosensors that were coated with the same composite but without dexamethasone-21 phosphate disodium displayed acute and chronic inflammation as well as fibrous encapsulation in both normal and diabetic rats. On the other hand, tissues that were incorporated the dummy biosensors coated with dexamethasone containing composites remained normal (i.e. similar to untreated tissues) with no inflammatory reaction or fibrous encapsulation transpiring over the one-month period in both the normal and diabetic rats (Figure 7.7). This polymeric composite together with the active release of drug represent an innovative approach to control the foreign body reaction at the tissue–biosensor interface to extend the lifetime of implanted biosensors.

Schoenfish *et al.* had earlier demonstrated that the adherence of proteins is limited when the electrochemical oxygen biosensor is coated with a polymer that

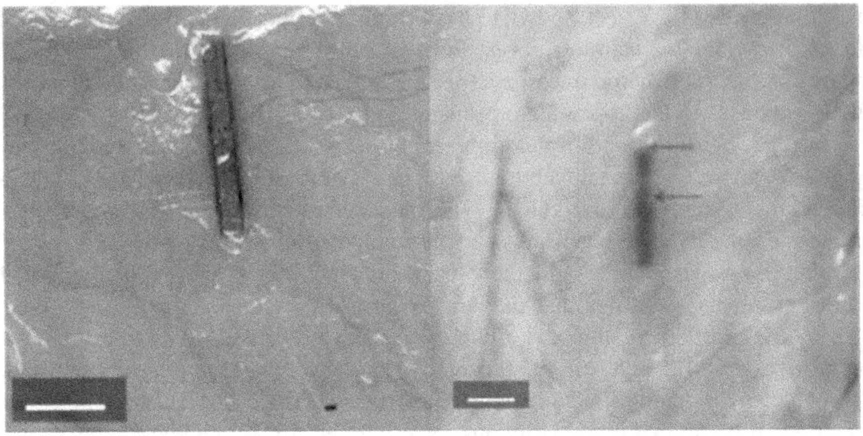

Figure 7.7 Subcutaneous tissue containing dummy biosensors without (left) and with (right) composite coating. Scale bar = 2 mm. Reproduced with permission from Reference 91

slowly releases physiological levels of NO [92]. Subsequently, sol–gel outer coatings with NO releasing chemistry for glucose biosensors have been developed. Recently, this group developed a NO-releasing dendrimer doped electrospun polyurethane fibres as porous outermost glucose biosensor membranes [93]. Again, such approach demonstrated the ability to combine both active (i.e. NO-release) and passive (i.e. porous) strategies within a single outer biosensor coating.

However, this kind of active release feature may bring in additional complications, complexity and uncertainty to the design of implantable biosensors and may cause problems to the efficacy and safety of the biosensors. In addition, because the inflammatory response is an essential part of healing that help to kill any bacteria that may be in the wound. Drugs or reagents which may undermine this otherwise normal aspect of wound healing might endanger the patient. Colvin *et al.* reported a unique catalytic strategy to mediate the biological protection benefit from normal *in vivo* oxidative inflammatory response with the realistic need to protect the performance and stability of a glucose sensitive material used within an implantable glucose biosensor [94]. It was reported that a 3-nm thick layer of plasma-sputtered metallic platinum onto the porous surface of the hydrogel exhibits immediate protection from biosensor signal loss due to oxidation both *in vitro* and *in vivo* and this considerably extends the beneficial lifetime of the implantable glucose biosensor from 1 day to ~6 months (Figure 7.8). This finding may serve as a new strategy to protect an implanted material and/or device from *in vivo* oxidative damage that is a necessary part of the inflammation process, leading to much improved overall stability and reliability for long-term applications.

Biofouling can also be minimised by using a self-cleaning membrane. This is another type of strategy to improve the biocompatibility without introducing additional substance into the living system and it can physically remove adsorbed cells. Hydrogels that are thermos-responsive, namely poly(N-isopropylacrylamide)

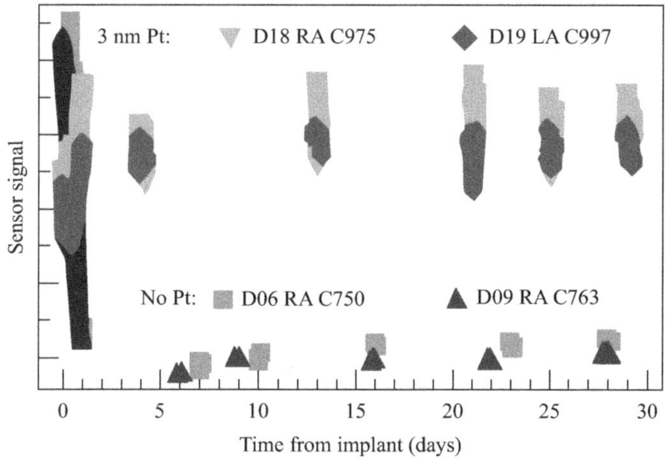

Figure 7.8 Platinum protection in vivo. (a) exemplary biosensor signal from diabetes patient for biosensors without (D06, right arm, C750 and D09, right arm, C763) and with (D18, right arm, C975and D19, left arm, C997) 3 nm Pt. Reproduced with permission from Reference 94

(PNIPAAm), nanocomposite hydrogels are possible self-cleaning active membranes for implantable glucose biosensors since they undergo de-swelling and re-swelling when heated above and cooled below their volume phase transition temperature (~33–35 °C), respectively. Basically, a membrane in the 'off-state' will be fully swollen for optimal glucose diffusion. When performing self-cleaning (on-state), the membrane would begin to de-swell via transdermal heating. This process has been demonstrated to cause the removal of cultured cells *in vitro* [95, 96]. In addition, the self-cleaning may be able to perform well via transdermal thermal cycling. Unfortunately, PNIPAAm hydrogels are limited by their poor mechanical strength. Gant *et al.* [97] and Abraham and co-workers [98] reported the use of a double network nanocomposite hydrogel composed of an interpenetrating, asymmetrically cross-linked PNIPAAm matrix with polysiloxane nanoparticles (~200 nm) (Figure 7.9). In their studies, unique thermos-responsive nanocomposite hydrogels were developed to create tough and strong self-cleaning biosensor membranes for implantable biosensors.

This hydrogel was shown to have significantly improved thermos-sensitivity in terms of both the rate and the extent of de-swelling and re-swelling versus a conventional PNIPAAm. The volume phase transition temperature was also adjusted to ~38 °C with N-vinylpyrrolidone co-monomer such that the membrane would be swollen (off-state) and becomes hydrophobic at body temperature (~35 °C, wrist subcutaneous tissue) to maximise glucose diffusion. Thus, when heated about the volume phase transition temperature, the membrane would then undergo reversible de-swelling (on-state) and becomes hydrophilic, which should detach adhered cells from its surface. In addition, PNIPAAm hydrogels are non-degradable and this would be advantageous to maintain membrane functionality and to endure containment of sensing materials [99].

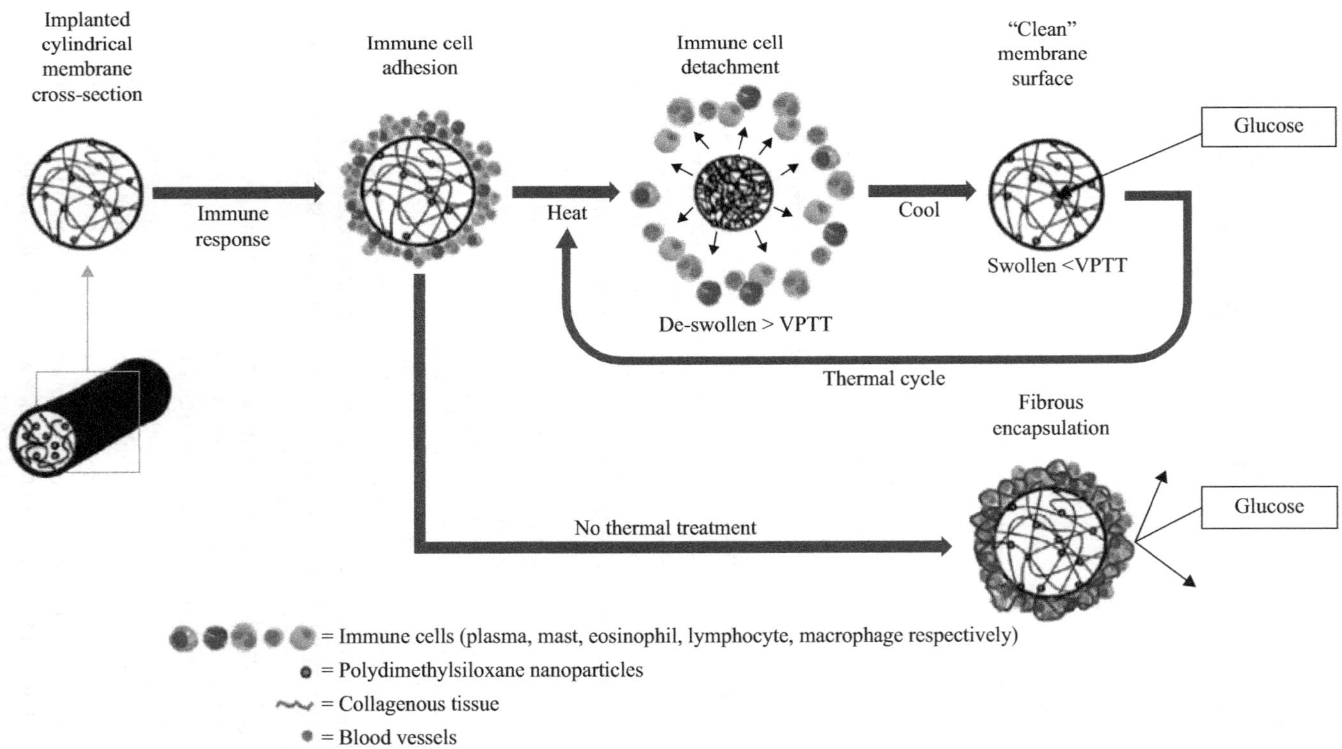

Figure 7.9 Biofouling of a membrane surrounding an implanted biosensor compromises analyte diffusion. The double network nanocomposite membrane is designed to exhibit self-cleaning when thermally cycling above its volume phase transition temperature. Reproduced with permission from Reference 98

7.5 Conclusion and future prospects

Enzyme-based amperometric microbiosensors are presently the dominant biosensors for monitoring and detection of biomolecules and have already shown great potentials to be translated into implantable for diseases like diabetes. The future outlooks of implantable microbiosensors and especially metabolic monitoring will continue to be bright if they can more readily be implanted and explanted without the need for complicated surgery. The synergy between implantable biosensors and nanotechnology is crucial in the areas of miniaturisation and post-implantation inflammation. Since the degree of inflammation is largely dependent on the size of the implanted device, nanotechnology has been used to decrease not only the inflammation but also the size of the implants [100]. In addition, ultrasensitive devices are also highly valued such as the recently fabricated lacate microbiosensor based on lactate oxidase and oxygen-rich platinum doped cerium oxide nanoparticles [101]. It was shown that platinum in the platinum doped cerium oxide nanoparticles are electrocatalytic for the detection of the enzymatically produced hydrogen peroxide and the cerium oxide nanoparticles serve as an intrinsic oxygen source for lactate oxidase, thus empowering lactate monitoring even in an oxygen-depleted tissue. The results in the study successfully demonstrated that the platinum doped cerium oxide nanoparticles are a versatile material for use in implantable enzyme-based biosensors [101]. Enzyme immobilisation methods are also one area in which efforts could be spent on and this could help lower the cost of biosensor fabrication since some commercially available enzymes are expensive and scarce. However, for a long-term implantable biosensor to be feasible, the foreign body response still poses enormous challenges. Toward the goal of longer continuous monitoring, researchers have very recently reported a novel biosensor that comprises a stack of different gels (xerogels) and polymer films in a layer-by-layer assembled manner that can detect slight concentration changes in glucose in real-time [102]. One of the xerogel layers was not immobilised with GOx and it is able to reduce glucose flow rate. This could be important for continuous use since it permits the enzyme to reset before the next influx of glucose. This specific combination of layers yields a composite film material that could act as an effective first-generation biosensor with adjustable properties. In the case of CGM, Dexcom and the University of Padova have recently developed an advanced CGM, called G4AP, to particularly address the intensive performance requirements for future artificial pancreas studies. The G4AP employed the same biosensor and transmitter as the G4 platinum but contains updated de-noising and calibration algorithms for improved accuracy and reliability [103]. According to Facchinetti, accuracy is determined not only by the biosensor design and materials but also by the algorithms used to convert the raw biosensor signal into a calibrated glucose value [104]. In the near future, GlySens will be coming up with a CGM system for people with diabetes. It is good to mention that this system will include a long-lived (18 months) fully implantable biosensor which is also a dual enzyme-based (GOx and catalase) amperometric biosensor. The GlySens device touted to be a potentially major technological leap. Development of this implantable biosensor would require a multidisciplinary team. Indeed, the future development of implantable micro-biosensors and devices will require the combination of multidisciplinary areas like chemistry, solid state physics, bioengineering and medicine.

Acknowledgement

This work is supported by the Ministry of Education, Republic of Singapore.

References

[1] Meyerhoff M.E. 'In vivo blood-gas and electrolyte sensors: progress and challenges.' *Trends Anal. Chem.* 1993, vol. 12 (6), pp. 257–265.
[2] Koschinsky T., Heinemann L. 'Sensors for glucose monitoring: technical and clinical aspects.' *Diabetes/Metab. Res. Rev.* 2001, vol. 17 (2), pp. 113–123.
[3] Vashist S.K. 'Non-invasive glucose monitoring technology in diabetes management: a review.' *Anal. Chim. Acta.* 2012, vol. 750, pp. 16–27.
[4] Klonoff D.C. 'The benefits of implanted glucose sensors.' *J. Diabetes Sci. Technol.* 2007, vol. 1 (6), pp. 797–800.
[5] Karube I., Sode K., Tamiya E. 'Microbiosensors.' *J. Biotechnol.* 1990, vol. 15 (3), pp. 267–281.
[6] Jaffari S.A., Turner A.P. 'Recent advances in amperometric glucose biosensors for in vivo monitoring.' *Physiol. Meas.* 1995, vol. 16 (1), pp. 1–15.
[7] Frost M.C., Meyerhoff M.E. 'Implantable chemical sensors for real-time clinical monitoring: progress and challenges.' *Curr. Opin. Chem. Biol.* 2002, vol. 6 (5), pp. 633–641.
[8] Frost M., Meyerhoff M.E. 'In vivo chemical sensors: tackling biocompatibility.' *Anal. Chem.* 2006, vol. 78 (21), pp. 7370–7377.
[9] Ganter M., Zollinger A. 'Continuous intravascular blood gas monitoring: development, current techniques, and clinical use of a commercial device.' *Br. J. Anaesth.* 2003, vol. 91 (3), pp. 397–407.
[10] Lim C., Slack S., Ufer S., Lindner E. 'Protein adsorption to planar electrochemical sensors and sensor materials.' *Pure Appl. Chem.* 2004, vol. 76 (4), pp. 753–764.
[11] Wu Y., Rojas A.P., Griffith G.W., *et al.* 'Improving blood compatibility of intravascular oxygen sensors via catalytic decomposition of S-nitrosothiols to generate nitric oxide in situ.' *Sens. Actuators, B.* 2007, vol. 121 (1), pp. 36–46.
[12] Mahutte C.K. 'On-line arterial blood gas analysis with optodes: current status.' *Clin. Biochem.* 1998, vol. 31 (3), pp. 119–130.
[13] Reach G., Wilson G.S. 'Can continuous glucose monitoring be used for the treatment of diabetes?' *Anal. Chem.* 1992, vol. 64 (6), pp. 381A–386A.
[14] Cunningham D.D., Stenken J.A. (eds.). *In Vivo Glucose Sensing*. Vol. 174. Hoboken, New Jersey, John Wiley & Sons; 2009.

[15] Ertefai S., Gough D.A. 'Physiological preparation for studying the response of subcutaneously implanted glucose and oxygen sensors.' *J. Biomed. Eng.* 1989, vol. 11 (5), pp. 362–368.
[16] Gifford R., Kehoe J.J., Barnes S.L., Kornilayev B.A., Alterman M.A., Wilson G.S. 'Protein interactions with subcutaneously implanted biosensors.' *Biomaterials.* 2006, vol. 27 (12), pp. 2587–2598.
[17] Onuki Y., Bhardwaj U., Papadimitrakopoulos F., Burgess D.J. 'A review of the biocompatibility of implantable devices: current challenges to overcome foreign body response.' *J. Diabetes Sci. Technol.* 2008, vol. 2 (6), pp. 1003–1015.
[18] Stefan R., Baiulescu G.E., Aboul-Enein H.Y., van Staden J.F. 'Estimation of uncertainties in clinical analysis.' *Accredit. Qual. Assur.* 1999, vol. 4 (6), pp. 225–229.
[19] Linko S. 'Automated ion-selective measurement of lithium in serum. a practical approach to result-level verification in a two-way method validation.' *Accredit. Qual. Assur.* 2001, vol. 6 (1), pp. 31–36.
[20] Bakker E., Qin Y. 'Electrochemical Sensors.' *Anal. Chem.* 2006, vol. 78 (12), pp. 3965–3983.
[21] Stefan R.I., van Staden J.F., Aboul-Enein H.Y. 'Estimation of uncertainties for the application of electrochemical sensors in clinical analysis.' *Accredit. Qual. Assur.* 2003, vol. 8 (2), pp. 86–89.
[22] Mataveli L.R.V., Antunes N.d.J., Brigagao M.R.P.L, Schmidt de Magalhaes C., Wisniewski C., Luccas P.O. 'Evaluation of a simple and low cost potentiometric biosensor for pharmaceutical and in vivo adrenaline determination.' *Biosens. Bioelectron.* 2010, vol. 26 (2), pp. 798–802.
[23] Ponmozhi J., Frias C., Marques T., Frazão O. 'Smart sensors/actuators for biomedical applications: review.' *Measurement.* 2012, vol. 45 (7), pp. 1675–1688.
[24] Lee D., Cui T. 'Layer-by-layer self-assembled single-walled carbon nanotubes based ion-sensitive conductometric glucose biosensors.' *IEEE Sens. J.* 2009, vol. 9 (4), pp. 449–456.
[25] Cui X., Liu G., Lin Y. 'Amperometric biosensors based on carbon paste electrodes modified with nanostructured mixed-valence manganese oxides and glucose oxidase.' *Nanomedicine.* 2005, vol. 1 (2), pp. 130–135.
[26] Shichiri M., Kawamori R., Yamasaki Y., Hakui N., Abe H. 'Wearable artificial endocrine pancrease with needle-type glucose sensor.' *Lancet.* 1982, vol. 2 (8308), pp. 1129–1131.
[27] Wang J. 'Electrochemical glucose biosensors.' *Chem. Rev.* 2008, vol. 108 (2), pp. 814–825.
[28] Palmisano F., Zambonin P.G., Centonze D. 'Amperometric biosensors based on electrosynthesised polymeric films.' *Fresenius' J. Anal. Chem.* 2000, vol. 366 (6–7), pp. 586–601.
[29] O'Neill R.D., Lowry J.P., Mas M. 'Monitoring brain chemistry in vivo: voltammetric techniques, sensors, and behavioral applications.' *Crit. Rev. Neurobiol.* 1998, vol. 12 (1&2), pp. 69–127.

[30] Newman J.D., Turner A.P.F. 'Home blood glucose biosensors: a commercial perspective.' *Biosens. Bioelectron.* 2005, vol. 20 (12), pp. 2435–2453.

[31] Yoo E.-H., Lee S.-Y. 'Glucose biosensors: an overview of use in clinical practice.' *Sensors.* 2010, vol. 10 (5), pp. 4558–4576.

[32] Wilson G.S., Ammam M. 'In vivo biosensors.' *FEBS J.* 2007, vol. 274 (21), pp. 5452–5461.

[33] Felice A.K.G., Sygmund C., Harreither W., Kittl R., Gorton L., Ludwig R. 'Substrate specificity and interferences of a direct-electron-transfer-based glucose biosensor.' *J. Diabetes Sci. Technol.* 2013, vol. 7 (3), pp. 669–677.

[34] Turner A.P.F., Chen B., Piletsky S.A. 'In vitro diagnostics in diabetes: meeting the challenge.' *Clin. Chem.* 1999, vol. 45 (9), pp. 1596–1601.

[35] Schuhmann W., Wohlschlaeger H., Lammert R., *et al.* 'Leaching of dimethylferrocene, a redox mediator in amperometric enzyme electrodes.' *Sens. Actuators, B.* 1990, vol. 1 (1–6), pp. 571–575.

[36] Chaubey A., Malhotra B.D. 'Mediated biosensors.' *Biosens. Bioelectron.* 2002, vol. 17 (6–7), pp. 441–456.

[37] Palmisano F., Zambonin P.G., Centonze D., Quinto M. 'A disposable, reagentless, third-generation glucose biosensor based on overoxidized poly (pyrrole)/tetrathiafulvalene-tetracyanoquinodimethane composite.' *Anal. Chem.* 2002, vol. 74 (23), pp. 5913–5918.

[38] Liu Y., Wang M., Zhao F., Xu Z., Dong S. 'The direct electron transfer of glucose oxidase and glucose biosensor based on carbon nanotubes/chitosan matrix.' *Biosens. Bioelectron.* 2005, vol. 21 (6), pp. 984–988.

[39] Kuila T., Bose S., Khanra P., Mishra A.K., Kim N.H., Lee J.H. 'Recent advances in graphene-based biosensors.' *Biosens. Bioelectron.* 2011, vol. 26 (12), pp. 4637–4648.

[40] Tsai T.-W., Heckert G., Neves L.F., *et al.* 'Adsorption of glucose oxidase onto single-walled carbon nanotubes and its application in layer-by-layer biosensors.' *Anal. Chem.* 2009, vol. 81 (19), pp. 7917–7925.

[41] Gierwatowska M., Kowalewska B., Cox J.A., Kulesza P.J. 'Multifunctional mediating system composed of a conducting polymer matrix, redox mediator and functionalized carbon nanotubes: integration with an enzyme for effective bioelectrocatalytic oxidation of glucose.' *Electroanalysis.* 2013, vol. 25 (12), pp. 2651–2658.

[42] Azevedo A.M., Martins V.C., Prazeres D.M.F., Vojinovic V., Cabral J.M.S., Fonseca L.P. 'Horseradish peroxidase: a valuable tool in biotechnology.' *Biotechnol. Annu. Rev.* 2003, vol. 9, pp. 199–247.

[43] Zafar M.N., Safina G., Ludwig R., Gorton L. 'Characteristics of third-generation glucose biosensors based on corynascus thermophilus cellobiose dehydrogenase immobilized on commercially available screen-printed electrodes working under physiological conditions.' *Anal. Biochem.* 2012, vol. 425 (1), pp. 36–42.

[44] Guiseppi-Elie A. 'An implantable biochip to influence patient outcomes following trauma-induced hemorrhage.' *Anal. Bioanal. Chem.* 2011, vol. 399 (1), pp. 403–419.

[45] Spehar-Deleze A., Anastasova S., Popplewell J., Vadgama P. 'Extreme physiological state: development of tissue lactate sensor.' *2012 Ninth International Conference on Wearable and Implantable Body Sensor Networks (BSN)*; London, UK, May 2012 (IEEE, 2012), pp. 17–21.
[46] Qin S., van der Zeyden M., Oldenziel W.H., Cremers T.I.F.H., Westerink B. H.C. 'Microsensors for in vivo measurement of glutamate in brain tissue.' *Sensors.* 2008, vol. 8 (11), pp. 6860–6884.
[47] Burmeister J.J., Gerhardt G.A. 'Self-referencing ceramic-based multisite microelectrodes for the detection and elimination of interferences from the measurement of L-glutamate and other analytes.' *Anal. Chem.* 2001, vol. 73 (5), pp. 1037–1042.
[48] Guerrieri A., Lattanzio V., Palmisano F., Zambonin P.G. 'Electrosynthesized poly(pyrrole)/poly(2-naphthol) bilayer membrane as an effective anti-interference layer for simultaneous determination of acethylcholine and choline by a dual electrode amperometric biosensor.' *Biosens Bioelectron.* 2006, vol. 21 (9), pp. 1710–1718.
[49] Wahono N., Qin S., Oomen P., Cremers T.I.F., de Vries M.G., Westerink B.H.C. 'Evaluation of permselective membranes for optimization of intracerebral amperometric glutamate biosensors.' *Biosens. Bioelectron.* 2012, vol. 33 (1), pp. 260–266.
[50] Swamy B.E.K., Venton B.J. 'Carbon nanotube-modified microelectrodes for simultaneous detection of dopamine and serotonin in vivo.' *Analyst.* 2007, vol. 132 (9), pp. 876-884.
[51] Hernandez G., Shizgal P. 'Dynamic changes in dopamine tone during self-stimulation of the ventral tegmental area in rats.' *Behav. Brain Res.* 2009, vol. 198 (1), pp. 91–97.
[52] Robinson D.L., Venton B.J., Heien M.L.A.V., Wightman R.M. 'Detecting subsecond dopamine release with fast-scan cyclic voltammetry in vivo.' *Clin. Chem.* 2003, vol. 49 (10), pp. 1763–1773.
[53] Zou X., Luo L., Ding Y., Wu Q. 'Chitosan incorporating cetyltrimethylammonium bromide modified glassy carbon electrode for simultaneous determination of ascorbic acid and dopamine.' *Electroanalysis.* 2007, vol. 19 (17), pp. 1840–1844.
[54] Njagi J., Chernov M.M., Leiter J.C., Andreescu S. 'Amperometric detection of dopamine in vivo with an enzyme based carbon fiber microbiosensor.' *Anal. Chem.* 2010, vol. 82 (3), pp. 989–996.
[55] Cannon R.O., III. 'Role of nitric oxide in cardiovascular disease: focus on the endothelium.' *Clin. Chem.* 1998, vol. 44 (8, Pt. 2), pp. 1809–1819.
[56] Zhang L., Zhao G.-C., Wei X.-W., Yang Z.-S. 'A nitric oxide biosensor based on myoglobin adsorbed on multi-walled carbon nanotubes.' *Electroanalysis.* 2005, vol. 17 (7), pp. 630–634.
[57] Gifford R., Batchelor M.M., Lee Y., Gokulrangan G., Meyerhoff M.E., Wilson G.S. 'Mediation of in vivo glucose sensor inflammatory response via nitric oxide release.' *J. Biomed. Mater. Res., Part A.* 2005, vol. 75A (4), pp. 755–766.

[58] Koh W.C.A., Rahman M.A., Choe E.S., Lee D.K., Shim Y.-B. 'A cytochrome C modified-conducting polymer microelectrode for monitoring in vivo changes in nitric oxide.' *Biosens. Bioelectron.* 2008, vol. 23 (9), pp. 1374–1381.

[59] Dikalov S., Grigor'ev I.A., Voinov M., Bassenge E. 'Detection of superoxide radicals and peroxynitrite by 1-hydroxy-4-phosphonooxy-2,2,6,6-tetramethylpiperidine: quantification of extracellular superoxide radicals formation.' *Biochem. Biophys. Res. Commun.* 1998, vol. 248 (2), pp. 211–215.

[60] Orrenius S. in Poli G., Albano E., Dianzani M.U. (ed.). *Free Radicals: From Basic Science to Medicine*. Basel: Birkhauser Verlag; 1993, pp. 47.

[61] Stohs S.J., Bagchi D. 'Oxidative mechanisms in the toxicity of metal ions.' *Free Radical Biol. Med.* 1995, vol. 18 (2), pp. 321–336.

[62] Di J., Bi S., Zhang M. 'Third-generation superoxide anion sensor based on superoxide dismutase directly immobilized by sol-gel thin film on gold electrode.' *Biosens. Bioelectron.* 2004, vol. 19 (11), pp. 1479–1486.

[63] Ganesana M., Erlichman J.S., Andreescu S. 'Real-time monitoring of superoxide accumulation and antioxidant activity in a brain slice model using an electrochemical cytochrome C biosensor.' *Free Radical Biol. Med.* 2012, vol. 53 (12), pp. 2240–2249.

[64] Kondepati V.R., Heise H.M. 'Recent progress in analytical instrumentation for glycemic control in diabetic and critically ill patients.' *Anal. Bioanal. Chem.* 2007, vol. 388 (3), pp. 545–563.

[65] Rocchitta G., Secchi O., Alvau M.D., *et al.* 'Simultaneous telemetric monitoring of brain glucose and lactate and motion in freely moving rats.' *Anal. Chem.* 2013, vol. 85 (21), pp. 10282–10288.

[66] Cordeiro C.A., de Vries M.G., Ngabi W., Oomen P.E., Cremers T.I.F.H., Westerink BHC 'In vivo continuous and simultaneous monitoring of brain energy substrates with a multiplex amperometric enzyme-based biosensor device.' *Biosens. Bioelectron.* 2015, vol. 67, pp. 677–686.

[67] Vashist S.K. 'Continuous glucose monitoring systems: a review.' *Diagnostics.* 2013, vol. 3 (4), pp. 385–412, 28.

[68] Bode B.W., Gross T.M., Thornton K.R., Mastrototaro J.J. 'Continuous glucose monitoring used to adjust diabetes therapy improves glycosylated hemoglobin: a pilot study.' *Diabetes Res. Clin. Pract.* 1999, vol. 46 (3), pp. 183–190.

[69] Vaddiraju S., Burgess D.J., Tomazos I., Jain F.C., Papadimitrakopoulos F. 'Technologies for continuous glucose monitoring: current problems and future promises.' *J. Diabetes Sci Technol.* 2010, vol. 4 (6), pp. 1540–1562.

[70] Mastrototaro J.J. 'The minimed continuous glucose monitoring system.' *Diabetes Technol. Ther.* 2000, vol. 2 (Suppl. 1), pp. S/13–S/18.

[71] Bode B., Gross K., Rikalo N., *et al.* 'Alarms based on real-time sensor glucose values alert patients to hypo- and hyperglycemia: the guardian continuous monitoring system.' *Diabetes Technol. Ther.* 2004, vol. 6 (2), pp. 105–113.

[72] Pandit K. 'Continuous glucose monitoring.' *Indian J. Endocrinol. Metab.* 2012, vol. 16 (Suppl 2), pp. S263–S266.

[73] Heineman W., Karube I., Schmid R., Turner A. *Biosensors 92 Proceedings: The Second World Congress on Biosensors*. Burlington: Elsevier; 2014.

[74] Rebrin K., Sheppard N.F., Jr., Steil G.M. 'Use of subcutaneous interstitial fluid glucose to estimate blood glucose: revisiting delay and sensor offset.' *J. Diabetes Sci. Technol.* 2010, vol. 4 (5), pp. 1087–1098.

[75] Rossetti P., Bondia J., Vehi J., Fanelli C.G. 'Estimating plasma glucose from interstitial glucose: the issue of calibration algorithms in commercial continuous glucose monitoring devices.' *Sensors.* 2010, vol. 10, pp. 10936–10952.

[76] Degani Y., Heller A. 'Direct electrical communication between chemically modified enzymes and metal electrodes. I. electron transfer from glucose oxidase to metal electrodes via electron relays, bound covalently to the enzyme.' *J. Phys. Chem.* 1987, vol. 91 (6), pp. 1285–1289.

[77] McGarraugh G. 'The chemistry of commercial continuous glucose monitors.' *Diabetes Technol. Ther.* 2009, vol. 11 (Suppl. 1), pp. S17–S24.

[78] Damiano E.R., El-Khatid F.H., Zheng H., Nathan D.M., Russell S.J. 'A comparative effectiveness analysis of three continuous glucose monitors.' *Diabetes Care.* 2013, vol. 36 (2), pp. 251–259.

[79] Fraser D.M. 'An introduction to in vivo biosensing: progress and problems.' in Fraser, D.M. (ed.). *Biosensors in the Body: Continuous in Vivo Monitoring.* Chichester; New York, John Wiley & Sons; 1997.

[80] Williams D.F. 'On the mechanisms of biocompatibility.' *Biomaterials.* 2008, vol. 29 (20), pp. 2941–2953.

[81] Thevenot D.R., Toth K., Durst R.A., Wilson G.S. 'Electrochemical biosensors: recommended definitions and classification.' *Biosens. Bioelectron.* 2001, vol. 16 (1–2), pp. 121–131.

[82] Yu B., Long N., Moussy Y., Moussy F. 'A long-term flexible minimally-invasive implantable glucose biosensor based on an epoxy-enhanced polyurethane membrane.' *Biosens. Bioelectron.* 2006, vol. 21 (12), pp. 2275–2282.

[83] Yu B., Wang C., Ju Y.M., *et al.* 'Use of hydrogel coating to improve the performance of implanted glucose sensors.' *Biosens. Bioelectron.* 2008, vol. 23 (8), pp. 1278–1284.

[84] Koschwanez H.E., Yap F.Y., Klitzman B., Reichert W.M. 'In vitro and in vivo characterization of porous poly-L-lactic acid coatings for subcutaneously implanted glucose sensors.' *J. Biomed. Mater. Res., Part A.* 2008, vol. 87A (3), pp. 792–807.

[85] Koschwanez H.E., Reichert W.M. 'In vitro, in vivo and post explantation testing of glucose-detecting biosensors: current methods and recommendations.' *Biomaterials.* 2007, vol. 28 (25), pp. 3687–3703.

[86] Ju Y.M., Yu B., Koob T.J., Moussy Y., Moussy F. 'A novel porous collagen scaffold around an implantable biosensor for improving biocompatibility. I. in vitro/in vivo stability of the scaffold and in vitro sensitivity of the glucose sensor with scaffold.' *J. Biomed. Mater. Res., Part A.* 2008, vol. 87A (1), pp. 136–146.

[87] Wang N., Burugapalli K., Wijesuriya S., *et al.* 'Electrospun polyurethane-core and gelatin-shell coaxial fibre coatings for miniature implantable biosensors.' *Biofabrication.* 2014, vol. 6 (1), pp. 015002/1--015002/18.

[88] Patil S.D., Papadmitrakopoulos F., Burgess D.J. 'Concurrent delivery of dexamethasone and vegf for localized inflammation control and angiogenesis.' *J. Controlled Release*. 2007, vol. 117 (1), pp. 68–79.

[89] Moussy Y., Hersh L., Dungel P. 'Distribution of [3h]dexamethasone in rat subcutaneous tissue after delivery from osmotic pumps.' *Biotechnol. Prog.* 2006, vol. 22 (3), pp. 819–824.

[90] Galeska I., Kim T.-K., Patil S.D., *et al.* 'Controlled release of dexamethasone from PLGA microspheres embedded within polyacid-containing PVA hydrogels.' *AAPS J.* 2005, vol. 7 (1), pp. E231–E240.

[91] Wang Y., Papadimitrakopoulos F., Burgess D.J. 'Polymeric "smart" coatings to prevent foreign body response to implantable biosensors.' *J. Controlled Release*. 2013, vol. 169 (3), pp. 341–347.

[92] Schoenfisch M.H., Mowery K.A., Rader M.V., Baliga N., Wahr J.A., Meyerhoff M.E. 'Improving the thromboresistivity of chemical sensors via nitric oxide release: fabrication and in vivo evaluation of no-releasing oxygen-sensing catheters.' *Anal. Chem.* 2000, vol. 72 (6), pp. 1119–1126.

[93] Koh A., Lu Y., Schoenfisch M.H. 'Fabrication of nitric oxide-releasing porous polyurethane membranes-coated needle-type implantable glucose biosensors.' *Anal. Chem.* 2013, vol. 85 (21), pp. 10488–10494.

[94] Colvin A.E., Jiang H. 'Increased in vivo stability and functional lifetime of an implantable glucose sensor through platinum catalysis.' *J. Biomed. Mater. Res., Part A.* 2013, vol. 101A (5), pp. 1274–1282.

[95] Okano T., Yamada N., Okuhara M., Sakai H., Sakurai Y. 'Mechanism of cell detachment from temperature-modulated, hydrophilic-hydrophobic polymer surfaces.' *Biomaterials.* 1995, vol. 16 (4), pp. 297–303.

[96] Kobayashi J., Okano T. 'Fabrication of a thermoresponsive cell culture dish: a key technology for cell sheet tissue engineering.' *Sci. Technol. Adv. Mater.* 2010, vol. 11 (1), pp. 1–12.

[97] Gant R.M., Hou Y., Grunlan M.A., Cote G.L. 'Development of a self-cleaning sensor membrane for implantable biosensors.' *J. Biomed. Mater. Res., Part A.* 2009, vol. 90A (3), pp. 695–701.

[98] Abraham A.A., Fei R., Cote G.L., Grunlan M.A. 'Self-cleaning membrane to extend the lifetime of an implanted glucose biosensor.' *ACS Appl. Mater. Interfaces*. 2013, vol. 5 (24), pp. 12832–12838.

[99] Patenaude M., Hoare T. 'Injectable, mixed natural-synthetic polymer hydrogels with modular properties.' *Biomacromolecules.* 2012, vol. 13 (2), pp. 369–378.

[100] Vaddiraju S., Tomazos I., Burgess D.J., Jain F.C., Papadimitrakopoulos F. 'Emerging synergy between nanotechnology and implantable biosensors: a review.' *Biosens. Bioelectron*. 2010, vol. 25 (7), pp. 1553–1565.

[101] Sardesai N.P., Ganesana M., Karimi A., Leiter J.C., Andreescu S. 'Platinum-doped ceria based biosensor for in vitro and in vivo monitoring of lactate during hypoxia.' *Anal. Chem.* 2015, vol. 87 (5), pp. 2996–3003.

[102] Poulos N.G., Hall J.R., Leopold M.C. 'Functional layer-by-layer design of xerogel-based first-generation amperometric glucose biosensors.' *Langmuir.* 2015, vol. 31 (4), pp. 1547–1555.

[103] Garcia A., Rack-Gomer A.L., Bhavaraju N.C., *et al.* 'Dexcom G4ap: an advanced continuous glucose monitor for the artificial pancreas.' *J. Diabetes Sci. Technol.* 2013, vol. 7 (6), pp. 1436–1445.

[104] Facchinetti A., Sparacino G., Guerra S., *et al.* 'Real-time improvement of continuous glucose monitoring accuracy – the smart sensor concept.' *Diabetes Care.* 2013, vol. 36 (4), pp. 793–800.

Chapter 8

Nanomaterials based biosensors: a smart approach towards on-site clinical diagnosis

Renu Singh[1] and Jaesung Jang[1]

8.1 Introduction

A biosensor device is defined by its biological receptor unit with unique specificities toward corresponding analytes of biological origin like nucleic acids (NA; DNAs, RNAs of bacteria or viruses, or proteins which are generated from the immune system (antibodies, antigens) of infected living organisms. One of many other challenges in biosensor development is the efficient signal capture of the biological transduction event by translating the interaction of analyte with the biological element into electrochemical, electrochemiluminescent, magnetic, electrical, and optical signals. Considering that most biological systems, including viruses, bacteria, membranes, and protein complexes, are naturally nanostructured materials (~1–100 nm diameter) and that molecular interactions take place on a nanometer scale, nanomaterials are intuitive candidates for integration into biomedical devices [1,2]. Nanomaterials are being promising candidates due to the possibility to immobilize an enhanced quantity of bioreceptor units at minute volumes and even itself as transduction element in order to increase sensitivities and to lower down the limit of detection (LOD) down to even individual molecules. Moreover, this can be attributed to the ability to tailor the size and structure, and hence the properties of nanomaterials, thus opening up excellent prospects for designing novel biosensing systems and enhancing the performance of biomedical devices [3]. Newly developed nanomaterials i.e., nanowires, nanotubes, nanoparticles, nanorods, nanocrystals, and nanocomposites having large variety of functional groups, including metal nanoparticles (MNPs)-gold (Au), silver (Ag) NPs, quantum dots (QDs)-cadmium selenide (CdSe), cadmium telluride (CdTe), zinc sulphide (ZnS), magnetic nanoparticles (MGNPs)-iron oxide (Fe_3O_4), carbon nanostructures-carbon nanotubes (CNT), graphene oxide (GO), nanostructured conducting polymers (NCPs)-polyaniline (PANI), polypyrrole (PPY), and nanostructured metal oxide (NMO)-zirconium dioxide (ZrO_2) have attained great

[1]School of Mechanical and Nuclear Engineering, Ulsan National Institute of Science and Technology (UNIST), Ulsan 689-798, Republic of Korea

attention as they are promising building blocks for the realization of nanoscale biosensors due to their biocompatibility and technologically important combination of properties, i.e., high surface area, good electrical properties, and chemical stability (Figure 8.1). The chemical, electronic, and optical properties of nanomaterials generally depend on both their dimensions and their morphology [4]. They can

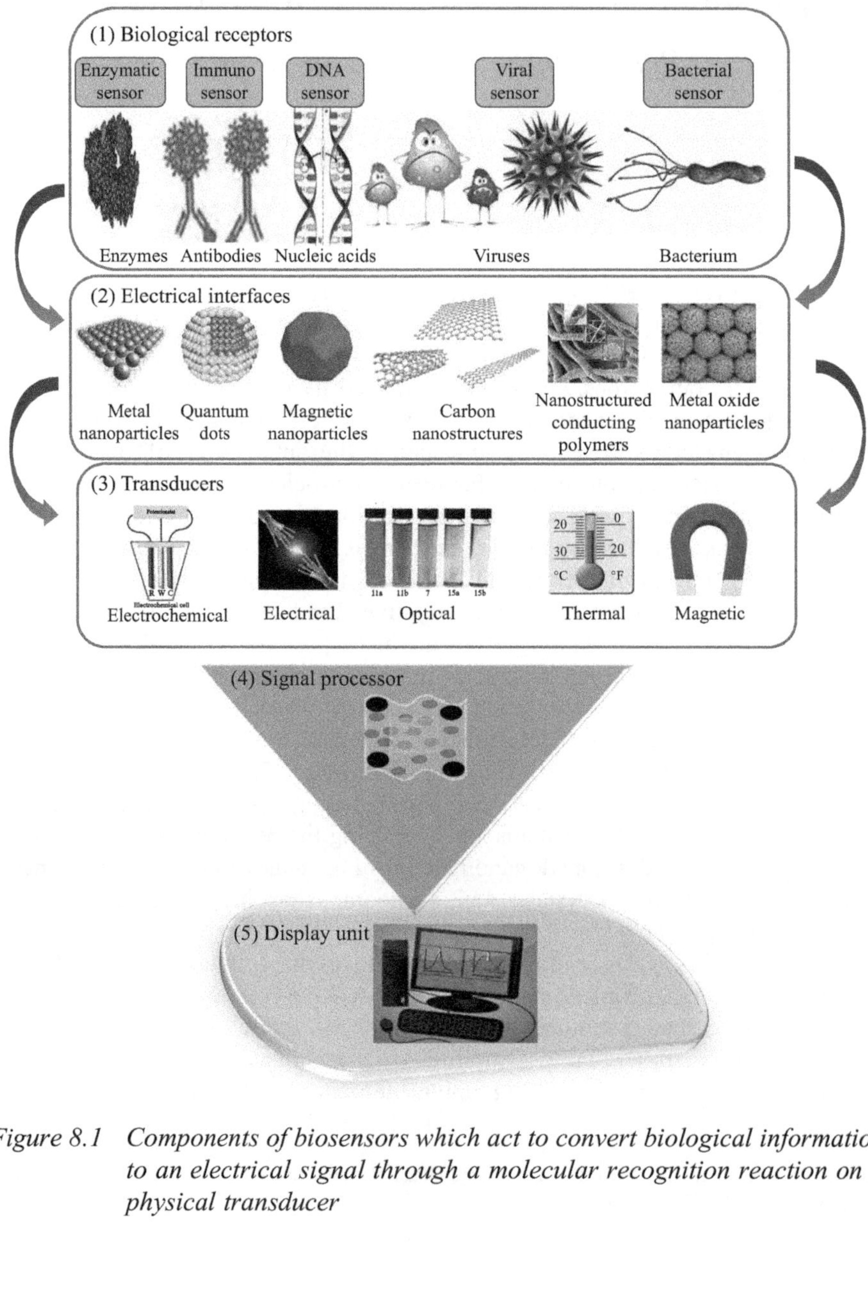

Figure 8.1 Components of biosensors which act to convert biological information to an electrical signal through a molecular recognition reaction on a physical transducer

create the way for the miniaturization of biosensing devices with nanometer dimensions, easy-to-use, and inexpensive sensors in order to obtain better sensitivity, specificity, and faster rates of recognition compared to current solutions. Due to the immense advancement of nanobiotechnology interdisciplinary research field, this book chapter summarizes the importance of variety of nanomaterials by focusing on nano-objects which provide many further constructive properties.

8.2 Conventional techniques for clinical diagnosis

The conventional techniques for clinical diagnosis include microscopy; simple, easy to use and a versatile technique, culture; gold standard for diagnosis, and serology. These conventional techniques are inexpensive but protracted methods. In case of microscopy the interpretation may be subjective but it has limited sensitivity. The other technique culture comes with the possibility of reduced viability during transportation and risk of contamination with commensal flora and moreover, choice of culture media and interpretation of culture results requires skillful technical. Serology has the disadvantage of the occurrence of false-positive results due to cross-reaction with other organisms and the requirement of convalescent sera. Another growth independent strategy from last two decades; molecular methods include the non-amplification methods, e.g., hybridization using probes as well as amplification based methods and particularly suited for unculturable organisms, e.g., *Treponema pallidum*; difficult to grow organisms, e.g., Human immunodeficiency virus (HIV), Hepatitis B virus (HBV), *Bordetella pertussis;* slow growing organisms, e.g., *Mycobacterium tuberculosis*; and dangerous to culture organisms, e.g., *Coxiella burnetti*. The nucleic acid amplification techniques have taken an irreversible position in diagnostics. These include polymerase chain reaction (PCR), ligase chain reaction (probe amplification), loop-mediated isothermal amplification (isothermal amplification), transcription based amplification (target amplification), and branch DNA technology (signal amplification) [5]. These methods result in both qualitative and quantitative analysis of the test and are known to be sensitive but are time consuming and expensive.

8.3 Nanomaterials for clinical diagnosis

Nanomaterials became important components in bioanalytical devices since they clearly enhance the performances in terms of sensitivity and LOD down to single molecules detection through new signal transduction technologies. The development of tools and processes used to fabricate, measure and image nanoscale objects, has led to the development of sensors that interact with extremely small molecules that need to be analyzed. These advances are particularly exciting in the context of biosensing, where the requirements are for low concentration detection and high specificity.

For the fabrication of high performance biosensor, the role of immobilization of the desired biomolecule onto a matrix (Figure 8.2) is very much crucial and

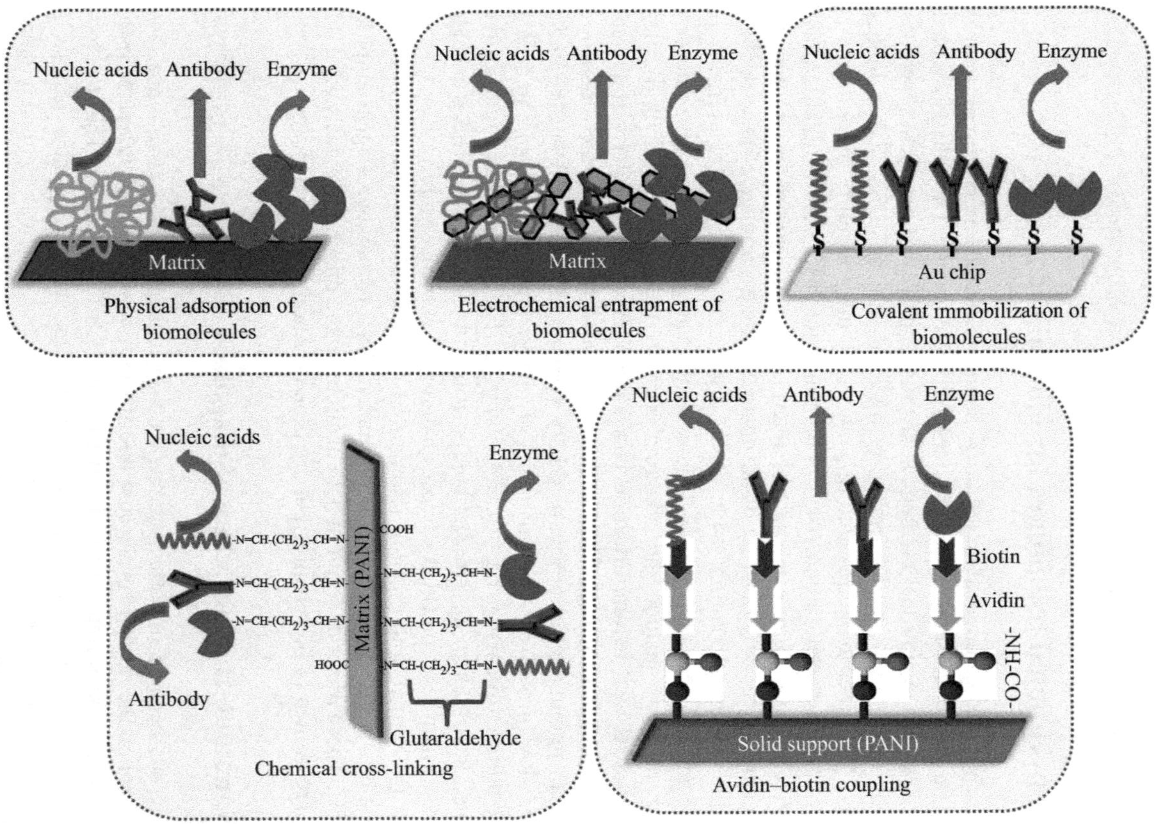

Figure 8.2 Schematic showing the immobilization of various biomolecules (DNA, antibody, enzyme) onto solid support via different immobilization methods

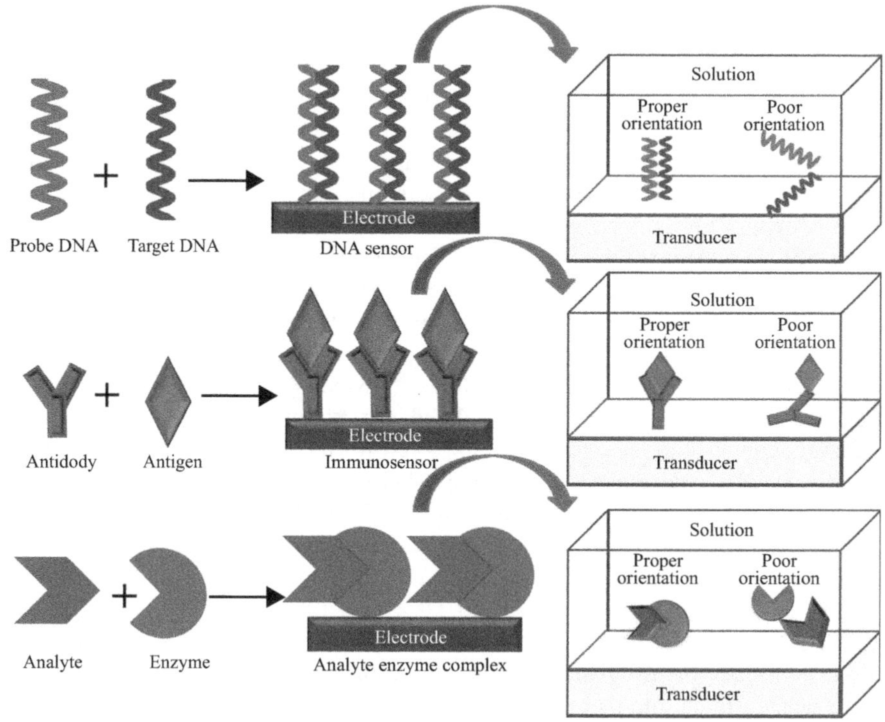

Figure 8.3 Illustration of proper vs poor orientation of various biomolecules (DNA, antibody, enzyme)

requires complete retention of their biological recognition properties in the active state. The covalently attached biomolecules at one terminus onto the nanomaterials surface has an advantage in terms of stability and reproducibility of the surface functionalization and allows for the highest degree of thermodynamic freedom that significantly speeds up the attachment rate (Figure 8.3). The microenvironment provided by a nanomaterial may help a biomolecule to retain its conformation with maximum biological activity, resulting in enhanced signal transduction and stability. Nanomaterials are being explored due to their exceptional optical and electrical properties owing to electron and phonon confinement, high surface-to-volume ratio, modified surface work function, high surface reaction activity, high catalytic efficiency and strong adsorption ability. In particular, nanomaterials with engineered morphology, size, functionality, adsorption capability and high biomolecule loading capacity have been found to provide enhanced electron transport between a biomolecule and electrode. These unique properties of nanomaterials can be utilized for interfacing biological recognition events with electronic signal transduction and for designing new generation of bioelectronics devices which exhibits novel functions.

8.3.1 Metal nanoparticles

MNPs are interesting materials with unique electronic and electrocatalytic properties depending on their size and morphology [6,7]. In particular, AuNPs are real jewels beyond its nano-size and are much explored materials as components for biosensors development due to the capability to greatly improve electron transfer when a biological component is maintained in contact with nanostructured surface owing to its fascinating features such as ease-of-synthesis, high bio-compatibility and non-cytotoxicity [8]. Their optical properties can change upon binding to certain molecules, permitting the recognition and quantification of analyte. The sensitive detection can be exploited by property to change absorption spectra drastically of AuNPs when several particles come close to each other [9]. Most biological molecules can be labeled with MNPs without compromising their biological activities [10]. On the other hand, Ag, platinum (Pt), palladium, copper (Cu), and cobalt (Co) have also been explored for the biosensors development.

Zhang *et al.* developed a sensitive label-free bio-barcode assay using two-component oligonucleotide-modified with AuNPs and magnetic beads (MBs) for quantitative detection, based on the redox activity of guanine (G) and adenine (A) nucleobases, of two NA targets Human T-lymphotropic virus (I-II) simultaneously and detected in the range from 4.4×10^{-11} to 2.0×10^{-9} M with LOD of 1.71×10^{-12} M for T_1-DNA and 1.55×10^{-12} M for T_2-DNA [11]. Cheong *et al.* fabricated microfluidic sensor using the longitudinal resonance of Au nanorods that transforms near-infrared into thermal energy hence resulting heat causes pathogen lysis. Consequently, the DNA was extracted out of the cell body and transferred to PCR system. Two different Au rods AR 3 and AR 15 exhibits efficient lysis of *Escherichia coli* cells and quick pathogen detection by real-time PCR using SYBR Green I without any optical hindrance (Ct values, 21.60 and 22.07, respectively). When a different Taq polymerase is used without hot start, they obtained better Ct values (17.31 and 18.67 for AR 3 and 15, respectively) with the Au nanorods, suggesting that Au nanorods are also compatible with different Taq polymerases. This has led to successful demonstration of a one-step real-time PCR system for clinical diagnosis without removal or changing of reagents [12]. Chua *et al.* fabricated the glass fiber-based lateral flow DNA biosensor that uses capture reagents coupled to carrier beads and detector reagent bioconjugated to AuNps, for the detection of food borne pathogen, *Vibrio cholerae*. The DNA biosensor contained a test line that captured the target PCR amplicons, an internal amplification control (IC) line which captures IC amplicons and a control line that acted as membrane control to validate the functionality of this device. The test line captured biotin labeled DNA, while the IC line captures digoxigenin labeled DNA. The detector reagent recognized the fluorescein haptens of the amplified DNA and produces visual red lines having the LOD of 5 ng target DNA and did clinical evaluation with 174 strains of *V. cholerae* and non-*V. cholerae* bacteria with 100 percent sensitivity and specificity [13]. Hao *et al.* developed a quartz crystal microbalance (QCM) biosensor to detect *Bacillus anthracis* based on the recognition of its specific DNA sequences, i.e., the 168 bp fragment of the Ba813 gene in chromosomes and the

340 bp fragment of the pag gene in plasmid pXO1 via the ssDNA immobilization onto Au QCM electrode to hybridize with the target ssDNA sequence obtained by asymmetric PCR. Thiol-DNA fragment complementary to the other end of the target DNA was functionalized with AuNPs for amplification of signal and showed LOD 3.5×10^2 CFU ml^{-1} of *B. anthracis* vegetative cells just after asymmetric PCR amplification, but without culture enrichment [14]. Optical-affinity biosensors based on surface-plasmon resonance (SPR) allow label-free qualitative and quantitative measurements of biomolecular interactions between a biomolecule immobilized on a metal surface and the analyte in solution [15]. Despite being such a powerful technique, the sensitivity of SPR biosensors is sometimes limited by inability to measure small changes in refractive index. AuNPs have demonstrated their potential to amplify SPR detection [16]. Hence, Joung *et al.* employed AuNPs in a signal-amplification method for high-sensitivity detection of *E. coli* 16s rRNA using peptide nucleic-acid probes with an SPR biosensor system [17]. An ultra-trace voltammetric method was developed by Wang *et al.* using CNT loaded with silver nanoparticles, placed on a gold microelectrode, for early detection of HIV-1 to prevent the spreading of the disease effectively and revealed the LOD of 0.5 pM within the detection range of 1.0–100 pM [18]. Chen *et al.* demonstrated an ultrasensitive electrochemical biosensor for the detection of influenza A virus based on glucose oxidase (GOx)-catalyzed deposition of Cu hexacyanoferrate (HCF) nanoparticles and exhibited the LOD of 1.0 fM within the range of 1.0 fM to 10 pM, due to the high catalytic activity of GOx, and cumulative nature of the formation of CuHCF nanoparticles catalyzed by GOx attached to the hybridized DNA [19].

8.3.2 Quantum dots

Nanostructured materials are interesting tools with specific physical and chemical properties because of their quantum-size effects when compared to bulk materials [20]. QDs are spherical, fluorescent nanocrystals made up of semiconductor materials of intermediate size typically between 2 and 8 nm in diameter; are indebted to unique properties such as, narrow sized tunable emission spectra, broad excitation spectra, negligible photo bleaching, high sensitivity and stable fluorescence with simple excitation without the need of laser and hence can improve the sensitivity of biosensor. Bioconjugated QDs have the potential to be used in cancer diagnosis due to its bright and stable fluorescent light emission and sensitivity of fluorescence imaging and hence may be used in the future for locating cancer tumors in patients [21]. Fan *et al.*, developed a facile ethanolamine/glucose mixed solution route for the controllable synthesis of CdSe hollow nanostructures and consequently used it for the fabrication of electrochemical DNA sensor for Avian Influenza Virus (AIV) [22]. Roh *et al.* developed RNA biosensor for hepatitis C virus (HCV) NS3 protein detection. They previously stated that quantum dots-conjugated RNA oligonucleotide can recognize the HCV NS3 protein specifically and sensitively. At a concentration of 0.01 $\mu g \cdot ml^{-1}$, 7,8,4'-trihydroxyisoflavone and 6,7,4'-trihydroxyisoflavone showed more than a 30 percent inhibition activity of a nanoparticle-based RNA oligonucleotide biochip system [23]. Alvi *et al.* fabricated a potentiometric biosensor for detection of cholesterol based on bio-chemically functionalized InN QDs by utilizing the substantial advantages of high surface charge density and low-dimensionality of the InN QDs to generate highly sensitive and rapid response within the range from 1×10^{-6} to 1×10^{-3} M [24] (Figure 8.4). Liu *et al.* demonstrated the feasibility of detecting 250 zM *E. coli* O157:H7 *eae*A target DNA by using magnetic bead-based DNA detection assay with multi-layers QDs labeling strategy within 40–60 min [25].

8.3.3 Magnetic nanoparticles

MGNPs are powerful and versatile diagnostic tools in biology and medicine as it is manipulated using external magnetic field and always were traditionally used for concentration, separation, purification and identification of specific cells. MGNPs consist of magnetic element, i.e., iron, nickel, and their derivatives are employed in fabrication of biosensors. Magnetic sensors, such as magnetic relaxation switch assay sensors, magneto-resistive sensors, and magnetic particle relaxation sensors have been developed [26]. Superparamagnetic Fe_3O_4 nanoparticles are versatile agent for early diagnosis of cancer and are being used as contrast agents for MRI imaging and as an in-vitro application in bioassay by means of a vehicle for the detection of biomarkers [27].

In recent years, the magnetic properties of some NPs have also been used as labels in biosensing [28,29]. Koets *et al.* developed a magneto-resistant sensor using superparamagnetic particles for *E. coli* and *Salmonella* detection having 4–250 pM LOD using a one-step format with total assay times of less than 3 min. MNPs detected by a Giant Magneto Resistance (GMR) sensor were shown to be very powerful, since the magnetic particles speed up the assay by reducing diffusion limitations. Moreover, the absence of magnetic materials in biological samples means that background signals are low [30]. Several immunomagnetic biosensors were developed for label-free detection of *E. coli.* Mujika *et al.* reported a magnetoresistive immunosensor for the analysis of *E. coli* O157:H7 in food and clinical samples and this sensor was capable of detecting and quantifying small magnetic field variations caused by the presence of superparamagnetic beads bound to the antigens previously immobilized on the sensor surface [31]. Singh *et al.* recently utilized chitosan (CH)–Fe_3O_4 nanobiocomposite for detection of *Neisseria gonorrhoeae* and observed that the presence of Fe_3O_4 nanoparticles ($\sim$18 nm) increased the electro-active surface area of nanobiocomposite that provided desirable environment for loading of DNA with better conformation leading to increased electron transfer kinetics between the medium and electrode. This biosensor was capable to accurately discriminate complementary sequence from mismatch sequences having LOD of 1×10^{-15} M within range of 1×10^{-16} M to 1×10^{-6} M [32]. Haseen *et al.* fabricated streptavidin modified MGNPs based DNA biosensor by functionalizing nanoparticles onto bare Au electrode using a magnet for detection of HBV via non-faradic impedance spectroscopy to detect 50 pmol of HBV DNA and 160 pmol of HIV DNA on sample of 20 μl [33]. Tran *et al.* fabricated CH/Fe_3O_4

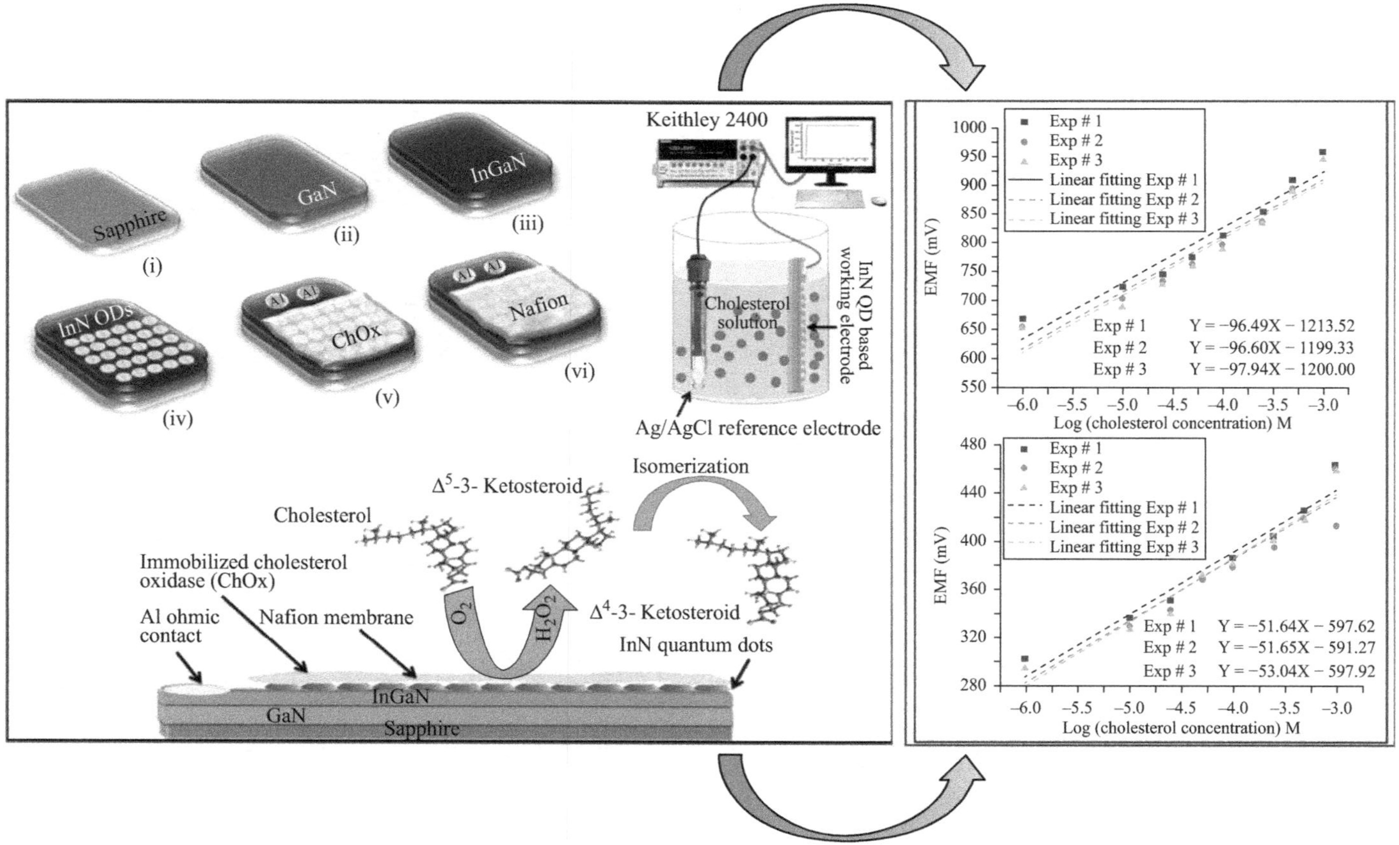

Figure 8.4 QDs based potentiometric biosensor for clinical diagnosis of cholesterol depicting electrochemical cell voltage sensing response as a function of the logarithmic cholesterol concentrations [24]

nanobiocomposite-based sensor for electrochemical HIV-1 detection and stated that suitable microenvironment provided by Fe_3O_4 nanoparticles contributes to higher electron transfer and enhanced sensitivity and low LOD (50 pM) [34]. Electrically active polyaniline-coated magnetic NPs were employed as a magnetic concentrator and biosensor transducer in one system to detect *B. anthracis* spores from food matrices [35].

8.3.4 Carbon nanostructures

CNTs and graphene are the most promising nanostructured carbon materials for biosensing applications where each allotrope has its particular advantage as transducer element. They have received great attention in the last decades with the emergence of nanoscience area due to the capability of increment in the charge transfer which finally leads to improve the LOD [36]. CNTs exceptional properties (e.g., small size, great strength, high electrical and thermal conductivity, and large specific surface area) make them excellent amplification platforms to increase the number of signal-generating molecules [37,38]. Graphite is the simplest form of C–C bond with sp2 hybridization with weak bond energy between adjacent layers and r bond with and out of plane of p orbitals. Viswanathan *et al.* used liposome-coated CNTs for electrochemical detection of the cholera toxin at ultratrace levels [39]. *E. coli* was determined with an LOD of 10 CFU ml^{-1} using tyrosinase biosensor to determine phenol, by employing Fe_3O_4 MGNPs-coated CNTs and was based on the principle of determination of the phenol produced by an enzymatic reaction in the bacteria-containing solution [40]. Using horseradish peroxidase-labeled *Staphylococcus aureus* enterotoxin B antibodies immobilized onto nanoAu/CH-multi-walled (MW) CNTs, *S. aureus* enterotoxin B was detected with a conductometric immunobiosensor in the linear range 0.5–83.5 ng ml^{-1} [41]. Field-effect transistors (FETs) fabricated by using SWCNTs can monitor direct charge-transfer reaction between analyte and CNT. The CNT structure allows the accumulation of carriers in the bulk of the nanodiameter structure and increases the sensitivity to the point that single-molecule detection is possible [42]. Vilamizar *et al.* reported the development of CNT-FET for the detection of *S. infantis* at 100 CFU ml^{-1} in 1 h [43]. Similarly, *E. coli* was detected using an aptamer functionalized CNT-FET [44]. Shiraishi *et al.* observed that the incorporation of fullerene into polymeric structure dramatically improves the surface coverage of the immobilized probe specific to *E. coli* extracted from 16S rDNA [45]. Wang *et al.* utilized reduced GO platform for the fabrication of highly sensitive and selective NA sensor for the detection of *S. aureus* and observed that the sensor can be used to detect upto 100 fM target concentration [46]. In view of the recent revelations and potential applications of CNT-DNA nanobiohybrid, the core-shell structural biowire comprising of CNT and DNA was fabricated via electrophoretic deposition technique by Das *et al.* They postulated the wrapping mechanism and revealed that the peripheral wrapping of DNA along the length of CNT in nanoscale may act as a single nanowire enhancing the electron transport capability [47]. MWCNT were used as a platform by Tam *et al.* for the detection of influenza virus and detected as low as 0.5 nM of target DNA with the response time of ~4 min [48]. AIV was detected using MWCNT–cobalt phthalocyanine (CoPc) nanocomposite and poly (amidoamine) (PAMAM) dendrimer as a platform onto glassy carbon electrode based on oxidation signals of G without any external labels and detected 1.0 pg ml^{-1} within range from 0.01 to 500 ng ml^{-1} [49]. Zuo *et al.* used a simple strategy to integrate the aptamer-functionalized GO biosensor in the microfluidic biochip through the novel use of porous chromatography paper as a simple 3D storage substrate to detect microorganisms directly, without cumbersome sample preparation procedures and made it feasible for field detection [50]. Singh *et al.* fabricated a label-free electrical immunosensor for the detection of swine influenza virus based on dielectrophoretically deposited SWCNTs by varying the channel length from 2 to 10 μm with binding of the influenza viruses to the antibodies deposited into the channels and postulated LOD of 1 PFU ml^{-1} having linear behavior within the range from 1 to 10^4 PFU ml^{-1} with response time of 30 min [51] (Figure 8.5).

8.3.5 Nanostructured conducting polymers

Researchers are continuously evaluating several NCPs for the fabrication of biosensors for clinical diagnosis. Among them, the thin films of polymers like PANI, PPY are two of the widely used materials in present age. Since the biotin-strept (avidin) system has high binding capacity for NA immobilization due to the high affinity constant (Ka $= 10^{15}$ M^{-1}) between avidin and biotin, it is also widely used to immobilize NA on solid support interface to construct biosensors for bacterial detection. Arora *et al.* fabricated voltammetric biosensors utilizing avidin-modified nanostructured PANI electrochemically deposited onto Pt disk electrode for direct detection of *E. coli* by immobilizing a 5′-biotin-labeled *E. coli* probe, in the presence of methylene blue as a DNA hybridization indicator (Figure 8.6) and postulated LOD of complementary target probe (0.009 ng μl^{-1}), *E. coli* genomic DNA (0.01 ng μl^{-1}) and 11 *E. coli* cells ml^{-1} with the response time of 60 s to 14 min without using PCR [52]. Sheng *et al.* reported PANI based ultrasensitive biosensor for detection of the amplified target syphilis DNA and showed 0.5 pM LOD having the linear behavior within the range from 1.0 pM to 1.0 nM with correlation coefficient of 0.998 [53]. Singh *et al.* fabricated DNA sensor based on NA probe (from *Opa*, a multi-copy gene of *N. gonorrhoeae*) functionalized using avidin–biotin as cross-linking agent onto PANI matrix and detected 0.5×10^{-15} M of complementary target within 60 s of hybridization time at 25 °C by DPV using MB [54]. In order to amplify the detection signal and to achieve improved LOD, incorporated MWCNT into PANI that provided conducting channels facilitating faster charge transfer via electrons from one polymer chain to other and finally to the electrode surface and improved LOD 1.2×10^{-17} M [55]. Singh *et al.* explored PANI–nFe_3O_4-CNT trio matrix having LOD 1×10^{-19} M and tested STD sensor with positive and negative PCR amplicons of gonorrhoea affected patient samples [56]. PANI-Fe_3O_4 nanocomposite based biosensor was developed for the clinical diagnosis and exhibited good specificity for *N. gonorrhoeae* species against nongonorrhoeae type of *Neisseria* species and other gram-negative bacterias and showed the improved affinity constant 3.39×10^8 M^{-1} for hybridization calculaed via Langmuir adsorption isotherm model [57].

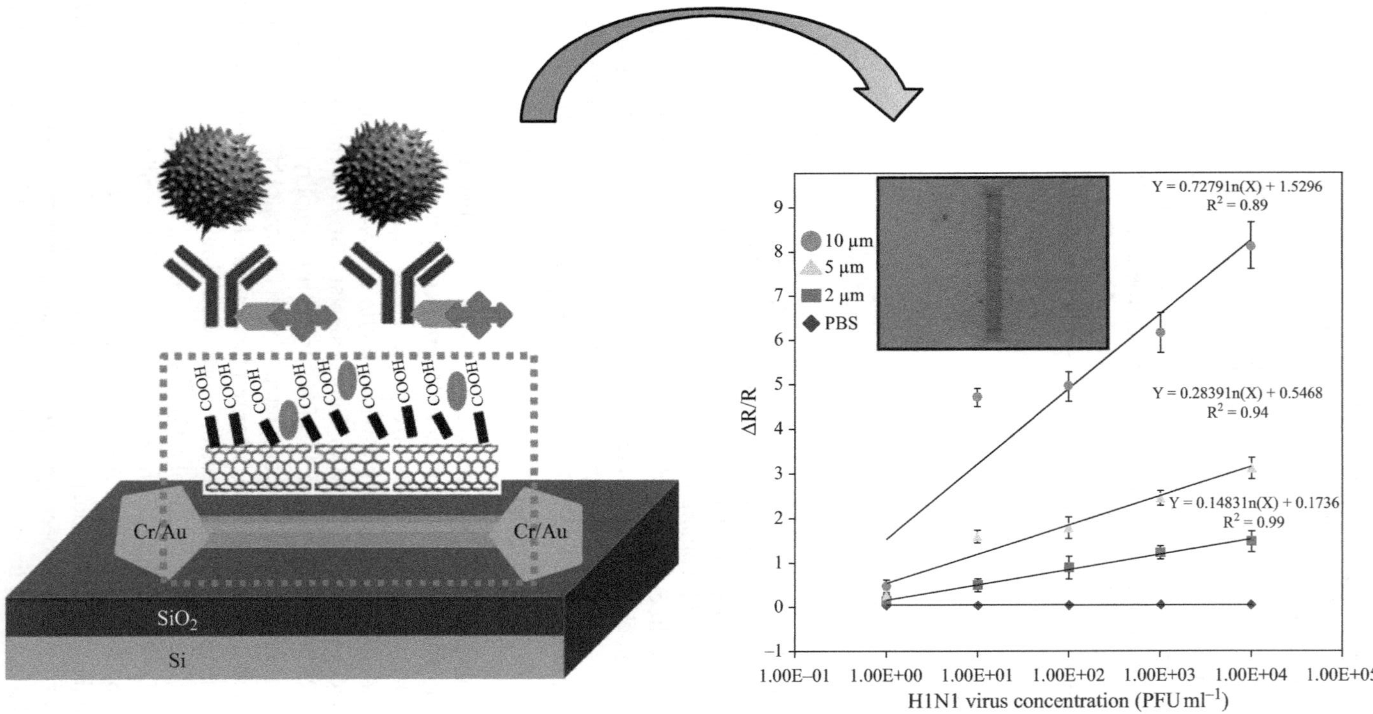

Figure 8.5 Carbon nanostructures based immunosensor for clinical diagnosis of H1N1 influenza virus [51]

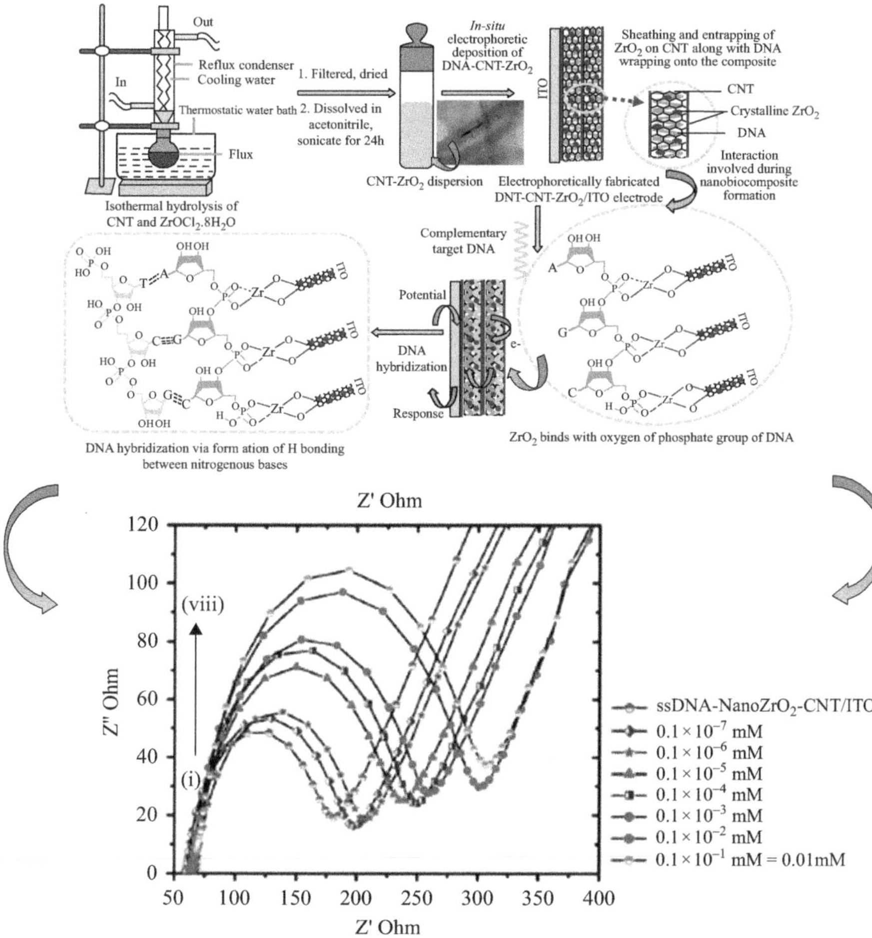

Figure 8.6 Nanostructured metal oxide based DNA biosensor for Mycobacterium tuberculosis *diagnosis [58]*

8.3.6 Nanostructured metal oxide

NMO and their composites are of utmost research interest due to the enhanced surface coverage, electrical and mechanical properties. Considering the synergy between biocompatible ZrO_2 and electrochemically superior CNT, ZrO_2 grafted CNT, obtained via isothermal hydrolysis of zirconium oxychloride in presence of CNT, were electrophoretically deposited onto indium-tin-oxide for detection of *M. Tuberculosis* upto 1×10^{-8} mM DNA [58] (Figure 8.6). Solanki *et al.* exploited sol–gel derived nanostructured ZrO_2 which provided more surface area for detection of *E. coli* and revealed the LOD of 10^{-6} to 10^{6} pM [59]. Sol–gel derived nanostructured zinc oxide nanoparticles were also exploited for clinical diagnosis [60]. Various types of nanoparticles based biosensors for clinical diagnosis has been shown in Table 8.1.

Table 8.1 Various types of nanoparticles based biosensors for clinical diagnosis

Nanomaterials	Clinical diagnosis of microorganism	Method of immobilization	Measurement conditions	Type of biosensor	Detection limit	Detection range	Correlation coefficient	Detection time	Technique used	[Reference] (Year)
AuNPs and two-component oligonucleotide-modified MBs	HTLV-I, HTLV-II	Covalent binding	–	Electrical bio-barcode assay	1.71×10^{-12} M for T_1-DNA and 1.55×10^{-12} M for T_2-DNA	4.4×10^{-11} to 2.0×10^{-9} M	0.9955 and 0.9975	–	DPV	[11] (2009)
Au nanoparticle	*Escherichia coli*	–	PBS buffer	Optothermal biosensor	10000 cells μl^{-1}	–	30 s	–	Real-time PCR	[12] (2008)
AuNps	*Vibrio cholera*	Covalent binding	50 μl 10 mM PBS, pH 7.4 with 0.5% Tween-20, 24 °C	Disposable lateral flow-based DNA biosensor	5 ng	1 to 100 ng	–	10 min	Glass fiber membrane carrier bead system	[13] (2011)
AuNPs coated QCM electrode	*Bacillus anthracis*	Au–SH bond	0.3M NaCl, 1 0mM PB with pH 7.4, 200 μl min^{-1} of buffer, 30 °C	DNA biosensor	3.5×10^2 CFU ml^{-1}	3.5×10^2 to 3.5×10^7 CFU ml^{-1}	–	30 min	QCM	[14] (2011)
AuNPs coated SPR gold chip	*E. coli*, *Staphylococcus aureus*	Avidin–biotin coupling	30 mM Tris buffer, pH 7.4	Surface plasmon resonance biosensors	58.2 ± 1.37 pg ml^{-1}, 7×10^5 CFU	–	–	–	SPR	[17] (2008)
CNT loaded with silver nanoparticles	HIV-1	Au–SH bond	0.10 M PBS, pH 7.4, pulseamplitude, 20 mV; pulse width, 60 ms; scan rate, 20 $mV.s^{-1}$, RT	–	0.5 pM	1.0×10^{-12} to 1.0×10^{-10} M	0.9956	60 min	DPV	[18] (2011)
CuHCF nanoparticles onto Au electrode	HIV	Avidin–biotin coupling	Potential, 4 mV–1.0 V; step potential, 4 mV; amplitude, 50 mV; pulse,0.05 s; and pulse period, 0.2 s; electrolyte solution, 0.10 M KNO_3, RT	–	1.0 fM	1.0 fM to 10 pM	0.98	2 h	DPV	[19] (2010)

CdSe hollow nanostructures onto GCE	AIV	Physical adsorption	B–R buffer, pH 7.0, containing2.0 × 10^{-5} mol l^{-1} MB with 0.02 mol l^{-1} NaCl, Scan rate 50 mV s^{-1}, 40 °C	–	1.0 × 10^{-12} mol l^{-1}	–	–	60 min	DPV	[22] (2010)
Carboxyl-terminated QDs605	HCV	Covalent binding	Phosphate buffer pH 7.2, RT	Inhibitor screening on a biochip	0.01 μg·ml^{-1}	0.1 to 0.5 μg·ml^{-1}	–	–	Emission wavelength as the optical imaging probe	[23] (2012)
InN QDs grown on an InGaN layer	Cholesterol oxidase	Electrostatic binding	phosphate buffer (pH 7.0)	Quantum dot based electrochemical biosensor	–	1 × 10^{-6} to 1 × 10^{-3} M	–	–	Electro-chemical cell voltage (EMF)	[24] (2013)
Magnetic bead with multi-layers quantum dots labeling	*E. coli*	–	20 mM Tris–HCl, pH 7.5, 1.0 M LiCl, 2 mMEDTA, RT	Fluorescence-based assay	250 zM	500–250 zM	–	40–60 min	QCM	[25] (2008)
Fe_3O_4 magnetic nanoparticles		Avidin–biotin coupling	phosphate buffer solution	–	100 nM	–	–	–	–	[28] (2008)
Streptavidin coated magnetic particles	*Salmonella*	Physical adsorption	–	Giant magneto-resistance (GMR) detection	4:00 PM	4–250 pM	–	–	GMR method	[30] (2009)
Superparamagnetic microspheres	E. coli O157:H7	Physical adsorption	–	Magnetoresistive immunosensor	10^5 CFU ml^{-1}	–	–	–	Magneto-resistance	[31] (2009)
CH-Fe_3O_4 Nanocomposite onto ITO electrode	*Neisseria gonorrhoeae*	Avidin–biotin coupling	Methylene blue at pulse height of 50 mV, pulse width of 70 ms in 0.05 M phosphate buffer of pH 7.0 containing 0.153 M NaCl, 25 °C	–	1 × 10^{-15} M	1 × 10^{-16} to 1 × 10^{-6} M	0.99	–	DPV	[32] (2011)

(Continues)

Table 8.1 (Continued)

Nanomaterials	Clinical diagnosis of microorganism	Method of immobilization	Measurement conditions	Type of biosensor	Detection limit	Detection range	Correlation coefficient	Detection time	Technique used	[Reference] (Year)
Streptavidin modified magnetic nanoparticles onto Au electrode	HIV	Streptavidin-biotin coupling	PBS buffer pH 7; frequency range between100 mHz and 100 kHz under a potential value of −300 mV, RT	–	50 pmol of HBV DNA and 160 pmol of HIV DNA	2.53–50.6 nmol ml^{-1}	–	–	EIS	[33] (2008)
CH/Fe_3O_4 nanobio-composite onto SPE	HIV-1	Covalent binding	CV: scan rate: 50 mV s^{-1}; potential range: −0.5 V to +0.2 V vs. SCE. SWV: frequency: 12.5 Hz; start potential: −0.6 V; end potential: +0.4 V; step: 8 mV; amplitude: 25 mV EIS: frequency range from 200 kHz to 10 mHz using 5 mV	–	50 pM	50–300 pM	–	–	EIS, SWV	[34] (2011)
Polyaniline-coated magnetic (EAPM) nanoparticle	*B. anthracis*	Physical adsorption	–		4.2×10^2 spores ml^{-1}	–	–	16 min	Resistance	[35] (2009)
Liposomes and Poly(3,4-ethylenedioxy-thiophene)-coated carbon nanotubes	Cholera	Covalent binding	PBS buffer, SWV	Electrochemical immunosensor	10^{-16} g/100 μl of 10^{-15} g ml^{-1}	10^{-14} to 10^{-7}g ml^{-1}		60 s	Square-wave voltammetry	[39] (2006)
Fe_3O_4 nanoparticles-coated carbon nanotubes nanocomposite	*E. coli*	Glutaraldehyde cross-linking	PBS (0.02 M, pH 7.0) with operating potential of −200 mV, CV, Scan rate: 100 mV s^{-1}	Amperometric tyrosinase biosensor	5.0×10^{-9} M	1.0×10^{-8} to 3.9×10^{-5} M	0.994	4 h		[40] (2009)

Carbon nanotube	*Salmonella infantis*,	Physical-dsorption	–	Field-effect transistors based immunosensor	100 CFU ml^{-1}	–	–	1 h	I–V measurement	[43] (2008)
Single walled carbon-nanotube	*E. coli*	Biotin–avidin coupling	–	Aptamer-based Field-Effect Transistors		10^5 to 10^7 CFU ml^{-1}	–	20 min	FET arrays combined with the most probable number (MPN) method	[44] (2008)
Fullerene into poly(methyl-methacrylate)	*E. coli*	Physical adsorption	0.02 M Tris–HCl buffer, pH 7.0, room temperature (RT)	–	–	–	–	–	DPV	[45] (2007)
Reduced graphene oxide	methicillin-resistant *S. aureus*	Electrostatic interaction	0.1 Hz to 100,000 Hz in the pH 7.4 phosphate buffer with 5 mV amplitude, RT	–	10^{-13} fM	10^{-6} to 10^{-14} M	–	30 min	EIS	[46] (2011)
CNT–DNA core-shell	*Mycobacterium tuberculosis*	Covalent binding	PBS; 0.05 M, pH 7.0, 10 ml 20 μM MB, 30 °C,	–	0.1 nM	0.2 mM to 0.1 nM	0.994	–	DPV	[47] (2012)
MWCNT onto SiO_2 grown Si wafer	Influenza virus A	Covalent binding	PBS, pH 7.5	–	0.5 nM	1–10 nM	–	4 min	EIS	[48] (2009)
(MWNTs–CoPc) and PAMAM	AIV	Covalent binding	TBS (20 mM Tris–HCl buffer solution, pH 7.0, 20 mM NaCl +0.30 V to +1.20 V pulse amplitude 0.1 V, pulse width 0.05 s, and pulse period 0.2 s	–	1.0 pg ml^{-1}	0.01–500 ng ml^{-1}	0.998	20 min	DPV	[49] (2009)

(Continues)

Table 8.1 (Continued)

Nanomaterials	Clinical diagnosis of microorganism	Method of immobilization	Measurement conditions	Type of biosensor	Detection limit	Detection range	Correlation coefficient	Detection time	Technique used	[Reference] (Year)
A PDMS/paper/glass hybrid microfluidic biochip	*Lactobacillus acidophilus, S. aureus* and *Salmonella enterica.*	Covalent binding	Fluorescence intensities, Cy3 optical filters (Ex = 550 nm; Em = 570 nm). 37° C	Aptamer Microfluidic sensor	11.0 CFU ml^{-1}, 61 CFU ml^{-1}, 800 CFU ml^{-1},	9.4–150.0 CFU ml^{-1}, 10^4 to 10^6 CFU ml^{-1}, 42.2–675.0 CFU ml^{-1}		99.7, 99.5, 99.3	Fluorescence	[50] (2013)
CNT deposited onto Si/SiO_2 substrate	Swine influenza virus H1N1	Avidin–biotin coupling	–	Electrical immunosensor	1 PFU ml^{-1}	1–1 × 10^4 PFU ml^{-1}	30 min	0.89, 0.94, 0.99	Resistance	[51] (2014)
PANI electrochemically deposited onto a Pt disk electrode	*E. coli*	Avidin–biotin coupling	20 μM MB pretreatment in phosphate buffer, 0.05 M, pH 7.0, at 0.1 V pulse height of 50 mV, and pulse width of 70 ms for 10 s , 30–45 °C	–	Artificial DNA-(0.009 ng μl^{-1}), *E. coli* genomic DNA-(0.01 ng μl^{-1}) and *E. coli* cells-11 cells ml^{-1}	0.0064–2.3 ngμl^{-1}	–	8–14 min, 60–360 s, 60 s	DPV	[52] (2007)
PANI	*Treponema pallidum*	Au–SH bond	5.0 mM $K_3Fe(CN)_6$/ $K_4Fe(CN)_6$ (1:1), 0.2 M KCl at a bias potential of +195 mV (vs. SCE), frequency range of 10^5–10^{-2} Hz	–	0.5 pM	1.0 pM and 1.0 nM	0.998	–	SWV, EIS	[53] (2010)
PANI/ITO	*N. gonorrhoeae*	Avidin–biotin coupling	Methylene blue at pulse height of 50 mV, pulse width of 70 ms in 0.05 M phosphate buffer of pH 7.0 containing 0.153 M NaCl, 25 °C	–	0.5 × 10^{-15} M	1 × 10^{-16} to 1 × 10^{-6} M	0.9974	60 s	DPV	[54] (2009)

PANI-MWCNT nanocomposite onto ITO electrode	*N. gonorrhoeae*	Covalent binding	Methylene blue at pulse height of 50 mV, pulse width of 70 ms in 0.05 M phosphate buffer of pH 7.0 containing 0.153 M NaCl, 25 °C	–	1.2×10^{-17} M	1×10^{-17} to 1×10^{-6} M	–	60 s	DPV	[55] (2010)
Polyaniline-iron oxide-carbon nanotubes nanobiocomposite	*N. gonorrhoeae*	Avidin–biotin coupling	20 μM methylene blue, pre-treatment at +0.1 V for 10 s, at step potential of 3 mV and modulation amplitude of 50 mV, 0.05 M PBS (pH 7.0, 0.9% NaCl)	DNA electro-chemical biosensor	1×10^{-19} M	1×10^{-19} M to 1×10^{-6} M	0.997	45 s	DPV	[56] (2012)
Polyaniline-iron oxide nanocomposite	*N. gonorrhoeae*	Glutaraldehyde as cross-linker	20 μM methylene blue, pre-treatment at +0.1 V for 10 s, at step potential of 3 mV and modulation amplitude of 50 mV, 0.05 M PBS (pH 7.0, 0.9% NaCl)	DNA electro-chemical biosensor	1×10^{-15} M, 1×10^{-17} M	1×10^{-16} M to 1×10^{-6} M, 1×10^{-18} M to 1×10^{-6} M	–	–	EIS, DPV	[57] (2012)
NanoZrO_2-CNT/ITO electrode	*M. tuberculosis*	Electrostatic interaction	$[Fe(CN)_6]^{3-/4-}$ in PBS pH 7.0	–	1×10^{-8} mM	1×10^{-2} to 1×10^{-8} mM	0.9 95	20 min	EIS	[58] (2011)
Sol–gel derived nano ZrO_2	*E. coli*	Electrostatic interaction	PBS, 50 mM, pH 7.0 and 0.7% NaCl, 20 μM MB	–	10^{-6} pM	10^{-6} to 10^{6} pM	0.993	–	DPV	[59] (2009)

8.4 Challenges and future prospects

The management of clinical diagnosis via pathogen detection using a simple, rapid and cost-effective method presents a major challenge to the biological safety of the world. The field of clinical diagnosis is nascent and therefore, faces a dynamic set of challenges as the field evolves. One of the major challenges in clinical diagnosis using electrochemical, electrochemiluminescent, magnetic, gravimetric, or optical biosensor design is to immobilize biomolecules onto an electrode substrate for effective signal transduction. Detecting pathogens using biosensors is a relatively new concept and many of the techniques discussed, are still in their infancy. Existing clinical diagnosis methods are time consuming and expensive, and consequently, demand for accurate clinical diagnosis via pathogenic biosensors by rapid detection systems is increasing. The electrochemical and optical techniques will probably become more popular as microelectronics and microfluidics also progress. Some techniques are restricted due to non-suitability in-field and requirement of highly trained personnel. Many of these methods currently have limitations involving sensor surface formation, reproducibility, renewability and necessary sample preparation. The immense efforts are needed to develop this comprehensive library of core techniques into practical diagnostic applications. The general basis of methods to detect binding pathogenic analytes to specific bioreceptors are available but require refinement and in some cases further miniaturization. The use of biomolecule-functionalized surfaces can drastically boost the specificity of the detection system, but may also pose reproducibility problems and increased complexity. Several nanobiosensor architecture-based mechanical devices, optical resonators, functionalized nanoparticles, nanowires, nanotubes, and nanofibers have been in use. As nanobiosensor technology becomes more refined and reliable, it will eventually make lab-on-a-chip devices for rapid screening of a wide variety of analyses at low cost. In particular, nanomaterials such as gold metal nanoparticles, carbon nanotubes, graphene, magnetic nanoparticles, and quantum dots have been actively investigated for their applications in biosensors, which have become a new interdisciplinary frontier for the application of clinical diagnosis.

The commercial biosensors for clinical diagnosis via pathogen detection are tips of the iceberg compared to the vast literature on academic research. The intrinsic disadvantages (slow response, low sensitivity, and poor selectivity) using bacteria and virus as the biosensing element limit the widespread interest of biosensors for pathogen detection on the market. Fortunately, with the amalgamation of biotechnology, nanotechnology, physics, chemistry, electronics, bioengineering, and novel immobilization strategy in the past years, biosensors for pathogen detection are becoming more powerful in the field of analytical chemistry.

8.5 Conclusions

In summary, recent developments of nanomaterials based biosensors for clinical diagnosis by detecting several pathogens as infectious diseases management at an early stage is currently of prime interest so as to circumvent the delay in diagnosis.

The incorporation of nanomaterial transducer with collaborative transducing elements opens up a new era for further development of novel biosensors for detecting a broad range of target analytes. Hence, the advantages of nanomaterials based biosensors over existing detection methodologies and the role of various immobilization matrices used for fabrication of nanomaterials based biosensors are discussed. The conventional pathogen detection methods are sensitive but still lag behind the analytical methods due to long response time and decreasing in the response time is a needle in a haystack problem. Besides this, efforts have been made to discuss the various techniques used for biosensor construction, the analytical performance of these biodevices for bacterial and viral pathogens for their applications to medical diagnosis. Recent developments in the buzzword 'nanotechnology' and material science can be advantageously used to obtain engineered and customerized nanomaterials that could provide novel platforms for immobilization of biorecognition component that may lead to the development of useful and reliable biosensor devices. And the use of microarray for simultaneous measurement with integrated microfluidic system may provide solution for the fabrication of smart low cost point-of-care devices in reliable pathogen detection. Efforts should be directed towards the synthesis of novel nanomaterials for the fabrication of electrochemical, optical and other biosensors on a large scale so as to benefit the mankind. With exposure of the commercial market the applications of the biosensor technology can be greatly enhanced and with time, miniaturized biosensor for pathogen detection may become available that could be used near a patient's bedside, a doctor's clinic or even home use.

Acknowledgments

This work was supported by Basic Science Research Program through the National Research Foundation of Korea (NRF) funded by the Ministry of Education, Science and Technology (2012R1A2A2A01012528).

References

[1] Wang J., Chen G., Jiang H., Li Z., Wang, X. 'Advances in nano-scaled biosensors for biomedical applications'. *Analyst.* 2013;**138**(16):4427–4435.

[2] Alharbi K.K., Al-sheikh, Y.A. 'Role and implications of nanodiagnostics in the changing trends of clinical diagnosis'. *Saudi Journal of Biological Sciences*. 2014;**21**(2):109–117.

[3] Hayat A., Catanante G., Marty, J.L. 'Current trends in nanomaterial-based amperometric biosensors'. *Sensors (Basel)*. 2014;**14**(12):23439–23461.

[4] Sajanlal P.R., Sreeprasad T.S., Samal A.K., Pradeep, T. 'Anisotropic nanomaterials: structure, growth, assembly, and functions'. *Nano Reviews*. 2011;**2**:5883–1–5883–62.

[5] Reid C.M., Mark L.S., Feinstein, A.R. 'Use of methodological standards in diagnostic test research. Getting better but still not good'. *The Journal of American Medical Association*. 1995;**274**(8):645–651.

[6] Park K.W., Choi J.H., Kwon B.K., Lee S.A., Sung, Y.E. 'Chemical and electronic effects of Ni in Pt/Ni and Pt/Ru/Ni alloy nanoparticles in methanol electrooxidation'. *Journal of Physical Chemistry B.* 2002;**106**(8):1869–1877.

[7] El-Deab M.S., Ohsaka, T. 'An extraordinary electrocatalytic reduction of oxygen on gold nanoparticles-electrodeposited gold electrodes'. *Electrochemistry Communications.* 2002;**4**(4):288–292.

[8] Liu T., Tang J., Jiang, L. 'The enhancement effect of gold nanoparticles as a surface modifier on DNA sensor sensitivity'. *Biochemical and Biophysical Research Communications.* 2005;**313**(1):3–7.

[9] Sperling R.A., Rivera Gil P., Zhang F., Zanella M., Parak, W.J. 'Biological applications of gold nanoparticles'. *Chemical Society Reviews.* 2008;**37** (9):1896–1908.

[10] Hrapovic S., Liu Y., Male K.B., Luong, J.H. 'Electrochemical biosensing platforms using platinum nanoparticles and carbon nanotubes'. *Analytical Chemistry.* 2004;**76**(4):1083–1088.

[11] Zhang X., Su H., Bi S., Li S., Zhang, S., 'DNA-based amplified electrical bio-barcode assay for one-pot detection of two target DNAs'. *Biosensors and Bioelectronics.* 2009;**24**(8):2730–2734.

[12] Cheong K.H., Yi D.K., Lee J.G., *et al.* 'Gold nanoparticles for one step DNA extraction and real-time PCR of pathogens in a single chamber'. *Lab on a Chip.* 2008;**8**(5):810–813.

[13] Chua A.L., Yean C.Y., Ravichandran M., Lim B.H., Lalitha, P. 'A rapid DNA biosensor for the molecular diagnosis of infectious disease'. *Biosensors and Bioelectronics.* 2011;**26**(9):3825–3831.

[14] Hao R.Z., Song H.B., Zuo G.M., *et al.*, 'DNA probe functionalized QCM biosensor based on gold nanoparticle amplification for Bacillus anthracis detection'. *Biosensors and Bioelectronics.* 2011;**26**(8):3398–3404.

[15] Hoa X.D., Kirk A.G., Tabrizian, M. 'Towards integrated and sensitive surface plasmon resonance biosensors: a review of recent progress'. *Biosensors and Bioelectronics.* 2007;**23**(2):151–160.

[16] Wang, J. 'Amplified transduction of biomolecular interactions based on the use of nanomaterials'. *Advances in Biochemical Engineering/Biotechnology.* 2008;**109**:239–254

[17] Joung H.A., Lee N.R., Lee S.K., *et al.*, 'High sensitivity detection of 16s rRNA using peptide nucleic acid probes and a surface plasmon resonance biosensor'. *Analytica Chimica Acta.* 2008;**630**(2):168–173

[18] Wang R., Xue C., Gao M., Qi H., Zhang, C. 'Ultratrace voltammetric method for the detection of DNA sequence related to human immunodeficiency virus type 1'. *Microchimica Acta.* 2011;**172**(3–4):291–297.

[19] Chen X., Xie H., Seow Z.Y., Gao, Z. 'An ultrasensitive DNA biosensor based on enzyme-catalyzed deposition of cupric hexacyanoferrate nanoparticles'. *Biosensors and Bioelectronics.* 2010;**25**(6):1420–1426.

[20] Luz R.A.S., Iost R.M., Crespilho, F.N. 'Nanomaterials for biosensors and implantable biodevices'. *Nanobioelectrochemistry* (Springer-Verlag Berlin Heidelberg). 2013;27–48.

[21] Xing Y., Rao, J. 'Quantum dot bioconjugates for in vitro diagnostics & in vivo imaging'. *Cancer Biomarker.* 2008;**4**(6):307–319.
[22] Fan H., Ju P., Ai, S. 'Controllable synthesis of CdSe nanostructures with tunable morphology and their application in DNA biosensor of Avian Influenza Virus'. *Sensors and Actuators B.* 2010;**149**(1):98–104.
[23] Roh, C. 'Facile inhibitor screening of hepatitis C virus NS3 protein using nanoparticle-based RNA'. *Biosensors.* 2012;**2**(4):427–432.
[24] Alvi N.H., Gomez V.J., Soto Rodriguez P.E.D., *et al.*, 'An InN/InGaN quantum dot electrochemical biosensor for clinical diagnosis'. *Sensors.* 2013;**13**(10):13917–13927.
[25] Liu Y.J., Yao D.J., Chang H.Y., Liu C.M., Chen, C. 'Magnetic bead-based DNA detection with multi-layers quantum dots labeling for rapid detection of *Escherichia coli* O157:H7'. *Biosensors and Bioelectronics.* 2008;**24** (4):558–565.
[26] Koh I., Josephson, L. 'Magnetic nanoparticle sensors'. *Sensors* (Basel). 2009;**9**(10):8130–8145.
[27] Hofmann-Amtenbrink M., Hofmann H., Montet, X. 'Superparamagnetic nanoparticles-a tool for early diagnostics'. *Swiss Medical Weekly.* 2010;**140** (w13081):1–8.
[28] Shen W., Schrag B.D., Carter M.J., Xiao, G. 'Quantitative detection of DNA labeled with magnetic nanoparticles using arrays of MgO-based magnetic tunnel junction sensors'. *Applied Physics Letters.* 2008;**93**:033903.
[29] Lowery T.J., Palazzolo R., Wong S.M., Prado P.J., Taktak, S. 'Single-coil, multisample, proton relaxation method for magnetic relaxation switch assays'. *Analytical Chemistry.* 2008;**80**(4):1118–1123.
[30] Koets M., van der Wijk T., van Eemeren J.T.W.M., van Amerongen A., Prins, M.W.J. 'Rapid DNA multi-analyte immunoassay on a magneto-resistance biosensor'. *Biosensensors and Bioelectronics.* 2009;**24** (7):1893–1898.
[31] Mujika M., Arana S.Castaño E., *et al.*, 'Magnetoresistive immunosensor for the detection of Escherichia coli O157:H7 including a microfluidic network'. *Biosensensors and Bioelectronics.* 2009;**24**(5):1253–1258.
[32] Singh R., Verma R., Kaushik A., *et al.*, 'Chitosan-iron oxide nano-composite platform for mismatch-discriminating DNA hybridization for detection of *Neisseria gonorrhoeae* causing sexually transmitted disease'. *Biosensensors and Bioelectronics.* 2011;**26**(6):2967–2974.
[33] Hassen W.M., Chaix C., Abdelghani A., Bessueille F., Leonard D., Jaffrezic-Renault, N. 'An impedimetric DNA sensor based on functionalized magnetic nanoparticles for HIV and HBV detection'. *Sensors and Actuators B.* 2008;**134**(2) 755–760.
[34] Tran L.D., Nguyen B.H., Hieu N.V., Tran H.V., Nguyen H.L., Nguyen, P.X. 'Electrochemical detection of short HIV sequences on chitosan/Fe_3O_4 nanoparticle based screen printed electrodes'. *Materials Science and Engineering C.* 2011;**31**(2):477–485.

[35] Pal S., Alocilja, E.C. 'Electrically active polyaniline coated magnetic (EAPM) nanoparticle as novel transducer in biosensor for detection of Bacillus anthracis spores in food samples'. *Biosensensors and Bioelectronics.* 2009;**24**(5):1437–1444.

[36] Rivas G.A., Rubianes M.D., Rodriguez M.C., *et al.* 'Carbon nanotubes for electrochemical biosensing'. *Talanta.* 2007;**74**(3):291–307.

[37] Sinha N., Ma J., Yeow, J.T. 'Carbon nanotube-based sensors'. *Journal of Nanoscience and Nanotechnology.* 2006;**6**(3):573–590.

[38] Wang, J. 'Nanomaterial-based electrochemical biosensors'. *Analyst* (Cambridge, UK). 2005;**130**(4):421–426.

[39] Viswanathan S., Wu L.C., Huang M.R., Ho, J.A. 'Electrochemical immunosensor for cholera toxin using liposomes and poly(3,4-ethylenedioxythiophene)-coated carbon nanotubes'. *Analytical Chemistry.* 2006;**78**(4):1115–1121.

[40] Cheng Y., Liu Y., Huang J., *et al.*, 'Amperometric tyrosinase biosensor based on Fe_3O_4 nanoparticles-coated carbon nanotubes nanocomposite for rapid detection of coliforms'. *Electrochimica Acta.* 2009;**54**(9):2588–2594.

[41] Chen, Z.G. 'Conductometric immunosensors for the detection of staphylococcal enterotoxin B based bio-electrocalytic reaction on micro-comb electrodes'. *Bioprocess and Biosystems Engineering.* 2008;**31**(4):345–350.

[42] Gruner, G. 'Carbon nanotube transistors for biosensing applications'. *Analytical and Bioanalytical Chemistry.* 2006;**384**(2):322–335.

[43] Villamizar R.A., Maroto A., Rius F.X., Inza I., Figueras, M.J. 'Fast detection of Salmonella Infantis with carbon nanotube field effect transistors'. *Biosensensors and Bioelectronics.* 2008;**24**(2):279–283.

[44] So H.M., Park D.W., Jeon E.K., *et al.*, 'Detection and titer estimation of *Escherichia coli* using aptamer-functionalized single-walled carbon-nanotubes field-effect transistors'. *Small.* 2008;**4**(2):197–201.

[45] Shiraishi H., Itoh T., Hayashi H., *et al.*, 'Electrochemical detection of *E. coli* 16S rDNA sequence using air-plasma-activated fullerene-impregnated screen printed electrodes'. *Bioelectrochemistry.* 2007;**70**(2):481–487.

[46] Wang Z., Zhang J., Chen P., *et al.*, 'Label-free, electrochemical detection of methicillin-resistant staphylococcus aureus DNA with reduced graphene oxide-modified electrodes'. *Biosensensors and Bioelectronics.* 2011;**26**(9):3881–3886.

[47] Das M., Dhand C., Sumana G., Srivastava A.K., Nagarajan R., Malhotra, B.D. 'Electrophoretically fabricated core-shell CNT-DNA biowires for biosensing'. *Journal of Material Chemistry.* 2012;**22**(1):2727–2732.

[48] Tam P.D., Hieu N.V., Chien N.D., Le A.T., Tuan, A.T. 'DNA sensor development based on multi-wall carbon nanotubes for label-free influenza virus type A detection'. *Journal of Immunological Methods.* 2009;**350**(1–2):118–124.

[49] Zhu X., Ai S., Chen Q., Yin H., Xu, J. 'Label-free electrochemical detection of Avian Influenza Virus genotype utilizing multi-walled carbon

nanotubes–cobalt phthalocyanine–PAMAM nanocomposite modified glassy carbon electrode'. *Electrochemistry Communication.* 2009;**11**(7):1543–1546.

[50] Zuo P., Li X., Dominguez D., Ye, B.C. 'A PDMS/paper/glass hybrid microfluidic biochip integrated with aptamer-functionalized graphene oxide nano-biosensors for one-step multiplexed pathogen detection'. *Lab on a Chip.* 2013;**13**(19):3921–3828.

[51] Singh R., Sharma A., Hong S., Jang, J. 'Electrical immunosensor based on dielectrophoretically-deposited carbon nanotubes for detection of influenza virus H1N1'. *Analyst.* 2014;**139**(21):5415–5421.

[52] Arora K., Prabhakar N., Chand S., Malhotra, B.D. '*Escherichia coli* genosensor based on polyaniline'. *Analytical Chemistry.* 2007;**79**(16): 6152–6158.

[53] Sheng Q., Wang J., Zheng J., Xu Z., Zhang, H., 'Ultrasensitive electrical biosensing of syphilis DNA using target-guided formation of polyaniline based on enzyme-catalyzed polymerization'. *Biosensors and Bioelectronics.* 2010;**25**(9):2071–2077.

[54] Singh R., Prasad R., Sumana G., *et al.*, 'STD sensor based on nucleic acid functionalized nanostructured polyaniline'. *Biosensors and Bioelectronics.* 2009;**24**(7):2232–2238.

[55] Singh R., Dhand C., Sumana G., *et al.*, 'Polyaniline/carbon nanotubes platform for sexually transmitted disease detection'. *Journal of Molecular Recognition.* 2010;**23**(5):472–479.

[56] Singh R., Verma R., Sumana G., *et al.*, 'Nanobiocomposite platform based on polyaniline-iron oxide-carbon nanotubes for bacterial detection'. *Bioelectrochemistry.* 2012;**86**:30–37.

[57] Singh R., Matharu Z., Srivastava A.K., Sood S., Gupta R.K., Malhotra, B.D. 'Nanostructured platform for the detection of *Neisseria gonorrhoeae* using electrochemical impedance spectroscopy and differential pulse voltammetry'. *Microchim Acta.* 2012;**177**(1–2):201–210.

[58] Das M., Dhand C., Sumana G., *et al.*, 'Zirconia grafted carbon nanotubes based biosensor for *M. Tuberculosis* detection'. *Applied Physics Letters.* 2011;**99**:143702–143703.

[59] Solanki P.R., Kaushik A., Chavhan P.M., Maheshwari S.N., Malhotra, B.D. 'Nanostructured zirconium oxide based genosensor for *Escherichia coli* detection'. *Electrochemistry Communication.* 2009;**11**(12):2272–2277.

[60] Ansari A.A., Singh R., Sumana G., Malhotra, B.D. 'Sol–gel derived nanostructured zinc oxide film for sexually transmitted disease sensor'. *Analyst.* 2009;**134**(5):997–1002.

Chapter 9

Optical waveguide-based biosensor for label-free monitoring of living cells

N. Orgovan[1,2], B. Szabó[1,2] and R. Horvath[1]

Abstract

Here, we briefly discuss the past, present, and possible future of label-free optical biosensors in cell research, especially focusing on the kinetic monitoring of cellular adhesion. Currently available optical biosensors possess outstanding potentials still not rightfully recognized and still waiting to be fully exploited in the field of cell science. Thus, during the description we give special emphasis to the advantages that the state-of-the-art optical cell-based biosensors possess as compared to microscope- or force measurement-based techniques widely used to characterize cell adhesion. To name here only a few, they enable label-free detection close to a planar sensor surface, have high sensitivity, and generate superior quality kinetic data. Such information-rich kinetic data, in turn, can be analyzed in-depth and comparatively. To exemplify the importance of in-depth kinetic analysis, we review a recent study, in which the Epic BenchTop high-throughput optical biosensor was used to measure the dependence of cancer cell adhesion kinetics on the surface density of integrin ligands. Based on the kinetic data, a model enabling the label-free determination of the dissociation constant of the adhesion ligands bound to their native cell membrane receptors has been constructed. As an outlook, the perspectives of the technology is briefly discussed.

9.1 Label-free optical biosensors in cell adhesion research

Cell adhesion is a fundamental biological process during which a cell anchors itself to a suitable surface and spreads on it, obtaining a well-spread morphology characteristic to the cell type. Cell adhesion plays cardinal roles on the level of individual cells – e.g. in intracellular signaling [1, 2], migration [3], proliferation [4], differentiation [5],

[1]Nanobiosensorics Group, Hungarian Academy of Sciences for Energy Research, Institute for Technical Physics and Materials Science, H-1120 Budapest, Hungary
[2]Department of Biological Physics, Eötvös University, H-1117 Budapest, Hungary

gene expression [6], and in general, cell fate determination [7] – as well on the level of multicellular organisms – e.g. in cell–cell communication [8], immune function [9, 10], cancer development [11, 12], or in the initiation and pathogenesis of bacterial [13] and viral diseases [14]. For decades the phenomenon of cell adhesion has thus been enjoying the ever-increasing scientific interest of various inter-disciplinary fields, including materials science, pharmacology, biophysics, and more, both in basic and applied research. This prominent attention has stimulated many technological developments which gave rise to new techniques or modified already existing ones, all to enable a more detailed characterization of cell adhesion. Based on the approach they use, these can be classified into three main groups.

First, a class of techniques attempts to characterize cell adhesion in the most direct manner: by quantifying cell-exerted forces. Some of these techniques measure the adhesion force by actually detaching the cell from its substrate (e.g. flow chamber [15, 16], variants of atomic force microscopy [17, 18], or micropipette [19]), while others characterize cell-exerted forces through the cell-caused deformations of an elastic substrate (variants of cell traction force microscopy and their predecessors [20, 21]).

In contrast, another class of techniques focuses on the visualization and/or tracking of the cell and its adhesion-associated subcellular structures (e.g. those of filamentous actin, or focal adhesion components) [22]. Visualization is performed under a microscope (e.g. wide-field, confocal, electron, or total internal reflection microscope), which is subsequently followed by in-depth image analysis [22].

Surface-sensitive label-free optical biosensors constituting the third class of techniques are relative newcomers to cell adhesion science [23]. (Although impedance-based label-free biosensors can also be used to measure cell adhesion, space limitations force us to omit them from this discussion. For references, see [24, 25].) Several members of the family have been shown to be able to measure cell adhesion, including surface plasmon resonance (SPR) [26, 27], optical waveguide lightmode spectroscopy (OWLS) [28–31], photonic crystal (PC) biosensors [32], and resonant waveguide grating (RWG, or more commonly recognized as Epic) biosensors [33, 34]. Albeit they have been on the horizon for a considerable time, and albeit they offer promising potentials to the field, their introduction to cell adhesion research has been long delayed. This was partially due to the aversion that encompassed their unselective detection mechanism [35]; they are sensitive to any process which is accompanied by refractive index (RI) changes in a thin layer closest to the sensor surface [28]. For this, they have often been referred as black boxes, and their signal has been considered obscure and difficult to interpret [35]. However, with an appropriate surface chemistry and rigorous experimental controls in hand, such biosensors can readily and specifically measure the adherency of a population of cells. Indeed, the biosensor signal integrates changes in both the size of the sensor area covered by cells and the optical density therein (i.e. it depends on the density of filamentous actin near the surface, and on the number and size of focal adhesions), which makes the signal an excellent single measure of cell adherency. Further reasons for the delay in permeation of optical biosensorics to cell science have been (i) the lack of high-throughput in the case of the first-generation and (ii) the high cost in the case of the second-generation instruments

(SPR, OWLS, and PC, Epic systems, respectively). Accordingly, first-generation platforms were not suitable for cutting-edge cell (adhesion) research, since single measurements conducted hours apart could be hardly compared due to the inter-experimental variability inherent to living cells. In contrast, second-generation systems were microplate-based high-throughput biosensors, but the first of their kind was an expensive platform with integrated robotics, and hence predominantly only some pharmaceutical companies could afford to buy it.

With the recent commercialization of the small-footprint next-generation optical biosensor, the Epic BenchTop (Epic BT) [33, 36] (and with the permeation of the EnSpire benchtop multimodal microtiter plate reader, which combines Epic label-free technology with labeling technologies), we expect the long-stand *status quo* to change soon, i.e. the potentials of label-free biosensorics to be rightfully recognized and exploited in cell science. In particular, Epic BT offers the following set of advantages: it (i) detects RI changes only in an approximately 150 nm thick layer closest to a planar sensor surface (which is the most relevant in cell adhesion) [28, 36]; (ii) produces an integrated signal which is an excellent single measure of cell adherence [31, 37]; (iii) does not require labeling of any kind to monitor cell behavior; (iv) as a microplate-based system, offers high-throughput detection; (v) yields superior quality kinetic data, which can be subjected to in-depth kinetic analysis [34]. This latter feature in itself is such that the microscope- or force measurement-based techniques can hardly compete with. At the same time, however, it is becoming increasingly evident that kinetic analysis is the key to a more detailed characterization of the effect of e.g. substrate modifications or drug treatments on cellular behavior, including cell adhesion. Given their high sensitivity, surface-sensitive evanescent field-based techniques can detect not only large-scale, but also tiny variations during adhesion, thus molecular movements and rearrangements in the basal membrane of the adhered cells can be monitored in real time. These dynamic changes are often termed as dynamic mass redistribution (DMR) in the literature [23, 33, 38–40]. The conceptually different types of DMRs are briefly summarized in Figure 9.1.

The forthcoming years may bring further innovations to commercially available label-free optical biosensors, so they could e.g. (i) measure the adhesion and signaling of single cells; (ii) combine high-throughput detection with multi-mode waveguides enabling depth profiling of cell RI variations [30]; or (iii) use flow-through microfluidics in a high-throughput arrangement [38, 41].

9.2 The Epic BenchTop optical biosensor

The Epic BT system (Corning Incorporated, Corning, NY, USA) is an evanescent field-based optical biosensor [42] enabling high-throughput label-free detection at a solid–liquid interface [23, 33, 36, 40]. It accepts 96- or 384-well *Society for Biomolecular Screening* (SBS) standard format biosensor microplates. The bottom of an Epic microplate serves as a planar optical waveguide – i.e. a thin, high refractive-index, transparent dielectric layer (waveguide layer, made of the biocompatible material niobium pentoxide [43]) on a thicker substratum. At the

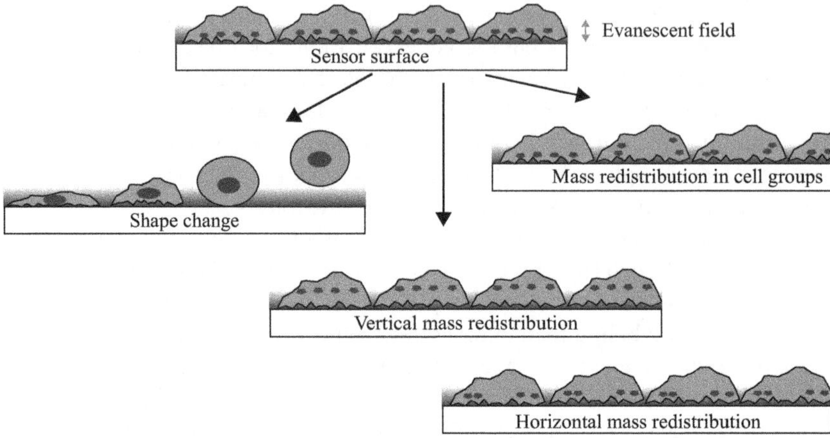

Figure 9.1 Schematic illustration of cell activity detection with label-free optical biosensors. Practically, all types of cellular activities are accompanied by dynamic mass redistributions (DMRs), which in turn generally cause a net change in the local refractive index. A detectable change occurring in the sensing layer of the biosensor (evanescent field, illuminating only the bottom ~150 nm high portion of cells) provokes a biosensor response (e.g. a spreading curve). Conceptually, four types of mass redistributions can be distinguished. Considerable changes in cell shape involve large-scale DMRs in directions both vertical and horizontal to the planar sensor surface. This is the case during cell spreading when spherical cells enter the sensing layer, which is followed by cell attachment to, and cell spreading on the appropriately prepared sensor surface. In contrast, cells already spread on the sensor surface can exhibit intracellular DMR which is dominant in either the vertical or horizontal direction, while the cell shape does not change considerably. Typically this is the case when spread cells are stimulated or treated with highly specific effector molecules. The detection of horizontal DMR within cells requires a high spatial-resolution biosensor, a kind which is currently not commercially available. Still, biosensors with modest spatial resolution are already successfully used to detect larger scale spatial variances in DMR responses (e.g. when a group of cells respond to a treatment, others not)

position of each well, an optical grating is embedded into the waveguide layer to enable the incoupling of the illuminating light; thus separate biosensors are created. Incoupled light beams undergo total internal reflections at the inner surfaces of the waveguide layer, and gain a phase shift upon each reflection. The extent of the acquired phase shift depends on the RI of the medium being closest to the reflecting surface (because an exponentially decaying electromagnetic field, called an evanescent field, penetrates into a ~150 nm thick layer of the neighboring medium and probes the local RI [28, 44]). Light beams incoupled by the same grating interfere with each other, but only positive interference results in wave-guiding. This criterion is met only at a certain illuminating wavelength, called the resonant wavelength (λ). Any process accompanied by RI-variations in the ~150 nm thick layer over the biosensor surface alters the acquired phase shift when the beams undergo reflections at the waveguide layer–sample interface. This untunes the resonance, but waveguiding can resume at an illuminating wavelength $\lambda' \neq \lambda$. The primary signal output by the Epic BT system is the shift of the resonant wavelength ($\Delta\lambda = \lambda' - \lambda$) in each well.

In practice, all wells of an Epic microplate are simultaneously read out every 3 s by sweeping the illuminating wavelength through a range of 15000 pm with 0.25 pm precision [42]. The guided wavelength is outcoupled by the same grating used for incoupling, and the resonant wavelength distribution within each well is imaged with a spatial resolution of ~90 μm using a complementary metal-oxide semiconductor (CMOS) camera. The small footprint and tolerance to high temperatures of the Epic BT allows it to be placed into a non-humidified cell incubator and, therefore, a better approximation of the *in vivo* environmental conditions can be provided for the investigated cells.

9.3 Cell adhesion on tailored surfaces

In a work described previously, we aimed at measuring and characterizing the dependence of cell adhesion kinetics on the surface density of adhesion ligands in a label-free manner [34]. As such, the work fitted into a hot multidisciplinary research topic concerned with the relative relevance of individual substrate properties in cell behavior determination. Tailoring of a given substrate property – either biochemical (e.g. the density, orientation, or variability of adhesion ligands) or physical (e.g. elasticity, hidrophobicity, or topography) – without affecting all the others is generally a challenging task. Similarly so is the proper and detailed quantitative characterization of the effects of this modification on cell behavior.

Given the relative ease it can be accomplished with, many have tuned the surface density of adhesion ligands (especially that of the RGD tripeptide) and investigated how the cells respond [45–49]. Various approaches enable the average surface density of the RGD motif (arginine-glycine-aspartic acid, a minimal integrin recognition sequence present in several key proteins of the extracellular matrix [50, 51]) to be tuned at will [45–49]. However, one of the most intriguing recent studies has relied on an advanced technique, called block copolymer micelle nanolithography, to enable the RGD motifs to be positioned in a *strict nanoscale order* on a planar surface [52]. As it has turned out, the degree of ordering has a substantial impact on cell spreading. Cell attachment and spreading on an *ordered* nanopattern of ligands were highly restricted when the ligand spacing was increased beyond ~70 nm. In contrast, *randomly* distributed ligands with an average interligand distance of more than 92 nm were still able to promote marked cell spreading [52]. It has been claimed that the failure of cell spreading in the former case was due to the overly large interligand distances restricting effective integrin clustering, and the spreading observed in the latter case could be attributed to locally higher ligand densities that were sufficient to promote clustering.

Notwithstanding the impressive work done in the field, it seems like most investigations got stuck at the level of quantifying cell adhesion and spreading at a single time point and, therefore, could only imperfectly describe the effect of substrate modifications (e.g. adhesion-enhancing or -inhibitory). The dynamic aspects of adhesion and spreading have hitherto very rarely been considered [45, 46, 53, 54], mainly because only few techniques enable these processes to be monitored with adequate data quality, especially without the incorporation of labels that may potentially perturb cellular behavior.

9.4 The dependence of cell adhesion kinetics on the surface density of integrin ligands, as measured with the Epic BT biosensor

As mentioned earlier, surface-sensitive label-free biosensors are inherently capable of generating good quality kinetic data. Thus, we used Corning's next-generation high-throughput optical biosensor, the Epic BT, to measure the dependence of cell adhesion kinetics on the average surface density of RGD motifs (for the original report, see Reference [34]). The protocol and workflow for a typical label-free cell adhesion assay utilizing the Epic BT is detailed in a recent book chapter [55].

To tune the average surface density of RGD motifs, we used two copolymers, the biologically inactive PLL-*g*-PEG (poly(L-lysine)-graft-poly(ethylene glycol)), and its RGD-functionalized counterpart, PLL-*g*-PEG-RGD. If immobilized on a surface, the former functions as a protein-resistant and cell-repellent agent [56], while the latter is selectively recognized by a subgroup of adhesion receptor integrins [57], and thus induces cell adhesion [48]. The copolymers were immobilized on the biosensors (Epic microplate wells) via room-temperature physisorption from coating solutions. Coating solutions were obtained by mixing the stock solutions of PLL-*g*-PEG and PLL-*g*-PEG-RGD (both dissolved to a final concentration of 1 mg ml^{-1}) in the desired ratios. As described earlier [34], the surface density of RGD motifs was tuned by varying the volume percent Q of the PLL-*g*-PEG-RGD solution in the mixed solution of copolymers. The average surface density of RGD ligands (ν_{RGD}), as well as the average RGD-to-RGD distance ($d_{RGD-RGD}$) could be easily calculated using Q and the molecular quantities characterizing the composition of the copolymers [34, 49]. (When discussing trend-like effects of RGD-tuning, ν_{RGD} and $d_{RGD-RGD}$ are freely interchanged in further text.) In the work described in Reference [34], ν_{RGD} was tuned over four orders of magnitude.

Having the surfaces prepared, the microplate wells were given assay buffer (HBSS with 20 mM HEPES). Next, we established a baseline with the biosensor, then introduced the suspension of HeLa cells into the wells. All experiments were done in triplicates. After 2 h, the biosensor signals saturated and thus the biosensor experiment was terminated. A single set of obtained signals is shown in Figure 9.2. As it is seen, surfaces with an average interligand distance of 147 nm were already able to mildly induce cell adhesion (Figure 9.2). Maximum biosensor responses ($\Delta\lambda_{max}$) increased as a response to decreasing the interligand distance until saturation was reached at around $d_{RGD-RGD} \approx 10$ nm. The saturation is not surprising considering that the diameter of an integrin in the cell membrane is 8–12 nm [52], thus ligands closer to each other than this cannot be simultaneously bound.

Given the high resolution of the data set, it could be subjected to kinetic analysis. All the obtained spreading curves followed a symmetrical sigmoid shape, which can be described by the following logistic equation [58]:

$$\Delta\lambda(t) = \frac{\Delta\lambda_{max}}{1 + \exp(-r(t-m))}, \tag{9.1}$$

where $\Delta\lambda_{max}$ is the signal value at the maximum (plateau) of the spreading curve, r is the rate constant of spreading, and m is the time at which the ordinate is exactly $\Delta\lambda_{max}/2$. We used (9.1) to fit each individual data sequence (and not the averaged

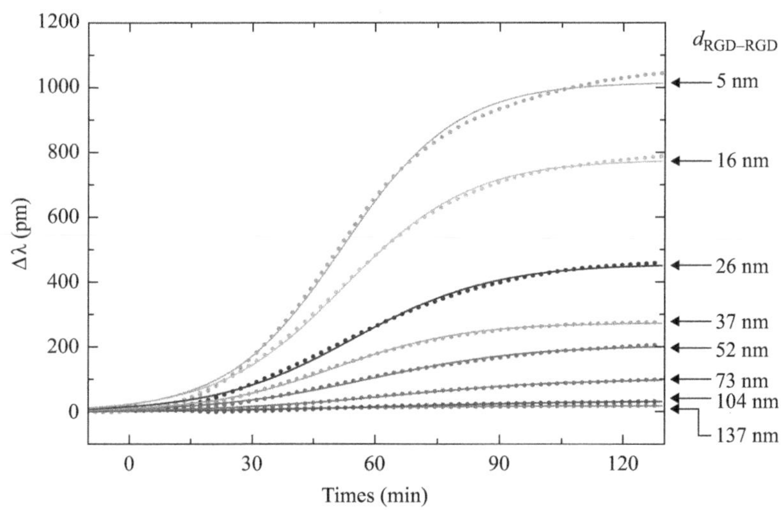

Figure 9.2 Spreading curves (the resonant wavelength shift Δλ as a function of time) provoked by HeLa cells, as was measured with the Epic BT at different RGD surface densities. The average interligand distances are indicated on the right side of the figure: cells on higher RGD-density surfaces induced higher biosensor signals. Dots: individual spreading curves registered by the Epic BT. Solid curves: fits. Note, that only one series of curves is shown, and some data and the corresponding fits have been omitted from this figure to avoid crowding and overlaps. Figure is replotted from Reference [34]

curves of triplicates, Figure 9.2), then the fitting parameters ($\Delta\lambda_{max}$ and r) of triplicates were averaged and their mean values were plotted against ν_{RGD} and $d_{RGD-RGD}$.

r was found to be practically independent of the surface density of RGD motifs (not shown) [34]. This was in accordance with a previous report [46], where substrata were coated with varying amounts of fibronectin, and the rate of contact area increase of isotropically spreading fibroblasts was measured with TIRFM. We have proposed that r most probably depended on the growth of the filopodia governed by actin polymerization and was therefore naturally independent from ν_{RGD} [34].

In contrast to r, the maximum biosensor response ($\Delta\lambda_{max}$) did depend on the average surface density of RGD motifs (ν_{RGD}) (Figure 9.3) [59]. The backgrounds of this dependency can be understood in the light of previous findings [52, 60]. It has earlier been shown that if the RGD surface density is decreased, cell adhesion diminishes either abruptly (there is a critical interligand distance) or successively, depending on whether the RGD motifs are positioned in a strict nanoscale order or at random. In our case, the nanoscale distribution of the RGD motifs was disordered, but not completely random: the adsorption of the PLL-*g*-PEG-RGD molecules corresponded to a random deposition of islands, each with an average of 3 RGD motifs. Still, this dispersion resulted in a highly disordered RGD distribution, and thus the observed successive decrease of cell adhesion with decreasing ν_{RGD} is in nice

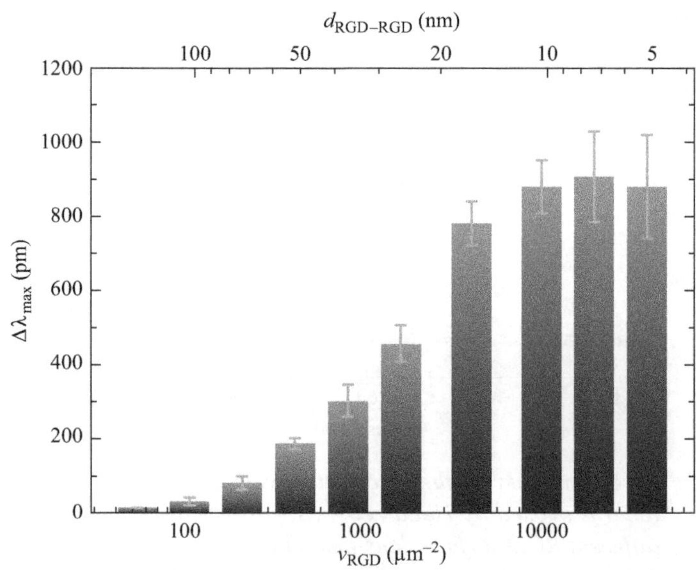

Figure 9.3 Maximum biosensor response ($\Delta\lambda_{max}$) as a function of the average surface density of RGD motifs (ν_{RGD}, bottom axis) and as a function of the average interligand distance ($d_{RGD-RGD}$, top axis). Error bars represent the standard deviation from the mean. Figure is replotted from Reference [34]

agreement with expectations [52]. In further accordance with previous findings [52], we obtained the maximum biosensor response at around an average interligand distance of 10 nm–indeed, separation distances smaller than the diameter of an integrin in the cell membrane (8–12 nm) cannot possibly increase the biosensor response further.

To further analyze the dependence of $\Delta\lambda_{\max}$ on ν_{RGD}, we assumed that the receptor–ligand interaction can be described as a monovalent binding reaction [34]. Denoting the surface concentrations of the unbound receptor (integrin), unbound ligand (RGD), and that of their bound form as R, L and B, respectively, the receptor–ligand reaction can be described as:

$$R + L \underset{k_{\mathrm{d}}}{\overset{k_{\mathrm{a}}}{\rightleftharpoons}} B. \tag{9.2}$$

According to the kinetic mass action law (KMAL), in equilibrium the attachment and detachment reactions (characterized by two-dimensional rate coefficients k_{a} and k_{d}, respectively) have equal rates:

$$B_{\mathrm{eqm}} = \frac{L_0 R_0}{L_0 + {}^{2D}K_{\mathrm{d}}}, \tag{9.3}$$

where $L_0 = L + B$ and $R_0 = R + B$ (i.e. $R_0 = \nu_{\mathrm{RGD}}$), and ${}^{2D}K_{\mathrm{d}} = k_{\mathrm{d}}/k_{\mathrm{a}}$ is the two-dimensional dissociation constant. Supposing that B_{eqm} was directly proportional to the optical response measured at saturation ($\Delta\lambda_{\max}$), and fitting the data plotted as $\Delta\lambda_{\max}$ *vs.* ν_{RGD} (Figure 9.4) with (9.3), we found that ${}^{2D}K_{\mathrm{d}} = 1753 \pm 243\ \mu\mathrm{m}^{-2}$.

The relationship between the two- and three-dimensional dissociation constants is given as:

$${}^{3D}K_{\mathrm{d}} = \frac{{}^{2D}K_{\mathrm{d}}}{l_{\mathrm{c}}}, \tag{9.4}$$

where l_{c} is a characteristic length of the interacting system, often referred to as confinement length [61, 62]. We proposed l_{c} to be the average cell-substrate separation distance [34]. The extent of separation is the result of the combined effect of nonspecific repulsion and specific bonding forces between the cell and the underlying substrate [61]. Various techniques have been utilized to determine the separation distance, and the obtained average values are typically in the range of 40–160 nm [63–65]. Lacking more precise information, we assumed an average separation distance and an equivalent confinement length of $l_{\mathrm{c}} = 100$ nm.

Using (9.4), the estimated value of the three-dimensional dissociation constant is ${}^{3D}K_{\mathrm{d}} \approx 30\ \mu\mathrm{M}$. In comparison, $\alpha IIb\beta3$ integrins incorporated into a lipid planar bilayer have shown to have an affinity of 1.7 μM for an RGD-containing linear peptide (having a very similar amino acid sequence to that used to functionalize the PEG-chains) [66]. The roughly twentyfold discrepancy between this value and ours can be attributed to differences between the investigated systems. First, the platelet integrin $\alpha IIb\beta3$ is unlikely to have the exact same affinity for the same linear

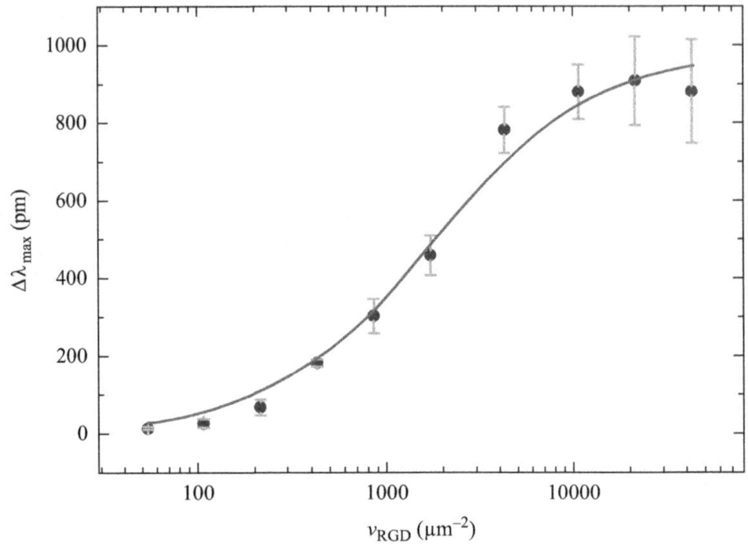

Figure 9.4 *The maximum wavelength shift provoked by cells ($\Delta\lambda_{max}$) as a function of the surface density of RGD motifs (ν_{RGD}), and the fit performed to derive the two-dimensional dissociation constant. Fitting (9.3) (solid line) describing the equilibrium of single-step monovalent binding to the data yielded a 2D dissociation constant of* $^{2D}K_d = 1753 \pm 243 \mu m^{-2}$ *for the binding between integrins embedded in their native (cell) membrane and the RGD motifs. Error bars on the dots represent the standard deviation from the mean. Figure is replotted from Reference [34]*

RGD-sequence as the RGD-specific integrins of HeLa. Second, platelet integrins isolated with a detergent and grafted uniformly into planar lipid bilayers have been claimed to be all activated, thus showing maximum affinity for their ligands [67]. In contrast, affinity regulation is an intrinsic property of $\alpha IIb\beta 3$ integrins in platelets (they are able to switch from a low affinity "inactive" to a high affinity "activated" state upon induction) [68]; thus, they are expected to show a larger dissociation constant (smaller affinity) for a certain ligand when they are in their native environment compared to when embedded into a model cell membrane system.

In summary, the simplest model described by (9.3) seems to be sufficient to characterize the integrin–ligand interaction; it fitted our data remarkably well and yielded a dissociation constant with a reasonable value.

In a recent book chapter [55], we described how the dissociation constant for the interaction between adhesion ligands and their native cell membrane receptors can be determined with the help of the Epic BT. Exceeding the limitations of most of the regular scientific articles, therein we also provide an extensive list of helpful notes and hints about the technique and all stages of the workflow; a description that will hopefully prompt and encourage future applications.

9.5 Outlook

As a continuation of the experimental work described earlier and published previously (see Reference [34]), we wish to further exploit the potentials of the Epic BT. Accumulating preliminary data show that cell adhesion and spreading do not always follow trivial kinetics (i.e. cannot be described by a symmetrical sigmoid). For the first time this became evident in the case of drug-treated cells. For example, varying concentrations of a small molecule adhesion inhibitor severely altered the kinetics of cell spreading, while the maximal biosensor responses were completely unaffected by it. Surprisingly, spread cell morphology showed a striking dependence on the concentration of the same drug in the assay medium, but nonetheless, the biosensor responses at saturation were the very same, i.e. they were independent of the presence of the drug (preliminary data). In a separate study, we monitored the adhesion and spreading kinetics of unstimulated, untreated human primary monocytes, dendritic cells, and macrophages. The biosensor signal invoked by these immune cells followed nontrivial, non-monotonic kinetics [69], which was unexpected, because if untreated and unperturbed, all the other tested cell types induced a biosensor signal which could be described with a symmetrical sigmoid [29, 58].

All these findings emphasize the fundamental importance of kinetic monitoring in cell (adhesion) studies. Using more sophisticated models, kinetic data analysis may then shed light on the governing and limiting intracellular processes during cell adhesion.

Acknowledgment

The support of the Hungarian Scientific Research Fund (OTKA-PD 73084) is gratefully acknowledged. This work was supported by the Lendület program of the Hungarian Academy of Sciences, the ERC_HU project of NKFIH to RH, the Bolyai Scholarship, and the MedinProt grant of the Hung. Acad. Sci. to B.Szabó.

Used symbols λ: resonant wavelength; $\Delta\lambda$: resonant wavelength shift; $\Delta\lambda_{max}$: maximum recorded shift in resonant wavelength; r: rate constant of spreading, m: constant of integration; t: time; Q: volume percent of the PLL-g-PEG-RGD solution in the mixed solution of copolymers; ν_{RGD} : average surface density of RGD motifs; $d_{RGD-RGD}$: average interligand distance; L: surface concentration of unbound ligand; R: surface concentration of unbound receptor; B: surface concentration of the integrin-ligand complex; k_a: two-dimensional association rate constant; k_d: two-dimensional dissociation rate constant; ${}^{2D}K_d$: two-dimensional dissociation constant; ${}^{3D}K_d$: three-dimensional dissociation constant; l_c: confinement length.

References

[1] R. O. Hynes, "Integrins: bidirectional, allosteric signaling machines," *Cell*, vol. 110, pp. 673–687, 2002.

[2] R. O. Hynes, "Integrins: versatility, modulation, and signaling in cell adhesion," *Cell*, vol. 69, no. 1, pp. 11–25, Apr. 1992.

[3] P. W. Wiseman, C. M. Brown, D. J. Webb, *et al.*, "Spatial mapping of integrin interactions and dynamics during cell migration by image correlation microscopy," *J. Cell Sci.*, vol. 117, no. Pt 23, pp. 5521–5534, Nov. 2004.

[4] A. E. Aplin, A Howe, S. K. Alahari, R. L. Juliano, and C. Hill, "Signal transduction and signal modulation by cell adhesion receptors: the role of integrins, cadherins, immunoglobulin-cell adhesion molecules, and selectins," *Pharmacol. Rev.*, vol. 50, no. 2, pp. 198–263, 1998.

[5] C. Shi and D. I. Simon, "Integrin signals, transcription factors, and monocyte differentiation," *Trends Cardiovasc. Med.*, vol. 16, no. 5, pp. 146–152, Jul. 2006.

[6] N. Wang, J. D. Tytell, and D. E. Ingber, "Mechanotransduction at a distance: mechanically coupling the extracellular matrix with the nucleus," *Nat. Rev. Mol. Cell Biol.*, vol. 10, pp. 75–82, 2009.

[7] C. H. Streuli, "Integrins and cell-fate determination," *J. Cell Sci.*, vol. 122, no. Pt 2, pp. 171–177, Jan. 2009.

[8] D. A. Goodenough, J. A. Goliger, and D. L. Paul, "Connexins, connexons, and intercellular communication," *Annu. Rev. Biochem.*, vol. 65, pp. 475–502, 1996.

[9] E. S. Harris, T. M. McIntyre, S. M. Prescott, and G. A. Zimmerman, "The leukocyte integrins," *J. Biol. Chem.*, vol. 275, no. 31, pp. 23409–23412, Aug. 2000.

[10] T. A. Springer, "Adhesion receptors of the immune system," *Nature*, vol. 346, pp. 425–434, 1990.

[11] J. S. Desgrosellier and D. A. Cheresh, "Integrins in cancer: biological implications and therapeutic opportunities," *Nat. Rev. Cancer*, vol. 10, no. 1, pp. 9–22, Jan. 2010.

[12] C. Wai Wong, D. E. Dye, and D. R. Coombe, "The role of immunoglobulin superfamily cell adhesion molecules in cancer metastasis," *Int. J. Cell Biol.*, vol. 2012, p. 340296, Jan. 2012.

[13] E. C. Boyle and B. B. Finlay, "Bacterial pathogenesis: exploiting cellular adherence," *Curr. Opin. Cell Biol.*, vol. 15, no. 5, pp. 633–639, Oct. 2003.

[14] P. L. Stewart and G. R. Nemerow, "Cell integrins: commonly used receptors for diverse viral pathogens," *Trends Microbiol.*, vol. 15, no. 11, pp. 500–507, Nov. 2007.

[15] E. Décavé, D. Garrivier, Y. Bréchet, B. Fourcade, and F. Bruckert, "Shear flow-induced detachment kinetics of Dictyostelium discoideum cells from solid substrate," *Biophys. J.*, vol. 82, no. 5, pp. 2383–2395, May 2002.

[16] A. George and T. L. Proulx, "Relationship between 3T3 cell spreading and the strength of adhesion on glass and silane surfaces," vol. 14, no. 4, pp. 243–254, 1993.

[17] E. Potthoff, O. Guillaume-Gentil, D. Ossola, *et al.*, "Rapid and serial quantification of adhesion forces of yeast and mammalian cells," *PLoS One*, vol. 7, no. 12, p. e52712, Jan. 2012.

[18] G. Sagvolden, I. Giaever, E. O. Pettersen, and J. Feder, "Cell adhesion force microscopy," *Proc. Natl. Acad. Sci. USA*, vol. 96, no. 2, pp. 471–476, Jan. 1999.

[19] R. Salánki, C. Hős, N. Orgovan, *et al.*, "Single cell adhesion assay using computer controlled micropipette," *PLoS One*, vol. 9, no. 10, p. e111450, Jan. 2014.
[20] S. S. Hur, Y. Zhao, Y-S. Li, E. Botvinick, and S. Chien, "Live cells exert 3-dimensional traction forces on their substrata," *Cell. Mol. Bioeng.*, vol. 2, no. 3, pp. 425–436, Sep. 2009.
[21] JH-C. Wang and J-S. Lin, "Cell traction force and measurement methods," *Biomech. Model. Mechanobiol.*, vol. 6, no. 6, pp. 361–371, Nov. 2007.
[22] D. C. Worth and M. Parsons, "Advances in imaging cell-matrix adhesions," *J. Cell Sci.*, vol. 123, no. Pt 21, pp. 3629–3638, Nov. 2010.
[23] Y. Fang, "Label-free cell-based assays with optical biosensors in drug discovery," *Assay Drug Dev. Technol.*, vol. 4, no. 5, pp. 583–595, 2006.
[24] J. Wegener, C. R. Keese, and I. Giaever, "Electric cell-substrate impedance sensing (ECIS) as a noninvasive means to monitor the kinetics of cell spreading to artificial surfaces," *Exp. Cell Res.*, vol. 259, no. 1, pp. 158–166, Aug. 2000.
[25] J. M. Atienza, J. Zhu, X. Wang, X. Xu, and Y. Abassi, "Dynamic monitoring of cell adhesion and spreading on microelectronic sensor arrays," *J. Biomol. Screen.*, vol. 10, no. 8, pp. 795–805, Dec. 2005.
[26] A. W. Peterson, M. Halter, A. Tona, K. Bhadriraju, and A. L. Plant, "Using surface plasmon resonance imaging to probe dynamic interactions between cells and extracellular matrix," *Cytometry. A*, vol. 77, no. 9, pp. 895–903, Sep. 2010.
[27] V. Yashunsky, V. Lirtsman, M. Golosovsky, D. Davidov, and B. Aroeti, "Real-time monitoring of epithelial cell-cell and cell-substrate interactions by infrared surface plasmon spectroscopy," *Biophys. J.*, vol. 99, no. 12, pp. 4028–4036, Dec. 2010.
[28] K. Tiefenthaler and W. Lukosz, "Sensitivity of grating couplers as integrated-optical chemical sensors," *J. Opt. Soc. Am. B*, vol. 6, no. 2, p. 209, Feb. 1989.
[29] N. Orgovan, R. Salánki, N. Sándor, *et al.*, "In-situ and label-free optical monitoring of the adhesion and spreading of primary monocytes isolated from human blood: dependence on serum concentration levels," *Biosens. Bioelectron.*, vol. 54, pp. 339–344, Apr. 2014.
[30] R. Horvath, K. Cottier, H. C. Pedersen, and J. J. Ramsden, "Multidepth screening of living cells using optical waveguides," *Biosens. Bioelectron.*, vol. 24, no. 4, pp. 805–810, Dec. 2008.
[31] J. J. Ramsden and R. Horvath, "Optical biosensors for cell adhesion," *J. Recept. Signal Transduct. Res.*, vol. 29, no. 3–4, pp. 211–223, Jan. 2009.
[32] S. M. Shamah and B. T. Cunningham, "Label-free cell-based assays using photonic crystal optical biosensors," *Analyst*, vol. 136, no. 6, pp. 1090–1102, Mar. 2011.
[33] Y. Fang, A. M. Ferrie, N. H. Fontaine, J. Mauro, and J. Balakrishnan, "Resonant waveguide grating biosensor for living cell sensing," *Biophys. J.*, vol. 91, no. 5, pp. 1925–1940, Sep. 2006.

[34] N. Orgovan, B. Peter, S. Bősze, J. J. Ramsden, B. Szabó, and R. Horvath, "Dependence of cancer cell adhesion kinetics on integrin ligand surface density measured by a high-throughput label-free resonant waveguide grating biosensor," *Sci. Rep.*, vol. 4, p. 4034, Jan. 2014.

[35] J. Comley, "Progress in the implementation of label-free detection part I: cell-based assays," *Drug Discov. World Summer 2008*, 2008.

[36] N. Orgovan, B. Kovacs, E. Farkas, *et al.*, "Bulk and surface sensitivity of a resonant waveguide grating imager," *Appl. Phys. Lett.*, vol. 104, no. 8, p. 083506, Feb. 2014.

[37] R. Horvath, H. C. Pedersen, N. Skivesen, D. Selmeczi, and N. B. Larsen, "Monitoring of living cell attachment and spreading using reverse symmetry waveguide sensing," *Appl. Phys. Lett.*, vol. 86, no. 7, p. 071101, 2005.

[38] V. Goral, Q. Wu, H. Sun, and Y. Fang, "Label-free optical biosensor with microfluidics for sensing ligand-directed functional selectivity on trafficking of thrombin receptor," *FEBS Lett.*, vol. 585, no. 7, pp. 1054–1060, Apr. 2011.

[39] Y. Fang, "Label-free receptor assays," *Drug Discov. Today. Technol.*, vol. 7, no. 1, pp. e5–e11, Jan. 2011.

[40] R. Schröder, J. Schmidt, S. Blättermann, *et al.*, "Applying label-free dynamic mass redistribution technology to frame signaling of G protein-coupled receptors noninvasively in living cells," *Nat. Protoc.*, vol. 6, no. 11, pp. 1748–1760, Nov. 2011.

[41] N. Orgovan, D. Patko, C. Hos, *et al.*, "Sample handling in surface sensitive chemical and biological sensing: a practical review of basic fluidics and analyte transport," *Adv. Colloid Interface Sci.*, vol. 211C, pp. 1–16, Sep. 2014.

[42] A. M. Ferrie, Q. Wu, and Y. Fang, "Resonant waveguide grating imager for live cell sensing," *Appl. Phys. Lett.*, vol. 97, no. 22, p. 223704, Nov. 2010.

[43] Y. Fang, "Label-free biosensors for cell biology," *Int. J. Electrochem.*, vol. 2011, pp. 1–16, 2011.

[44] J. J. Ramsden, S. Y. Li, E. Heinzle, and J. E. Prenosil, "Optical method for measurement of number and shape of attached cells in real time," *Cytometry*, vol. 19, no. 2, pp. 97–102, Feb. 1995.

[45] C. A. Reinhart-King, M. Dembo, and D. A. Hammer, "The dynamics and mechanics of endothelial cell spreading," *Biophys. J.*, vol. 89, no. 1, pp. 676–689, Jul. 2005.

[46] B. J. Dubin-Thaler, G. Giannone, H-G. Döbereiner, and M. P. Sheetz, "Nanometer analysis of cell spreading on matrix-coated surfaces reveals two distinct cell states and STEPs," *Biophys. J.*, vol. 86, no. 3, pp. 1794–1806, Mar. 2004.

[47] B. F. Bell, M. Schuler, S. Tosatti, M. Textor, Z. Schwartz, and B. D. Boyan, "Osteoblast response to titanium surfaces functionalized with extracellular matrix peptide biomimetics," *Clin. Oral Implants Res.*, vol. 22, no. 8, pp. 865–872, Aug. 2011.

[48] S. VandeVondele, J. Vörös, and J. A. Hubbell, "RGD-grafted poly-L-lysine-graft-(polyethylene glycol) copolymers block non-specific protein adsorption

while promoting cell adhesion," *Biotechnol. Bioeng.*, vol. 82, no. 7, pp. 784–790, Jun. 2003.

[49] M. Schuler, G. R. Owen, D. W. Hamilton, *et al.*, "Biomimetic modification of titanium dental implant model surfaces using the RGDSP-peptide sequence: a cell morphology study," *Biomaterials*, vol. 27, no. 21, pp. 4003–4015, Jul. 2006.

[50] E. Ruoslahti, "RGD and other recognition sequences for integrins," *Annu. Rev. Cell Dev. Biol.*, vol. 12, pp. 697–715, Jan. 1996.

[51] U. Hersel, C. Dahmen, and H. Kessler, "RGD modified polymers: biomaterials for stimulated cell adhesion and beyond," *Biomaterials*, vol. 24, no. 24, pp. 4385–4415, Nov. 2003.

[52] J. Huang, S. V. Gra, F. Corbellini, *et al.*, "Impact of order and disorder in RGD nanopatterns on cell adhesion," *Nano Lett.*, vol. 9, pp. 1111–1116, 2009.

[53] E. A. Cavalcanti-Adam, T. Volberg, A. Micoulet, H. Kessler, B. Geiger, and J. P. Spatz, "Cell spreading and focal adhesion dynamics are regulated by spacing of integrin ligands," *Biophys. J.*, vol. 92, no. 8, pp. 2964–2974, Apr. 2007.

[54] T. Frisch and O. Thoumine, "Predicting the kinetics of cell spreading," *J. Biomech.*, vol. 35, no. 8, pp. 1137–1141, Aug. 2002.

[55] N. Orgovan, B. Peter, S. Bosze, J. J. Ramsden, B. Szabó, and R. Horvath, "Label-free profiling of cell adhesion: determination of the dissociation constant for native cell membrane adhesion receptor-ligand interaction," in *Label-Free Biosensor Methods in Drug Discovery*, Y. Fang, Ed. Springer, 2015, pp. 327–338.

[56] G. L. Kenausis, J. Vo, D. L. Elbert, *et al.*, "Poly(L-lysine)-g-poly(ethylene glycol) layers on metal oxide surfaces: attachment mechanism and effects of polymer architecture on resistance to protein adsorption," pp. 3298–3309, 2000.

[57] M. Barczyk, S. Carracedo, and D. Gullberg, "Integrins," *Cell Tissue Res.*, vol. 339, no. 1, pp. 269–280, Jan. 2010.

[58] A. Aref, R. Horvath, and J. J. Ramsden, "Spreading kinetics for quantifying cell state during stem cell differentiation," *J. Biol. Phys. Chem.*, vol. 10, no. November, pp. 1–7, 2010.

[59] AÁ. Rauscher, Z. Simon, G. J. Szöllosi, L. Gráf, I. Derényi, and A. Malnasi-Csizmadia, "Temperature dependence of internal friction in enzyme reactions," *FASEB J.*, vol. 25, no. 8, pp. 2804–2813, Aug. 2011.

[60] M. Arnold, E. A. Cavalcanti-Adam, R. Glass, *et al.*, "Activation of integrin function by nanopatterned adhesive interfaces," *Chemphyschem*, vol. 5, no. 3, pp. 383–388, Mar. 2004.

[61] G. I. Bell, M. Dembo, and P. Bongrand, "Cell adhesion. Competition between nonspecific repulsion and specific bonding," *Biophys. J.*, vol. 45, no. 6, pp. 1051–1064, Jun. 1984.

[62] M. L. Dustin, S. K. Bromley, M. M. Davis, and C. Zhu, "Identification of self through two-dimensional chemistry and synapses," *Annu. Rev. Cell Dev. Biol.*, vol. 17, pp. 133–157, Jan. 2001.

[63] C. S. Izzard and L. R. Lochner, "Cell-to-substrate contacts in living fibroblasts: an interference reflexion study with an evaluation of the technique," *J. Cell Sci.*, vol. 21, no. 1, pp. 129–159, Jun. 1976.
[64] K-F. Giebel, C. Bechinger, S. Herminghaus, *et al.*, "Imaging of cell/substrate contacts of living cells with surface plasmon resonance microscopy," *Biophys. J.*, vol. 76, no. 1, pp. 509–516, Jan. 1999.
[65] C. M. Lo, M. Glogauer, M. Rossi, and J. Ferrier, "Cell-substrate separation: effect of applied force and temperature," *Eur. Biophys. J.*, vol. 27, no. 1, pp. 9–17, Jan. 1998.
[66] M. Pfaff, K. Tangemann, B. Muller, *et al.*, "Selective recognition of cyclic RGD peptides of NMR defined conformation by alpha(II)beta(3), alpha(V)beta(3), and alpha(5)beta(1) integrins," *J. Biol. Chem.*, vol. 269, no. 82, pp. 20233–20238, 1994.
[67] B. Müller, H. G. Zerwes, K. Tangemann, J. Peter, and J. Engel, "Two-step binding mechanism of fibrinogen to alpha(IIb)beta(3) integrin reconstituted into planar lipid bilayers," *J. Biol. Chem.*, vol. 268, no. 9, pp. 6800–6808, Mar. 1993.
[68] H. Ginsberg, X. De, and F. Plow, "Inside-out integrin signaling," *Curr. Opin. Cell Biol.*, vol. 4, pp. 766–771, 1992.
[69] N. Orgovan, U-S. Rita, N. Sándor, *et al.*, "Label -free kinetic monitoring of the adhesion kinetics of human primary monocytes, dendritic cells, and macrophages on fibrinogen- and PLL-g-PEG-RGD- coated surfaces," *in press*.

Chapter 10

Optical biosensors for the detection of food borne pathogens

Nawfal Adam Mungroo[1] *and Suresh Neethirajan*[1]

10.1 Introduction

Contagious illnesses are responsible for approximately 20 million deaths annually in the world [1]. In the US alone, 48 million cases, 128,000 hospitalisations, and 3,000 deaths from food borne diseases were reported in 2011 [2]. Some examples of these bacterial and viral agents are *Listeria monocytogenes, Staphylococcus aureus, Salmonella sp, Escherichia coli 0157:H7, Norovirus, Hepatitis A, Hepatitis E, Adenovirus (Enteric),* and *Rotaviruses* [3].

Salmonella is one of the most common bacteria responsible for food borne diseases. *Salmonella* has over 2,463 serotypes and the most prevalent strains are *Salmonella typhimurium* and *Salmonella enteritidis* [5]. *Salmonella* originates from animal intestines and can end up on beef and poultry by contamination during the process of slaughter. It is also found in other animal derived products namely milk and eggs [4]. Vegetable products can also be contaminated with *Salmonella* through the industrial process. Salmonellosis is a pathology which involves acute fever, diarrhoea, gastroenteritis, and vomiting. The symptoms usually occur within 6–72 h after ingestion and the disease can last up to 7 days [5]. Gastroenteritis is primarily caused by the *typhimurium* serotype; there have been 1.3 billion cases of *typhimurium* gastroenteritis which lead to 3 million reported annual deaths. The mortality rate in advanced countries is approximately 1 percent compared to 24 percent in developed countries. *Salmonella enteric* infection leads to typhoid fever and is less common compared to *typhimurium.* As evidenced, 17 million cases which lead to 500,000 annual deaths have been reported [6].

Escherichia coli (E. coli) is a bacterium commonly found in the intestines of warm-blooded animals. Most serotypes of *E. coli* are harmless with the exception of *E. coli O157:H7*. The primary sources of *E. coli O157:H7* include undercooked poultry, meat, and hamburgers and milk-based products such as cheese and yogurt. Additional sources may consist of contaminated vegetables and water. The clinical symptoms associated with *E. coli O157:H7* include severe abdominal pain, bloody

[1]BioNano Laboratory, School of Engineering, University of Guelph, Guelph, ON N1G 2W1

diarrhoea, renal failure, and vomiting amongst other complications. The duration of this disease is about 8 days [7]. Approximately 10 percent of patients infected with *E. coli* progress towards haemolytic uraemic syndrome with a mortality rate of 3–5 percent [8].

Calicivirus (including *Norovirus*) is a ribonucleic acid (RNA) virus which is responsible for abdominal pain, vomiting, nausea, diarrhoea, headaches, and low-grade fever. The difference between *calicivirus* and bacteria is that the former spreads primarily from infected individuals. Annually, *Norovirus* contributes to around 21 million illnesses, 71,000 hospitalisations, and 800 deaths in the US [9].

Food borne illnesses have emerged as a growing concern in the world today [10]. Aside from the human casualties, they are also responsible for economic losses. The cost associated with food borne illnesses can be tracked using the cost-of-illness methodology which measures the individual and societal resources consumed as a result of an adverse illness [11]. While direct costs associated at an individual level include the diagnosis, treatments and management of the illness, indirect costs include operational expenditures for healthcare facilities and personnel [12, 13]. Data show that food borne illnesses cost annually around $10–83 billion [14], $86 million [12], $1.289 billion [15], $171 million [13], and $2 million [10], in the US, New Zealand, Australia, Sweden, and Croatia, respectively. In short, food borne pathogens not only affect the health of billions of individuals but also cause significant economic losses worldwide.

Current detection practices have been established by governments and regulatory organisations to limit the economic impact and provide a safer platform for consumers. The established protocols for food borne pathogens detection are divided into safety, shelf-life prediction, adulteration, and process monitoring. Through the subsequent stages of testing, different threshold levels have been established that make the detection process more difficult [16]. Conventional processes commonly involve cultivating sample cells in highly specialised laboratories making the procedure time consuming and costly. Additionally, since the transport of food samples to the testing laboratory can take several hours to days, the sample cells may possibly become stressed leading to false negative results [17].

10.2 Current technologies for pathogen detection

The most common techniques used in clinical and food industries for the detection of pathogens are Enzyme-Linked Immunosorbent Assay (ELISA) and Polymerase Chain Reaction (PCR). A brief description of each technique and their benefits and drawbacks are discussed in Sections 10.3 and 10.4.

10.3 Enzyme-linked immunosorbent assay (ELISA)

ELISA is a biochemical technique used for the detection of target pathogens through the recognition of their corresponding antigens. The mechanism behind ELISA involves combining the specificity of antibodies with the sensitivity of enzyme assays. After immobilisation of target antigens, detection antibodies bind to them. Enzymes linked to detection antibodies act as catalysts and this ultimately results in a detectable colourimetric signal [18]. The colour obtained is directly proportional to the amount of antibody bound to the target pathogens [18, 19].

Three types of ELISA techniques namely competitive, direct, and sandwich are used. While the competitive method involves mixing antigens with primary antibodies and adding those antibodies to immobilised antigens and later adding secondary antibodies for colour generation, the direct method involves the addition of enzyme conjugated antibodies directly to the immobilised target antigens. As for the sandwich technique, capture antibodies are initially added to immobilise target antigens on the substrate [18, 19]. Although these techniques are highly sensitive with detection limits as low as tens of picogram proteins per mL of sample [21], they are widely considered to be costly [22, 23], labour intensive, and time consuming which make them impractical for onsite pathogens detection [20].

10.4 Polymerase chain reaction (PCR)

PCR is a molecular technique used for in vitro amplification of deoxyribonucleic acid (DNA) fragment using enzymatic replication [19]. The principle behind PCR detection entails lysing the target pathogen and extracting its genetic component (DNA or RNA). Following this step, enzymes, primers, and other reagents are added and the content is cycled through three different temperatures. This process is repeated 20–40 times. Through this process, the specific genetic sequence in a target pathogen is amplified and detected through gel electrophoresis [21]. Several variants of the PCR technique namely multiplex, nested, reverse, semi-quantitative, and real-time methods are used, with the latest having the advantages of being fast, reducing contamination risk, and compatibility with fluorescence [25]. As is the case for ELISA, while PCR has excellent sensitivity and selectivity, it is considered to be a costly, labour intensive, and time consuming technique [21, 24], leading to biosensors being an appealing competitive alternative for onsite pathogens detection.

10.5 Biosensors

10.5.1 Overview

Biosensors have been a growing tool for the detection of pathogens in the medical and food processing industry. The first biosensor was a glucose sensing device, invented by Professor Clark in 1962. A biosensor is defined as an analytical device used for the detection of target analytes. It consists of biorecognition and transducer elements which transform a biochemical signal into a measurable signal. Biosensors can be classified into optical, piezoelectric, and electrochemical. The characteristics of an optimal biosensor are high efficiency, superior selectivity and sensitivity, fast response, and biocompatibility [26].

10.5.2 Biorecognition techniques

Since the selectivity and sensitivity of biosensors depend on the characteristics of their biorecognition component, different recognition elements have been developed and will be discussed here. These chiefly include antibodies, enzymes, and nucleic acids [26]. Other examples include aptamer- and cell-based biorecognition elements. Aptamers are synthetic strands of nucleic acids used to detect oligosaccharides, amino acids, peptides, and proteins [31]. Aptamers are adaptable to different chemical tags and can be produced at lower costs to antibodies [32]. Cell-based biorecognition takes advantage of the capability of living cells to recognise the intracellular and extracellular microenvironment, and to ultimately create a response upon contact between a stimulus and the cell [33]. The main drawback of cell-based biosensors is their low selectivity and stability [31].

10.5.3 Antibodies

Antibodies are one of the most commonly utilised recognition elements in biosensors due to their highly specific nature. The structure of an antibody consists of four polypeptides (two heavy chains and two light chains) joined in a "Y" shape. The specificity of antibodies originates from the interaction between the distinctive recognition structure on the antigen surface and the antibody binding site that is made up of 110–130 amino acids present in the Fab fragment [28]. Antibodies are classified as monoclonal or polyclonal. While monoclonal antibodies are produced from a single clone antibody molecule and subsequently interact only with specific epitope on the antigen, polyclonal antibodies are formed by multiple clones of antibody-producing molecules and interact with multiple epitopes on the antigen. The selection between the two antibodies depends on the types of pathogens that need to be detected [1].

10.5.4 Enzymes

Enzymes have been used with the first generation of biosensors in 1962. They are appropriate for short-term use due to their selectivity, sensitivity, and cost effectiveness. Their selectivity originates from the complementary structures of the binding sites with the respective substrates [30]. The primary drawback with enzymes is their fragility and instability. As a result, this can cause a decrease in the performance of the biosensors and limit their practical use. The most common enzymes used for biosensing applications are glucose oxidase and horseradish peroxidase [31].

10.5.5 Nucleic acids

DNA-based biosensors are an emerging method in areas such as pathogen classification, genotyping, drug discovery, sequencing and molecular diagnostics. These biosensors depend on the interaction between a single stranded DNA probe and the analyte. This interaction causes the hybridisation of complementary single stranded DNA to form double stranded DNA, and subsequently to produce a biochemical reaction allowing the amplification of electrical signal by the transducer [31]. Unlike antibody-antigen complexes where bonding occurs at a few specific sites, bonding for nucleic acids occurs at regular nucleotide intervals along the length of the nucleic acid duplex. As a result, there is a higher possibility for bonding ultimately leading to higher specificity and detection of pathogens [19]. However, the drawback to high sensitivity is that contaminated DNA-based biosensors often increase the risk of false positives [31].

10.6 Transduction techniques

Non-optical based biosensors are categorised as electrochemical and piezoelectric biosensors. They are equally important for pathogen detection when compared to optical based biosensors in terms of practicality, selectivity, and sensitivity. This section provides a brief overview of non-optical biosensors, and below section discusses the main types of optical biosensors.

10.6.1 Electrochemical

Electrochemical biosensors are based on target analytes modulating the chemical reactions that involve transfer of electrons and use reduction and oxidation (redox) catalyzing enzymes. They are generally composed of a reference, working, and counter electrodes. While electrochemical biosensors are generally simple to use, require minimal pre-treatment of sample and are inexpensive to manufacture, they usually lack effective discrimination between different pathogens and their sensitivity is not consistent with different analyte concentrations. Electrochemical biosensors can be categorised as amperometric [29], impedimetric [34], potentiometric, and conductimetric biosensors. The fundamental principles of those sensors are very similar except for the units of measurements (current v/s impedance v/s voltage v/s resistance, respectively) [16, 35, 37, 38, 40].

10.6.2 Piezoelectric

Piezoelectric biosensors are an example of mass-based biosensors that measure the changes in mass due to biomolecular binding between two entities such as antibody/antigen and enzyme/substrate interactions. Quartz crystal microbalance (QCM) is the most common label free piezoelectric biosensor. While the benefits of piezoelectric biosensors include low cost, real-time monitoring and practicality, their response is not as specific and sensitive due to a high possibility of interference [27]. Their quality depends on parameters such as the type of biomaterials immobilised on the crystal, their frequency shift and surface properties of the quartz crystal [29]. Table 10.1 shows different limit of detection (LOD) values of QCM for pathogens in food and clinical settings [36].

10.7 Sample preparation

Sample preparation is the first step towards obtaining a highly sensitive measurement. The objective behind sample preparation involves concentrating the target cells so that they are within the operating spectrum of the detection technique to

Table 10.1 Summary of QCM Limit of Detection (LOD) for different bacteria [36]

Bacteria	Limit of Detection (LOD) (CFU/mL)	Matrix	Time per assay (min)
S. typhimurium (this study)	10–20	PBS	12
S. typhimurium	10^2	BHY broth/chicken meat solution	60
S. paratyphi	1.7×10^2	PBS	50
M. tuberculosis	2.0×10^2	Sputum	30
S. typhimurium	10^3	Chicken exudates	Not available
S. typhimurium	10^3	PBS	30
E. coli	10^3	BHY broth	30–50
Salmonella spp	10^4	PBS	10
S. enteritidis	10^5	Saline solution	35
E. coli	1.7×10^5	Food samples	20–30
F. tularensis	5×10^6	PBS	35
S. typhimurium	10^7	Not stated	40
P. aeruginosa	1.3×10^7	Nutrient broth	20
L. monocytogenes	10^7	Tris buffer	30

obtain consistent measurements for repeated sampling [19]. The sampling process consists of three key steps: sample collection, sample handling, and sample preparation. Immunomagnetic separation is considered the most appropriate method for bacterial immobilisation in clinical and food samples. Its principle involves coating paramagnetic particles with organism specific ligands in the liquid solution to be analysed. A magnetic field is then applied and the bacteria are separated as illustrated in Figure 10.1.

10.8 Optical biosensors

Optical based biosensors are categorised into surface plasmon resonance (SPR), fluorescence based biosensors, Raman spectroscopy, and others.

10.8.1 Surface plasmon resonance (SPR)

SPR is a label-free technique commonly used in the detection of pathogens. The mechanism behind SPR entails sending initial rays of polarised light through a thin conducting film, which consists of two transparent media with different refractive indexes. Consequently, there is absorption of some of the photons by the conducting film and the remaining attenuated light is reflected at a specific angle (SPR angle) because of the different refractive indexes. Upon binding of affinity partners (e.g. antigen/antibody, enzyme/substrates, etc.) this leads into a change in the reflective index which is detected by the SPR biosensors and displayed on a sonogram. The information is then translated into mass concentrations as illustrated

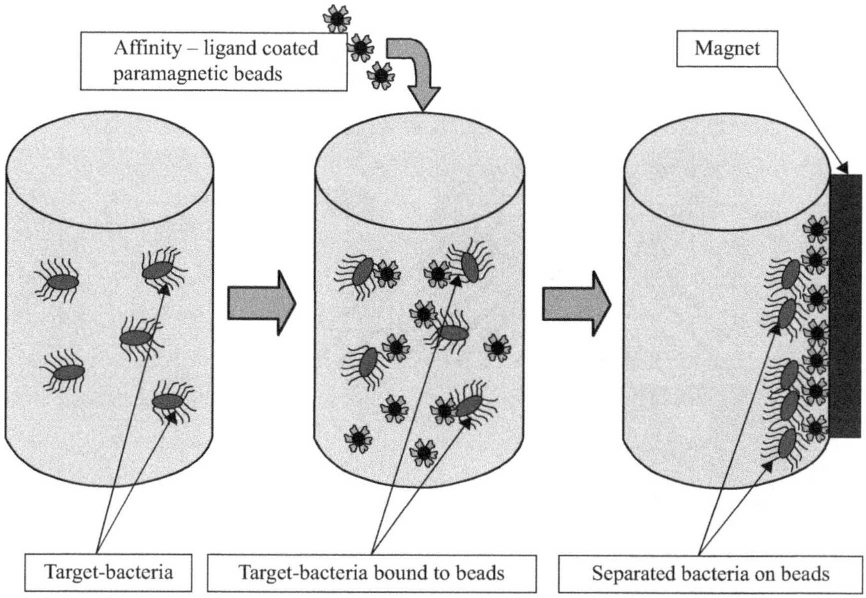

Figure 10.1 Illustration of immunomagnetic separation. Reproduced from Reference 19 with permission from Springer

in Figure 10.2. The unit response on a sonogram is defined as a resonance unit, which is equal to approximately 1 picogram (pg)/mm^2 of material bound of surface area [42]. The advantages of SPR based biosensors include fast response since it is a label-free system, increased sensitivity and selectivity through the use of nanoparticles, and practicality for onsite detection of pathogens.

To ensure optimal use of SPR biosensors, molecular recognition elements (MREs) must be immobilised onto the metal surface. A self-assembled monolayer, which is formed through spontaneous adsorption of either thiols or disulphides on the metal surface, strengthens the binding of the MREs on the metal surface [19].

Even though the SPR approach provides very accurate sensitivity, it is limited in terms of its practicality for industry and clinical use. For example, culturing the bacteria is a lengthy process that can take several hours. Additionally, there is no clear indication about how SPR is able to quickly and effectively discriminate between different types of pathogens. A few studies proposed coating different types of antibodies on the SPR surface such that different bacteria can bind to their respective antibodies. However, it is unclear whether the sonogram measurement would be precise enough to be able to discriminate between the different types of bacteria. Lastly, this detection technique involves expensive and complicated pre-treatment such as coating the required antibodies on the surface. In conclusion, SPR technology is an emerging optical sensing tool for the detection of pathogens.

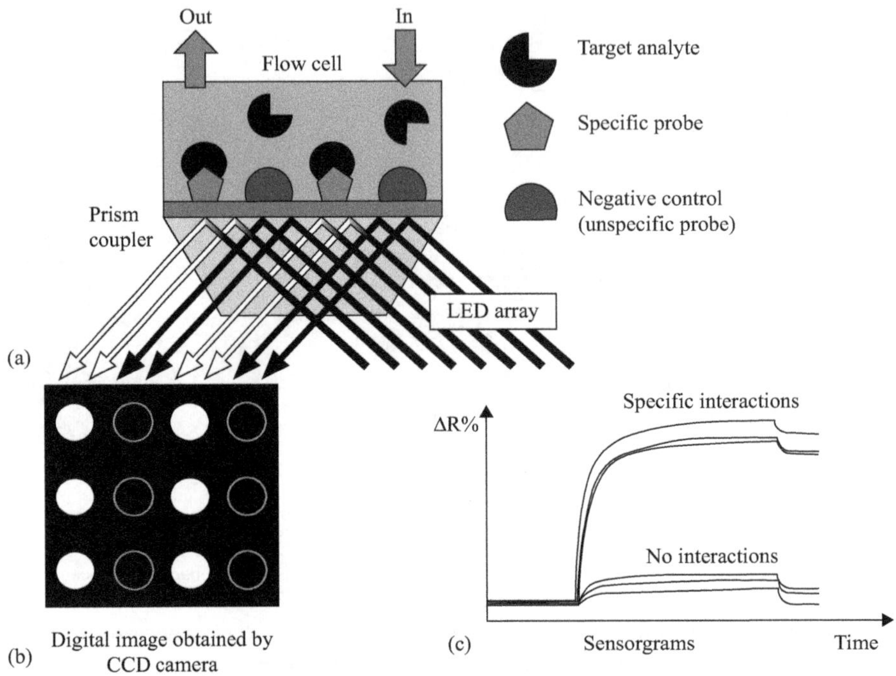

Figure 10.2 Surface plasmon resonance (SPR) principles and sonogram representation. (a) A high refractive index prism is in contact with the detection cell and couples the incident light to the surface plasmon by evanescent waves. p-polarised light is directed to the prism, on which the biomolecular probe is tethered, and a CCD camera collects the output signal as variations in reflectivity. (b) Data are recorded as intensity variation of the reflected light at a fixed angle for each ROI selected. (c) Sensorgrams corresponding to the interactions of the analyte with the spots on the surface. Reproduced from Reference 37 with permission from Elsevier Ltd

10.9 Fluorescence

Fluorescence based detection is the most utilised technique for biomolecular imaging. Properties of fluorescent based biosensors include increased sensitivity and selectivity, acceptable spatial and temporal resolution, and low cost. There are two essential steps in the design of a fluorescent based biosensor. The first stage involves identifying a macromolecular receptor with strong affinity and specificity to the target analyte. The second stage entails binding the receptor element to the signal transducing component. However, since the signal produced from this binding will be weak, an in-between stage comprising of incorporating foreign report moieties such as synthetic fluorophore or auto-fluorescent protein (AFP) is required to enhance the resulting signal [42].

10.9.1 Auto-fluorescent protein (AFP)

The most common type of AFP is the green fluorescent protein (GFP) from jellyfish. The working principle of AFP entails producing a spontaneous fluorescent emission in cells through the autocatalytic formation of the chromophore after translation. There exist two techniques which can be used to design AFP-based biosensors: analyte-sensitive sensors and conformation-sensitive sensors. While analyte-sensitive sensors depend on AFP variants' fluorescent properties which are directly affected upon interaction of the target analyte and a chromophore moiety element in AFP, conformation-sensitive sensors depend on conformational changes of the receptor which are associated with the ligand binding event and are responsible for creating a fluorescent signal response from AFPs which allow for more versatility [42].

The conformational sensitive sensors can be categorised into dual AFP-fused fluorescent resonance energy transfer (FRET)-based biosensors, single circularly permuted (CP) AFP-based biosensors and split AFP-based biosensors. FRET is defined as a physicochemical event occurring upon two conditions: close proximity between two fluorophores (<10 nm) and overlapping emission spectrum of the donor and the excitation spectrum of the acceptor. Two AFPs in combination with the receptor protein allow a FRET-based biosensor protein that responds to dynamic fluctuation of intracellular ligand concentration by a ratiometric fluorescence change. On the other hand, CP-AFPs are designed for targeting Ca^{2+}, cGMP, H_2O_2, Zn^{2+} by attaching a short peptide linker and regenerating the novel N and C termini at a specific position [68]. This method may not be adequate for pathogen detection since it is not able to sense small conformational changes upon binding with the substrate. Finally, unlike the above mentioned two methods, split AFP-based biosensors completely suppress the initial fluorescence resulting from the binding to the substrate by splitting AFP into two fragments [42].

10.9.2 Bioluminescence resonance energy transfer

Bioluminescence resonance energy transfer (BRET) mechanism is determined by the biochemical energy generated when bioluminescent proteins excite fluorophores. The principle behind bioluminescence assay depends on the measurement of emitted light from the intercellular components of the pathogens. The first stage involves the lysis of the bacteria/viral cell to remove intercellular components and the latter is measured using a bioluminescent reaction with luciferase [52]. The bioluminescent signal is then converted to measurable electrical by PMT and it is further detected. The concentration of the intracellular ATP is proportional to the bioluminescence intensity [53]. Growing interest is shown for BRET-based biosensors for quick and easy detection of pathogens for their improved response time, sensitivity and simplicity. However, there is still work to be done to optimise BRET-based biosensors in terms of selectivity and sensitivity which ultimately limit their applications [54].

10.9.3 Quantum dots

To remediate the discrepancies of fluorescence based techniques, quantum dots (QDs) have been introduced. QDs are semiconductor nanoparticles constructed from elements of Groups II–VI, III–V and IV–VI of the periodic table [25, 26]. The optical characteristics of QDs can be customised by changing the size of the QDs. As a result, QD's spectrum ranges from ultraviolet to the infrared light. Examples of QDs include CdS, CdSe, GaAs, InP, PbS, PbSe amongst others [43]. Other QDs advantages over fluorescent dyes include improvement in resistance to photobeaching (could be 100 times larger), increase in brightness (up to 20 times), availability of more colours through multistaining methods by incorporating organic probes and achieving further discrimination by the fluorescence lifetime using fluorescence lifetime imaging (FLIM) [44]. These benefits of QDs not only improve the sensitivity of biosensors, but also discriminate between different pathogens.

In one QDs study [45], three food-borne pathogenic bacteria (*S. enteritidis, S. aureus,* and *E. coli*) were detected using multicolour QD probes based on multiplex fluoroimmunoassay in food samples. The procedure involved conjugating multicolour QDs of different emissions (504 nm, 557 nm, and 604 nm) to antibodies of *S. enteritidis, S. aureus,* and *E. coli* as illustrated in Figures 10.3 and 10.4. The results showed three distinct peaks confirming that three different pathogens can be detected simultaneously in less than 2 h (Table 10.2) [45].

When comparing QD based detection to other techniques, it can be observed that the LOD is equally as sensitive as illustrated in Table 10.1. QD based detection is highly sensitive and selective. The disadvantages of QD based recognition are

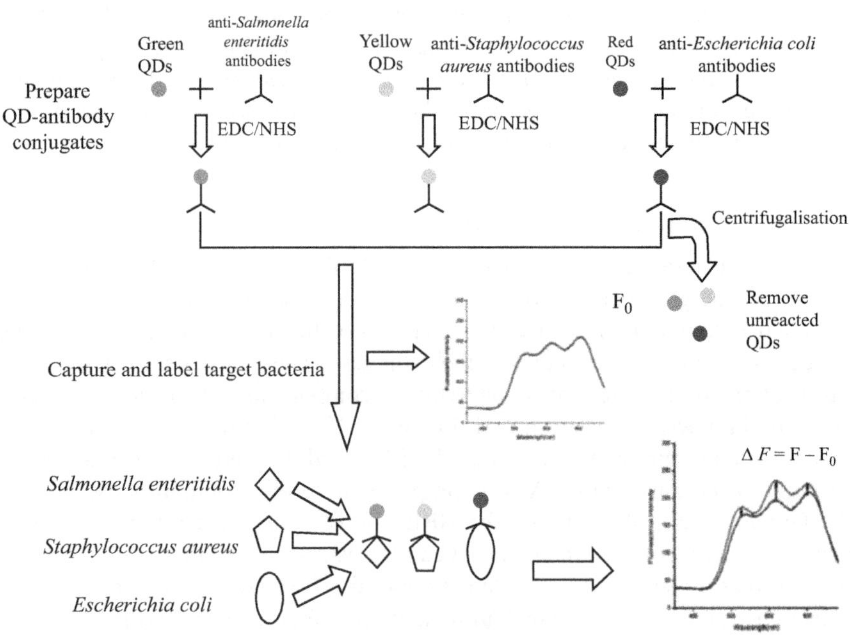

Figure 10.3 Schematic representing the conjugation of three pathogenic bacteria with QDs. Reproduced from Reference 45 with permission from Elsevier Ltd

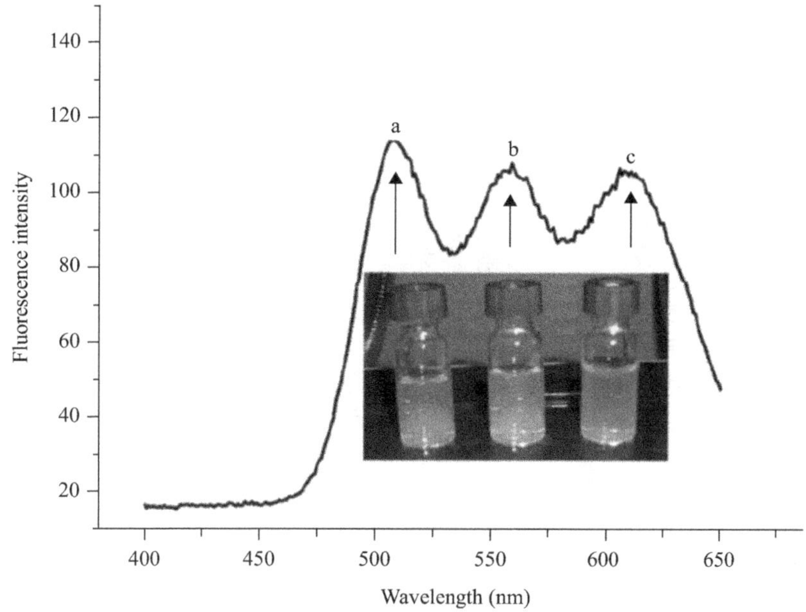

Figure 10.4 *Fluorescence spectra of three QDs with three emission wavelength. Reproduced from Reference 45 with permission from Elsevier Ltd*

Table 10.2 *Comparisons of different techniques as compared to this study (adapted from [45])*

Salmonella		***Staphylococcus aureus***		***Escherichia coli***	
Technique	**LOD (CFU/mL)**	**Technique**	**LOD (CFU/mL)**	**Technique**	**LOD (CFU/mL)**
This Study	10^2	This Study	10^2	This Study	10^2
Fluorescence method based on CdSe/ZnS QDs	10^2	Surface plasmon resonance	10^5	Insertion/ deletion-based approach	10^2
Flow cytometry	10^4	Fluorescence method using QDs	10^2	Capture-cum-detection	10^2

the duration of the pre-treatment process and the cost associated with it. Therefore, the current trends in QD based detection involve finding a less expensive method to incorporate QD for the detection of pathogens. Additional trends include reducing the testing time. Table 10.3 summarises the current developments with QD based pathogen detection focusing on performance and practicality.

Table 10.3 Summary of recent QD based detection of pathogens

Objective of study	Methods and Justification	LOD	Remarks	References
Detection of *E. coli O157:H7* and *Salmonella* in ground beef	A bead-free quantum dot-facilitated isolation method has been implemented to remediate to autofluorescence emitted by the magnetic beads which strongly interferes with the target detection signal	Detection signals were increased fourfold. 10 CFU/g *E. coli O157:H7* and *Salmonella* from artificially contaminated ground beef	Preparation including enrichment accounts for 27 h. The cost of QD was estimated to be US $35/mL which is fairly expensive	[46]
Quantum dot-based array for sensitive detection of *E. coli*	A proof of concept method in an antibody microarray detects *E. coli O157:H7* at concentrations below 10 CFU/mL without bacteria pre-enrichment	Improved performance (three orders of magnitude) in terms of LOD as compared to ELISA	Cross-reactivity studies show little interference of other bacteria when working at concentrations of 100 CFU/mL	[47]
Detection of pathogenic mycobacteria based on functionalised quantum dots coupled with immunomagnetic separation	Development of two prototypical diagnostic assays designed for use at point-of-care. These methods incorporate gold nanoparticles and a combination of magnetic beads and CdSe QDs for the detection of conserved genomic regions of DNA belonging to *Mycobacterium spp.* without the need for amplification	The minimum detection limit of the assay was defined to 10^4 bacteria/mL, which could be further decreased by a 1 log when fluorescence was measured with a spectrofluorometer	This technique can be further applied to other proteins and implemented in clinical or food safety industry	[48]

Exploring the feasibility of using quantum dot nanoparticles to rapidly detect pathogenic *Salmonella*	Selective detection was achieved with anti-*Salmonella* polyclonal antibodies immobilised by streptavidin–biotin binding or covalent binding to the QD surface. Superparamagnetic particles were used to separate and concentrate cells from each sample	*Salmonella* detection limits were 1.4×10^3 CFU/mL in PBS–BSA and 4×10^3 CFU/mL in food extracts	[49]
Using bioconjugated CdTe QDs as fluorescent label for rapid, technically simple and efficient detection of *S. Enteritidis*	Highly fluorescent and water-soluble CdTe quantum dots were prepared by using thioglycolic acid and 1-thioglycerol as ligands and were then conjugated with anti-*Salmonella* antibodies	The low detection limit was 1×10^2 CFU/mL without sample enrichment	[50]

Microfluidics are becoming more and more attractive option due to their portability, small volume requirements, lower detection limits, and effective waste management capabilities. The fabrication of microfluidics coupled with QD-FRET is fairly simple and involves the following stages: the first step involves depositing biotinylated surface ligands for immobilising the QD. The next procedure entails assembling the solid-phase assay within each channel by administrating streptavidin-functionalised QDs (SAv-QDs) and biotinylated oligonucleotide probe successively through electro-osmotic flow and electrophoretic force, respectively. The sample solution containing oligonucleotide targets is introduced and after a few minutes, it is consumed as the plug moves in the channel. A cyanine dye 3 (Cy3) tag on the target oligonucleotide is carried into close proximity to the immobilised QD donor by hybridisation to the probe. A 405 nm laser is then excited, enabling FRET from the QD. The length of this FRET-sensitised Cy3 spatial profile from the channel interior is used to quantify the amount of nucleic acid present in a sample as illustrated in Figure 10.5 [44].

A study by Kim and colleagues implemented the design of a portable fluorometer using QDs and a microfluidic platform to measure the amount of *Salmonella* in chicken extract as shown in Figure 10.6. The detection limit of the sensor was 10^3 CFU/mL *Salmonella* in the chicken extract. In conclusion, QDs provide a framework to satisfy both the selectivity and sensitivity aspects of detection. Lastly, QDs can also be integrated with other non-fluorescent based techniques and more complex microfluidic designs.

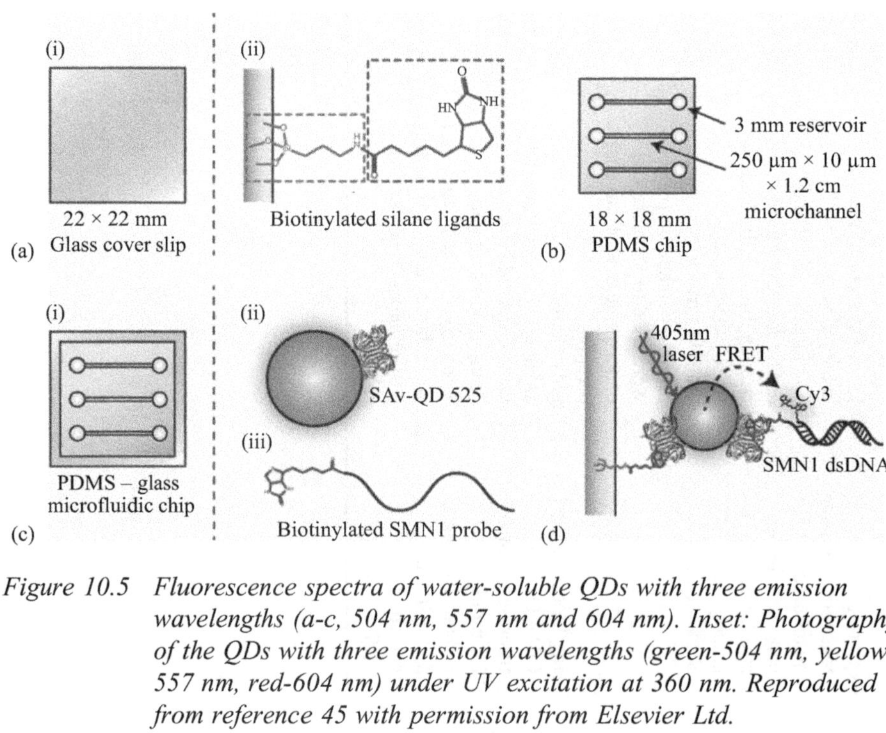

Figure 10.5 Fluorescence spectra of water-soluble QDs with three emission wavelengths (a-c, 504 nm, 557 nm and 604 nm). Inset: Photography of the QDs with three emission wavelengths (green-504 nm, yellow-557 nm, red-604 nm) under UV excitation at 360 nm. Reproduced from reference 45 with permission from Elsevier Ltd.

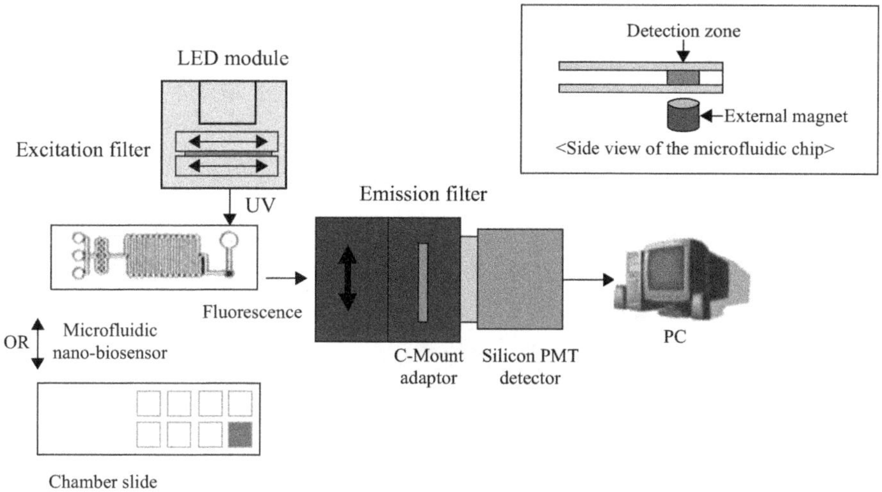

Figure 10.6 *Schematic illustrating the application of QDs with a microfluidic platform. Reproduced from Reference 51 with permission from Elsevier Ltd*

10.10 Surface enhanced Raman spectroscopy (SERS)

Surface Enhanced Raman Spectroscopy (SERS) is a surface spectroscopy technique which amplifies Raman signals by several degrees of magnitude. Raman spectroscopy is an inelastic process whereby the frequency of the scattered photon differs from that of the incident photon as illustrated in Figure 10.7. When subjected to molecules, Raman signals provide information about their chemical structures. In SERS, the excitation laser is in resonance with the surface plasmon of a metal substrate (typically gold or silver) in the form of a roughened metal film, colloids or colloidal solution immobilised on a surface. When an analyte is in close proximity to the metal, the energy from the plasmon resonance may be coupled into bonds of the analyte, causing a significant increase in the Raman signal. Under ideal conditions, SERS is able to detect a single molecule using the intrinsic vibrational fingerprint of the detected analytes [19, 56]. Additionally, Raman spectroscopy performance is not affected by the surrounding water making this system adequate for pathogen detection [57].

There has been consensus among researchers that metal colloids (gold and silver) improve SERS measurements. This is because the metal colloids create an enhancement effect when single nanoparticles form aggregates of two or more, due to coupling of the electromagnetic field. SERS can be modelled as follows:

$$E_s = gE_o$$

E_s is the average magnitude of the field radiated by a metal particle and it is dependent on the relationship between the field enhancement averaged over a surface particle g and the magnitude of the incident field E_o. Hence, the

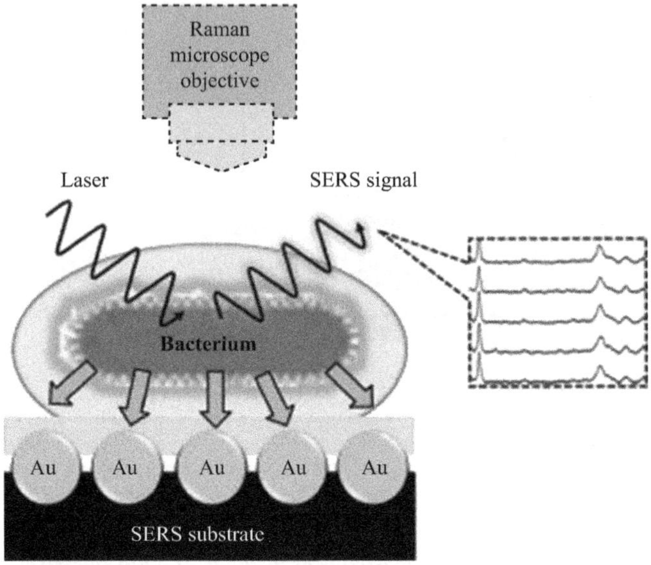

Figure 10.7 SERS based detection of bacteria. Specific probes are immobilised on the sensor surface interacting with the bacteria and producing shifts in the SERS spectra. Reproduced from Reference 58 with permission from Elsevier Ltd

Raman-scattered light depicted by the molecule consists of a field strength E_R which is directly proportional to the magnitude of the field radiated by the metal particle E_s and α_R which is an appropriate combination of the Raman tensor components as shown in the following relation:

$$E_R \propto \alpha_R E_s \propto \alpha_R g E_o$$

Using the same principle, the metal particle can scatter light at the *Raman shifted* wavelength enhanced by a factor g'.

$$E_{SERS} \propto \alpha_R g g' E_o$$

The SERS intensity I_{SERS} (where I_o is the initial intensity) can ultimately be modelled as follows:

$$I_{SERS} \propto |\alpha_R|^2 * |gg'|^2 I_o$$

Finally, SERS enhancement G can be defined as the ratio of the Raman-scattered intensity in the presence of the metal particle to its value in the absence of the metal particle and defining α_{R_o} as the Raman polarisability of the isolated molecule.

$$G = \left|\frac{\alpha_R}{\alpha_{R_o}}\right| |gg'|^2$$

The following example highlights the importance of silver nanoparticle (AgNPs) in a stepwise fashion: the first step involves assembling linker bonded silver nanospheres clusters on the surface (a) followed by the deposition of AgNPs (b). As observed, only a single Si substrate Raman peak is present in the spectrum without any trace of the aminosilane (c). The dithiol linker, 1,4-benzenedithiol, is allowed to bind to the silver nanoparticles (d), and the surface is again exposed to a dilute silver nanoparticle solution to form nanoparticle clusters. As observed from the Raman spectrum, it is evident that dithiol is present as illustrated from the multiple peaks [59].

Due to its high specificity, SERS can be applied to pathogen detection in the food industry and the clinical environment. A study by Wang and colleagues confirmed that SERS was effective for recognising *S. typhimurium and S. aureus* in complex food matrices. The procedure involved immobilising antibody specific to the pathogens on a silica coated magnetic probes which in turn was bound to the protein on the surface of the bacteria. Gold nanoparticles were used as probes. The results (Figure 10.8) showed the SERS was able to discriminate between the two types of bacteria and that lowest cell concentration detected in spinach solution was 10^3 CFU/mL. A blind test conducted in peanut butter validated the LOD [20].

Another study used SERS alongside a microfluidic platform to discriminate between *S. aureus, E. coli,* and *P. aeruginosa* in a blood sample. The motive behind this research was to utilise a hybrid electrokinetic mechanism (dielectrophoresis, electrophoresis, electrohydrodynamics simultaneously) to concentrate and isolate the bacteria from the sample. A SERS-active roughened electrode was used to rapidly and effectively detect bacteria. The electrokinetic approach was able to isolate and concentrate the concerned bacteria within 3 min ensuring a LOD of 5×10^3 CFU/mL [62].

A similar study integrating SERS nanoprobes and microfluidics dielectrophoresis device has been used to detect other types of bacteria such as *Salmonella enterica serotype Choleraesuis* and *Neisseria lactamica*. Similarly, the SERS nanoprobes were immobilised using specific antibody onto the surface of nanoaggregate-embedded beads (NAEBs), coated with silica and dye-induced aggregates of gold nanoparticles (AuNPs). The purpose of the NAEB was to enhance the Raman signals due to the presence of well-defined plasmonic hot spots at junctions between AuNPs as illustrated in Figure 10.9. The detection time for this set up was 10 min with a LOD of 70 mL^{-1}. When compared to ELISA, the SERS nanoprobe-based biosensing method excelled in sensitivity and required lower amount of antibody in the assay (100-fold less). The total assay time comprising of sample pre-treatment was estimated to be less than 2 h. In conclusion, this particular technique is promising in terms of robustness of results, response time, and practicality for the detection of pathogens [63].

In conclusion, SERS combines high sensitivity and selectivity with practicality through the use of microfluidics. SERS based techniques are cost effective and rapid which makes them an ideal biosensor for the detection of pathogens.

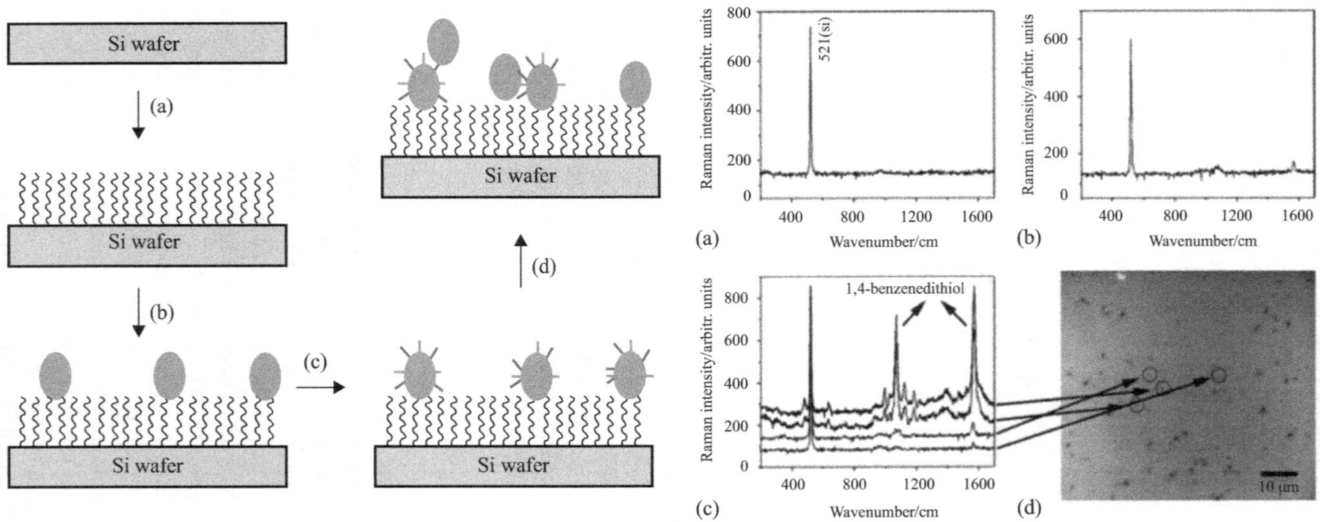

Figure 10.8 Schematic representation of the importance of nanoparticles in SERS enhancements. Reproduced from Reference 59 with permission from Wiley Publishers

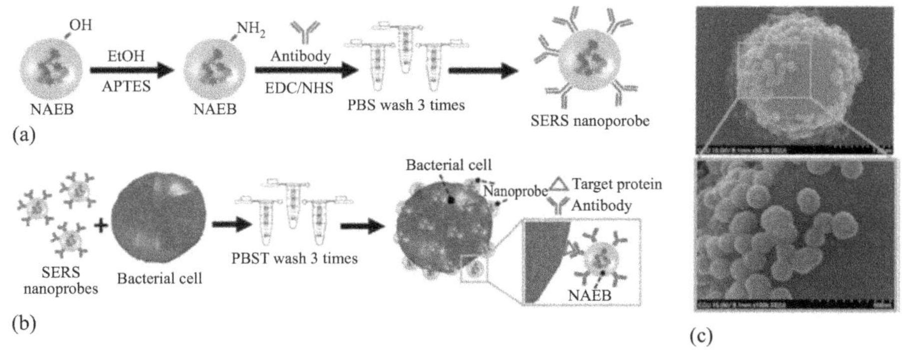

Figure 10.9 Schematic illustrating the process for generating antibody-conjugated NAEBs as novel probes. Reproduced from Reference 63 with permission from Wiley Publishers

10.11 Other methods

10.11.1 Interferometry

Interferometry based biosensors measure the phase change of a guided wave when its evanescent field reacts with a sample. This change in phase can be related to the concentration of analyte in the sample. There exists four types of interferometry based biosensors namely Mach-Zehnder interferometer, Young's interferometer, Hartman interferometer, and Backscattering interferometer [39]. Mach-Zehnder interferometer is made up of a beam splitter which separates a coherent, polarised single frequency of a laser beam into two branches as seen in Figure 10.10. The first branch consists of a window which ensures an interaction of the evanescent field with the sample while keeping the reference arm protected from the sample. The two branches recombine at the output causing an interference [43, 44]. Young's interferometer differs in that it involves having the two branches combine at the interference fringes on a CCD detector. On the other hand, the Hartman interferometer positions the optical elements over a planar waveguide and arranges them in strips. Finally, backscattering interferometers use a simple optical arrangement consisting of a microfluidic path, phototransducer, and a coherent light source [39].

10.11.2 Optical fibre

Fibre-optic biosensors utilise the reflective properties of light to sense numerous analytes simultaneously. Fibre-optic biosensors consist of a core, cladding, and jacket, each with their respective refractive indexes. The core and cladding are necessary for light transmission as illustrated in Reference 27.

Optical fibres are classified as Fibre Bragg's grating and long-term grating. The difference between each type of grating is their construction. The Fibre Bragg method involves etching the fibre surface followed by drawing the physical pattern on the surface. On the other hand, the long-term grating depends on periodic grating of 100 μm to 1 mm which provides extensive sensing abilities to refractive

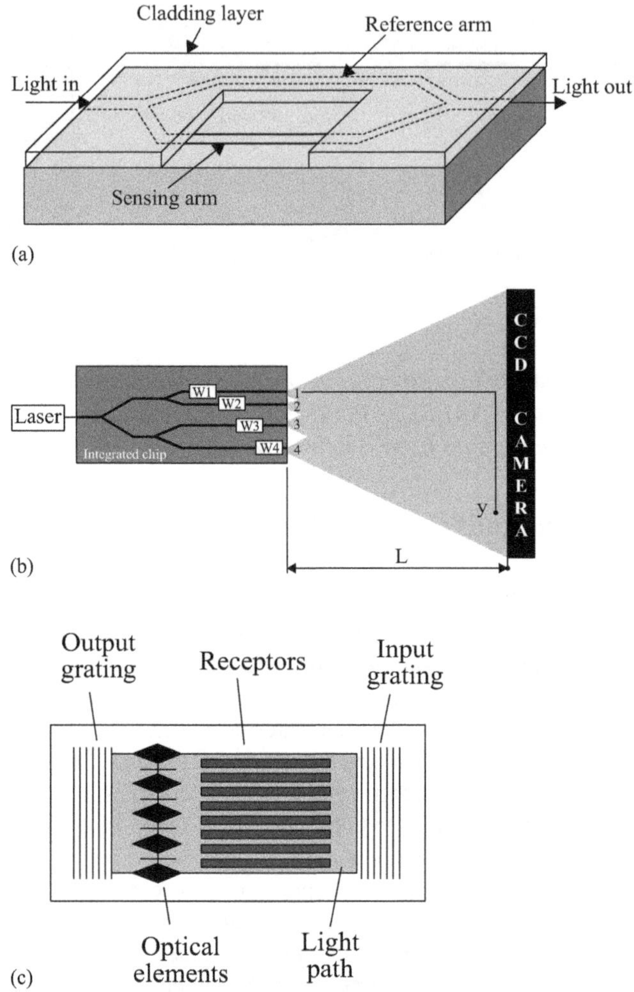

Figure 10.10 (a) Mach-Zehnder interferometer sensor. (b) Young's interferometer (c) Hartman interferometer. Reproduced from Reference 40 with permission from Elsevier Ltd

indexes. Hence, the benefits are high sensitivity with minimal loss of light and low detection limits [39]. Some of the drawbacks of fibre-optic biosensors include a short lifespan of reagents under incident light and slow response time as a result of the diffusion of analytes [14].

10.11.3 Carbon nanotubes

Carbon nanotubes (CNT) and graphene have had tremendous interest in the biosensing field. The intrinsic characteristics of CNT such as semiconductivity, photophysical capabilities, and band gap fluorescence and strong resonance Raman

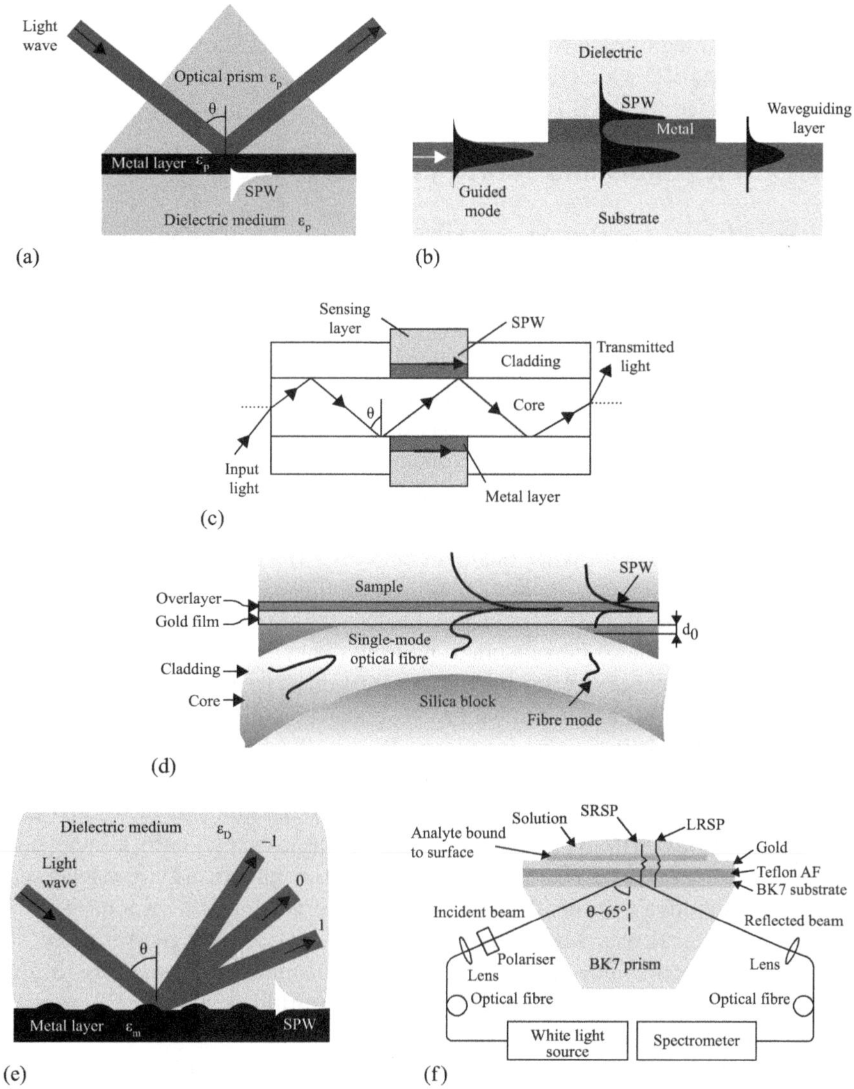

Figure 10.11 Various SPR sensor configurations. (a) Prism coupling (b) Waveguide coupling (c) Optical fibre coupling (d) Side-polished fibre coupling (e) Grating coupling (f) Long-range and short-range surface plasmon. Reproduced from Reference 40 with permission from Elsevier Ltd

scattering (Figure 10.11) make CNT a viable option for biosensing use. A study by Chen and colleagues proposed a sensitive method to detect multiplex protein using functionalised single-walled carbon nanotubes as multicolour Raman labels. Through this method, they stated that CNT provided improved sensitivity as compared to conventional fluorescence based and Raman techniques. Part of the study involved integrating CNT with SERS and the results showed a detection limit of 1×10^{-15} Mol/L, which is three orders of magnitude less in comparison to fluorescence-based methods [41].

10.12 Conclusions and future prospects

Food borne illnesses pose an important threat to the health of billions of individuals across the world. This problem is also responsible for economic losses worth billions of dollars. Part of the solution involves detecting the pathogens at an early stage in the food processing chain. Conventional methods such as ELISA and PCR are limited in terms of their practicality. Hence there is an immense need to use biosensors as a superior alternative. The field of biosensors is broad and can be categorised as optical and non-optical based. The main drawback with non-optical based biosensors is inconsistent measurements and limited sensitivity. On the other hand, optical based biosensors such as ones using fluorescence and SERS provide high sensitive and consistent readings. The future of optical based biosensors is trending towards a field with deployable, cost effective, and sensitive units. Microfluidics provides an excellent platform to allow this transition from in lab testing to onsite detection. In conclusion, biosensors are excellent for the detection of pathogens. The type of biosensors to be used depends on the given application.

The future of biosensors for pathogen detection is trending towards improved selectivity, sensitivity, and practicality. To enhance the performance metrics of biosensors, more sensitive biorecognition elements such as biomemtics are being established. Other researchers are investigating label free recognition techniques. Additionally, novel detection techniques such as combinations of SERS and QCM, or application of QD with fluorescence are being researched with the aim for higher selectivity and lower false positive results. In terms of practicality, the tendency is towards field deployable units that can provide accurate and fast responses for both industry and clinical use. Microfluidics serves as an excellent platform for rapid and accurate detection due to their miniaturised channels for reactions to occur. Furthermore there is less wastage of reagents ensuring cost effectiveness when being used in mass scale production [64].

A study by Dastider and colleagues looked into developing an affordable and simple biosensor for accurate detection of *Salmonella typhimurium.* A microfluidic device was also designed to ensure a fast response and its performance was compared to a non-microfluidic setting. Monoclonal anti-*Salmonella* antibodies were first immobilised on the high density interdigitated electrode surface to recognise the *Salmonella typhimurium* as illustrated in Figure 10.12. The response signal was captured using an impedance analyzer. The detection time without any enrichment was about 3 h and the detection limit for the microfluidic platform was 3×10^3 CFU/mL compared to the 3×10^4 CFU/mL for the nonmicrofluidic biosensor. This confirmed that the presence of microfluidics could result in a 10-fold increase in sensitivity. Additionally the impedance response was also higher by a factor of 2–2.9 compared to the non microfluidic techniques [65].

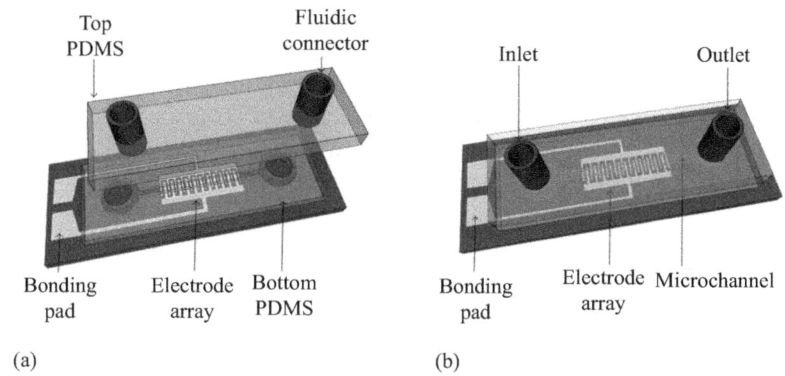

Figure 10.12 Schematic of impedance biosensor with the microfluidic platform. Reproduced from Reference 65 with permission from Hindawi Publishing Corporation

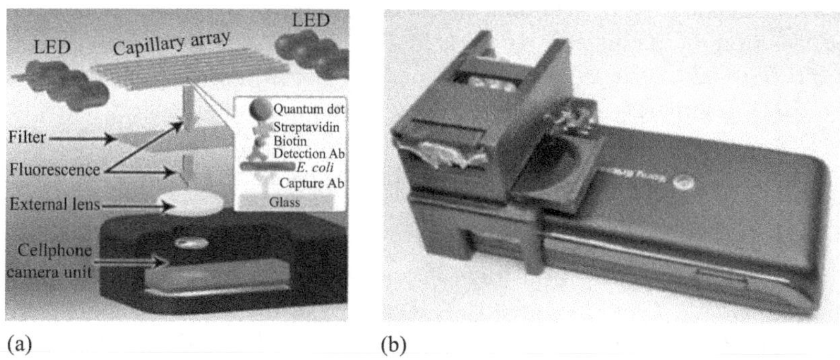

Figure 10.13 Schematic representing the experimental set up of cell phone based biosensor. Reproduced from Reference 66 with permission from the Royal Society of Chemistry

To ensure onsite detection, several approaches using the camera light of cell phones or the computational power of smart phones have been developed for the recognition of pathogens. Hongying and colleagues attempted to integrate an antibody functionalised glass capillaries with QDs as signal reporters to specifically detect *E. coli* particles in liquid samples using a light-weight (~28 g) and compact (3.5 cm × 5.5 cm × 2.4 cm) attachment to the existing camera unit of the cell-phone. The set up involves exciting the QDs using the LED light as illustrated in Figure 10.13. To acquire the appropriate wavelength, an inexpensive long pass glass filter (cut-off wavelength ~610 nm) was used to eliminate the scattered UV and in the process a dark background was obtained for fluorescent imaging. The captured fluorescent response was then imaged by the cell-phone camera unit through an additional lens. The detection limit when tested in food matrix (e.g. fat free milk) was of ~5–10 CFU/mL per sample [66].

The combination of smart and active packaging with biosensors is an innovative approach with regards to food safety. The idea of intelligent packaging, with self-healing properties (able to repair tears), working in synergy with biosensors would ensure improved safety at the customer level. One possible approach is to promote a user-friendly biosensor kit with a smart packaging such that the customers can easily test their own safety prior to consumption [16].

Acknowledgements

The authors thank the Natural Sciences and Engineering Research Council of Canada and the Ontario Ministry of Research and Innovation for funding this study.

References

[1] D. Ivnitski, I. Abdel-Hamid, P. Atanasov, and E. Wilkins, "Biosensors for detection of pathogenic bacteria," *Biosens. Bioelectron.*, vol. 14, no. 7, pp. 599–624, Oct. 1999.

[2] "2011 Estimates of Foodborne Illness in the United States," *Centers for Disease Control and Prevention*, 15-Apr-2011. [Online]. Available: http://www.cdc.gov/Features/dsFoodborneEstimates/.

[3] T. Duque, A. C. Chaves Ribeiro, H. S. de Camargo, P. A. da Costa Filho, H. P. Mesquita Cavalcante, and D. Lopes, "New Insights on Optical Biosensors: Techniques, Construction and Application," in *State of the Art in Biosensors – General Aspects*, T. Rinken, Ed. InTech, 2013.

[4] "Salmonella," *Public Health Agency of Canada*, 06-May-2014. [Online]. Available: http://phac-aspc.gc.ca/fs-sa/fs-fi/salmonella-eng.php.

[5] "World Health Organisation," *Salmonella (non-typhoidal)*, Aug-2013. [Online]. Available: http://www.who.int/mediacentre/factsheets/fs139/en/.

[6] "Public Health Agency of Canada," *Salmonella enterica spp.*, 18-Feb-2011. [Online]. Available: http://www.phac-aspc.gc.ca/lab-bio/res/psds-ftss/salmonella-ent-eng.php.

[7] "US Food and Drug Administration," *Foodborne Pathogenic Microorganisms and Natural Toxins Handbook Escherichia coli O157:H7, 16-Dec-2014.* [Online]. Available: http://www.fda.gov/Food/FoodborneIllnessContaminants/CausesOfIllnessBadBugBook/ucm071284.htm.

[8] "Enterohaemorrhagic Escherichia coli (EHEC)," *World Health Organization*, 2011. [Online]. Available: http://www.who.int/mediacentre/factsheets/fs125/en/.

[9] "Centres for Disease Control and Prevention," *Norovirus*, 26-Jul-2013. [Online]. Available: http://www.cdc.gov/norovirus/about/overview.html.

[10] T. McLinden, J. M. Sargeant, M. Thomas, A. Papadopoulos, and A. Fazil, "Component costs of foodborne illness: a scoping review," *BMC Public Health*, vol. 14, no. 1, p. 509, 2014.

[11] J. Toljander, A. Dovarn, Y. Andersson, S. Ivarsson, and R. Lindqvist, "Public health burden due to infections by verocytotoxin-producing Escherichia coli (VTEC) and Campylobacter spp. as estimated by cost of illness and different approaches to model disability-adjusted life years," *Scand. J. Public Health*, vol. 40, no. 3, pp. 294–302, May 2012.

[12] M. McPherson, M. D. Kirk, J. Raupach, B. Combs, and J. R. G. Butler, "Economic costs of shiga toxin–producing *Escherichia coli* infection in Australia," *Foodborne Pathog. Dis.*, vol. 8, no. 1, pp. 55–62, Jan. 2011.

[13] "Public Health Agency of Canada," *Economic Burden of Illness in Canada*. [Online]. Available: http://www.phac-aspc.gc.ca/ebic-femc/index-eng.php. [Accessed: 20-Mar-2015].

[14] D. G. Nyachuba, "Foodborne illness: is it on the rise?" *Nutr. Rev.*, vol. 68, no. 5, pp. 257–269, Apr. 2010.

[15] R. J. Lake, P. J. Cressey, D. M. Campbell, and E. Oakley, "Risk ranking for foodborne microbial hazards in New Zealand: burden of disease estimates," *Risk Anal.*, vol. 30, no. 5, pp. 743–752, May 2010.

[16] K. Warriner, S. M. Reddy, A. Namvar, and S. Neethirajan, "Developments in nanoparticles for use in biosensors to assess food safety and quality," *Trends Food Sci. Technol.*, vol. 40, no. 2, pp. 183–199, Dec. 2014.

[17] "New Sensor to Detect Harmful Bacteria on Food Industry Surfaces," *University of Southampton*, 11-Jun-2014. [Online]. Available: http://www.southampton.ac.uk/biosci/news/2014/06/11_new_sensor_to_detect_harmful_bacteria_on_food_surfaces.page.

[18] S. D. Gan and K. R. Patel, "Enzyme immunoassay and enzyme-linked immunosorbent assay,"*J. Invest. Derm.*, vol. 133. no. 9, pp. 1–3, 2013.

[19] M. Zourob, S. Elwary, and A. Turner, *Principles of bacterial detection biosensors, recognition receptors, and microsystems*. New York: Springer, 2008.

[20] "ELISA Mechanism." [Online]. Available: http://www.mercodia.se/uploads/images/learning%20center/ELISA%20tech%20Sandwich%20800x588.jpg. [Accessed: 08-Mar-2015].

[21] J.-Y. Yoon and B. Kim, "Lab-on-a-chip pathogen sensors for food safety," *Sensors*, vol. 12, no. 12, pp. 10713–10741, Aug. 2012.

[22] "Life Technologies," 09-Mar-2015. [Online]. Available: http://igene.lifetechnologies.com/products/selector/immunoassays.

[23] V. Velusamy, K. Arshak, O. Korostynska, K. Oliwa, and C. Adley, "An overview of foodborne pathogen detection: in the perspective of biosensors," *Biotechnol. Adv.*, vol. 28, no. 2, pp. 232–254, Mar. 2010.

[24] O. Lazcka, F. J. D. Campo, and F. X. Muñoz, "Pathogen detection: a perspective of traditional methods and biosensors," *Biosens. Bioelectron.*, vol. 22, no. 7, pp. 1205–1217, Feb. 2007.

[25] J. E. Hardingham, A. Chua, J. W. Wrin, A. Shivasami, I. Kanter, N. C. Tebbutt, and T. J. Price, "Polymerase chain reaction: types, utilities and limitations," in *Mutation Detection Using High Resolution Probe Melting Analysis, Polymerase Chain Reaction*, InTech, 2012.

[26] R. Ramasamy, N. Gopal, V. Kuzhandaivelu, and S. Murugaiyan, "Biosensors in clinical chemistry: an overview," *Adv. Biomed. Res.*, vol. 3, no. 1, p. 67, 2014.

[27] N. Mungroo and S. Neethirajan, "Biosensors for the detection of antibiotics in poultry industry—a review," *Biosensors*, vol. 4, no. 4, pp. 472–493, Nov. 2014.

[28] W. Wang, S. Singh, D. L. Zeng, K. King, and S. Nema, "Antibody structure, instability, and formulation," *J. Pharm. Sci.*, vol. 96, no. 1, pp. 1–26, Jan. 2007.

[29] B. Byrne, E. Stack, N. Gilmartin, and R. O'Kennedy, "Antibody-based sensors: principles, problems and potential for detection of pathogens and associated toxins," *Sensors*, vol. 9, no. 6, pp. 4407–4445, Jun. 2009.

[30] B. D. Leca-Bouvier and L. J. Blum, "Enzyme for biosensing applications," in *Recognition Receptors in Biosensors*, M. Zourob, Ed. New York, NY: Springer New York, 2010, pp. 177–220.

[31] V. Perumal and U. Hashim, "Advances in biosensors: principle, architecture and applications," *J. Appl. Biomed.*, vol. 12, no. 1, pp. 1–15, Jan. 2014.

[32] C. Feng, S. Dai, and L. Wang, "Optical aptasensors for quantitative detection of small biomolecules: a review," *Biosens. Bioelectron.*, vol. 59, pp. 64–74, Sep. 2014.

[33] P. Wang and Q. Liu, *Cell-based biosensors principles and applications*. Boston: Artech House, 2010.

[34] A.-C. Huet, P. Delahaut, T. Fodey, S. A. Haughey, C. Elliott, and S. Weigel, "Advances in biosensor-based analysis for antimicrobial residues in foods," *TrAC Trends Anal. Chem.*, vol. 29, no. 11, pp. 1281–1294, Dec. 2010.

[35] Y. Song, H. Zhang, C. H. Chon, S. Chen, X. Pan, and D. Li, "Counting bacteria on a microfluidic chip," *Anal. Chim. Acta*, vol. 681, no. 1–2, pp. 82–86, Nov. 2010.

[36] F. Salam, Y. Uludag, and I. E. Tothill, "Real-time and sensitive detection of Salmonella Typhimurium using an automated quartz crystal microbalance (QCM) instrument with nanoparticles amplification," *Talanta*, vol. 115, pp. 761–767, Oct. 2013.

[37] S. Scarano, M. Mascini, A. P. F. Turner, and M. Minunni, "Surface plasmon resonance imaging for affinity-based biosensors," *Biosens. Bioelectron.*, vol. 25, no. 5, pp. 957–966, Jan. 2010.

[38] S. Bouguelia, Y. Roupioz, S. Slimani, *et al.*, "On-chip microbial culture for the specific detection of very low levels of bacteria," *Lab. Chip*, vol. 13, no. 20, p. 4024, 2013.

[39] T. Duque, A. C. Chaves Ribeiro, H. S. de Camargo, P. A. da Costa Filho, H. P. Mesquita Cavalcante, and D. Lopes, "New insights on optical biosensors: techniques, construction and application," in *State of the Art in Biosensors – General Aspects*, T. Rinken, Ed. InTech, 2013.

[40] X. Fan, I. M. White, S. I. Shopova, H. Zhu, J. D. Suter, and Y. Sun, "Sensitive optical biosensors for unlabeled targets: a review," *Anal. Chim. Acta*, vol. 620, no. 1–2, pp. 8–26, Jul. 2008.

[41] Z. Chen, S. M. Tabakman, A. P. Goodwin, *et al.*, "Protein microarrays with carbon nanotubes as multicolor Raman labels," *Nat. Biotechnol.*, vol. 26, no. 11, pp. 1285–1292, Nov. 2008.

[42] K. Tainaka, R. Sakaguchi, H. Hayashi, S. Nakano, F. F. Liew, and T. Morii, "Design strategies of fluorescent biosensors based on biological macromolecular receptors," *Sensors*, vol. 10, no. 2, pp. 1355–1376, Feb. 2010.

[43] J. Li and J.-J. Zhu, "Quantum dots for fluorescent biosensing and bioimaging applications," *The Analyst*, vol. 138, no. 9, p. 2506, 2013.

[44] A. Fontes and B. S. Santos, Quantum *dots: applications in biology*. Springer Publishing, 2014.

[45] B. Wang, Q. Wang, Z. Cai, and M. Ma, "Simultaneous, rapid and sensitive detection of three food-borne pathogenic bacteria using multicolor quantum dot probes based on multiplex fluoroimmunoassay in food samples," *LWT - Food Sci. Technol.*, Dec. 2014.

[46] L. Wang, C.-S. Wu, X. Fan, and A. Mustapha, "Detection of Escherichia coli O157:H7 and Salmonella in ground beef by a bead-free quantum dot-facilitated isolation method," *Int. J. Food Microbiol.*, vol. 156, no. 1, pp. 83–87, May 2012.

[47] N. Sanvicens, N. Pascual, M. T. Fernández-Argüelles, *et al.*, "Quantum dot-based array for sensitive detection of Escherichia coli," *Anal. Bioanal. Chem.*, vol. 399, no. 8, pp. 2755–2762, Mar. 2011.

[48] E. Liandris, M. Gazouli, M. Andreadou, L. A. Sechi, V. Rosu, and J. Ikonomopoulos, "Detection of pathogenic mycobacteria based on functionalized quantum dots coupled with immunomagnetic separation," *PLoS ONE*, vol. 6, no. 5, p. e20026, May 2011.

[49] L. Yang and Y. Li, "Simultaneous detection of Escherichia coli O157:H7 and Salmonella typhimurium using quantum dots as fluorescence labels," *The Analyst*, vol. 131, no. 3, p. 394, 2006.

[50] B. Wang, X. Huang, M. Ma, Q. Shi, and Z. Cai, "A simple quantum dot-based fluoroimmunoassay method for selective capturing and rapid detection of Salmonella Enteritidis on eggs," *Food Control*, vol. 35, no. 1, pp. 26–32, Jan. 2014.

[51] G. Kim, J.-H. Moon, C.-Y. Moh, and J. Lim, "A microfluidic nano-biosensor for the detection of pathogenic Salmonella," *Biosens. Bioelectron.*, Aug. 2014.

[52] A. Singh, S. Poshtiban, and S. Evoy, "Recent advances in bacteriophage based biosensors for food-borne pathogen detection," *Sensors*, vol. 13, no. 2, pp. 1763–1786, Jan. 2013.

[53] J. Luo, X. Liu, Q. Tian, *et al.*, "Disposable bioluminescence-based biosensor for detection of bacterial count in food," *Anal. Biochem.*, vol. 394, no. 1, pp. 1–6, Nov. 2009.

[54] Z. Xia and J. Rao, "Biosensing and imaging based on bioluminescence resonance energy transfer," *Curr. Opin. Biotechnol.*, vol. 20, no. 1, pp. 37–44, Feb. 2009.

[55] A. Koyun, E. Ahlatcıoğlu, and Y. Koca İpek, "Biosensors and Their Principles," in *A Roadmap of Biomedical Engineers and Milestones*, InTech, 2012.

[56] E. C. Le Ru and P. G. Etchegoin, *Principles of surface-enhanced Raman spectroscopy and related plasmonic effects*. Amsterdam, Boston: Elsevier, 2009.

[57] D. Kim, A. R. Campos, A. Datt, *et al.*, "Microfluidic-SERS devices for one shot limit-of-detection," *The Analyst*, vol. 139, no. 13, p. 3227, 2014.

[58] S. C. B. Gopinath, T.-H. Tang, Y. Chen, M. Citartan, and T. Lakshmipriya, "Bacterial detection: From microscope to smart phone," *Biosens. Bioelectron.*, vol. 60, pp. 332–342, Oct. 2014.

[59] M. Moskovits, "Surface-enhanced Raman spectroscopy: a brief retrospective," *J. Raman Spectrosc.*, vol. 36, no. 6–7, pp. 485–496, Jun. 2005.

[60] S. Schlücker, Ed., *Surface enhanced Raman spectroscopy: analytical, biophysical and life science applications*. Weinheim, Germany: Wiley-VCH Verlag, 2011.

[61] Y. Wang, S. Ravindranath, and J. Irudayaraj, "Separation and detection of multiple pathogens in a food matrix by magnetic SERS nanoprobes," *Anal. Bioanal. Chem.*, vol. 399, no. 3, pp. 1271–1278, Jan. 2011.

[62] I-Fang Cheng, H.-C. Chang, T.-Y. Chen, C. Hu, and F.-L. Yang, "Rapid (<5 min) identification of pathogen in human blood by electrokinetic concentration and surface-enhanced Raman spectroscopy," *Sci. Rep.*, vol. 3, Aug. 2013.

[63] H.-Y. Lin, C.-H. Huang, W.-H. Hsieh,. "On-line SERS detection of single bacterium using novel SERS nanoprobes and a microfluidic dielectrophoresis device," *Small*, vol. 10, no. 22, pp. 4700–4710, Nov. 2014.

[64] C. Rivet, H. Lee, A. Hirsch, S. Hamilton, and H. Lu, "Microfluidics for medical diagnostics and biosensors," *Chem. Eng. Sci.*, vol. 66, no. 7, pp. 1490–1507, Apr. 2011.

[65] S. Ghosh Dastider, S. Barizuddin, N. S. Yuksek, M. Dweik, and M. F. Almasri, "Efficient and rapid detection of *Salmonella* using microfluidic impedance based sensing," *J. Sens.*, vol. 2015, pp. 1–8, 2015.

[66] H. Zhu, U. Sikora, and A. Ozcan, "Quantum dot enabled detection of Escherichia coli using a cell-phone," *The Analyst*, vol. 137, no. 11, p. 2541, 2012.

[67] T. S. Park, W. Li, K. E. McCracken, and J.-Y. Yoon, "Smartphone quantifies Salmonella from paper microfluidics," *Lab. Chip*, vol. 13, no. 24, p. 4832, 2013.

[68] C. Ricciardi, G. Canavese, R. Castagna, *et al.*, "Online portable microcantilever biosensors for Salmonella enterica serotype enteritidis detection," *Food Bioprocess Technol.*, vol. 3, no. 6, pp. 956–960, Dec. 2010.

Chapter 11

Generation and optimisation of antibodies for biosensor applications

H. Ma[1] *and R. O'Kennedy*[1]

11.1 Antibody generation for use in biosensors

Antibodies are widely applied in biosensors for detection of various diseases, food and environmental contaminants and biological warfare agents [1]. The efficacy, sensitivity and specificity of antibody-based biosensors are mainly dependent on the antibody. Therefore, how the antibody is generated, isolated, purified and optimised before incorporation into the biosensor is crucial. This chapter focuses on the generation, and purification of antibodies and their optimisation for use in biosensors.

Antibodies are also known as immunoglobulins (Igs) and possess antigen binding specificity. There are three main types of antibodies applied in biosensors, namely, polyclonal, monoclonal and recombinant antibodies. Polyclonal antibodies are derived from multiple B lymphocyte clones and they recognise multiple epitopes. Unlike polyclonal antibodies, monoclonal antibodies are generated from a single B lymphocyte (B cell) and react with a single antigenic epitope. A recombinant antibody does not exist naturally but is assembled from recombinant DNA by combining antibody heavy chain and light chain gene sequences [2].

Igs are produced by B-lymphocyte-derived plasma cells. Antibodies are found in serum, as well as in interstitial fluids and exocrine secretions. Antibodies can effectively identify, kill or neutralise invading bacteria, parasites, toxins or viruses and destroy other foreign entities [2]. Mammalian antibodies are classified into five isotypes IgM, IgD, IgG, IgE and IgA based on five different heavy polypeptide chains μ, δ, γ, ε and α, respectively [3]. There are two types of light chains in mammalian antibodies, namely, lambda (λ) and kappa (κ). However, each antibody possesses either a λ or κ. Both heavy and light chains contain two main regions: i.e. the variable (V) region at the N-terminal end and the constant (C) region at the C-terminal end. The amino acid sequence of the variable regions is responsible for the specificity of the antibody, and it is this region that is used for antigen-specific

[1]Biomedical Diagnostics Institute, Dublin City University, Dublin 9, Ireland

binding. For each isotype, the constant domain remains the same with the same amino acid consensus sequence [4].

The synonymous 'Y' shape associated with a basic immunoglobulin unit (Ig) monomer (or subunit) (Figure 11.1) consists of two light (V_L) and two heavy (V_H) chains, which are connected by disulphide bonds [5]. All five isotypes, IgM, IgD, IgG, IgE and IgA, are composed of this basic structure with specific modifications. IgD, IgE and IgG are monomers, while IgA is either a monomer or a dimer and IgM is a pentamer [3]. However, heavy-chain antibodies which consist of two heavy chains and lack light chains are found in the members of the *Camelidae* family [6]. Immunoglobulin new antigen receptors (IgNAR) are heavy-chain antibodies found in cartilaginous fish. IgNARs contain only two heavy chains and each chain has one variable region and five constant regions (C_H1–5) [7] while among avian Igs, the major antibody IgY (the 180 kDa homologue of mammal IgG) consists of four constant Ig domains, like mammalian IgE, instead of three for mammalian IgG [8].

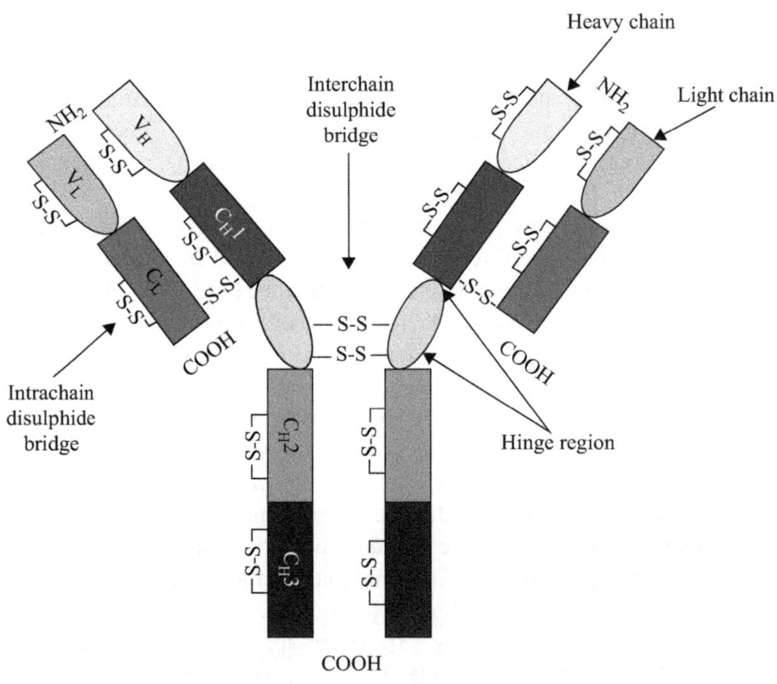

Figure 11.1 Structure of a basic IgG antibody. The basic antibody monomer consists of two light chains and two heavy chains which are connected by disulphide bonds. NH_2 = amino group; COOH = carboxylic acid group; V_H = variable region of antibody heavy chain; V_L = variable region of antibody light chain; C_L = constant region of antibody light chain; C_H1, 2, 3 = constant domains one, two and three of the antibody heavy chain and S–S = disulphide bond

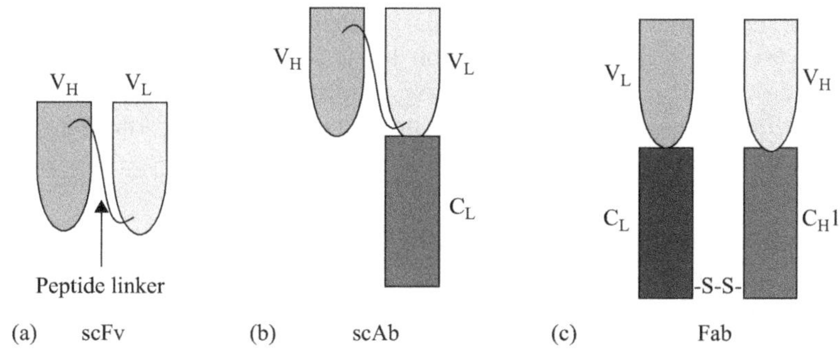

Figure 11.2 *Structures of a scFv (a), a scAb (b) and a Fab fragment (c). V_H = variable region of antibody heavy chain; V_L = variable region of antibody light chain; C_L = constant region of antibody light chain; C_H1 = constant domain one of antibody heavy chain and S–S = disulphide bond*

Various formats for recombinant antibodies exist. The single chain variable fragment (scFv) consists of the variable (binding) regions of antibody V_L and V_H, which are linked by a short peptide chain (Figure 11.2a). The popularity achieved by the scFv fragment is due to its short generation time, capacity to be expressed in *Escherichia coli* (*E. coli*), high antigen affinity and structural stability [9]. A single-chain antibody (scAb) consists of a scFv region fused to a light chain constant domain (C_L) (Figure 11.2b), which was shown to significantly improve expression levels in *E. coli* [10]. The fragment antigen-binding (Fab) unit consists of a full antibody light chain, connected to a second antibody domain comprised of V_H and C_H1 regions connected by disulphide bonding (Figure 11.2c).

11.2 Polyclonal antibody generation

11.2.1 Process of adaptive immune response

Exposure to an antigens leads to the generation of an immune response and to immunological memory (the ability of the immune system to respond more rapidly and effectively to pathogens that have been encountered previously) which takes from several days (helper T-cell memory) to weeks (memory B-cell) to establish, and an enhancement of the immune response will be achieved by future exposure. Immunological memory ensures a quick and efficient immune response on later infection. The adaptive immune response is also classified as either a humoral or a cell-mediated immunity.

Humoral immunity, or antibody-mediated immunity, is mediated through B-cells by producing Igs which are specific to foreign antigens. The antigen-specific Ig-producing B cells then move from primary lymphoid organs (e.g. bone marrow, thymus and fetal liver) to secondary lymphoid organs, for instance, spleen, lymph nodes and small masses of lymph tissue [11]. Mature circulating B-cells have one type of Ig on their surface. Upon a second or subsequent encounter with their specific antigen the B cell rapidly proliferates and transforms into an antibody-secreting plasma cell [12].

11.2.2 Hosts for polyclonal antibody production

The production of polyclonal antibodies is usually conducted by carrying out several rounds of antigen immunisation of the host animal. Specific antibodies are then generated by B lymphocytes. Finally, polyclonal antibodies are extracted from the serum of animals, whereas for chickens, polyclonal antibodies can also be extracted from egg yolks. Polyclonal serum offers the advantage of broad reactivity. However, polyclonal sera also display variability in specificity, avidity, relative percentage of constituent antibodies generated and are produced in limited quantities. It may also be difficult to reproduce these characteristics in new batches [2].

Rabbits, mice, chickens, goats and sheep are among the most common host animals chosen for the generation of polyclonal antibodies for biosensors. However, llamas, alpacas and camels are also used. Both rabbits and chickens can generate large amounts of polyclonal antibodies with high specificity. Usually immunisation of at least two animals per antigen is recommended, as in some cases there may be little or no response to the target antigen. This often occurs as each animal has a unique immune system and, therefore, the immune response is highly variable. Further comparisons between human, rabbit, mouse, chicken, goat, sheep, llama and alpaca antibodies are shown in Table 11.1.

The generation of antibodies using a rabbit as the host for immunisation offers a number of advantages. It is a medium sized animal and is easier and cheaper to maintain than larger animals (e.g. goats and sheep). A rabbit is able to produce a large amount of polyclonal antibodies in serum with an antibody concentration of 7–15 mg/mL (~5 mL serum per week). Young adult female rabbits are preferred because young rabbits generate a better antibody response than older animals, and female rabbits are more docile and less aggressive in social interactions than males. There are more than twenty functional heavy chain germline genes in the rabbit immune system, two constant kappa light chain (Cκ) genes and multiple variable kappa light chain (Vκ) genes ($\kappa:\lambda = 10\sim20:1$) [26]. Enormous diversity is generated by re-arrangement of the V (variable), D (diversity) and J (joining) gene segments.

Use of the murine immune system for the generation of antibodies with high affinity to a vast array of specific antigens is extensively documented [27]. Bachmann *et al.* [28] reported that in the mouse, approximately 1,000 to 10,000 specific B-cells are produced in response to a complex antigen. Murine complementarity determining regions 1 and 2 (CDR1 and CDR2) of heavy and light chains are determined by V gene segments, while CDR3 is produced by inaccurate joining of V, D and J gene segments ensuring great structural antibody diversity.

Table 11.1 Comparison of human, rabbit, mouse, chicken, goat, sheep, llama and alpaca antibodies

Hosts/ Characteristics	**Structure**	**Primarily used antibody**	**Molecular weight (kDa)**	**Main source**	**Diversity**	**Examples of biosensor-based applications**
Human [13]	IgM/G/A/D/E	IgG	150	Serum (~10 mg/mL)	High	Detection of infectious diseases [14] and cardiovascular diseases [15]
Rabbit [16]	IgM/G/A/D/E	IgG	150	Serum (7–15 mg/mL)	High	*Listeria monocytogenes* detection [17]
Mouse [18]	IgM/G/A/D/E	IgG	150	Serum (7–15 mg/mL); Ascitic fluid (5–15 mg/mL)	High	*Neisseria meningitidis* detection [17]
Chicken [13]	IgY/A/M	IgY	180	Egg yolk (15–25 mg/mL); Serum (~5 mg/mL)	Low	Detection of colon, breast and ovarian cancers [19, 20]
Goat [21]	IgM/G/A/D/E	IgG	150	Serum (20–30 mg/mL)	High	*Salmonella typhimurium* and *Listeria monocytogenes* detection [17]
Sheep [22]	IgM/G/A/D/E	IgG	150	Serum (20–30 mg/mL)	High	Atrazine detection in drinking water [23]
Llama/Alpaca [24]	IgM/G/A/D/E	IgG	IgG1: 160 IgG2: 92 IgG3: 86	Serum (~20 mg/mL)	High	Human prostate-specific antigen (hPSA) detection [25]

In general, the larger the phylogenetic distance between the immunised animal (e.g. chicken) and the antigen source (e.g. human), the greater the antibody response produced. Thus, chickens, which are phylogenetically more distant from humans than rabbits and mice, are more likely to achieve better immune responses to certain human proteins. Female chickens (hens) are favoured for producing large amounts of IgY, as this can be harvested from egg yolk. This process is more convenient than producing antibodies from blood when large quantities of antibody are needed. The immunoglobulin locus of chickens consists of only one functional copy of the V and J segment for both the heavy and light chains of the antibody. The production of an antibody repertoire in the chicken immune system is derived by re-arrangement of the V and J segments, which makes the diversity of antibodies limited [29].

Goats, sheep, llamas and alpacas are relatively large animals compared to mice, rats, rabbits or chickens. They are useful hosts if very large amounts of polyclonal antibodies are needed. Each one of them is able to produce 250–400 mL of blood while each rabbit can only produce 25–30 mL of blood. Moreover, llamas and alpacas, members of *Camelidae* family, are able to produce heavy chain antibodies which are more robust and easier to transform into bacterial cells for large-scale production due to their smaller size [30].

11.2.3 Purification of polyclonal antibodies

11.2.3.1 Receptor-ligand-based affinity chromatographic purification

Affinity chromatographic purification is the most popular method for antibody purification based on receptor–ligand or antigen–antibody binding. The antibody-containing sample is initially dissolved in a mobile phase (buffer) which then carries the sample through the stationary phase (agarose resin with ligand or antigen attached) which is usually packed into a column. The specific antibodies will be bound onto the resin and the non-specific antibodies and other impurities will be removed by running wash buffer through the column. Finally, the specific antibodies will be eluted by application of an elution buffer (often with low pH or high salt) to the column [31]. If the antibodies are eluted using a low pH elution buffer, neutralisation buffer is always added to preserve reactivity of purified antibodies, as monoreactive antibodies may gain the ability to bind to multiple antigens after exposure to low pH [32].

IgG purifications are generally carried out by using protein A or G. These are the most popular Ig-binding proteins and bind through the fragment crystallisable (Fc) or Fab region. IgM, IgA, IgD, IgE, Fab and scFv isolation is widely performed by using protein L via its specific binding to Ig kappa light chains.

Thiophilic adsorption chromatography, which consists of protein-free immunosorbent resin (containing sulfone-thioether groups), can be used for purification of a broad range of Igs (e.g. IgG, IgM, IgA, IgD, IgE, and IgY) via their affinity for sulfone-thioether groups in high salt conditions. It provides mild binding (non-denaturing) and elution conditions (salt-free or very low salt at near neutral pH) for Ig purification, which leads to significant recovery of functional antibody.

11.2.3.2 Chicken IgY purification based on delipidation-and-precipitation techniques

IgY is not bound by typical IgG affinity resins (Protein A, G or L), therefore, IgY is usually purified by applying techniques of delipidation-and-precipitation. This method includes two major steps: (1) removal of lipids present in the egg and (2) the precipitation of IgY [33]. There are many IgY purification kits based on delipidation-and-precipitation commercially available (e.g. Pierce Biotechnology/Thermoscientific, Promega, Agro-Bio, GE Healthcare, Affiland and Gallus Immunotech). About 80–120 mg IgY per egg yolk can be obtained using this approach.

11.2.3.3 Polyclonal antibody purification using antigen-antibody binding-based affinity chromatographic strategies

Antigen-specific affinity purification is performed via antigen-antibody binding. The antigen can be immobilised to a solid support surface through a unique functional group (e.g. sulphydryl on a single terminal cysteine or C-terminal carboxyl amino acids in a peptide) or through streptavidin–biotin interactions (one of the strongest non-covalent interactions known in nature). After passing the antibody sample over the antigen, the antigen-specific antibody will be bound onto the solid support surface, while the non-specific antibodies and impurities are then washed away by the washing buffer. Finally, the antigen-specific antibodies are eluted by changing pH (low pH buffer is usually used and the eluted antibodies are then collected in neutralisation buffer to preserve reactivity of purified antibodies [32]) or by changing the salt concentration.

11.3 Monoclonal antibody generation

11.3.1 Hybridoma cell production

In order to produce monoclonal antibodies, which are monospecific, antibody-generating B cells (e.g. harvested from spleen) are initially fused with B cell-derived cancer cells (myelomas) and the specific hybrids, with the required antibody-secreting specificity, selected. These hybrid cell lines are called hybridomas. To generate monoclonal antibodies animals (e.g. mice and rabbits) are immunised using a specific antigen. Once an ideal immune response is achieved, the spleen is harvested for B-cell collection. The antibody-producing B-cells will then be fused with myeloma cells to form hybridomas by electrofusion or by the addition of polyethylene glycol (PEG). Hybridomas can be isolated using a selection medium which contains aminopterin. Myeloma cells lack the enzyme hypoxanthine-guanine-phosphoribosyl transferase (HGPRT), used for the salvage synthesis of nucleic acids, but will survive through the use of the *de novo* purine synthesis pathway. The *de novo* purine synthesis pathway can be blocked on exposure to aminopterin which inhibits dihydrofolate reductase thus disabling the replication of DNA. Therefore, the myeloma cells cannot survive when aminopterin is present. Unfused spleen cells will gradually die because of their restricted life-span. However, the fused hybridoma cells are able to survive as the spleen cells contribute HGPRT and the myeloma cells provide the capacity for continuous growth [34].

Each B-cell only synthesises antibodies with a single specificity. Once a single clone is selected, the hybridoma (grown in DMEM with 10 per cent (v/v) fetal bovine serum at 37 °C with 5 per cent (v/v) CO_2) is able to divide (characteristic of myelomas) and express the antibodies (characteristic of B-cells) which are specific for the immunised antigen. The monoclonal antibody, e.g. IgG, can then be easily purified from the culture medium.

11.3.2 Purification of monoclonal antibodies

Culture medium from tissue culture flasks derived from actively growing selected hybridomas, over a number of days, is centrifuged at 125 g for 5 min. The supernatant is then concentrated from approximately 500 to 5 mL using an Amicon® stir cell system (GE Healthcare) with an ultrafiltration membrane (100 kDa molecular weight 'cut-off'). The monoclonal antibody in the concentrated supernatant can be purified by applying receptor-ligand-based and antigen-antibody binding-based affinity chromatographic strategies, as described in Section 11.4.

11.3.3 Recombinant antibody generation

Use of recombinant antibodies has many advantages for applications with biosensors (Table 11.2). Recombinant antibody technology offers the possibility of production of antibodies with high sensitivity, specificity and stability for use in disease diagnosis, therapy and many other areas. The orientation, labelling and immobilisation of recombinant antibody can be easily achieved by using genetically and chemically insert tags (e.g. biotin, polyhistidine or hemagglutinin). Antibody expression in *E. coli* has several advantages, for instance, large quantities, can be produced quickly and at low cost [35]. Over the last twenty years, antibody genes have been cloned,

Table 11.2 Key advantages of recombinant antibodies [2, 35]

Advantages of recombinant antibodies
• Can be fully standardised in terms of performance
• Screening can be easily automated
• Range of natural and synthetic antibody libraries available
• Facilitate addition of tags to aid isolation and immobilisation
• Specificity can be altered to exact requirements (i.e. highly specific for one target or for class of targets)
• Can reduce dependence on animals for antibody production
• Can be tailored to a range of antibody-based formats e.g. scFv, Fv, scAb etc.
• Stability can be enhanced by genetic engineering
• Tags can be added by fusion or chemically to aid correct orientation on sensor surfaces
• Relative costs of production are continually reducing

genetically manipulated and expressed in *E. coli* to produce antigen-binding proteins for various biosensor applications (e.g. detection of human prostate-specific antigen, morphine-3-glucuronide, aflatoxin B1, simazine and diphenylurea) [36].

11.3.4 Generation of recombinant antibodies

Host animals are immunised and subsequently boosted using the required antigen. After a suitable antibody titre (usually $\geq$ 1:10,000) is achieved, the animals are sacrificed. RNA is extracted from the spleen and bone marrow, followed by cDNA synthesis. The antibody genes are amplified from cDNA using specifically designed primers and are cloned into a phage display vector (e.g. pComb3H or pComb3X) [37]. The recombinant genes are then transformed into electro-competent bacteria (e.g. XL1-Blue or Top10F′) to produce the antibody phage library [38]. Each bacterium from this library will express a single individual recombinant antibody on the surface of a phage particle. Finally, the extraction and selection of highly specific antibody is performed generally using phage display technology with several rounds of bio-panning (Figure 11.3). The most widely applied formats of recombinant antibodies used in sensors are scFv and Fabs (Figure 11.2a and b).

Phage, a type of virus that infects bacteria, can adopt foreign genes into the non-crucial regions of its genome. In phage display technology, foreign DNA (e.g. gene for scFv or Fab), is inserted into phage gene III, the gene that encodes one of the phage coat proteins, and is expressed as a fusion protein. After infecting Gram-negative bacteria (e.g. XL1-blue and Top10F′ *E. coli*) the phage starts the replication of coat protein genes, including gene III and the foreign DNA. Gene III and the foreign DNA is then expressed as a fusion protein and is displayed on the surface of phage [39].

11.3.5 Selection of recombinant antibodies through phage display

The phage (e.g. M13, T4, T7 and λ phage)-expressed antibodies are then screened via biopanning for antibodies which are specific to the target. Usually, several cycles (3–5) of biopanning are needed for enrichment of the required antibodies, as increasing rounds of biopanning are more likely to result in higher enrichment for specific antibodies [40].

Each cycle of biopanning includes three basic steps. Firstly, this involves selection of specific phage which bind to the target. At this step, the prepared phage clones are added to tubes or microwells coated with a defined amount of the target antigen. The coating antigen concentration is usually decreased with each round of biopanning. Secondly, removal of non-specific phage from the solid surface of the well or tube is achieved by washing 5–10 times using phosphate-buffered saline (PBS) with 0.1 per cent (v/v) Tween-20 (PBST) and with PBS. The number of washings is usually increased with each round of biopanning. Finally, specific phage is collected by eluting phage remaining bound to the immobilised antigen using a freshly prepared trypsin solution. The eluted phage can be kept at 4 °C for long-term storage and are analysed initially for specificity by a polyclonal phage enzyme-linked immunosorbent assay (ELISA). If specific binding to the target antigen is detected, single colonies will be selected for analysis of specific antibody expression. However, if no specific binding is detected by polyclonal phage ELISA, the eluted phage will be re-infected into *E. coli* and the next round of biopanning performed [2]. A typical bio panning cycle is illustrated in Figure 11.3.

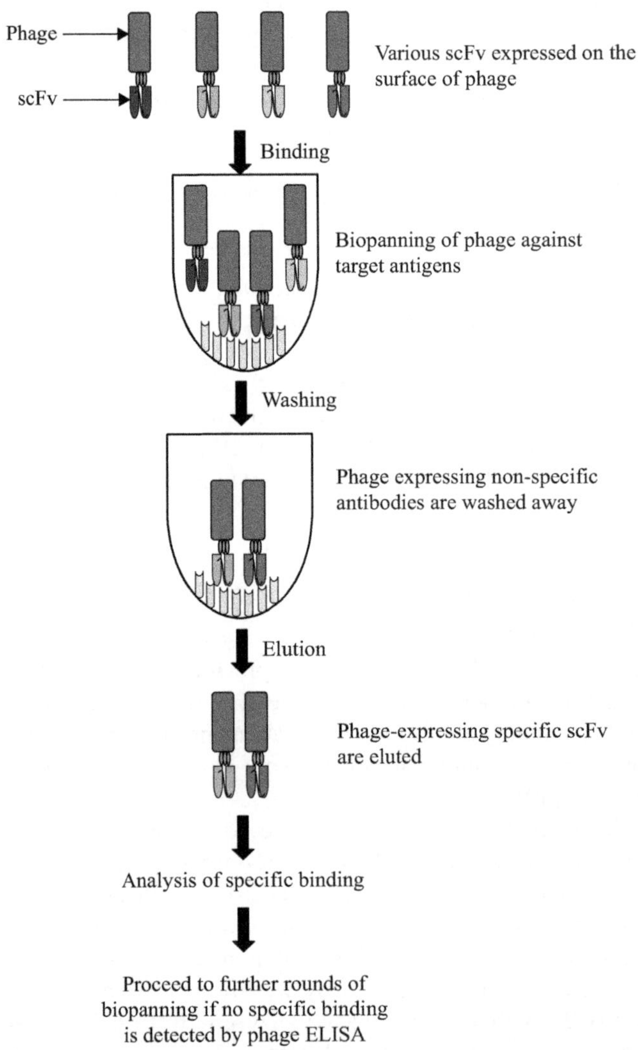

Figure 11.3 Illustration of a typical biopanning cycle

11.3.6 DiCAST, a novel technology of direct clone analysis and selection

A novel direct clone analysis and selection technology, called DiCAST, provides single-cell and real-time analysis and characterisation and can be very efficiently applied for antibody screening [41]. DiCAST is a microtool which enables the identification of monospecific antibodies from 0.95 to 15 million individual bacterial or mammalian cells using capillary plates of highly densely packed micro-capillary flow-through arrays. The process involves single antibody-secreting cell, capture. The antibody of interest binds the specific antigen, and is then detected by fluorescently-labelled secondary antibody. A high resolution image is generated and the microcapillary with the desired cells corresponding to the fluorescent spot can be located and the required cells recovered (Figure 11.4) [41].

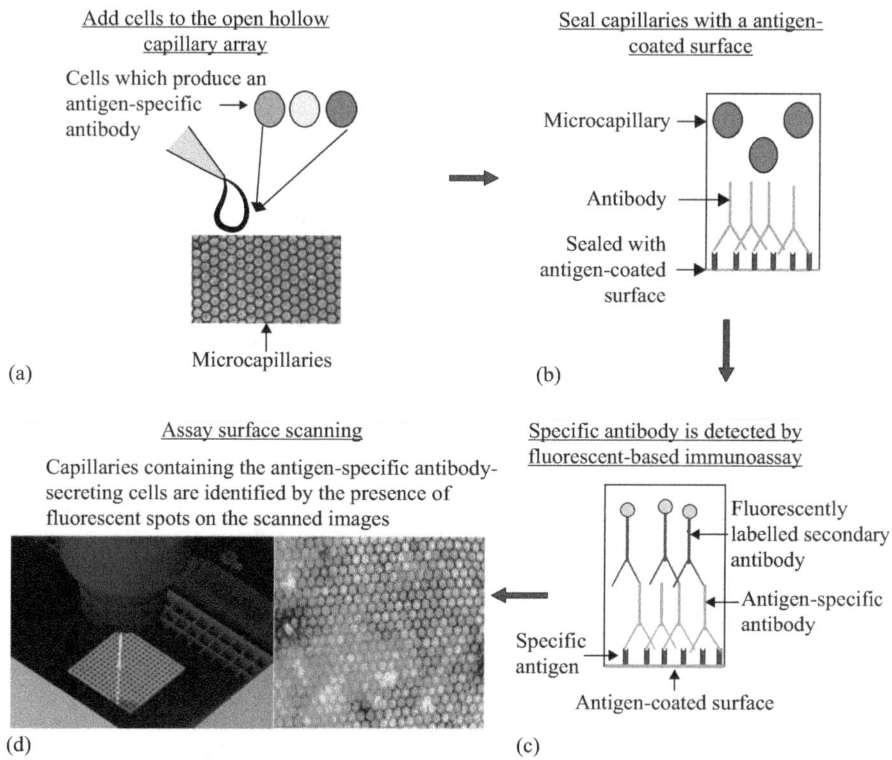

Figure 11.4 The DiCAST process. It involves a number of stages. (a) Capture and culturing of single cells in densely packed microcapillary arrays. (b) Antibody-antigen specific binding occurs on an antigen-coated surface. (c) Detection of antigen-specific antibody is demonstrated using a fluorescence-based immunoassay. (d) Detection of a positive assay signal is achieved by scanning. Cells are then recovered using an automated collection system

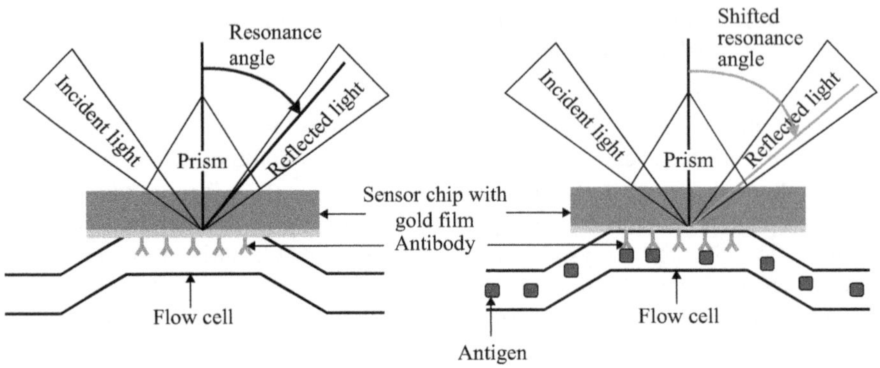

Figure 11.5 Biacore detection system. Antibodies are immobilised onto the sensor chip surface of the flow cell. Specific antigens are then passed over the antibody surface. The binding of antibody and antigen will cause a mass change, which leads to a shift of resonance angle that is proportional to the concentration of the binding antigen

11.3.7 Selection of recombinant antibodies using Biacore 4000

Biacore 4000 is a surface plasmon resonance (SPR)-based analytical instrument, which offers several advantages including high sensitivity, label-free and 'real-time' analysis of interactions between proteins and other molecules and it is ideal for use in antibody selection. Antibody-antigen binding on the gold sensor surface will result in an increase of mass at the sensor surface due to binding events (e.g. an antibody with its cognate antigen), which will lead to a change of refractive index. This change will cause the shift of the resonance angle, which is recorded and converted to resonance units (RU) in real time (Figure 11.5). A change in surface protein concentration of about 1 ng/mm^2 corresponds to a 0.1° shift of resonance angle and represents approximately 1,000 RU [42]. Biacore 4000 has multiple detection spots (20 detection spots in 4 flow cells for parallel analysis) enabling high capacity unattended sample-handling [43]. Therefore, Biacore 4000 provides a promising selection system for recombinant antibodies. Conroy and his colleagues have successfully selected scFv with high affinity and specificity from over 300 individual colonies from the output of the fourth round of biopanning for application in biosensors for human cardiovascular disease diagnostics [44].

11.3.8 Expression of soluble recombinant antibodies

11.3.8.1 Expression of soluble recombinant antibody fragments in *E. coli*

The most widely applied expression system for small recombinant antibody fragments (e.g. for scFv, Fab and bispecific antibodies) is *E. coli*. In this system, the functional antibody fragments are transported to an oxidising environment to ensure that the required disulphide bonds are generated with attendant protein folding. This is achieved by attaching the bacterial leader peptide sequences to the N terminus of the antibody [45]. The antibody chains are usually transported to the periplasmic space containing the disulphide bond family of enzymes of type A (DsbA) and of type C (DsbC), protein disulphide isomerase (PDI) and the seventeen kilodalton proteins (skp) that are crucial to the formation of disulphide bonds, and for folding and assembly of antibodies [46]. The antibody expression level in the periplasm is usually not very high [47].

11.3.9 Purification of recombinant antibodies

11.3.9.1 Recombinant antibody purification using metal-charged affinity resins

Immobilised metal ion affinity chromatography (IMAC) is one of the most popular recombinant antibody purification techniques and is based on the coordinate covalent bonding of specific groups (e.g. histidine) to metals (e.g. nickel, copper, zinc and cobalt ions). The specific groups are usually located on the C-terminal end of the scFv or Fab to prevent purification of truncated proteins. After incubating recombinant antibody (e.g. scFv or Fab)-containing samples with the metal-charged resin, the specific group tagged-recombinant antibodies will be bound onto the resin, while non-tagged antibodies and most impurities are then washed away with washing buffer. Finally, the specific group tagged-recombinant antibodies are eluted by changing pH (low pH buffer is usually used and the eluted antibodies are then collected in neutralisation buffer to preserve reactivity of purified antibodies [32]); or elution is achieved by adding a competitive molecule (e.g. 250 mM imidazole) [31].

11.3.9.2 Recombinant antibody purification using antigen-antibody binding-based affinity chromatographic strategies

Recombinant antibodies can be purified by applying antigen-antibody binding-based affinity chromatographic strategies described in Section 11.4.

11.4 Antibody optimisation for biosensor applications

Antibody specificity, sensitivity, affinity, stability, immobilisation (related to antibody labelling) and working dilution are key factors for antibody-based biosensors [48]. In this section, various antibody optimisation strategies for these elements are described.

11.4.1 Optimisation of antibody specificity, sensitivity and affinity for biosensors through genetic modification

In order to improve antibody specificity, sensitivity and affinity, gene mutations can be applied to the recombinant antibody DNA sequence. The most popular and effective mutation methods are error-prone polymerase chain reactions (PCR) and chain shuffling [49].

Error prone PCR is a method to directly target (point mutation) or randomly change, delete or insert one or several gene bases into a wild-type DNA. For untargeted error prone PCR, a polymerase that has a high amplification error rate (up to 2 per cent) can be used. The PCR error rate can also be enhanced by

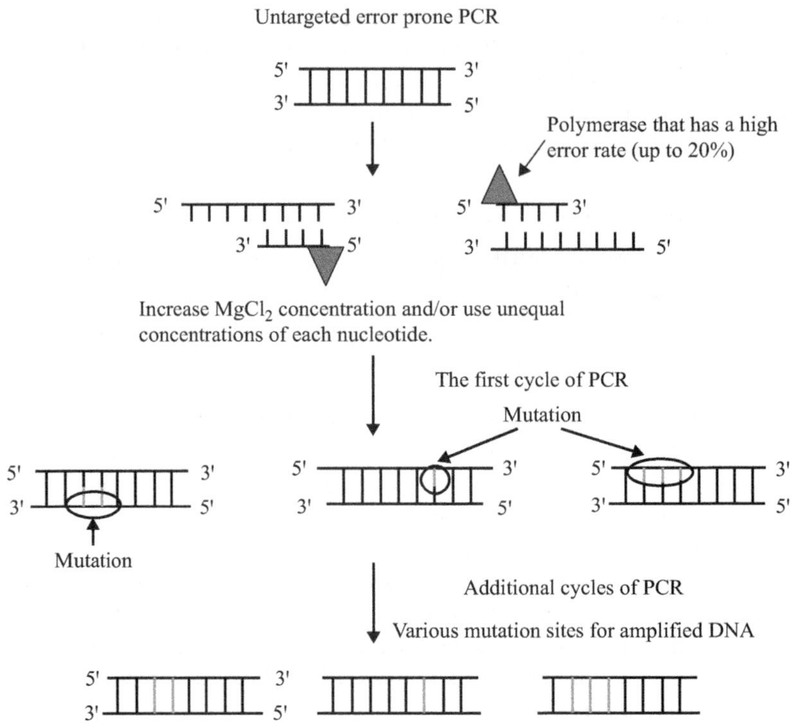

Figure 11.6 Illustration of untargeted error prone PCR

increasing the concentration of $MgCl_2$ in the reaction or using unequal concentrations of each nucleotide (Figure 11.6). For targeted error prone PCR, specific PCR primers can be designed for deleting or replacing one or more gene bases to induce the desired mutation at the required point(s) (Figure 11.7) [50]. After PCR amplification (untargeted and targeted), the library containing mutant DNA sequences will then be cloned into a suitable vector, and expressed (described in Section 11.3.4), followed by selection of desired antibodies using ELISA, Western blotting, immunofluorescent staining and SPR.

It was reported that the chain shuffling resulted in greater affinity improvement when compared to error-prone PCR [51]. Chain shuffling is an *in vitro* recombination method which is frequently used as a tool for antibody modification and is illustrated in Figure 11.8 [52]. It was successfully and widely used on *in vitro* antibody fragment affinity maturation. For scFv antibody light chain shuffling, the variable heavy chain gene would be recombined with a wide variety of light-chain variable genes. For heavy chain shuffling, the original variable light chain gene would be recombined with a variable domain library of heavy chain genes [53]. The outcome is a selection of antibodies with different binding characteristics, ideally including the required properties.

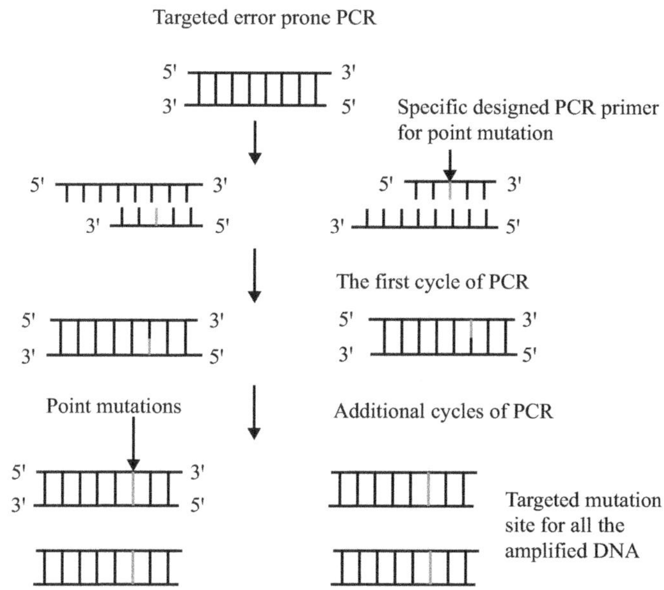

Figure 11.7 Illustration of targeted error prone PCR

11.4.2 Optimisation of antibody stability for biosensor applications

Antibody storage and working conditions (e.g. pH, temperature and constituents of the solution in which the antibody is dissolved or used) are highly crucial to antibody stability and should be optimised to maximise biosensor performance [54]. For most commercial antibodies, the storage pH is between 7.0 and 8.0, the storage buffer is usually PBS or TBS containing 0.02–0.09 per cent (w/v) sodium azide (used as a preservative to inhibit microbial growth) and 2–10 mg/mL BSA to aid stability, and the storage temperature is from 4 to −20 °C [55]. However, the working pH can be further optimised by comparing the antibody activity and affinity at various pHs [54, 56]. Different biosensors are required to work in various environments, for example, in different temperature zones and seasons, inside the body or in the ocean. The temperatures in these environments can vary dramatically. Therefore, the stability of antibodies must be analysed at the expected temperatures based on the projected working environment of the biosensors used for deployment. The components of the working buffer are very important. For instance, in the Biacore system no primary amine groups or other strong nucleophilic groups (e.g. Tris, sodium azide, glycine and BSA, which are usually present in storage buffers) should be present in the working buffer as they will compete with the immobilisation ligand for active esters on the surface of the sensor chip [43].

It is also possible to improve the stability of antibodies, particularly recombinant antibodies, by structural enhancement or generating a larger and more robust format. For instance, scFv can be converted to scAb, Fab or even IgG to achieve higher

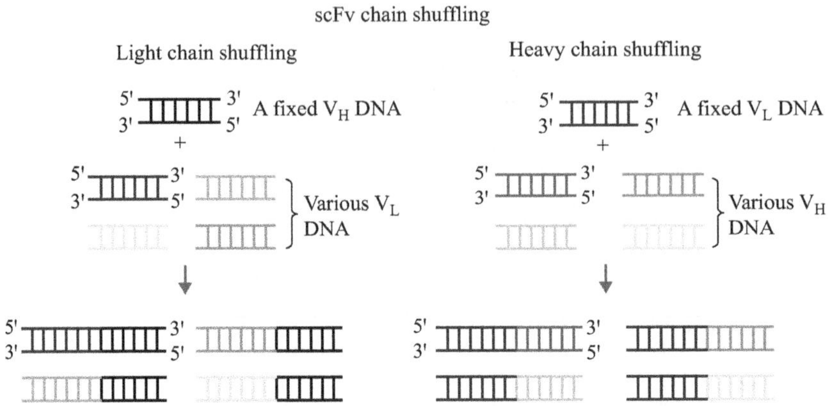

Figure 11.8 Strategy for scFv antibody chain shuffling. This involves recombination of the original variable heavy or light chain gene with a wide variety of light-chain variable genes or heavy-chain variable genes

stability. Quintero-Hernández *et al.* showed that after converting a scFv to a Fab format the *in vivo* stability improved significantly [57]. However, it was reported that some of the antibodies lost affinity after conversion to IgG [58]. Bivalent and trivalent antibodies (e.g. $(scFv)_2$, Fab-scFv, $(Fab)_2$ and $[(scFv)_2]_2)$ were shown to be more stable and effective than monospecific antibodies [59], and this approach may provide additional potential antibodies for use in biosensor applications.

A method was developed and patented for systematic control of antibody stability, which is based on screening a limited number of amino acid variations found in functional antibody variable domains. This was used to optimise the stability of scFv for biosensors, which successfully maintain function after incubation for more than 2 h at 70 °C [60].

11.4.3 Optimisation of antibody immobilisation strategies for biosensors

There are several antibody immobilisation strategies applied with biosensors, including random immobilisation, covalent immobilisation, orientated immobilisation and covalent-orientated immobilisation. The immobilisation strategy will be different for various biosensors, capture antibodies and sensor surfaces.

Random immobilisation is a strategy whereby antibody is bound to the biosensor surface in an irregular and uncontrolled manner typically by hydrophobic and electrostatic interactions. It usually gives low antibody immobilisation density and low antigen binding efficacy [61].

In a covalent immobilisation strategy, antibodies are bound to the sensor surface by covalent bonds, involving reactions with functional groups (e.g. amine, aldehyde and thiol) present on the protein surface and groups present on the sensor surface [62]. However, not all the antibodies may be correctly orientated for maximal binding thus limiting performance.

An orientated immobilisation strategy can improve activity of the antibody by providing the best functional orientation whereby the antibody is capable of optimised binding. Orientated immobilisation can be achieved by chemically attaching protein A, protein G or a small ligand, which is specific for the antibody Fc region, therefore, ensuring that the Fab region is available for interaction with the antigen. Orientated immobilisation of antibodies may play a valuable role in the performance of SPR immunoassays [63]. Lee *et al.* [64] demonstrated that the orientated immobilisation strategy increases the antigen-binding capacity of antibodies significantly when compared to the direct random immobilisation method. For recombinant antibodies, genetic insertion of tags (e.g. FLAG octapeptide, streptavidin-tag, avidin-Di-tag and hemagglutinin-tag) for orientated immobilisation is useful and easy to achieve [48].

Covalent-orientated immobilisation strategy combines elements of both covalent and orientated strategies which can result in high efficacy for the capture antibody. Tsai *et al.* [65] designed a chemically modified short-chain peptide ligand, which exhibited high affinity for the antibody Fc region, followed by covalent binding to a chip surface. This covalent-oriented antibody immobilisation strategy results in up to fourfold improvements over surfaces with random immobilisation. The work by Walper *et al.* showed that the limit of detection was dramatically improved when utilising covalent-orientated immobilisation, in comparison to direct covalent and random immobilisation strategies, in a SPR-based assay [66].

11.5 Summary

In summary, antibodies are ideal recognition elements for use in many biosensor-based applications. The approaches used with all antibody types are described. In addition, using molecular biology-based techniques antibodies may be generated and altered, thereby maximising specificity, sensitivity, stability, orientation and other factors to achieve optimal overall performance in many applications.

Acknowledgements

This work was supported by Science Foundation Ireland under CSET Grant No. 05/CE3/B754 and 10/CE/B1821. Barry O'Donnell, Biomedical Diagnostics Institute, Dublin City University, Dublin, Ireland is thanked for providing some images from his work on DiCAST.

References

[1] Conroy P.J., Hearty S., Leonard P., O'Kennedy R.J. 'Antibody production, design and use for biosensor-based applications'. *Seminars in Cell & Developmental Biology*. 2009;**20**(1):10–26.

[2] Ma H. 'Targeted neurotherapeutics for chronic inflammatory pain'. PhD thesis. Dublin City University. 2013.

[3] Attaelmannan M., Levinson S.S. 'Understanding and identifying monoclonal gammopathies'. *Clinical Chemistry*. 2000;**46**(8):1230–1238.

[4] Sun Y., Liu Z., Ren L., *et al.* 'Immunoglobulin genes and diversity: what we have learned from domestic animals'. *Journal of Animal Science and Biotechnology*. 2012;**3**(1):18–22.

[5] Alberts B., Johnson A., Lewis J., Raff M., Roberts K., Walter P. (eds.). *Molecular Biology of the Cell*. New York: Garland Science; 2002.

[6] Shaker G.H. 'Evaluation of anti-diphtheria toxin nanobodies'. *Journal of Nanotechnology, Science and Applications*. 2010;**3**:29–35.

[7] Stanfield R.L., Dooley H., Verdino P., Flajnik M.F., Wilson, I.A. 'Maturation of shark single-domain (IgNAR) antibodies: evidence for induced-fit binding'. *Journal of Molecular Biology*. 2007;**367**(2):358–372.

[8] Warr G.W., Magor K.E., Higgins D.A. 'IgY: clues to the origins of modern antibodies'. *Immunology Today*. 1995;**16**(8):392–398.

[9] Townsend S., Finlay W.J.J., Hearty S., O'Kennedy R. 'Optimizing recombinant antibody function in SPR immunosensing. The influence of antibody structural format and chip surface chemistry on assay sensitivity'. *Biosensors and Bioelectronics*. 2006;**22**(2):268–274.

[10] Hayes C.J., Leonard P., O'Kennedy R. 'Overcoming antibody expression and screening limitations by smart design: applications to PSA immunoassay development'. *Protein Expression and Purification*. 2012;**83**(1):84–91.

[11] Hoebe K., Janssen E., Beutler B. 'The interface between innate and adaptive immunity'. *Nature Immunology*. 2004;**5**(10):971–974.

[12] Janeway C.A. Jr, Travers P., Walport M., Shlomchik M.J. (eds.). *Immunobiology: The Immune System in Health and Disease*. New York: Garland Science; 2001. Chapter 8.

[13] Yaragalla S., Jebaraj C.I. 'Alternative artificial immunotherapy for common snakebites'. *Journal of Science*. 2012;**2**(4):165.

[14] Huang C.Y.M., Mateus F.R.C., Foley E.J., Beatty R., Cunningham T.B., Chang-Hasnain J.C. 'VCSEL optoelectronic biosensor for detection of infectious diseases'. *IEEE Photonics Technology Letters*. 2008;**20**(6):443–445.

[15] Real-Fernández F., Passalacqua I., Peroni E., *et al.* 'Glycopeptide-based antibody detection in multiple sclerosis by surface plasmon resonance'. *Sensors (Basel)*. 2012;**12**(5):5596–5607.

[16] Quessy S., Dubreuil J.D., Caya M., Létourneau R., Higgins R. 'Comparison of pig, rabbit and mouse IgG response to *Streptococcus suis* serotype 2 proteins and active immunization of mice against the infection'. *Canadian Journal of Veterinary Research*. 1994;**58**(3):220–223.

[17] Byrne B., Stack E., Gilmartin N., O'Kennedy R. 'Antibody-based sensors: principles, problems and potential for detection of pathogens and associated toxins'. *Sensors (Basel)*. 2009;**9**(6):4407–4445.

[18] Klein-Schneegans A.S., Kuntz L., Fonteneau P., Loor F. 'Serum concentrations of IgM, IgG1, IgG2b, IgG3 and IgA in C57BL/6 mice and their

congenics at the lpr (lymphoproliferation) locus'. *Journal of Autoimmunity*. 1989;**2**(6):869–875.

[19] Tao L., Zhang K., Sun Y., Jin B., Zhang Z., Yang K. 'Anti-epithelial cell adhesion molecule monoclonal antibody conjugated fluorescent nanoparticle biosensor for sensitive detection of colon cancer cells'. *Biosensors and Bioelectronics*. 2012;**35**(1):186–192.

[20] Lemamy G.J., Roger P., Mani J.C., Robert M., Rochefort H., Brouillet J.P. 'High-affinity antibodies from hen's-egg yolks against human mannose-6-phosphate/insulin-like growth-factor-II receptor (M6P/IGFII-R): characterization and potential use in clinical cancer studies'. *International Journal of Cancer*. 1999;**80**(6):896–902.

[21] Micusan V.V., Borduas A.G. 'Biological properties of goat immunoglobulins G'. *Immunology*. 1977;**32**(4):373–381.

[22] Strain G.M., Barta O., Olcott B.M., Braun W.F. Jr. 'Serum and cerebrospinal fluid concentrations of immunoglobulin G in Suffolk sheep with scrapie'. *American Journal of Veterinary Research*. 1984;**45**(9):1812–1813.

[23] Guilbault G.G., Hock B., Schmid R. 'A piezoelectric immunobiosensor for atrazine in drinking water'. *Biosensors Bioelectron*. 1992;**7**(6):411–419.

[24] Bravo P.W., Garnica J., Fowler M.E. 'Immunoglobulin G concentrations in periparturient llamas, alpacas and their crias'. *Small Ruminant Research*. 1997;**26**(1)145–49.

[25] Saerens D., Frederix F., Reekmans G., *et al.* 'Engineering camel single-domain antibodies and immobilization chemistry for human prostate-specific antigen sensing'. *Analytical Chemistry*. 2005;**77**(23):7547–7555.

[26] Burton D.R. '*Antibody libraries*' in Barbas 3rd C.F., Burton D.R., Scott J.K., Silverman, G.J. (eds.). *Phage Display: A Laboratory Manual*. New York: Cold Spring Harbor Laboratory Press; 2001. p. 3.8.

[27] Hanly W.C., Artwohl J.E., Bennett B.T. 'Review of polyclonal antibody production procedures in mammals and poultry'. *Institute for Laboratory Animal Research Journal*. 1995;**37**(3):93–118.

[28] Bachmann M.F., Kündig T.M., Hengartner H., Zinkernagel R.M. 'Regulation of IgG antibody titers by the amount persisting of immune-complexed antigen'. *European Journal of Immunology*. 1994;**24**(10):2567–2570.

[29] Ratcliffe M.J. 'Antibodies, immunoglobulin genes and the bursa of Fabricius in chicken B cell development'. *Developmental & Comparative Immunology*. 2006;**30**(1–2):101–118.

[30] Ghannam A., Kumari S., Muyldermans S., Abbady A.Q. 'Camelid nanobodies with high affinity for broad bean mottle virus: a possible promising tool to immunomodulate plant resistance against viruses'. *Plant Molecular Biology*. 2015;**87**(4–5):355–369.

[31] Ma H., O'Kennedy R. 'The purification of natural and recombinant peptide antibodies by affinity chromatographic strategies' in Houen G. (ed.). *Peptide Antibodies*. New York: Humana Press; 2015.

[32] McMahon M.J., O'Kennedy R. 'Polyreactivity as an acquired artefact, rather than a physiologic property, of antibodies: evidence that monoreactive

antibodies may gain the ability to bind to multiple antigens after exposure to low pH'. *Journal of Immunological Methods*. 2000;**241**(2–1):1–10.

[33] Pauly D., Chacana P.A., Calzado , Brembs B., Schade R. 'IgY technology: extraction of chicken antibodies from egg yolk by polyethylene glycol (PEG) precipitation'. *Journal of Visualized Experiments*. 2011;(51):3084.

[34] Tomita M., Tsumoto K. 'Hybridoma technologies for antibody production'. *Immunotherapy*. 2011;**3**(3):371–380.

[35] Karu A.E., Bell C.W., Chin T.E. 'Recombinant Antibody Technology'. *Institute for Laboratory Animal Research Journal*. 1995;**37**(3):132–141.

[36] Zeng X., Shen Z., Mernaugh R. 'Recombinant antibodies and their use in biosensors'. *Analytical and Bioanalytical Chemistry*. 2012;**402**(10): 3027–3038.

[37] Andris-Widhopf J., Steinberger P., Fuller R., Rader C., Barbas 3rd C.F. '*Generation of antibody libraries: PCR amplification and assembly of light- and heavy-chain coding sequences*' in Barbas 3rd C.F., Burton D.R., Scott J. K., Silverman, G.J. (eds.). *Phage Display: A Laboratory Manual*. New York: Cold Spring Harbor Laboratory Press; 2001. p. 9.1–9.113.

[38] Ma H., Meng J., Wang J., Hearty S., Dolly J.O., O'Kennedy R. 'Targeted delivery of a SNARE protease to sensory neurons using a single chain antibody (scFv) against the extracellular domain of P2X(3) inhibits the release of a pain mediator'. *Biochemical Journal*. 2014;**462**(2):247–256.

[39] Smith G.P. 'Filamentous fusion phage: novel expression vectors that display cloned antigens on the virion surface'. *Science*. 1985;**228**(4705):1315–1317.

[40] McCafferty J., Griffiths A.D., Winter G., Chiswell D.J. 'Phage antibodies: filamentous phage displaying antibody variable domains'. *Nature (London)*. 1990;**348**(6301):552–554.

[41] Fitzgerald V., Manning B., O'Donnell B., *et al*. 'Exploiting highly ordered subnanoliter volume microcapillaries as microtools for the analysis of antibody producing cells'. *Analytical Chemistry*. 2015;**87**(2):997–1003.

[42] Nagata K., Handa H. (eds.). *Real-Time Analysis of Biomolecular Interactions*. Tokyo: Springer-Verlag; 2000. p. 26–27.

[43] GE Healthcare Life Sciences. *Biacore*™ *Assay Handbook* [online]. Available from http://www.gelifesciences.com/file_source/GELS/Service%20and%20Support/Documents%20and%20Downloads/Handbooks/pdfs/Biacore%20Assay%20Handbook.pdf [Accessed 15 May 2015].

[44] Conroy P.J., O'Kennedy R.J., Hearty S. 'Cardiac troponin I: a case study in rational antibody design for human diagnostics'. *Protein Engineering Design and Selection*. 2012;**25**(6):295–305.

[45] Rapoport T.A. 'Protein translocation. a bacterium catches up'. *Nature (London)*. 1991;**349**(6305):107–108.

[46] Bothmann H., Pluckthun A. 'The periplasmic *Escherichia coli* peptidylprolyl cis,trans-isomerase FkpA. I. Increased functional expression of antibody fragments with and without cis-prolines'. *The Journal of Biological Chemistry*. 2000;**275**(22):17100–17105.

[47] Chen C., Snedecor B., Nishihara J.C., *et al.* 'High-level accumulation of a recombinant antibody fragment in the periplasm of *Escherichia coli* requires a triple-mutant (degP prc spr) host strain'. *Biotechnology and Bioengineering.* 2004;**85**(5):463–474.

[48] Conroy P.J., Hearty S., Leonard P., O'Kennedy R.J. 'Antibody production, design and use for biosensor-based applications'. *Seminars in Cell and Developmental Biology.* 2009;**20**(1):10–26.

[49] Lewis L., Lloyd C. 'Optimisation of antibody affinity by ribosome display using error-prone or site-directed mutagenesis'. *Methods in Molecular Biology.* 2012;**805**:139–161.

[50] Pritchard L., Corne D., Kell D., Rowland J., Winson M.J. 'A general model of error-prone PCR'. *Journal of Theoretical Biology.* 2005;**234**(4): 497–509.

[51] Swers J.S., Yeung Y.A., Wittrup K.D. 'Integrated mimicry of B cell antibody mutagenesis using yeast homologous recombination'. *Molecular Biotechnology.* 2011;**47**(1):57–69.

[52] Christensen P.A., Danielczyk A., Ravn P., *et al.* 'Modifying antibody specificity by chain shuffling of V_H/V_L between antibodies with related specificities'. *Scandinavian Journal of Immunology.* 2009;**69**(1):1–10.

[53] Kang A.S., Jones T.M., Burton D.R. 'Antibody redesign by chain shuffling from random combinatorial immunoglobulin libraries'. *Proceedings of the National Academy of Sciences of the United States of America.* 1991;**88**(24):11120–11123.

[54] Jiskoot W., Beuvery E.C., de Koning A.A., Herron J.N., Crommelin D.J. 'Analytical approaches to the study of monoclonal antibody stability'. *Pharmaceutical Research.* 1990;**7**(12):1234–1241.

[55] Abcam. *Antibody storage guide* [online]. 2015. Available from http://www.abcam.com/protocols/antibody-storage-guide

[56] Zheng J.Y., Janis L.J. 'Influence of pH, buffer species, and storage temperature on physicochemical stability of a humanized monoclonal antibody LA298'. *International Journal of Pharmaceutics.* 2006;**308**(1–2):46–51.

[57] Quintero-Hernández V., Juárez-González V.R., Ortíz-León M., Sánchez R., Possani L.D., Becerril B. 'The change of the scFv into the Fab format improves the stability and *in vivo* toxin neutralization capacity of recombinant antibodies'. *Molecular Immunology.* 2007;**44**(6):1307–1315.

[58] Steinwand M., Droste P., Frenzel A., Hust M., Dübel S., Schirrmann T. 'The influence of antibody fragment format on phage display-based affinity maturation of IgG'. *MAbs.* 2014;**6**(1):204–218.

[59] Wittel U.A., Jain M., Goel A., *et al.* 'Engineering and characterization of a divalent single-chain Fv angiotensin II fusion construct of the monoclonal antibody CC49'. *Biochemical and Biophysical Research Communications.* 2005;**329**(1):168–176.

[60] Fred J.S. *Methods for Systematic Control of Protein Stability.* United States Patent 20110130324 A1. 2011.

[61] Tang Y., Mernaugh R., Zeng X. 'Nonregeneration protocol for surface plasmon resonance: study of high-affinity interaction with high-density biosensors'. *Analytical Chemistry*. 2006;**78**(6):1841–1848.

[62] Wong L.S., Khan F., Micklefield J. 'Selective covalent protein immobilization: strategies and applications'. *Chemical Reviews*. 2009;**109**(9):4025–4053.

[63] Vashist S.K., Dixit C.K., MacCraith B.D., O'Kennedy R. 'Effect of antibody immobilization strategies on the analytical performance of a surface plasmon resonance-based immunoassay'. *Analyst*. 2011;**136**(21):4431–4436.

[64] Lee J.E., Seo J.H., Kim C.S., *et al.* 'A comparative study on antibody immobilization strategies onto solid surface'. *Korean Journal of Chemical Engineering*. 2013;**30**(10):1934–1938.

[65] Tsai C.W., Jheng S.L., Chen W.Y., Ruaan R.C. 'Strategy of Fc-recognizable Peptide ligand design for oriented immobilization of antibody'. *Analytical Chemistry*. 2014;**86**(6):2931–2938.

[66] Walper S.A., Brozozog Lee P.A., Goldman E.R., Anderson G.P. 'Comparison of single domain antibody immobilization strategies evaluated by surface plasmon resonance'. *Journal of Immunological Methods*. 2013;**388**(1–2):68–77.

Chapter 12

Smartphone-based *in vitro* diagnostic technologies for personalized healthcare monitoring and management

Sandeep Kumar Vashist[1,2,], A.G. Venkatesh[3,*], Roland Zengerle[1,2], Felix von Stetten[1,2] and John H.T. Luong[4]*

12.1 Introduction

Smartphones (SPs) have become omnipresent as evinced by 6.8 billion cell phone subscribers, i.e., 94% of the world population [1] with over 70% from developing countries. The current generation of SPs is equipped with sophisticated features such as advanced processors, increased memory, high-resolution camera, high-end security via fingerprinting, numerous smart applications, and a variety of built-in sensors. Therefore, SPs have been transformed into a prospective personalized IVD system to deliver mobile healthcare (mH) to remote, resource-deficient, private and public settings [2]. Individuals can perform several important diagnostics at their personalized settings and receive the real-time feedback from healthcare professionals. Moreover, as the SP-IVD data can be tagged with spatio-temporal information, it will greatly facilitate the monitoring and management of epidemics and emergency scenarios [3]. Significant advances have been made to improve signal response, robustness, and cost-effectiveness, while considerable efforts are well underway to reshape the landscape of healthcare and bioanalytical sciences [4].

[1]Hahn-Schickard, Georges-Koehler-Allee 103, 79110 Freiburg, Germany
[2]Laboratory for MEMS Applications, Department of Microsystems Engineering – IMTEK, University of Freiburg, Georges-Koehler-Allee 103, 79110 Freiburg, Germany
[3]Department of Electrical and Computer Engineering, Jacobs School of Engineering, University of California San Diego, San Diego CA 92093, USA
[4]Innovative Chromatography Group, Irish Separation Science Cluster (ISSC), Department of Chemistry and Analytical, Biological Chemistry Research Facility (ABCRF), University College Cork, Cork, Ireland
[*]These authors contributed equally.

There are substantial efforts in the development of SP-IVD based on lateral flow assays (LFA) [5–9], microscopy [10–14], electrochemical sensing [15–18], immunoassays (IA) [19–22], surface plasmon resonance-based biosensing [23, 24], flow cytometry [12,25], and optical detection [26–29]. Several companies have emerged and most of the healthcare and diagnostic giants and SP manufacturers were also participating into this competitive and emerging field. Consequently, there are numerous commercially available SP-based devices for general healthcare and fitness, which are being used by millions of customers worldwide [30]. These devices are manufactured by iHealth, AliveCor, GENTAG, Mobile Assay, CellScope, Holomic, Runtastic, Nonin, etc. Based on the current trend, the forthcoming SP-based mH era will revolutionize personalized healthcare monitoring and management *via* highly efficient and cost-effective SP-IVDs. This chapter provides a critical overview of SP-IVD together with the technical challenges, the trends and future possibilities for the next-generation of personalized mH devices.

12.2 Signal detection in SP-based *in vitro* diagnostics

The SP high resolution rear camera, ranging from a few megapixels (MP) to 41 MP, can be transformed to a spectrophotometer or microscope using an interface with necessary optical components and a sample compartment. The reusable or disposable interface links the bioassay to the SP and holds the camera in alignment with the optical components. The light source is usually an internal LED or the phone flash [31].

12.2.1 Colorimetric, fluorescent and luminescent detection

Colorimetric detection-using SP-IVD uses an optically opaque attachment, consisting of light emitting diodes (LEDs) and diffusers to provide uniform illumination, apertures to provide the desired imaging field-of-view (FOV), and a sample chamber [20,32] (Figure 12.1a and b). The FOV is enhanced by placing a plano-convex lens in front of the camera [32]. This setup equipped with monochromatic filter is extended for imaging the fluorescent signal of a labeled dye [33] such as EvaGreen, a dye used in the polymerase chain reaction (PCR) [34]. The ultra-violet (UV) LEDs or UV trans-illuminators are also needed for the desired excitation wavelength as desired in case of QDs [21]. For luminescent detection, the measurement is simply performed in the dark [35] using a plano-convex lens in front of the camera for converging the field of view [36] (Figure 12.1a–c). In photo-luminescence-based SP-IVD using QDs and Förster resonance energy transfer, the setup requires a UV lamp (365 nm) for excitation, a long-pass (400 nm cut-off) and a short-pass filter (650 nm cut-off), inserted in front of the SP camera [37]. For multi-sample imaging, a microtiter plate (MTP) with 96 wells, is placed on the gadget's screensaver to provide uniform bottom illumination inside a dark hood. The SP is simply placed on top of the hood in containment with an aperture in alignment with the SP back camera [28] (Figure 12.1d).

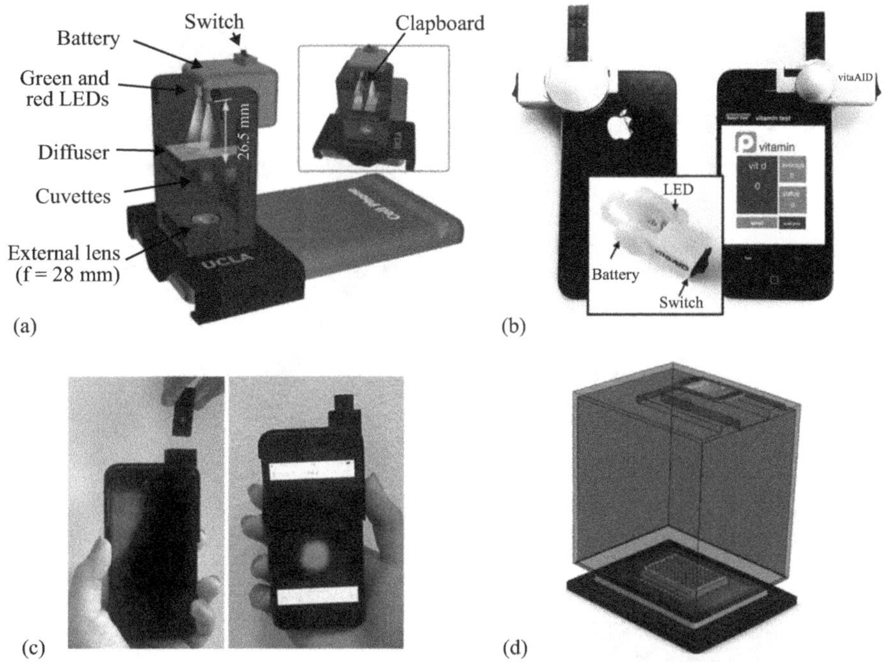

Figure 12.1 SP-IVD for colorimetric detection. (a) 3D schematic for colorimetric detection of Hg^{2+} [32]. Reproduced with permission from the American Chemical Society. (b) vitaAID accessory on an iPhone for colorimetric detection of vitamin D [43]. Reproduced with permission from the Royal Society of Chemistry. (c) Smartphone accessory and minicartridge for the biochemiluminescent detection of cholesterol [36]. Reproduced with permission from the American Chemical Society. (d) A smartphone-based colorimetric reader based on the screen-based bottom illumination provided by gadgets [28]. Reproduced with permission from Elsevier B.V.

A SP fluorimeter for measurement of a full emission spectrum of any light emitter [38] uses a cradle that incorporates a diffraction grating, cylindrical lens and a collimator (Figure 12.2). The transmission diffraction grating is placed in front of the camera with optics integrated to collimate light emitted from the sample onto the grating. The SP camera measures the emission spectrum.

12.2.2 SPR detection

In an angle-resolved SPR-based SP-IVD [23], a disposable SPR coupler is attached to the SP screen (Figure 12.3a). A red triangle displayed on the screen acts as a light source, while a white frame guides the placement of the SPR coupler. The Au-coated glass on top of the coupler serves as the sensing surface. The polydimethoxysilane (PDMS) plano-cylindric element collects the illumination

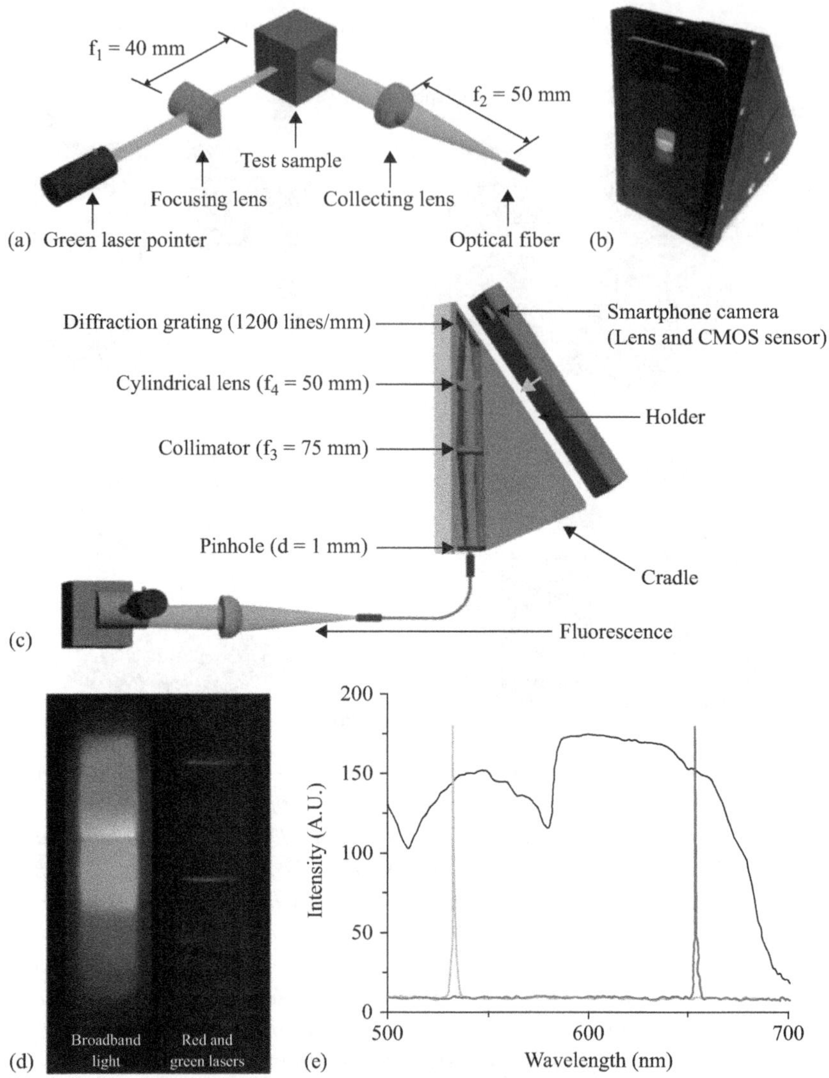

Figure 12.2 A smartphone fluorimeter [38]. (a) The excitation laser (532 nm) illuminates a cuvette containing the probe-target duplexes. Fluorophores linked to one end of the molecular beacon probes are excited to emit fluorescence in all directions. A portion of the emission is gathered by a collecting lens oriented perpendicular to the laser and enters the cradle, where it is further collimated before incidence upon a diffraction grating placed in front of the camera. (b and c) An optical cradle installed on the smartphone. The screen of the smartphone shows a spectrum of the transmitted light dispersed by the grating. (d) Images of broadband light, (upper line in left image) and (lower line in left image) laser beams. (e) Light intensity distributions of two lasers (solid light grey line near the X-axis with $\lambda_{green} = 532$ nm and solid dark grey line near the X-axis with $\lambda_{red} = 653$ nm) and a broadband light source (solid black line located away from the X-axis) measured by the smartphone fluorimeter. Reproduced with permission from the American Chemical Society

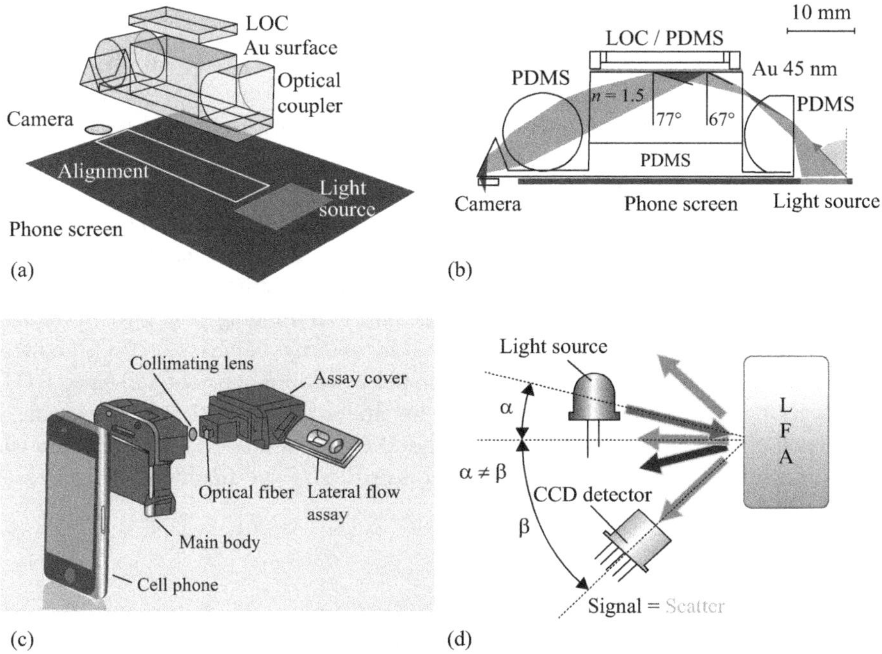

Figure 12.3 (a) A representative setup for an angle-resolved SPR using smartphone's screen illumination and front camera detection optically coupled by a disposable device and (b) raytrace of the experimental arrangement showing the light path from screen to camera [23]. Reproduced with permission from Wiley-VCH Verlag GmbH & Co. KGaA, Weinheim. (c) An exploded view of a smartphone-based LFA reader showing the placement of collimating lens and an optical fiber set at specific angles in reference to the LFA cassette [5]. (d) The detector is oriented at angle, β, that is optimized for decreased light scattering from a nitrocellulose membrane, as well as differs from the angle of light source to surface, α, which provides an improved signal-to-noise ratio [5]. Reproduced with permission from Elsevier B.V.

from the red triangle and directs it to the Au interface to reflect the light containing the angle-resolved SPR signal (Figure 12.3b). The reflected light is steered by total internal reflection inside a PDMS prism to the SP's front camera. The custom-made SPR chip has three channels: two calibration channels for high and low concentrations and the test channel. An iOS 5-based smart application is employed for image acquisition to control the camera exposure, i.e., exposure time and ISO number (sensitivity), so that the signals are measured under identical conditions.

12.2.3 Lateral flow assays

A SP-based lateral flow IA (LFIA) format (Figure 12.3c) is based on the signal detection at an optimized angle to maximize Mie scattering from a nitrocellulose membrane [18], resulting in maximal Rayleigh scattering from gold nanoparticles (Au NPs) in the LFIA bands (Figure 12.3d). The LFIA is illuminated by the SP embedded flash via an optical fiber and a collimating lens. Similarly, a compact and light-weight (~65 g) SP-based universal rapid diagnostic test (RDT) reader [6] has been developed to read various LFIAs. The RDT reader has an inexpensive plano-convex lens, three LED arrays (two located underneath the RDT tray for reflection imaging and one at the top for transmission imaging) and a cost-effective microcontroller. The RDT reader is powered by external batteries or the SP battery *via* a USB connection, and analyzes the sample in various types of LFIAs or RDTs in reflection or transmission imaging modes under diffused LED illumination. It provides highly accurate and repeatable digital evaluation of RDTs to differentiate even some minor color signal variation that is difficult to be quantified and assessed by the human eye.

12.2.4 Microscopy

Figure 12.4a and b shows a ~28 g SP attachment for the wide-field fluorescent and dark field imaging [39]. The device employs battery-powered LEDs, a plastic color filter to create a dark background, and an additional lens in front of the camera to image the fluorescent emission. The dark field imaging is acquired using the same setup but without the filter. A portable (~186 g) SP attachment for fluorescence microscopy has also been developed, which enables imaging of 100 nm nanoparticles and individual human cytomegalo viruses [40] (Figure 12.4c and d). It consists of a compact diode-laser (450 nm) and an optical setup with a long-pass interference filter; a low numerical aperture lens and a coarse mechanical translation stage (Figure 12.4d). Highly dense samples in the transmission mode are imaged [41] by a contact microscopic platform (76 g) using a glass-based tapered fiber array illuminated by a LED (Figure 12.4e and f). The sample transmission image is delivered from the taper's top-to-bottom with 3X magnification in each direction. The image is projected on the CMOS sensor of the SP via two lenses. A "shift and add" algorithm is used for the digital fusion of multi-frame images to improve resolution and obviate spatial artefacts.

12.2.5 Electrochemical detection

A compact SP-based electrochemical detection system [15] is based on a compact embedded circuit for signal processing and data analysis using a disposable SIM card-size microfluidic chip for fluidic handling and sensing; a sample loading capillary and processing and pumping (Figure 12.5). The sample is loaded by a pipette but subsequently driven by the flow capillary. The microfluidic chip (measuring 25 mm × 15 mm) has a modified PDMS surface coating that enables an autonomous capillary-driven flow with a constant flow rate. It has 2 inlets and an outlet (1 mm in diameter), and a 2 mm chamber downstream to merge the

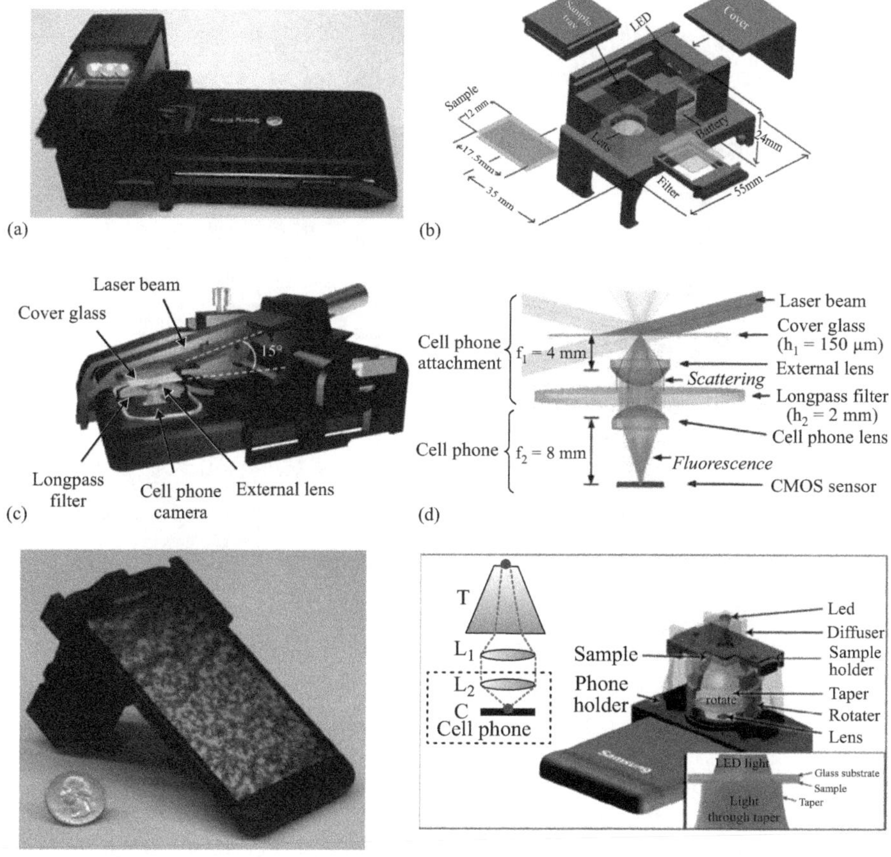

Figure 12.4 (a) Compact and lightweight (~28 g) smartphone attachment for wide-field fluorescent and darkfield imaging and (b) its schematic [39]. Reproduced with permission from The Royal Society of Chemistry. (c) Schematic of the smartphone-based fluorescence microscope and (d) ray-tracing diagram: excitation and scattered beams and the fluorescent emission [40]. Reproduced with permission from the American Chemical Society. (e) Smartphone-based contact microscopy platform and (f) schematic illustration of the smartphone attachment [41]. Reproduced with permission from The Royal Society of Chemistry

appropriate volumes of the sample (0.5 μL) and reporter (2 μL) solutions before their entrance to a zigzag mixer. Thereafter, the serpentine channels, with a spacing of 40 μm, enable a uniform flow of a sample-reporter mixture over the electrochemical sensor. A secondary serpentine channel, (25 cm long, 400 μm in width and 100 μm in height), acts as a capillary pump and a waste reservoir. It accommodates

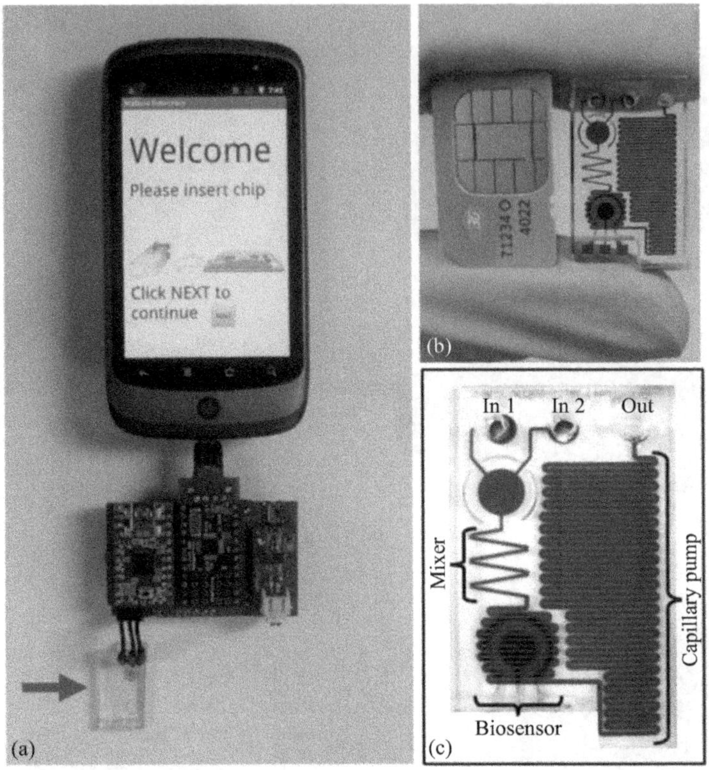

Figure 12.5 *(a) Smartphone-based electrochemical sensor with the arrow indicating the microfluidic chip [15]. (b) Comparison of the size of microfluidic chip with the smartphone SIM card. (c) Magnified view of dye-filled microfluidic chip with labeled components. Reproduced with permission from the Royal Society of Chemistry*

the tetramethylbenzidine/hydrogen peroxide (TMB/H_2O_2) substrate for washing as well as the enzymatic reaction for subsequent amperometric measurement. *Plasmodium falciparum* histidine-rich protein 2 (*Pf*HRP2) capture antibodies are uniformly bound to the polypyrrole-coated gold electrode surface. Without *Pf*HRP2, the antibodies cannot bind to the electrode and are washed away when the TMB/H_2O_2 substrate is loaded. In the presence of *Pf*HRP2, the detection antibodies bind to the electrode and result in electrochemical current, which is proportional to the *Pf*HRP2 concentration when the electrode is poised at a fixed potential. The user performs the measurement through a smart application that provides step-by-step instructions on the screen. After each measurement, the results are displayed on the SP's screen and stored in its memory for subsequent data transmission and analysis.

Similarly, iHealth Lab [42] has developed an iOS-enabled Wireless Smart Gluco-Monitoring System based on electrochemical detection. An audio jack-based miniaturized SP electrochemical sensing platform (~65 g), has also been

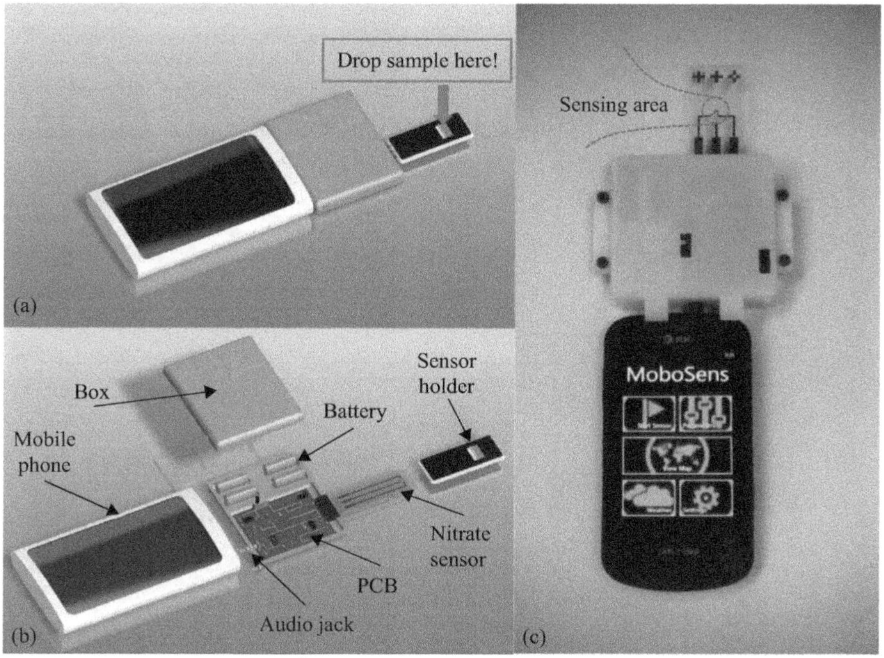

Figure 12.6 (a) Assembly view of audio jack-based electrochemical sensor, MoboSens, for the detection of nitrate concentration in water. (b) Detailed components of MoboSens. (c) Actual photograph of the complete MoboSens system. Reproduced with permission from Elsevier B.V.

demonstrated for analysis of nitrate in field water samples [18] (Figure 12.6). It comprises a microfabricated three-electrode sensor, a smart application and a circuit board to drive with the sensor.

12.2.6 Cytometry

A SP based optofluidic fluorescent imaging flow cytometer, in the form of a compact, lightweight (~18 g) and cost-effective SP attachment, has been developed for analyzing large sample volumes of >0.1 mL [11]. It employs an inexpensive lens, a plastic color filter (cost < 0.1 USD), two LEDs (cost ~0.6 USD) and coin cell batteries (cost ~0.5 USD). Using a syringe pump, the sample is continuously delivered to the imaging volume through a disposable microfluidic channel, which acts as a multi-layered opto-fluidic waveguide (Figure 12.7). The dark-field background is created by using an inexpensive plastic absorption filter as the guided excitation light propagates perpendicular to the detection path. The cell movement through the microfluidic channel is recorded and processed to determine the cell count and density. With a fluorescence resolution of ~2 μm, this platform can be

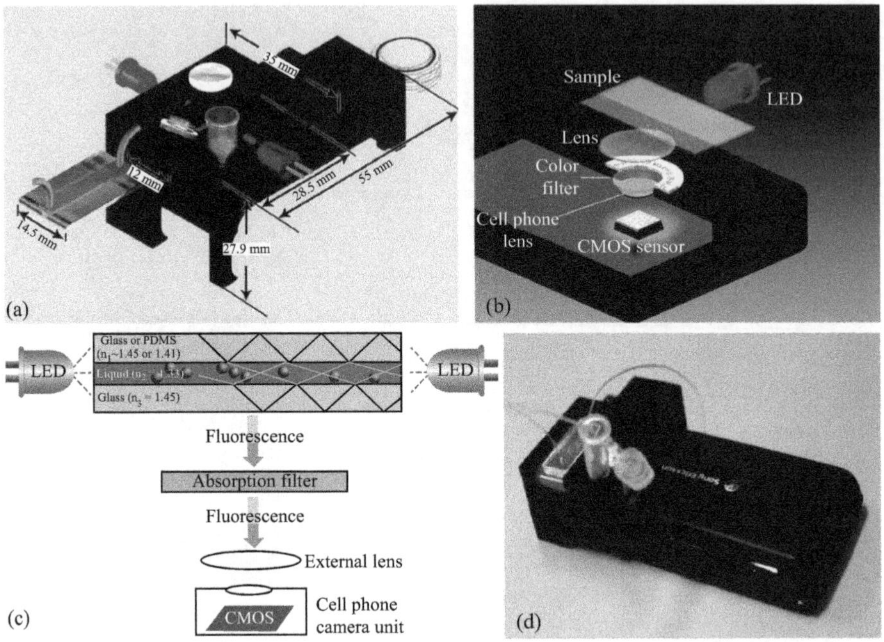

Figure 12.7 Smartphone-based flow cytometer [25]. (a–c) Schematics of the lightweight (~18 g) and compact (~35 × 55 × 27.9 mm³) optical attachment for optofluidic fluorescent imaging cytometry on a cell phone, which can be repeatedly attached or detached to the cell-phone body without the need for fine alignment. (d) Actual photograph of optofluidic fluorescent imaging cytometer on a cell phone. Reproduced with permission from the American Chemical Society

used for whole blood analysis and screening of waterborne parasites in drinking waters. Subsequently, the same group developed a miniaturized and low-cost SP imaging-based cytometry platform along with a smart application to measure the density of RBCs and WBCs that are imaged in bright-field and fluorescent modes. This platform can also simultaneously determine the hemoglobin (Hb) concentration in human blood samples [39] (Figure 12.8). The system for rapid blood analysis by using only ~10 μL of the sample provides a satisfactory analytical performance, as validated using a standard bench-top Sysmex KN21 hematology analyzer. Its universal base is attached to the cell phone camera unit and three "add-on" components for WBC/RBC counting and Hb density measurement. The desired "add-on" components can be clicked into the same port on the base attachment to perform the specific blood test via the smart application, running on the same cell phone for image analysis and cell counting.

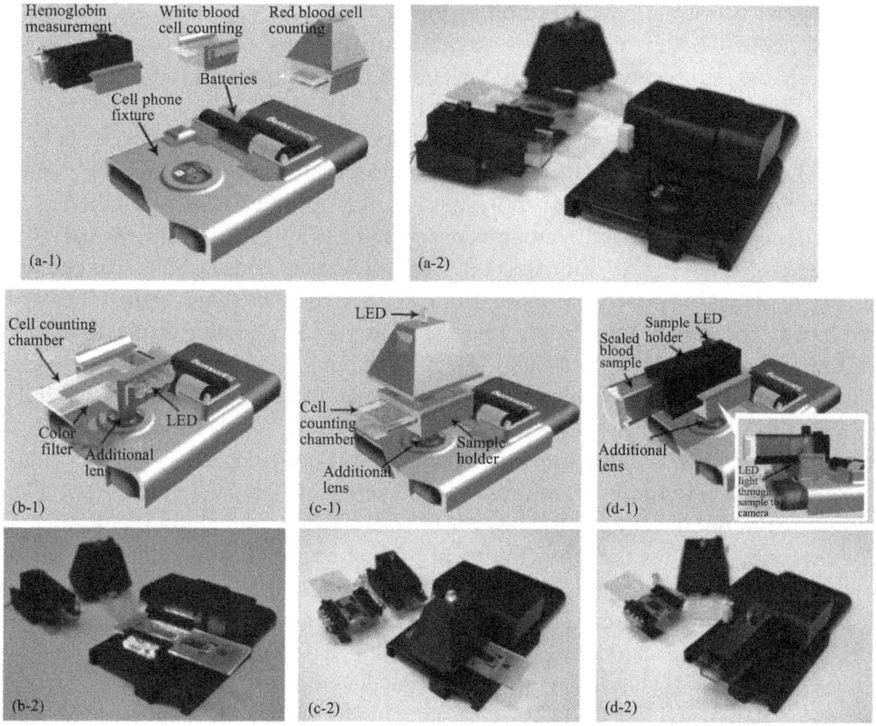

Figure 12.8 *Smartphone-based cytometry platform [12]. (a-1) and (a-2) Illustration and picture of smartphone-based blood analysis platform comprising a base attachment with two AA batteries and a universal port for adapting three different add-on components for WBC counting, RBC counting and hemoglobin measurements, respectively. (b-1) and (b-2) Illustration and picture of the WBC counting device. (c-1) and (c-2) Illustration and picture of the RBC counting device. (d-1) and (d-2) Illustration and picture of Hb measurement device. Reproduced with permission from the Royal Society of Chemistry*

12.3 Applications of smartphone-based *in vitro* diagnostics

12.3.1 Detection of biomolecules, metabolites and biomarkers

A colorimetric detection-based SP-IVD has been reported for 25-hydroxyvitamin D using an AuNP-based IA [43] (Figure 12.8b), the DNA sequences from Kaposi's sarcoma associated herpes virus (KSHV) using a microfluidic chip and an NP-based colorimetric assay [44], and the total blood cholesterol using the CardioCheck test strips [29]. A SP-based colorimetric reader (SPCR), based on the bottom illumination of a 96-well MTP by the gadget's screen, can estimate the chromogenic substrate concentration in an ELISA assay [28] (Figure 12.8d). For example, SPCR-based imaging of colorimetric product of C – reactive protein (CRP) IA has superior detection range and LOD compared to imaging by just placing the MTP on a white paper (Table 12.1).

A SP-IVD for the activity of trypsin, chymotrypsin and enterokinase, is based on a QD-based assay [37] with colorimetric detection. A compact optomechanical SP attachment using magnetic polystyrene microspheres and QD-labelled Ab detects recombinant bovine somatotropin (rBST) [45]. A different format is the paper microfluidic-based fluorescent IA of β-D-galactosidase [46]. Biochemiluminescent detection-based SP-IVD using a LFA minicartridge format has been developed for total bile acid [36] (Figure 12.1c), total cholesterol [36] (Figure 12.1c) and salivary cortisol [35]. A RDT reader (65 g) provides the readout of LFIAs for malaria, tuberculosis (TB) and human immunodeficiency virus (HIV) [6]. A SP-IVD for the Mie scattering optimized LFA was also reported for detecting thyroid stimulating hormone (TSH) [5] (Figure 12.3c).

A SP-based fluorescent microscope detects *Salmonella typhimurium* DNA using a paper microfluidics-based assay [47]. SP-IVD-based fluorescent detection has been conducted for the DNA fragment of the hepatitis B virus plasmid [48] and *Trypanosomacruzi* genomic DNA [34]. Unlabelled DNA is detected by monitoring electrochemical dissolution of a chromium electrode array in a microfluidic system [49]. A SP fluorimeter detects microRNA using a fluorescent molecular beacon assay [38]. A SP-IVD based on cytometry was developed for measuring Hb and the density of RBCs and WBCs [12]. A SP attachment (~28 g) is also used for fluorescent imaging of labeled WBCs in whole blood [39] (Figure 12.4a and b), whereas a SP-IVD based on angle-resolved SPR is for β_2-microglobulin [23] (Figure 12.3a and b). Imaging and sizing of single DNA molecules of λ and T7 bacteriophages using a compact and light-weight SP-based fluorescent microscope [50] was also demonstrated, with sizing accuracy of <1 kilobase-pairs over ~2 mm^2 field-of-view.

A SP-based electrochemical biosensor [15] was employed for the rapid, highly sensitive and specific detection of *Pf*HRP2 with LOD of 16 ng mL^{-1}. The procedure takes 15 min, uses two loading steps for the sample and reporter (*Pf*HRP2 detection antibodies conjugated to horse-radish peroxidase) solutions, and detects *Pf*HRP2 in human serum with LOD of 16 ng/mL.

The recently launched iHealth's Wireless Smart Gluco-Monitoring System [42] is a next-generation glucose monitoring device for diabetic monitoring and management, which can store up to 500 blood glucose test results, track the progress of the results and set up medication alerts. Moreover, it can automatically warn the user in case of the test strip expiry, to prevent potential false evaluation.

12.3.2 Detection of microorganisms

A SP-based fluorescent microscope was used for imaging *M. tuberculosis* bacilli in auramine O-stained sputum smears [14] and water-borne pathogenic *Giardia lamblia* cysts [39]. A compact SP attachment (~40 g) with fluorescent detection detects *Salmonella* and *E. coli* O157 without pre-enrichment [33].

Table 12.1 Bioanalytical applications of SP-IVD

Types of SP-IVD	Analytes detected	Characteristics of the bioanalytical application	Reference
Colorimetric detection	Peanut	Detects 1–25 ppm of peanut within 20 min	[20]
	Multi-analyte sensing arrays	An image processing algorithm for ascorbic acid, glucose, protein, ketones, urobilinogen, bilirubin and RBC in paper-based urine strips	[61]
	25-hydroxyvitamin D	Au NP-based IA, detection range: 15–110 nM	[43]
	Herpes virus nucleic acid	DNA sequences [1 mM] from KSHV using a NP assay in microfluidic chips	[44]
	CRP	CRP [0.035–0.182 μg mL^{-1}] with LOD of 0.026 μg mL^{-1}	[22]
	CRP	SBCR-based IA for CRP [0.3–81 ng mL^{-1}] with LOD of 0.4 ng mL^{-1}	[28]
	Cholesterol	The total cholesterol level in blood [140–400 mg dL^{-1}] within 60 s	[29]
	Proteases	A QD-based multiplex assay for the activity of trypsin, chymotrypsin and enterokinase [pM–nM]	[37]
	Cocaine	Au NP and aptamer-based assay for cocaine [0.2–0.8 mg mL^{-1}]	[53]
	HE4	Microchip ELISA for HE4 in urine with linearity of 19.5–1250 ng mL^{-1} and LOD of 19.5 ng mL^{-1}	[54]
	Hg	Plasmonic Au NP and aptamer-based assay for Hg^{2+} with LOD of ~3.5 ppb	[32]
Fluorescent detection	*M. tuberculosis*	*M. tuberculosis* bacilli in Auramine O-stained sputum smears	[14]
	Salmonella typhimurium DNA	A fluorescent microscope and a paper microfluidics-based assay for detecting *S. typhimurium* down to 10^4 CFU mL^{-1}	[47]
	DNA amplification	The DNA fragment of the Hepatitis B virus plasmid by cPCR	[48]
	rBST Abs	rBST Abs in milk extracts by an IA using magnetic polystyrene microspheres and QD-labeled detection Ab	[45]
	Salmonella and *E. coli O157*	LFIA strips for *Salmonella* and *E. coli O157* with LOD of 10^5 CFU mL^{-1}	[33]

(*Continues*)

Table 12.1 (*Continued*)

Types of SP-IVD	**Analytes detected**	**Characteristics of the bioanalytical application**	**Reference**
	β-D-galactosidase	A paper microfluidics-based IA for β-D-galactosidase, with linearity [0.7–12 nM] and LOD [0.7 nM]	[46]
	Single NPs & viruses	Fluorescent imaging of isolated 100 nM fluorescent NPs and human cytomegalo viruses	[40]
	microRNA	Using the fluorescent molecular beacon assay to detect microRNA with LOD of 10 pM	[38]
	RBCs, WBCs and Hb	A imaging cytometry platform for Hb concentration and the density of RBCs and WBCs	[12]
	E. coli	To detect *E. coli O157* by QD-based sandwich IA in glass capillaries with LOD of ~5–10 CFU mL^{-1}	[21]
	WBCs and *Giardia lamblia* cysts	Imaging labeled WBCs in whole blood and water-borne pathogenic *Giardia lamblia* cysts [resolution of 10 μm and FOV of 81 mm^2]	[39]
	Trypanosomacruzi	*T. cruzi* genomic DNA [0.1–100 fg μL^{-1}] with LOD of 9.6 ag	[34]
Luminescent detection	Bile acid	AnLFA minicartridge format for total bile acid in serum and oral fluid with linearity and LOD of 0.5–100 μM and 0.5 μM	[36]
	Cholesterol	Using a LFA minicartridge format for total cholesterol in serum with linearity and LOD of 20–386 mg dL^{-1} and 20 mg dL^{-1}	[36]
	Salivary cortisol	An LFIA for salivary cortisol [0.3–60 ng mL^{-1}] with LOD of 0.3 ng mL^{-1}	[62]
SPR detection	β2M	An angle-resolved SPR detection system for β2M with LOD of 0.1 μg mL^{-1}	[23]
Electro-chemical detection	*Pf*HRP2 biomarker for malaria	Detects *Pf*HRP2 in 15 min with LOD of 16 ng mL^{-1} using a compact embedded circuit, disposable microfluidic chip and capillary flow	[15]
	iHealth Wireless Smart Gluco-Monitoring System	Detects pathophysiological blood glucose concentrations using a miniaturized glucometer interfaced with SP via a smart application	[42]

Table 12.1 (*Continued*)

Types of SP-IVD	Analytes detected	Characteristics of the bioanalytical application	Reference
	Nitrate	An audio jack-based electro-chemical sensor that detects nitrate concentration in water with LOD of 0.2 ppm and linear detection range of 1.4–70 ppm within 1 min	[18]
Cytometry	Optofluidic fluor-escent imaging-based flow cytometer	Compact, light-weight and cost-effective SP-based flow cytometer with fluorescent resolution of ~2 μm and capability to analyze samples >0.1 mL	[25]
	RBCs, WBCs and Hb	Determines the density of RBCs, WBCs and Hb in blood using just 10 μL sample	[12]
Other detection techniques	Microscopy and spectroscopy	Stained and unstained blood smears, and transmission and fluores-cence spectroscopy of diffuse tissue	[13]
	Unlabelled DNA	Monitoring the electrochemical dissolution of chromium elec-trode array in a microfluidic system	[49]
	Malaria, TB, HIV	A SP-based integrated reader for malaria, TB and HIV.	[6]
	RBCs & WBCs	A glass-based tapered fiber-optic array and multi-frame imaging for RBCs and WBCs in transmission mode	[41]
	Salmonella and *E. coli*	A paper microfluidic device and a Mie scattering-based IA for *Salmonella* and *E. coli* [10^2–10^5 CFU mL^{-1}]	[51]
	P. falciparum-infec-ted and sickle RBCs	A smartphone-based microscope for the bright field imaging of *P. falciparum*-infected and sickle RBCs in blood smears	[14]
	TSH	A SP-based Mie scatter optimized LFA for TSH with LOD of 0.4 mIU L^{-1}	[5]
	AFB1	A reader and a LFIA using a com-petitive binding format for AFB1 with linearity of 5–1000 μg kg^{-1} and LOD of 5 μg kg^{-1}	[55]

A ~28 g attachment-based ISAP, based on a QD-based sandwich IA in a glass capillary, was employed for fluorescent detection of *E. coli* O157 [21]. Recently, a SP-IVD based on paper microfluidics together with the Mie scattering based IA was used for detecting *Salmonella* and *E. coli* [51]. A compact and light-weight (~205 g) opto-mechanical attachment coupled to a SP was developed for fluorescent microscopy (field-of-view ~0.8 cm^2) [52]. It detects *Giardia lamblia* cysts, with LOD of ~12 cysts per 10 mL, in disposable water sample cassettes comprising of absorbent pads and mechanical filter membranes.

12.3.3 Detection of other analytes

Peanut concentration has been detected by a SP-IVD employing a 40 g opto-mechanical SP attachment [20] compared to a 37 g battery-powered SP attachment for detecting Hg^{2+} using aplasmonic Au NP and aptamer-based assay [32] (Figure 12.1a). An AuNP and aptamer-based assay was used in SP-IVD for colorimetric detection of cocaine [53], whereas the HE4 cancer biomarker in urine was detected using SP-based microchip ELISA [54]. A SP-based reader for one-dot LFIA using a competitive binding format was reported for aflatoxin B1 (AFB1) [55]. An audio jack-based miniaturized and battery powered light-weight SP electrochemical sensor was employed for the detection of nitrate in water [18], with accuracy comparable to the standard methods.

12.3.4 Other bio-analytical applications

Two SP attachments were developed to transform a SP into a 350 X microscope and a visible-light spectrophotometer [13]. Of interest is a 78 g SP-based contact microscopy platform using a glass-based tapered fiber-optic array and multi-frame imaging [41] for RBCs and WBCs (Figure 12.4e and f). Another development is a SP-based high resolution microscope for bright field imaging of *P. falciparum*-infected and sickle RBCs in blood smears [14].

12.4 Conclusions, challenges and future trends

Hitherto, the developments have shown the excellent merger of various disciplines to create innovative SP-IVD tools. The SP-based devices with associated smart applications are being used for personalized general healthcare monitoring, notably analyses of blood glucose, weight, heart rate, etc., a major driving force in the creation of new enterprises such as iHealth LLC, Runtastic, AliveCor, GENTAG and Holomic LLC. The success of SP-based devices and smart applications together with improved diagnostic procedures [56, 57] will warrant further developments and applications of commercially-viable SP-IVD tools in the coming years. The SP-IVD, employing the FDA-cleared and/or CE-certified products such as LFIA strips, will have a higher market penetration compared to innovative concepts or technologies that require stringent clinical validation.

Considering the integration of various contributing technologies in SP, there will be continuous improvement in the SP-IVD's performance and features. Localized SPR (LSPR, interactions between the incident photons and the conduction band of a noble metal nanostructure) has a decay length of the electromagnetic field of ~6 nm [58], compared to 200 nm for SPR. The application of LSPR will minimize interference from solution refractive index fluctuations and increase sensitivity to refractive index changes on the surface. Another interesting aspect is the use of a photonic crystal that only reflects one wavelength of light to shift a shorter wavelength to a longer wavelength when biomolecules bind to the photonic crystal. The photonic crystal can be simply prepared by coating a common microscope slide with the photonic material. For handheld iPhone biosensor applications, a normal microscope slide is coated with the photonic material [59]. The coming years will witness the emergence of new biosensing concepts as well as the use of recently developed concepts such as Raman spectroscopy [60], for important and routine SP-IVD applications.

One major challenge is to identify relevant algorithms for highly reproducible imaging in a particular SP model or a specific application. Cloud computing significantly reduces healthcare costs, but is challenged by serious growing concern about the security and privacy of personal data. The national data security guidelines of most countries require confidential and sensitive data to be physically stored within their national boundaries. The cloud service providers, such as Amazon Web Services and Google, have started complying with these guidelines. Efforts are also underway to define an international cloud computing standard, e.g., the creation of EuroCloud and Google's Data Liberation Front [30]. Additionally, confidential data in personal health records (PHRs) must be encrypted to prevent any abuse.

References

[1] Measuring the Information Society Report 2014. Available from http://www.itu.int/en/ITU-D/Statistics/Pages/publications/mis2014.aspx. [Accessed Jan 04, 2015].

[2] Vashist S.K., Mudanyali O., Schneider E.M., Zengerle R., Ozcan A. 'Cellphone-based devices for bioanalytical sciences'. *Anal. Bioanal. Chem.* 2014;**406**(14):3263–77.

[3] Ozcan A. 'Mobile phones democratize and cultivate next-generation imaging, diagnostics and measurement tools'. *Lab. Chip.* 2014;**14**(17):3187–94.

[4] Erickson D., O'Dell D., Jiang L., *et al.* 'Smartphone technology can be transformative to the deployment of lab-on-chip diagnostics'. *Lab. Chip.* 2014;**14**(17):3159–64.

[5] You D.J., Park T.S., Yoon J.Y. 'Cell-phone-based measurement of TSH using Mie scatter optimized lateral flow assays'. *Biosens. Bioelectron.* 2013;**40**(1):180–5.

[6] Mudanyali O., Dimitrov S., Sikora U., Padmanabhan S., Navruz I., Ozcan A. 'Integrated rapid-diagnostic-test reader platform on a cellphone'. *Lab. Chip.* 2012;**12**(15):2678–86.

[7] Cooper D.C., Callahan B., Callahan P., Burnett L. 'Mobile image ratiometry: a new method for instantaneous analysis of rapid test strips'. *Nat. Preced.* 2012; doi: 10.1038/npre.2012.6827.1.

[8] Cadle B.A., Rasmus K.C., Varela J.A., *et al.* 'Cellular phone-based image acquisition and quantitative ratiometric method for detecting cocaine and benzoylecgonine for biological and forensic applications'. *Subst. Abuse.* 2010;**4**:21–33.

[9] Cooper D.C. 'Mobile image ratiometry for the detection of Botrytis cinerea (Gray Mold)'. *Nat. Preced.* 2012; doi: 10.1038/npre.2012.6989.1.

[10] Mudanyali O., Tseng D., Oh C., *et al.* 'Compact, light-weight and cost-effective microscope based on lensless incoherent holography for telemedicine applications'. *Lab. Chip.* 2010;**10**(11):1417–28.

[11] Bishara W., Sikora U., Mudanyali O., *et al.* 'Holographic pixel super-resolution in portable lensless on-chip microscopy using a fiber-optic array'. *Lab. Chip.* 2011;**11**(7):1276–9.

[12] Zhu H., Sencan I., Wong J., *et al.* 'Cost-effective and rapid blood analysis on a cell-phone'. *Lab. Chip.* 2013;**13**(7):1282–8.

[13] Smith Z.J., Chu K., Espenson A.R., *et al.* 'Cell-phone-based platform for biomedical device development and education applications'. *PLoS ONE.* 2011;**6**(3):e17150.

[14] Breslauer D.N., Maamari R.N., Switz N.A., Lam W.A., Fletcher D.A. 'Mobile phone based clinical microscopy for global health applications'. *PLoS ONE.* 2009;**4**(7):e6320.

[15] Lillehoj P.B., Huang M.C., Truong N., Ho C.M. 'Rapid electrochemical detection on a mobile phone'. *Lab. Chip.* 2013;**13**(15):2950–5.

[16] Geiger G.E., Oberding J.W., Ward R.N., White K.D. 'Blood glucose meter/modem interface arrangement'. U.S. Patent No. 7,181,350. 20 Feb. 2007; 2007.

[17] Peeters J.P. 'Diagnostic radio frequency identification sensors and applications thereof'. U.S. Patent No. 8,077,042. 13 Dec. 2011; 2011.

[18] Wang X., Gartia M.R., Jiang J., *et al.* 'Audio jack based miniaturized mobile phone electrochemical sensing platform'. *Sensor. Actuat. B: Chem.* 2014;**209**:677–5.

[19] Lu Y., Shi W., Qin J., Lin B. 'Low cost, portable detection of gold nanoparticle-labeled microfluidic immunoassay with camera cell phone'. *Electrophoresis.* 2009;**30**(4):579–82.

[20] Coskun A.F., Wong J., Khodadadi D., Nagi R., Tey A., Ozcan A. 'A personalized food allergen testing platform on a cellphone'. *Lab. Chip.* 2013; **13**(4):636–40.

[21] Zhu H., Sikora U., Ozcan A. 'Quantum dot enabled detection of Escherichia coli using a cell-phone'. *Analyst.* 2012;**137**(11):2541–4.

[22] McGeough C.M., O'Driscoll S. 'Camera phone-based quantitative analysis of C-reactive protein ELISA'. *IEEE T. Biomed. Circ. S.* 2013;**7**(5):655–9.

[23] Preechaburana P., Gonzalez M.C., Suska A., Filippini D. 'Surface plasmon resonance chemical sensing on cell phones'. *Angew. Chem.* 2012;**51**(46): 11585–8.

[24] Coskun A.F., Cetin A.E., Galarreta B.C., Alvarez D.A., Altug H., Ozcan A. 'Lensfree optofluidic plasmonic sensor for real-time and label-free monitoring of molecular binding events over a wide field-of-view'. *Sci. Rep.* 2014;**4**:6789.

[25] Zhu H., Mavandadi S., Coskun A.F., Yaglidere O., Ozcan A. 'Optofluidic fluorescent imaging cytometry on a cell phone'. *Anal. Chem.* 2011;**83**(17): 6641–7.

[26] Shen L., Hagen J.A., Papautsky I. 'Point-of-care colorimetric detection with a smartphone'. *Lab. Chip.* 2012;**12**(21):4240–3.

[27] Vashist S.K., Schneider E.M., Zengerle R., von Stetten F., Luong J.H.T. 'Graphene-based rapid and highly-sensitive immunoassay for C-reactive protein using a smartphone-based colorimetric reader'. *Biosens. Bioelectron.* 2015;**66**:169–76.

[28] Vashist S.K., van Oordt T., Schneider E.M., Zengerle R., von Stetten F., Luong J.H.T. 'A smartphone-based colorimetric reader for bioanalytical applications using the screen-based bottom illumination provided by gadgets'. *Biosens. Bioelectron.* 2015;**67**:248–55.

[29] Oncescu V., Mancuso M., Erickson D. 'Cholesterol testing on a smartphone'. *Lab. Chip.* 2014;**14**(4):759–63.

[30] Vashist S.K., Schneider E.M., Luong J.H.T. 'Commercial smartphone-based devices and smart applications for personalized healthcare monitoring and management'. *Diagnostics.* 2014;**4**(3):104–28.

[31] Lopez-Ruiz N., Curto V.F., Erenas M.M., *et al.* 'Smartphone-based simultaneous pH and nitrite colorimetric determination for paper microfluidic devices'. *Anal. Chem.* 2014;**86**(19):9554–62.

[32] Wei Q., Nagi R., Sadeghi K., *et al.* 'Detection and spatial mapping of mercury contamination in water samples using a smart-phone'. *ACS Nano.* 2014;**8**(2):1121–9.

[33] Rajendran V.K., Bakthavathsalam P., Jaffar Ali B.M. 'Smartphone based bacterial detection using biofunctionalized fluorescent nanoparticles'. *Microchim. Acta.* 2014;**181**(15–16):1815–21.

[34] Walker F.M., Ahmad K.M., Eisenstein M., Soh H.T. 'Transformation of personal computers and mobile phones into genetic diagnostic systems'. *Anal. Chem.* 2014;**86**(18):9236–41.

[35] Zangheri M., Cevenini L., Anfossi L., *et al.* 'A simple and compact smartphone accessory for quantitative chemiluminescence-based lateral flow immunoassay for salivary cortisol detection'. *Biosens. Bioelectron.* 2015;**64**:63–8.

[36] Roda A., Michelini E., Cevenini L., Calabria D., Calabretta M.M., Simoni P. 'Integrating biochemiluminescence detection on smartphones: mobile chemistry platform for point-of-need analysis'. *Anal. Chem.* 2014;**86**(15): 7299–304.

[37] Petryayeva E., Algar W.R. 'Multiplexed homogeneous assays of proteolytic activity using a smartphone and quantum dots'. *Anal. Chem.* 2014;**86**(6): 3195–202.

[38] Yu H., Tan Y., Cunningham B.T. 'Smartphone fluorescence spectroscopy'. *Anal. Chem.* 2014;**86**(17):8805–13.

[39] Zhu H., Yaglidere O., Su T.W., Tseng D., Ozcan A. 'Cost-effective and compact wide-field fluorescent imaging on a cell-phone'. *Lab. Chip.* 2011;**11**(2):315–22.

[40] Wei Q., Qi H., Luo W., *et al.* 'Fluorescent imaging of single nanoparticles and viruses on a smart phone'. *ACS Nano.* 2013;**7**(10):9147–55.

[41] Navruz I., Coskun A.F., Wong J., *et al.* 'Smart-phone based computational microscopy using multi-frame contact imaging on a fiber-optic array'. *Lab. Chip.* 2013;**13**(20):4015–23.

[42] Wireless Smart Gluco-Monitoring System. http://www.ihealthlabs.com/glucometer/wireless-smart-gluco-monitoring-system/. [Accessed Jan. 04, 2015].

[43] Lee S., Oncescu V., Mancuso M., Mehta S., Erickson D. 'A smartphone platform for the quantification of vitamin D levels'. *Lab. Chip.* 2014;**14**(8): 1437–42.

[44] Mancuso M., Cesarman E., Erickson D. 'Detection of Kaposi's sarcoma associated herpesvirus nucleic acids using a smartphone accessory'. *Lab. Chip.* 2014;**14**(19):3809–16.

[45] Ludwig S.K., Zhu H., Phillips S., *et al.* 'Cellphone-based detection platform for rbST biomarker analysis in milk extracts using a microsphere fluorescence immunoassay'. *Anal. Bioanal. Chem.* 2014;**406**(27):6857–66.

[46] Thom N.K., Lewis G.G., Yeung K., Phillips S.T. 'Quantitative fluorescence assays using a self-powered paper-based microfluidic device and a camera-equipped cellular phone'. *RSC Adv.* 2014;**4**(3):1334–40.

[47] Fronczek C.F., Park T.S., Harshman D.K., Nicolini A.M., Yoon J.-Y. 'Paper microfluidic extraction and direct smartphone-based identification of pathogenic nucleic acids from field and clinical samples'. *RSC Adv.* 2014; **4**(22):11103–10.

[48] Lee D., Chou W.P., Yeh S.H., Chen P.J., Chen P.H. 'DNA detection using commercial mobile phones'. *Biosens. Bioelectron.* 2011;**26**(11):4349–54.

[49] Huang Y.W., Ugaz V.M. 'Smartphone-based detection of unlabeled DNA via electrochemical dissolution'. *Analyst.* 2013;**138**(9):2522–6.

[50] Wei Q., Luo W., Chiang S., *et al.* 'Imaging and sizing of single DNA molecules on a mobile phone'. *ACS Nano.* 2014;**8**(12):12725–33.

[51] Park T.S., Li W., McCracken K.E., Yoon J.Y. 'Smartphone quantifies *Salmonella* from paper microfluidics'. *Lab. Chip.* 2013;**13**(24):4832–40.

[52] Koydemir H.C., Gorocs Z., Tseng D., *et al.* 'Rapid imaging, detection and quantification of *Giardia lamblia* cysts using mobile-phone based fluorescent microscopy and machine learning'. *Lab. Chip.* 2015; doi: 10.1039/C4LC01358A.

[53] Smith J.E., Griffin D.K., Leny J.K., Hagen J.A., Chavez J.L., Kelley-Loughnane N. 'Colorimetric detection with aptamer-gold nanoparticle conjugates coupled to an android-based color analysis application for use in the field'. *Talanta.* 2014;**121**:247–55.

[54] Wang S., Zhao X., Khimji I., *et al.* 'Integration of cell phone imaging with microchip ELISA to detect ovarian cancer HE4 biomarker in urine at the point-of-care'. *Lab. Chip.* 2011;**11**(20):3411–8.

[55] Lee S., Kim G., Moon J. 'Performance improvement of the one-dot lateral flow immunoassay for aflatoxin B1 by using a smartphone-based reading system'. *Sensors.* 2013;**13**(4):5109–16.

[56] Vashist S.K., Lam E., Hrapovic S., Male K.B., Luong J.H.T. 'Immobilization of antibodies and enzymes on 3-aminopropyltriethoxysilane-functionalized bioanalytical platforms for biosensors and diagnostics'. *Chem. Rev.* 2014; **114**(21):11083–130.

[57] Gubala V., Harris L.F., Ricco A.J., Tan M.X., Williams D.E. 'Point of care diagnostics: status and future'. *Anal. Chem.* 2012;**84**(2):487–515.

[58] Haes A.J., Van Duyne R.P. 'A unified view of propagating and localized surface plasmon resonance biosensors'. *Anal. Bioanal. Chem.* 2004; **379**(7–8):920–30.

[59] Gallegos D., Long K.D., Yu H., *et al.* 'Label-free biodetection using a smartphone'. *Lab. Chip.* 2013;**13**(11):2124–32.

[60] Ayas S., Cupallari A., Ekiz O.O., Kaya Y., Dana A. 'Counting molecules with a mobile phone camera using plasmonic enhancement'. *ACS Photonics.* 2014;**1**(1):17–26.

[61] Hong J.I., Chang B.Y. 'Development of the smartphone-based colorimetry for multi-analyte sensing arrays'. *Lab. Chip.* 2014;**14**(10):1725–32.

[62] Zangheri M., Cevenini L., Anfossi L., *et al.* 'A simple and compact smartphone accessory for quantitative chemiluminescence-based lateral flow immunoassay for salivary cortisol detection'. *Biosens. Bioelectron.* 2014;**64**:63–68.

Chapter 13
Lateral flow biosensors

Jia Li[1] *and Joanne Macdonald*[1,2]

13.1 Introduction

Over the last three decades, lateral flow biosensors have emerged as popular and practical tools toward point-of-care (POC) diagnostics, and have gained market share of more than a third of all POC tests [1]. The most famous example is the home pregnancy test that was commercialized in 1988 [2] into one of the most fundamentally successful products ever developed for onsite biomedical diagnosis. The US market alone is estimated at 20 million pregnancy tests per year, and the global market estimate is approximately 1.68 billion pregnancy tests sold each year [3].

A typical lateral flow biosensor employs a sandwich detection system and uses tracer(s) to generate detectable signal(s) (Figure 13.1). However, recent advances in nanomaterials offer a wide variety of improvement options, including new detection methodologies, signal transformation and improvements in sensitivity and specificity [4–6]. In this chapter, we describe the basic lateral flow detection system, the major components and their functions, critical parameters for successful lateral flow detection, and applications in biosensing. We also point out the hurdles facing commercial development of lateral flow biosensors. In particular, we consider future perspectives of lateral flow biosensors for personalized onsite biomedical diagnosis.

13.2 The mechanism of lateral flow immunoassay

A typical lateral flow immunoassay (LFIA) employs three antibodies and a tracer: a capture antibody (antibody 1) is coupled with a tracer; a detection antibody (antibody 2) is embedded in a test line; and a third antibody (antibody 3) that can directly bind to the capture antibody is immobilized at the control line (Figure 13.1a–c). The capture and detection antibodies can bind an analyte (antigen) at different epitopes. The control line indicates that the sample has migrated

[1]Inflammation and Healing Research Cluster, Genecology Research Centre, School of Science and Engineering, University of the Sunshine Coast, Qld, Australia
[2]Division of Experimental Therapeutics, Columbia University, New York, NY, USA

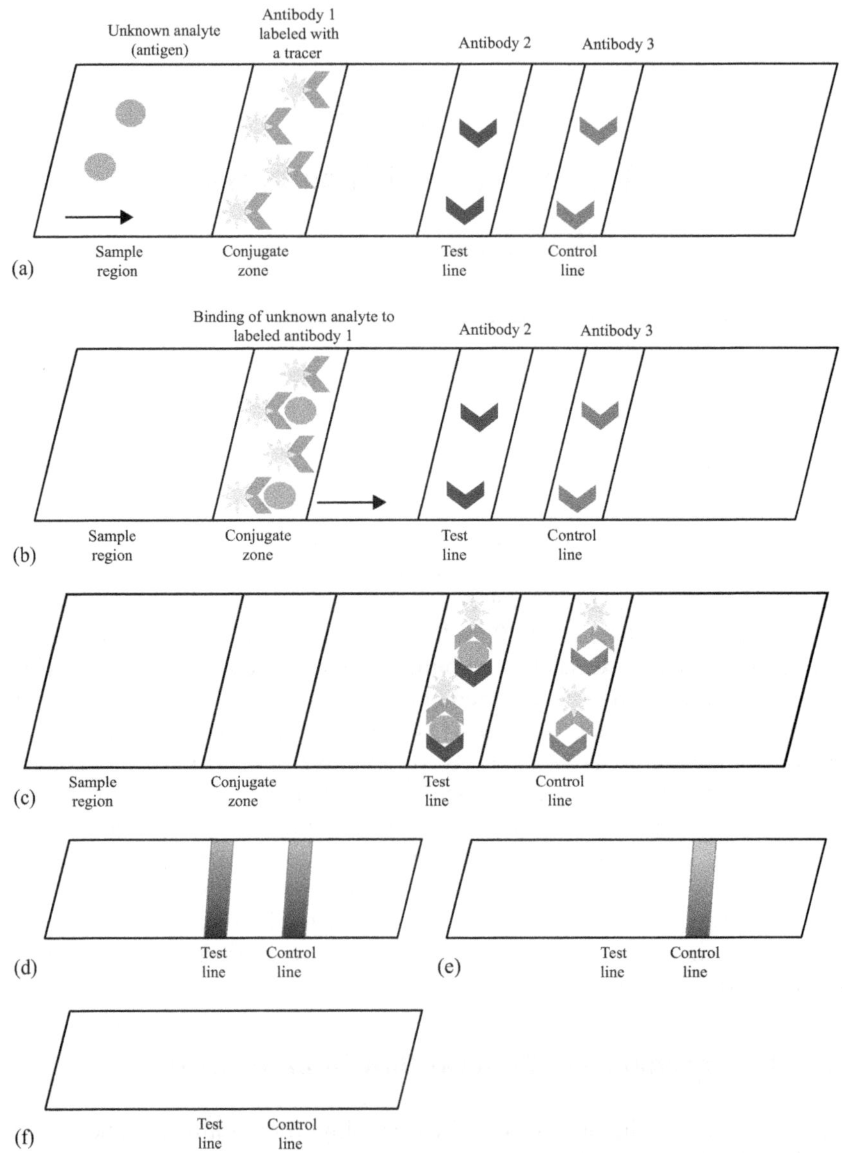

Figure 13.1 Mechanism of a lateral flow test conducted in sandwich assay format. On a reaction phase (e.g. nitrocellulose membrane): (a) The sample (grey circles) is loaded onto the sample region. (b) Binding of the unknown analyte to a labeled antibody (the conjugate, arrow with star) occurs in the conjugate zone. (c) The antigen/conjugate complexes and the unbound antigen and conjugates, travel to both the test and control lines, respectively. Binding of the labeled conjugate to either line results in the appearance of a colored stripe along that line. (d) A positive result. (e) A negative result. (f) Invalid results

across the membrane as intended, regardless of whether the analyte is present in the sample. Observation of both a colored test line and a colored control line on the membrane is a positive result (Figure 13.1d). A single line in the control zone is a negative result (Figure 13.1e). If no lines appear at all (Figure 13.1f) the result is invalid and must be repeated.

13.3 Types of LFIA

LFIAs can adopt different formats based on the type of analyte, which can involve direct detection without competition (noncompetitive immunoassay) or competing with known concentrations of analyte (competitive immunoassay). Both of these formats are useful for providing different information about analytes when performed in a LFIA format.

13.3.1 Noncompetitive immunoassay

The noncompetitive immunoassay is usually called a "sandwich assay," where the analyte is embedded between the capture and detection antibodies (Figure 13.1). In this format, the detection signal is proportional to the increasing concentration of the analyte [7]. However, a potential problem of the sandwich immunoassay is the detection of small molecules that contain only a single antigenic epitope. In addition, steric hindrance may prevent simultaneous binding of the analyte to both of the capture/tracer complex and the detection antibody.

13.3.2 Competitive immunoassay

The limitations of the noncompetitive assay can be compensated by using a competitive immunoassay. In the competitive format, the analyte (unknown concentration; denoted by a "U" in the circle in Figure 13.2) competes with a known concentration of analyte for binding to a single antibody; the detection signal is inversely proportional to the analyte (unknown concentration) (Figure 13.2b and c).

The competitive immunoassay has two manifestations, in which the known concentration of analyte is either pre-immobilized on the membrane (Figure 13.2b) or conjugated to the tracer (Figure 13.2c) [8, 9]. In both cases, a bright test line appears when the analyte in the sample is present in low concentrations, while a faint test line appears when the analyte in the sample is in high concentration (Figure 13.2b and c).

13.4 LFIA components

The outside simplicity of a lateral flow biosensor belies the underlying complexity of the internal workings. An understanding of the science behind how these devices are constructed is critical to understand and drive their successful implementation into new fields, such as personalized medicine. The materials used for construction of lateral flow biosensors are critical to the success of the final assays.

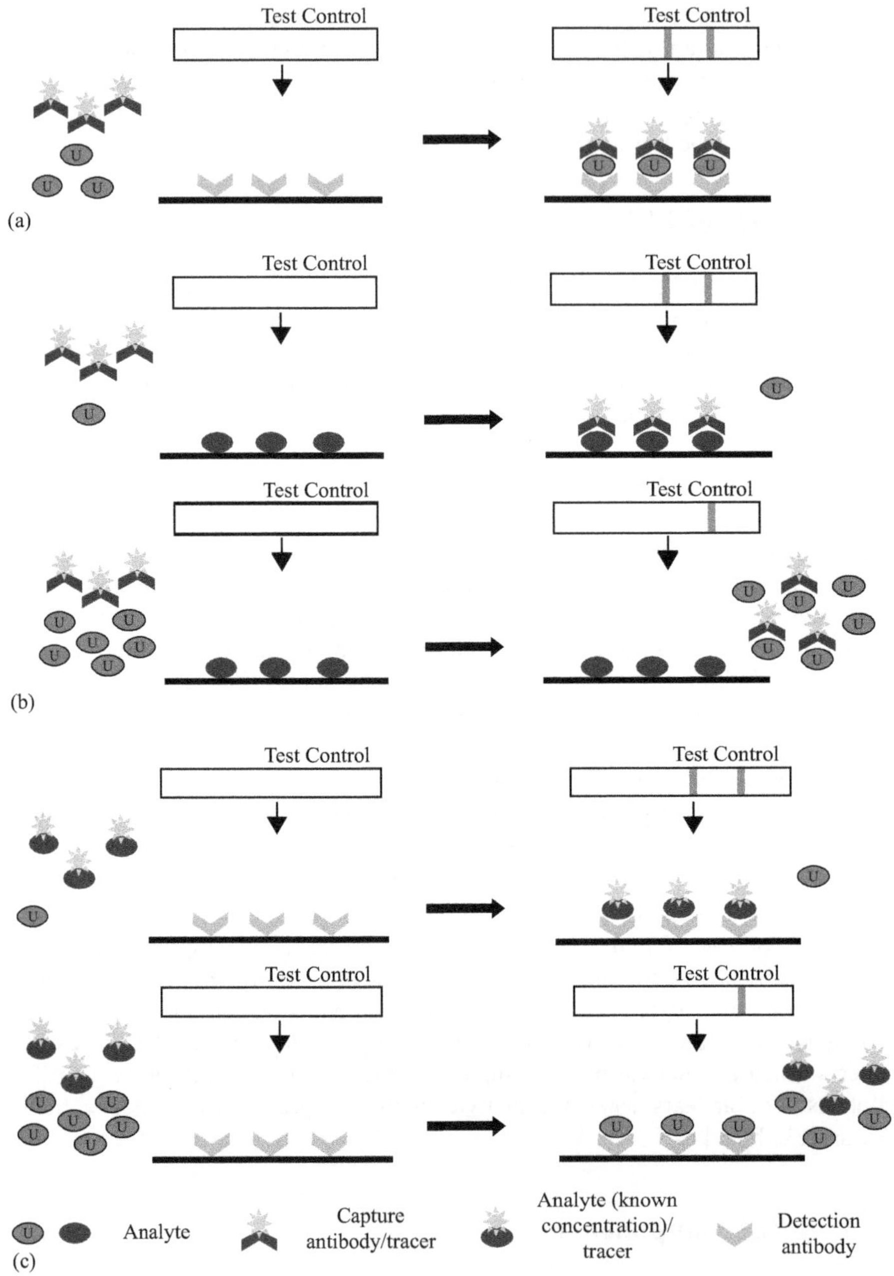

Figure 13.2 Types of LFIA. (a) Noncompetitive immunoassay. (b) Competitive immunoassay with known concentration of analyte being pre-immobilized to the membrane. (c) Competitive immunoassay with known concentration of analyte being pre-conjugated to the tracer

Here we explore in detail the four major materials: antibodies, membrane, tracer and pads. Emerging nanotechnology developments bestow some highly exciting elements for biosensor evolution. The application of nanomaterials allows easier sample concentration, higher molecular loading, and diverse detection methods and can boost the specificity and sensitivity. For lateral flow biosensors, the most common application of nanomaterials is within the transducer (tracer), which transforms the biomolecular interactions into a measurable signal. Different tracers that have been applied in lateral flow biosensors are discussed in Section 13.4.3.

13.4.1 Antibodies

In immunoassays, the most commonly employed antibodies are polyclonal and monoclonal antibodies [10]. Polyclonal antibodies are purified from whole serum, and as a collective can recognize multiple epitopes on any one antigen. Monoclonal antibodies are derived from hybridoma cell clones. Those generated from a single clone will thus possesses identical structure and reactivity, and only bind to one epitope on an antigen [10, 11]. The use of monoclonal antibodies in LFIAs is usually associated with improved detection sensitivity [12].

Apart from monoclonal and polyclonal antibodies that are produced in vivo, some "synthetic antibodies" have also been applied in the LFIA. One example is the recombinant antibody, which is translated from recombinant DNA by uniting target genes from multiple sources onto a vector, and are expressed as fusion proteins on the surfaces of cells or phage particles [13].Recombinant antibodies are often smaller than monoclonal and polyclonal antibodies, since only the antigen-binding part of the antibody (e.g. the Fab variable region) are expressed in most cases [10, 14]. The advantages of the recombinant antibody are that it has less lot-to-lot variation in comparison to the natural produced antibodies during production, and the antibody variable domains can be engineered more easily with desired affinity characteristics [12, 15]. However, recombinant antibodies often have lower affinity maturation than in vivo-produced antibodies, as animals immunized multiple times over a series of weeks create progressively stronger antibodies [16]. Additionally, the initial investment for creating a recombinant antibody library is costly and time consuming, and users need to become aware of relevant intellectual property protections surrounding the technology [17, 18].

Another example of "synthetic antibodies" is aptamers, which are single-stranded nucleic acids developed in vitro to bind protein or other nucleic acids [19]. Aptamers are usually produced by technique known as SELEX (systematic evolution of ligands by exponential enrichment) where a large amount of random single-stranded nucleic acids undergo screening to identify the most specific and high affinity binding candidates [20]. The advantages of aptamers are that they have equivalent or even higher binding affinity than many antibodies, and they are readily produced by chemical synthesis in vitro [21, 22]. However, a key concern of aptamers is their stability, as they can become inactivated by prevalent nucleases in biological samples. Stability of aptamers can be improved by modifying the backbone of the nucleotides (e.g. methylation of the 2' hydroxide groups on purine nucleosides) [23, 24], but this precludes their inclusion the screening selection process, and backbone modification subsequent to selection can affect antigen affinities.

Regardless of the antibody type, the interaction between the antibody and its corresponding antigen is pivotal for a sensitive immunoassay. This includes the strength of interaction between an antigen epitope and its corresponding antibody binding site (affinity) and the binding strength of an antigen-antibody complex (avidity) as influenced by the number of antibody binding sites and the geometry of the resulting antigen-antibody complexes [25]. Avidity is assay specific, and differs when the same antibody is used in different techniques [25]. In the development of new LFIAs, it is critical to obtain panels of antibodies to trial, in order to select an antibody that gives the best performance in the LFIA.

13.4.2 Membrane

In addition to antibodies, the texture of the membrane is also critical in a successful LFIA. The membrane serves as a stable binding surface to capture antibodies onto the test and control lines, and also to control the diffusive and capillary flow of the mobile phase (running buffer). The performance of the membrane is characterized by pore size, capillary flow rate, porosity and thickness (Figure 13.3) [26–28]. Indeed, the first two parameters are vital determinants for the assay sensitivity:

i. Pore size determines transportation of a particle through the membrane. Larger pores will decrease the sensitivity of the assay because the lines will spread out and be difficult to read. However, if the pores are too small, they will hinder the movement of reactants [29]. A variety of membrane pore sizes are available from manufacturers (ranging from 0.05 μm to about 12 μm) to cater for individual assay requirements.
ii. Capillary flow rate describes the membrane performance. With units of seconds per centimeter, the capillary flow rate defines the time required for liquid to migrate completely from the membrane front to the end. The one-dimensional transport of fluids in a porous substrate can be described by Washburn's theory, which defines the capillary flow rate as proportional to the square root of time [30]. Thus the further the test line is from the origin, the exponentially longer time it takes to wick to the test line. A slow flow rate allows sufficient interaction between antigen and antibody resulting in improved assay sensitivity, however, too slow flow rate increases assay time and is not favorable for rapid POC diagnostics [29].
iii. Porosity influences the surface area available for protein binding, and is associated with the pore size. The larger the pore size, the lower the surface area and the less protein binding capacity [27]. However, a small pore size can obstruct flow of reactants through the membrane.
iv. The membrane thickness determines the liquid absorption capacity of the membrane. Practically, it controls the width of test and control lines. If the membrane is very thick, then the width of these lines tends to be thinner, because only a narrow area is required to spread the same amount of solution, compared to a wider but thinner membrane.

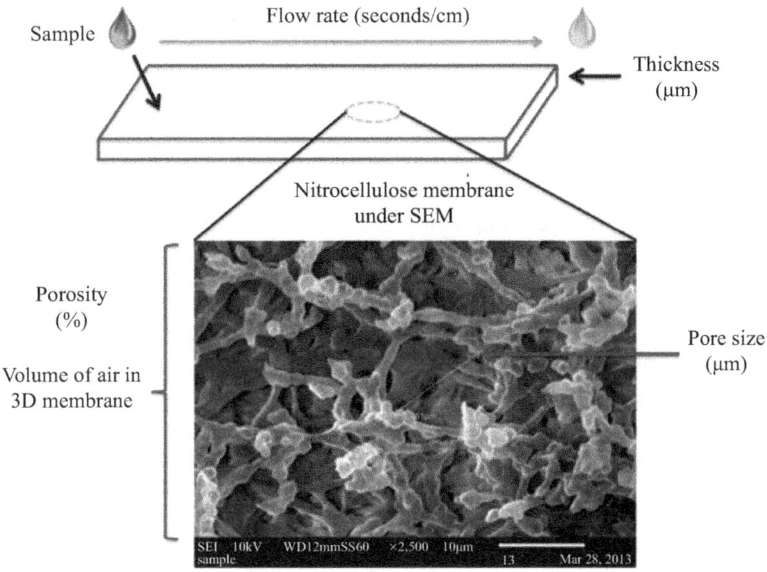

Figure 13.3 *Illustration of the four membrane parameters. An observation of the nitrocellulose membrane under the scanning electron microscope (SEM) is used as an example to illustrate the pore size and the porosity of the membrane*

Micro porous membranes for LFIA are produced from nitrocellulose, nylon, polyethersulfone, polyethylene, polyvinylidinedifluoride (PVDF) or fused silica [28, 3]. Among these, nitrocellulose is the most widely used, followed by nylon. Both nitrocellulose and nylon bind protein non-covalently, mainly through hydrophobic and electrostatic forces. However, nitrocellulose interacts with proteins more hydrophobic in nature, while nylon favors electrostatic interactions [32]. Although nitrocellulose has a lower protein binding capacity than nylon, it has better tolerability to blocking reagents (that block any other binding sites on the membrane other than the pre-deposited antibodies to prevent nonspecific binding), and thus allowing improved specificity and signal/noise ratios [27, 28]. Other advantages that account for the versatility of nitrocellulose include: (1) nitrocellulose can immobilize molecules in a near-quantitative fashion; (2) it can be cast to have pores sufficiently large to allow lateral flow of fluid in a reasonable time [33]; and (3) it has a long shelf-life for immobilized molecule storage [28]. In addition, the history of nitrocellulose use in molecular biology indicates that not only proteins but also nucleic acids can be immobilized onto it, as evidenced by Burnette's (Western blotting) and Southern's (Southern blotting) applications in detection of specific protein and DNA on nitrocellulose membranes, respectively [34, 35].

13.4.3 Tracers

Beyond the membranes and antibodies, the tracer is fundamentally important for transforming biomolecular recognition event(s) into a detectable signal. For POC lateral flow biosensors, a colorimetric visual signal is most favorable, since the results can be read directly via eye inspection. However, many different tracers have been applied in LFIA, such as enzymatic reactions, beads, particles or fluorescent dyes. In particular, the application of nanomaterials as tracers often bestows higher sensitivities.

i. Latex beads [36, 37] and colloidal gold particles are the most popular amongst the nanomaterial options, with colloidal gold particles being used most extensively. Both latex beads and colloidal gold particles can be manufactured with diverse size dimensions (from several nanometers to hundreds of micrometers), which empower their versatility in a number of different applications. On average, colloidal gold particles are smaller than latex beads, improving their mobility through membranes. However, latex beads have a wider color range corresponding to different particle sizes; whereas colloidal gold particles present mainly a lustrous cherry red color for the particle sizes from 5 nm to 250 nm in diameter [38, 39]. Attachment of latex beads and colloidal gold particles to the required antibody can be achieved either through physical or chemical means (also see Section 13.5.1) [40]. However, the conjugation of colloidal gold particles to the antibody is faster (e.g. 10 min) than the latex beads and is exceedingly stable, even in dried form [41], which may explain the prevalence of their use.
ii. An alternative to latex beads and colloidal gold particles is carbon particles. Their irregularity of shape and long conjugation time (one hour to several hours) to the antibody make them less popular, however their sensitivity in LFIA is comparable or even more sensitive to that of latex beads and colloidal gold particles. Additionally, carbon particles are relatively cheaper [42]. Carbon nanomaterials can adopt other formats. The uniform size format of carbon particles, known as carbon nanostrings (1D format), was first used as a tracer for LFIA by Lönnberg *et al.* for detecting the hormone – erythropoietin [43]. Kalogianni *et al.* applied it to detect polymerase chain reaction (PCR) products and visualize genotyping of single nucleotide polymorphisms (SNP) in human genomic DNA. Results depicted that as low as 2.5 fmol of amplified DNA could be detected [44]. Another 1D format of carbon nanomaterials is carbon nanotubes. The carbon nanotubes showed increasing binding efficiency to the analyte, and in turn enhanced the LFIA signal, due to its larger surface area for docking (bio)molecules. Yet, the movement of the carbon nanotubes/analyte complex was very slow, increasing the lateral flow detection time, as the carbon nanotubes are bulky in structure [45].
iii. Magnetic particles as colored labels have also been reported in LFIA. They can be adopted as either single particles or as particle aggregates [46, 47]. A 40-fold increase of sensitivity in LFIA through the use of Fe_3O_4 aggregates

compared to Fe_3O_4 particles was demonstrated by Liu *et al.* for the detection of paraoxon methyl [47].

iv. Enzymes are less popular because of substrate localization difficulties, as the products of enzymatic reactions are free to diffuse rapidly away from the tracer [38].

v. Liposomes have the ability to encapsulate high concentration of signals (e.g. fluorescent or bioluminescent dyes), and release them in a LFIA to yield visible lines, but their cumbersome requirements for drying and reconstitution, along with being susceptible to surfactant, have reduced their popularity [38, 48].

Other recently employed LFIA tracers include paramagnetic particles [49], quantum dots [50] and up-converting phosphorus (UP) [51]. Paramagnetic particles give off a nonvisual signal when subjected to a magnetic field; quantum dots emit visible light when exposed under ultra-violet light (UV); and UP become visible when excited with infrared light [49–51]. Although these particles demonstrate high amenability toward LFIA with easy manipulation of sizes, colors and signal intensities, these particular signals (nonvisual) can only be detected with the help of special instrumentations. However, the sensitivities of these tracers in LFIA are reported to be much higher than that of colloidal gold particles and latex beads [52–54].

13.4.4 Pads

One fundamental but often overlooked component of the LFIA is the series of interconnected pads that are mounted on a backing card within a plastic housing (Figure 13.4). Each pad serves one or more purposes, and the order and specific qualities of these pads are critical for successful functioning of the device:

i. The sample pad ensures even distribution of sample solution to upstream components. This pad can be made of cellulose or glass fiber, and is the site of sample loading. Reagents such as detergents (e.g. Tween or Triton) and blocking solution (e.g. bovine serum albumin, BSA or polyvinyl alcohol) can be impregnated within to enhance the flow rate [26, 31]. The sample pad may also serve to pretreat the sample to remove coarse materials (e.g. the whole cell) [31].

ii. The conjugate pad is adhered next to the sample pad, and is often the place where labeled antibody/tracer conjugates are deposited. Its main function is to control the release of reactants (e.g. analyte/antibody/tracer complexes) solution onto the membrane and hold the reactants stable over their entire shelf-life [26]. Conjugate pads can be made of glass fiber, polyester or synthetic nonabsorbent material (e.g. rayon).

iii. Incubation and detection pads are applied to the back of the membrane, to help stabilize the membrane, which can be very thin and fragile.

iv. Finally, the absorbent pad is used to enhance the capillary driving force and absorb all the unreacted substances. It is typically made of cotton and the absorbency rate varies from different thicknesses.

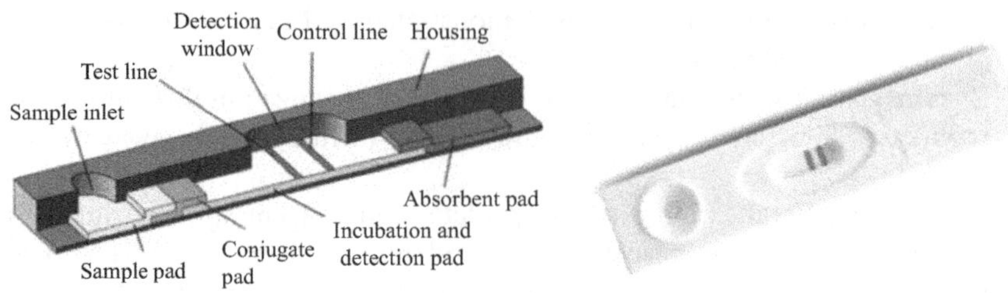

(a) (b)

Figure 13.4 A lateral flow device (LFD). (a) The components of the assembled LFD. Reproduced from Reference 55 with permission from The Royal Society of Chemistry. (b) A commercial LFD housed in a cassette with the inlet and the result windows. Courtesy of Valentina Razumova/Shutterstock.com

For commercial POC test kits, the whole lateral flow biosensor can be sealed within the plastic housing, except for the sample inlet window and a result reading window (Figure 13.4b).

13.5 Important parameters for LFIA

Beyond the physical compartments of the LFIA, several other parameters are critical for optimizing success. In particular, the antibody (or biomolecule) immobilization strategy and the coverage of the biomolecule on the tracer are core determinants for the sensitivity and specificity of the LFIA. In addition, nonbiological components such as the running buffer and pH also assist in the functioning of the assay.

13.5.1 Biomolecule immobilization

Biomolecule immobilization entails (1) the immobilization of biomolecule on the tracer and (2) the immobilization of biomolecule on the membrane. For a lateral flow immuno-biosensor, the two major biomolecules for immobilization are antibodies and nucleic acids (e.g. aptamers). The immobilization strategies for these two biomolecules share many common points, but also have differences due to their intrinsic properties.

Antibodies can be adsorbed onto tracer nanomaterials or membranes via electrostatic, hydrophobic, van der Waals and/or hydrogen forces [56, 57]. However, this physical absorption results in a random orientation during immobilization (Figure 13.5(i–iv)). Optimally, however, the antigenic binding sites should be fully exposed toward the analyte (Figure 13.5(i)). Two of the most effective ways to achieve this fashion are via bioaffinity or by chemically forming covalent bonds. Bioaffinity requires a strong ligand pair, such as biotin and avidin (dissociation constant of 10^{-15} M) [58]. This approach requires the antibody to be biotinylated in a site-specific manner (to the Fc region), before immobilization via

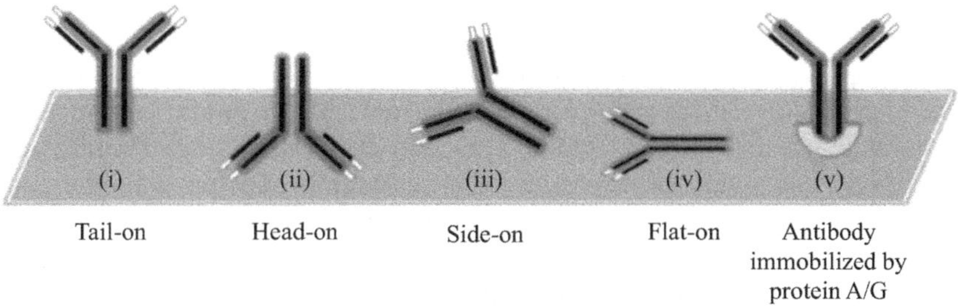

Figure 13.5 *Configurations of antibody immobilization. Antibody immobilized by physical absorption results in random orientations (i–iv). In contrast, immobilization using protein A or G leads to a maximized binding activity fashion (v)*

pre-immobilized avidin. The chemical approach can be performed by applying specific conjugation chemistries (e.g. carbodiimide and maleimide) between certain functional groups of the antibody (e.g. amine, carboxylate or sulfhydryl groups) and a functionalized surface of the nanomaterial or membrane [59, 60]. Notably, the carboxylate group in the Fc region and the sulfhydryl groups in the hinge and interchain regions of an antibody are ideal conjugation sites. Amine groups, on the other hand, can be distributed throughout the antibody and conjugation could potentially impede the antigen binding sites. In addition, some linkers (e.g. polyethylene glycol, PEG) are frequently applied in between the biomolecule and the surface of nanomaterials or membrane to minimize steric hindrance [61]. While chemical immobilization using the Fc region largely controls the orientation, it could still be tilted (instead of standing straight-up) in a partially active fashion (Figure 13.5(iii)). The use of protein A or G immobilization can effectively solve this issue, as protein A and G bind specifically to the Fc portion of immunoglobulin from many mammals [62, 63]. Immobilization of antibody using protein A or G may thus be the best option to maximize the binding activity of an antibody (Figure 13.5(v)).

In contrast to antibody immobilization, the immobilization of nucleic acids to nanomaterial or membrane surfaces is predominantly performed using surface chemistry. This is because (1) most nanomaterials have negatively-charged surfaces, causing repulsive interaction with nucleic acids and (2) nucleic acids cannot directly be immobilized onto the membrane except by UV cross-linking. Fortunately, chemical immobilization of nucleic acids is much easier than immobilizing antibodies, since issues of orientation are less of a problem. In addition, nucleic acids can be readily immobilized by forming dative bonds via amine, sulfhydryl or cyanide groups (tethered to one end of nucleic acid) [64]. Thus the surface chemistry described above for antibody immobilization can be similarly applied for nucleic acid immobilization. For both antibody and nucleic acids immobilized to the nanomaterials or membrane, blocking reagents such as Tween 20, BSA or casein are required to block nonspecific binding of the analyte, which is performed after immobilization.

13.5.2 Biomolecule coverage on the tracer

Another important consideration during biomolecule immobilization is the coverage of biomolecule on the nanomaterials. Biomolecule coverage can impacts the degree of biomolecule/tracer binding to the analyte and significantly affect immunoassay analytical sensitivity. Several research groups have shown that the proportion of biomolecule coverage does not have a linear relationship with analytical sensitivity [65–67]. Low biomolecule coverage can lead to low analytical sensitivity due to a low chance of binding to the analyte, and sometimes causes instability of the biomolecule/tracer conjugate. Conversely, high biomolecule coverage can also lead to low analytical sensitivity because of a steric hindrance effect [65–67]. The optimal biomolecule coverage lies in between and needs to be optimized for individual assays and analytes.

13.5.3 Buffer and pH

Another key factor for LFIA performance is the running buffer, since it interacts with all the molecules (analyte, detection molecules and capture/tracer molecules) involved in the LFIA. The buffer pH is critical for correct functionality of biomolecules during assay. Phosphate-buffered saline (PBS) and Tris-buffered saline (TBS) are the two commonly used buffers for LFIA. However, borate buffer has been reported to result in higher assay sensitivity than PBS and TBS; especially with the antigen-antibody detection modes. The best pH range is reported to be between 7.5 and 8.8 [42, 67, 68]. Lateral flow detection via oligonucleotide hybridizations frequently applies higher stringent buffers such as saline sodium citrate (SSC) [69]. SSC has been used for blotting, hybridization and stringency washes in Northern and Southern blots as well as DNA microarrays, and it maintains good stabilization of oligonucleotides. In nutshell, there is no universal buffer that applies to every LFIA; the buffer components and conditions need to be adjusted with respect to specific analytes and biomolecules to ensure a stable and active immunoassay performance.

13.6 Applications of lateral flow biosensors

The nature of LFIA devices is that their underlying complexity has lead to a revolution in operational simplicity. They are compact, portable in size and rapid POC result availability. Unipath first released their Clearview home pregnancy test for the detection of human Chorionic Gonadotropin (hCG) in 1988 [2]. Since then, LFIA have been applied to the detection of parasites [70], bacteria [71], cells [72], viruses [73], presence of toxins in food, [74] environmental samples [75], usage of illicit drugs [76], appearance of hormones [77] and biological markers [78]. Some well-established commercial lateral flow biosensors include the CardioDetect® FABP Rapid Test [79] for verifying acute myocardial infarction, DPP® HIV 1/2 Assay [80] for rapid diagnosis of HIV 1 and HIV 2 and NephroCheck® [81] for detecting acute kidney injury biomarkers.

One of the advantages of lateral flow biosensors is their utility for rapid deployment in response to disease outbreaks. Slomka *et al.* [82] demonstrated detection of H5N1 influenza virus in Egypt using two commercial lateral flow biosensors, Anigen and Quickvue. Similarly, a lateral flow biosensor was rapidly developed after the swine flu outbreak in 2013 [83].

LFIAs are also interesting in their potential for detection of nucleic acids, in a process named nucleic acid lateral flow (NALF). For NALF detection, nucleic acids can either be tagged with recognition labels, or act as the recognition molecules themselves [84, 85]. In the latter case, the recognition between two oligonucleotides is extremely sensitive, even down to a single base mismatch [86]. While not yet commercially available, this technique is particularly interesting for application in personalized medicine, since individualized assays for disease biomarkers could potentially be rapidly tailor-made based on physicians' recommendations.

Another interesting emerging technology is the multiplexed LFIA, which again has direct implications in personalized medicine, because it provides scope for detection of multiple disease biomarkers and could also theoretically be tailor-made to an individual's circumstance. Detection of multiple disease markers also improves diagnostic efficiency and precision, and reduces costs by replacing multiple individual assays with a single test kit. A few multiplexed lateral flow devices have been commercialized, such as the Milenia® QuickLine kits [87], the BD™ Directigen™ EZ Flu A+B kit [88] and RAID 8 and RAID TOX kits [89]. However, increased multiplexing remains a challenge for future development (e.g. greater than 5 analytes simultaneously), as there are issues with retaining sensitivity and specificity of detection without cross reactivity [90].

13.7 Major hurdles facing the lateral flow biosensors

Lateral flow biosensors are promising candidates for personalized and onsite biomedical diagnosis, with advantages over conventional diagnosis such as: (1) simplicity; (2) rapidness; (3) low cost; (4) reduction in testing sample volumes; (5) easier result interpretation by unskilled personnel. However, only a few lateral flow biosensors have been commercialized since the initial success of the home pregnancy test. Several hurdles are yet to be overcome before lateral flow biosensors become equivalent to conventional precision diagnostics.

Sensitivity is perhaps the biggest hurdle for lateral flow biosensors. Like a two-sided coin, the rapidness of a system where diagnosis occurs in only a few minutes by wicking analyte also proves to be the weakness, since ultra-sensitivity is hard to achieve during a short period of liquid movement that preclude equilibrium establishment between reaction molecules. However, many approaches have been applied to improve the sensitivity of the lateral flow biosensor and these can be achieved from both within and external to the device. The internal approach relies on improving the components of the lateral flow biosensor, such as the immunoassay format (noncompetitive or competitive; see Section 13.3), detection mode (antigen-antibody interaction or oligonucleotides hybridizations), using alternative tracers [91, 92] (see Section 13.4.3) and immobilization strategies (oriented and/or site-specific; see Section 13.5.1) [93]. In contrast, the external approach is more diverse, such as pre-concentration of analytes [94], thermal contrast [95], using wax pillars [96] or changing the architecture of the device [97]. However, the most common strategy for enhancing signals is amplification via enzymatic or chemical approaches [98, 99]. Most of these methods achieve more sensitive or even ultra-sensitive results.

Another major hurdle is to obtain quantitative results rather than the qualitative or semi-quantitative results. Quantitative results can be obtained with the help of extra equipment (e.g. lateral flow strip reader) or via image analysis. Yet, this is also a disadvantage, as the user cannot enjoy an equipment-free diagnosis experience. Ongoing research is looking for solutions to these issues, where perhaps a trade-off between diagnostic time, cost and sensitivity, could enable the possibility of quantification.

13.8 Future perspectives of lateral flow biosensors for personalized and onsite medicine

In the future, lateral flow biosensor can be integrated to more chemical processes. Ideally, integrating the lateral flow detection to the other two major diagnostics processes – sample preparation and amplification-completes an automated system or a micro total analysis system, which would even better serve the purpose of POC diagnosis. Developing such integration technology is a demanding job, because it is very hard to drive and direct reagent flow merely through capillary activity. Such demanding integration technology has a higher possibility of being realized by developing sophisticated microfluidic systems or "Lab-on-a-chip" [100, 101], but this will likely lead to an increased cost. Regardless, lateral flow biosensors are still incredibly promising POC candidates in terms of cost-effectiveness, and are capable of alleviating physical visits to hospitals and clinics for disease diagnosis.

The detection of nucleic acids in lateral flow biosensors reflects the trend that the traditional biochemical assays are being replaced by molecular testing. The underlying benefits are: (1) each living organism has certain unique nucleic acid sequences; (2) nucleic acid hybridization is highly specific and permits various combinations that can expand the detection capacity; and (3) nucleic acids can be pre-amplified before lateral flow detection, which allows low sample copy numbers to be detected. Understanding the natural nucleic acid amplification process in conjunction with molecular engineering and recombinant technology has lead to the advent of isothermal amplification as a replacement of the classical method – PCR [102]. Isothermal amplification performs nucleic acid replication at a single temperature and alleviates the usage of an expensive thermal cycler in PCR. For some isothermal amplification methods, a simple and portable heating device or even body heat will suffice for incubation [103, 104]. This allows incorporation with lateral flow detection as a facile diagnostic method conducted onsite or in resource-limited settings.

Result measurement, and in particular quantitative analysis, also needs consideration. Some portable devices (e.g. hand-held strip reader) are also available for quantitative result analysis [36]. In addition, the advancement of telecommunication devices, such as smartphones and Google Glass, can further assist lateral flow detection progression into telemedicine. These telecommunication devices can either immediately send the results to a well-equipped institution for data analysis or they can be used as an onsite analysis tool themselves [105, 106].

Finally, a major unrealized promise for lateral flow biosensors is the idea that devices could be tailor-made to an individual's needs. Many diseases require early prognosis so that immediate treatments can be implemented before disease progression and advancement of symptoms and morbidity. The Food and Drug Administration (FDA) approved an over-the-counter HIV lateral flow test for consumer use in 2012, which can deliver the results in as little as 40 min [107]. Similarly, a malaria home lateral flow test kit allows detection and/or confirmation of the four fatal species of *Plasmodium* within 10 min [108]. Sangeeta Bhatia from MIT has developed a urine sample-based lateral flow biosensor for cancer biomarker detection, and again the results are revealed within minutes [109]. The versatility of lateral flow biosensors for developing these pertinent detection kits is on the basis of identification of specific biomarkers of these diseases. As our knowledge of genetics and diseases in personalized medicine grows, there lies a tantalizing possibility that lateral flow biosensors could be ordered by individuals or their physicians to enable home monitoring of biomarkers related to their individual personal conditions. Literally, any disease-causing genes or biomarkers could be identified, and then lateral flow biosensors could be transformed to enable their detection and monitoring.

13.9 Conclusion

Research in lateral flow biosensors is accelerating, with an exponential increase in the number of published papers over the last three decades. The core reason of such rapid growth is that lateral flow biosensors are indeed catering for customer needs. There is no doubt that healthcare, especially with the emerging concept of onsite personalized biomedical diagnosis, is and will continue to be the most important area for the application of biosensors. In this field, lateral flow biosensors are one of the most promising candidates when leveraging by both the utility and cost. We predict that in less than a decade, systems that adopt lateral flow components will replace centralized laboratory facilities, with commercial enterprises providing custom-made individualized diagnostics available over the internet, as prescribed by doctors or simply requested by an individual wanting to monitor their own health.

References

[1] Marchant J. 'Next generation molecular and point-of-care diagnostics driving personalised healthcare'. Presented at Innovations in Diagnostics Conference; London, England, 2005.

[2] Chard T. 'Pregnancy tests: a review'. *Hum. Reprod.* 1992, vol. 7(5), pp. 701–10.

[3] Bio-Alternative Medical Devices. *Point of Care Diagnostic Market Expected to Be Worth over $20 Billion by 2014: Bio-Alternative Medical Devices* [online]. 2015. Available from: http://www.bioamd.com/investors [Accessed 22 Jun 2015].

[4] Song Y., Wei W., Qu X. 'Colorimetric biosensing using smart materials'. *Adv. Mater.* 2011, vol. 23(37), pp. 4215–36.

[5] Song S., Qin Y., He Y., Huang Q., Fan C., Chen H-Y. 'Functional nanoprobes for ultrasensitive detection of biomolecules'. *Chem. Soc. Rev.* 2010, vol. 39(11), pp. 4234–43.

[6] Tang D., Cui Y., Chen G. 'Nanoparticle-based immunoassays in the biomedical field'. *Analyst.* 2013, vol. 138(4), pp. 981–90.

[7] Brett G.M., Chambers S.J., Huang L., Morgan M.R.A. 'Design and development of immunoassays for detection of proteins'. *Food Control.* 1999, vol. 10(6), pp. 401–6.

[8] Esch M.B., Baeumner A.J., Durst R.A. 'Detection of cryptosporidium parvum using oligonucleotide-tagged liposomes in a competitive assay format'. *Anal. Chem.* 2001, vol. 73(13), pp. 3162–7.

[9] Ho J.A., Wauchope R.D. 'A strip liposome immunoassay for aflatoxin B1'. *Anal. Chem.* 2002, vol. 74(7), pp. 1493–6.

[10] Conroy P.J., Hearty S., Leonard P., O'Kennedy R.J. 'Antibody production, design and use for biosensor-based applications'. *Semin. Cell. Dev. Biol.* 2009, vol. 20(1), pp. 10–26.

[11] Köhler G., Milstein C. 'Continuous cultures of fused cells secreting antibody of predefined specificity'. *Nature.* 1975, vol. 256(5517), pp. 495–7.

[12] Andreotti P.E., Ludwig G.V., Peruski A.H., Tuite J.J., Morse S.S., Peruski L.F. Jr. 'Immunoassay of infectious agents'. *Biotechniques.* 2003, vol. 35(4), pp. 850–9.

[13] McCafferty J., Griffiths A.D., Winter G., Chiswell D.J. 'Phage antibodies: filamentous phage displaying antibody variable domains'. *Nature.* 1990, vol. 348(6301), pp. 552–4.

[14] Moore G.P. 'Genetically engineered antibodies'. *Clin. Chem.* 1989, vol. 35(9), pp. 1849–53.

[15] Krebs B., Rauchenberger R., Reiffert S., Rothe C., Tesar M., Thomassen E., *et al.* 'High-throughput generation and engineering of recombinant human antibodies'. *J. Immunol. Methods.* 2001, vol. 254(1–2), pp. 67–84.

[16] Ritter, M.A. *Methods in Molecular Medicine.* Diagnostic and Therapeutic Antibodies Series, no. 40 (Totowa, Humana Press, 2000).

[17] Swann P.G., Tolnay M., Muthukkumar S., Shapiro M.A., Rellahan B.L., Clouse K.A. 'Considerations for the development of therapeutic monoclonal antibodies'. *Curr. Opin. Immunol.* 2008, vol. 20(4), pp. 493–9.

[18] Shoemaker C.B. 'When will rAbs replace mAbs in labs?' *Vet. J.* 2005, vol. 170(2), pp. 151–2.

[19] Jayasena S.D. 'Aptamers: an emerging class of molecules that rival antibodies in diagnostics'. *Clin. Chem.* 1999, vol. 45(9), pp. 1628–5.

[20] Tuerk C., Gold L. 'Systematic evolution of ligands by exponential enrichment: RNA ligands to bacteriophage T4 DNA polymerase'. *Science.* 1990, vol. 249(4968), pp. 505–10.

[21] Brody E.N., Gold L. 'Aptamers as therapeutic and diagnostic agents'. *J. Biotechnol.* 2000, vol. 74(1), pp. 5–13.

[22] O'Farrell B. 'Lateral flow immunoassay systems: evolution from the current state of the art to the next generation of highly sensitive, quantitative rapid assays' in Wild D. (ed.). *The Immunoassay Handbook.* (Oxford, Elsevier Ltd, 2013), pp. 89–107.

[23] Eaton B.E., Pieken W.A. 'Ribonucleosides and RNA'. *Annu. Rev. Biochem.* 1995, vol. 64, pp. 837–63.

[24] Ruckman J., Green L.S., Beeson J., *et al.* '2′-Fluoropyrimidine RNA-based aptamers to the 165-amino acid form of vascular endothelial growth factor (VEGF165). Inhibition of receptor binding and VEGF-induced vascular permeability through interactions requiring the exon 7-encoded domain'. *J. Biol. Chem.* 1998, vol. 273(32), pp. 20556–67.

[25] Lipman N.S., Jackson L.R., Trudel L.J., Weis-Garcia F. 'Monoclonal versus polyclonal antibodies: distinguishing characteristics, applications, and information resources'. *ILAR J.* 2005, vol. 46(3), pp. 258–68.

[26] O'Farrell B. 'Evolution in lateral flow-based immunoassay systems' in Raphael C.W., Tse H.Y. (eds.). *Lateral Flow Immunoassay* (New York, Humana Press, 2009), pp. 1–34.

[27] Harvey M.A., Audette C.A., McDonogh R. 'The use of microporous polymer membranes in immunoassays'. *IVD Technology.* 1996, vol. 2, pp. 34–39.

[28] Tonkinson J.L., Stillman B.A. 'Nitrocellulose: a tried and true polymer finds utility as a post-genomic substrate'. *Front. Biosci.* 2002, vol. 7, pp. c1–12.

[29] Jones K.D. 'Troubleshooting protein binding in nitrocellulose membranes. Part 1: principles'. *IVD Technology.* 1999, vol. 5, pp. 32–41.

[30] Washburn E.W. 'The dynamics of capillary flow'. *Phys. Rev.* 1921, vol. 17(3), pp. 273–83.

[31] Posthuma-Trumpie G., Korf J., Amerongen A. 'Lateral flow (immuno)assay: its strengths, weaknesses, opportunities and threats. A literature survey'. *Anal. Bioanal. Chem.* 2009, vol. 393(2), pp. 569–82.

[32] Gershoni J.M., Palade G.E. 'Electrophoretic transfer of proteins from sodium dodecyl sulfate-polyacrylamide gels to a positively charged membrane filter'. *Anal. Biochem.* 1982, vol. 124(2), pp. 396–405.

[33] Mansfield M.A. 'The use of nitrocellulose membranes in lateral flow assays' in Wong R.C., Tse H.Y. (eds.). *Drugs of Abuse: Body Fluid Testing* (Totowa, Humana Press, 2005), pp. 71–85.

[34] Burnette W.N. '"Western Blotting": Electrophoretic transfer of proteins from sodium dodecyl sulfate-polyacrylamide gels to unmodified nitrocellulose and radiographic detection with antibody and radioiodinated protein A'. *Anal. Biochem.* 1981, vol. 112(2), pp. 195–203.

[35] Southern E.M. 'Detection of specific sequences among DNA fragments separated by gel electrophoresis'. *J. Mol. Biol.* 1975, vol. 98(3), pp. 503–17.

[36] Mao X., Wang W., Du T.E. 'Dry-reagent nucleic acid biosensor based on blue dye doped latex beads and lateral flow strip'. *Talanta.* 2013, vol. 114, pp. 248–53.

[37] Tian L., Sato T., Niwa K., Kawase M., Tanner A.C., Takahashi N. 'Rapid and sensitive PCR-dipstick DNA chromatography for multiplex analysis of the oral microbiota'. *Biomed. Res. Int.* 2014, vol. 2014, pp. 1–10.

[38] Chun P. 'Colloidal gold and other labels for lateral flow immunoassays' in Raphael C.W., Harley Y.T. (eds.). *Lateral Flow Immunoassay* (New York, Humana Press, 2009), pp. 75–90.

[39] Seal J., Braven H., Wallace P. 'Point-of-care nucleic acid lateral flow tests'. *IVD Technology*. 2006, vol. 8, pp. 41–54.

[40] Tomita N., Mori Y., Kanda H., Notomi T. 'Loop-mediated isothermal amplification (LAMP) of gene sequences and simple visual detection of products'. *Nat. Protoc.* 2008, vol. 3(5), pp. 877–82.

[41] Carney J., Braven H., Seal J., Whitworth E. 'Present and future applications of gold in rapid assays'. *IVD Technology*. 2006, vol. 12, pp. 41–49.

[42] Noguera P., Posthuma-Trumpie G.A., van-Tuil M., *et al.* 'Carbon nanoparticles in lateral flow methods to detect genes encoding virulence factors of Shiga toxin-producing Escherichia coli'. *Anal. Bioanal. Chem.* 2011, vol. 399(2), pp. 831–8.

[43] Lönnberg M., Drevin M., Carlsson J. 'Ultra-sensitive immunochromatographic assay for quantitative determination of erythropoietin'. *J. Immunol. Methods.* 2008, vol. 339(2), pp. 236–44.

[44] Kalogianni D., Boutsika L., Kouremenou P., Christopoulos T., Ioannou P. 'Carbon nano-strings as reporters in lateral flow devices for DNA sensing by hybridization'. *Anal. Bioanal. Chem.* 2011, vol. 400(4), pp. 1145–52.

[45] Qiu W., Xu H., Takalkar S., *et al.* 'Carbon nanotube-based lateral flow biosensor for sensitive and rapid detection of DNA sequence'. *Biosens. Bioelectron.* 2015, vol. 64, pp. 367–72.

[46] Sun J., Lei X., Wang W., *et al.* 'Development and evaluation of a paramagnetic nanoparticle based immunochromatographic strip for specific detection of 2009 H1N1 influenza virus'. *J. Nanosci. Nanotechnol.* 2013, vol. 13(3), pp. 1684–90.

[47] Liu C., Jia Q., Yang C., *et al.* 'Lateral flow immunochromatographic assay for sensitive pesticide detection by ssing Fe_3O_4 nanoparticle aggregates as color reagents'. *Anal. Chem.* 2011, vol. 83(17), pp. 6778–84.

[48] Edwards K.A., Baeumner A.J. 'Optimization of DNA-tagged dye-encapsulating liposomes for lateral-flow assays based on sandwich hybridization'. *Anal. Bioanal. Chem.* 2006, vol. 386(5), pp. 1335–43.

[49] Richardson J., Hawkins P., Luxton R. 'The use of coated paramagnetic particles as a physical label in a magneto-immunoassay'. *Biosens. Bioelectron.* 2001, vol. 16(9–12), pp. 989–93.

[50] Lingerfelt B.M., Mattoussi H., Goldman E.R., Mauro J.M., Anderson G.P. 'Preparation of quantum dot–biotin conjugates and their sse in immunochromatography assays'. *Anal. chem.* 2003, vol. 75(16), pp. 4043–9.

[51] Hampl J., Hall M., Mufti N.A., *et al.* 'Upconverting phosphor reporters in immunochromatographic assays'. *Anal. Biochem.* 2001, vol. 288(2), pp. 176–87.

[52] Zhang X., Li D., Wang C., *et al.* 'A CCD-based reader combined quantum dots-labeled lateral flow strips for ultrasensitive quantitative detection of anti-HBs antibody'. *J. Biomed. Nanotechnol.* 2012, vol. 8(3), pp. 372–9.

[53] Hampl J., Hall M., Mufti N.A., *et al.* 'Upconverting phosphor reporters in immunochromatographic assays'. *Anal. Biochem.* 2001, vol. 288(2), pp. 176–87.

[54] Wang Y., Xu H., Wei M., Gu H., Xu Q., Zhu W. 'Study of superparamagnetic nanoparticles as labels in the quantitative lateral flow immunoassay'. *Mater. Sci. Eng. C.* 2009, vol. 29(3), pp. 714–8.

[55] Mark D., Haeberle S., Roth G., von Stetten F., Zengerle R. 'Microfluidic lab-on-a-chip platforms: requirements, characteristics and applications'. *Chem. Soc. Rev.* 2010, vol. 39(3), pp. 1153–82.

[56] Arruebo M., Valladares M., González-Fernández Á. 'Antibody-conjugated nanoparticles for biomedical applications'. *J. Nanomater. 2009*, vol. 2009, pp. 1–24.

[57] Kong F., Hu Y.F. 'Biomolecule immobilization techniques for bioactive paper fabrication'. *Anal. Bioanal. Chem.* 2012, vol. 403(1), pp. 7–13.

[58] Diamandis E.P., Christopoulos T.K. 'The biotin-(strept)avidin system: principles and applications in biotechnology'. *Clin. Chem.* 1991, vol. 37(5), pp. 625–36.

[59] Kim D., Herr A.E. 'Protein immobilization techniques for microfluidic assays'. *Biomicrofluidics.* 2013, vol. 7(4), pp. 41501.

[60] Hermanson G.T. 'The reactions of bioconjugation' in Hermanson G.T. (ed.). *Bioconjugate Techniques* (Elsevier Inc., 2013), pp. 229–58.

[61] Eck W., Craig G., Sigdel A., *et al.* 'PEGylated gold nanoparticles conjugated to monoclonal F19 antibodies as targeted labeling agents for human pancreatic carcinoma tissue'. *ACS Nano.* 2008, vol. 2(11), pp. 2263–72.

[62] Goding J.W. 'Use of staphylococcal protein A as an immunological reagent'. *J. Immunol. Methods.* 1978, vol. 20, pp. 241–53.

[63] Akerstrom B., Brodin T., Reis K., Bjorck L. 'Protein G: a powerful tool for binding and detection of monoclonal and polyclonal antibodies'. *J. Immunol.* 1985, vol. 135(4), pp. 2589–92.

[64] Samanta D., Sarkar A. 'Immobilization of bio-macromolecules on self-assembled monolayers: methods and sensor applications'. *Chem. Soc. Rev.* 2011, vol. 40(5), pp. 2567–92.

[65] Safenkova I., Zherdev A., Dzantiev B. 'Factors influencing the detection limit of the lateral-flow sandwich immunoassay: a case study with potato virus X'. *Anal. Bioanal. Chem.* 2012, vol. 403(6), pp. 1595–605.

[66] Aveyard J., Mehrabi M., Cossins A., Braven H., Wilson R. 'One step visual detection of PCR products with gold nanoparticles and a nucleic acid lateral flow (NALF) device'. *Chem. Commun. (Camb).* 2007, vol. 7(41), pp. 4251–3.

[67] Li J., McMillan D., Macdonald J. 'Enhancing the signal of lateral flow immunoassays by using different developing methods'. *Sensor. Mater.* 2015, vol. 27(7), pp. 549–61.

[68] Thobhani S., Attree S., Boyd R., Kumarswami N., Noble J., Szymanski M., *et al.* Bioconjugation and characterisation of gold colloid-labelled proteins'. *J. Immunol. Methods.* 2010, vol. 356(1–2), pp. 60–9.

[69] Lie P., Liu J., Fang Z., Dun B., Zeng L. 'A lateral flow biosensor for detection of nucleic acids with high sensitivity and selectivity'. *Chem. Commun. (Camb).* 2012, vol. 48(2), pp. 236–8.

[70] Mens P.F., de Bes H.M., Sondo P., *et al.* 'Direct blood PCR in combination with nucleic acid lateral flow immunoassay for detection of plasmodium species in settings where malaria is endemic'. *J. Clin. Microbiol.* 2012, vol. 50(11), pp. 3520–5.

[71] Chua A., Yean C.Y., Ravichandran M., Lim B., Lalitha P. 'A rapid DNA biosensor for the molecular diagnosis of infectious disease'. *Biosens. Bioelectron.* 2011, vol. 26(9), pp. 3825–31.

[72] Wu W., Yu L., Fang Z., Lie P., Zeng L. 'A lateral flow biosensor for the detection of human pluripotent stem cells'. *Anal. Biochem.* 2013, vol. 436(2), pp. 160–4.

[73] Peng F., Wang Z., Zhang S., *et al.* 'Development of an immunochromatographic strip for papid detection of H9 subtype Avian Influenza viruses'. *Clin. Vaccine. Immunol.* 2008, vol. 15(3), pp. 569–74.

[74] Liu B-H., Tsao Z-J., Wang J-J., Yu F-Y. 'Development of a monoclonal antibody against Ochratoxin A and its application in enzyme-linked immunosorbent assay and gold nanoparticle immunochromatographic strip'. *Anal. Chem.* 2008, vol. 80(18), pp. 7029–35.

[75] Guo Y-R., Liu S-Y., Gui W-J., Zhu G-N. 'Gold immunochromatographic assay for simultaneous detection of carbofuran and triazophos in water samples'. *Anal. Biochem.* 2009, vol. 389(1), pp. 32–9.

[76] Li K., Liu L., Xu C., Chu X. 'Rapid determination of chloramphenicol residues in aquaculture tissues by immunochromatographic assay'. *Anal. Sci.* 2007, vol. 23(11), pp. 1281–4.

[77] Leung W., Chan P., Bosgoed F., *et al.* 'One-step quantitative cortisol dipstick with proportional reading'. *J. Immunol. Methods.* 2003, vol. 281(1–2), pp. 109–18.

[78] Xu Q., Xu H., Gu H., Li J., Wang Y., Wei M. 'Development of lateral flow immunoassay system based on superparamagnetic nanobeads as labels for rapid quantitative detection of cardiac troponin I'. *Mater. Sci. Eng. C.* 2009, vol. 29(3), pp. 702–7.
[79] VASOCARE Co., Ltd. *CardioDetect® Rapid Test* [online]. 2015. Available from: http://www.vasocare.co.kr/_ver01/_bbs_iw2000/?doc=bbs/board.php&bo_table=020201&page=1&wr_id=1&stext [Accessed 19 Dec 2015].
[80] Chembio Diagnostic Systems Inc. *DPP® HIV 1/2 Assay* [online]. 2015. Available from: http://chembio.com/products/human-diagnostics/dpp-hiv-12-assayx/ [Accessed 19 Dec 2015].
[81] Astute Medical Inc. *NephroCheck®* [online]. 2015. Available from: http://www.astutemedical.com/us/products/nephrocheck-test/ [Accessed 19 Dec 2015].
[82] Soliman M., Selim A., Coward V.J., *et al.* 'Evaluation of two commercial lateral flow devices (LFDs) used for flockside testing of H5N1 highly-pathogenic avian influenza infections in backyard gallinaceous poultry in Egypt'. *J. Mol. Genet. Med.* 2010, vol. 4, pp. 247–51.
[83] Ge Y., Wu B., Qi X., *et al.* 'Rapid and sensitive detection of novel Avian-Origin Influenza A (H7N9) virus by reverse transcription loop-Mediated isothermal amplification combined with a lateral-flow device'. *PLoS ONE.* 2013, vol. 8(8), pp. e69941.
[84] Glynou K., Ioannou P.C., Christopoulos T.K., Syriopoulou V. 'Oligonucleotide-functionalized gold nanoparticles as probes in a dry-reagent strip biosensor for DNA analysis by hybridization'. *Anal. Chem.* 2003, vol. 75(16), pp. 4155–60.
[85] Mao X., Xu H., Zeng Q., Zeng L., Liu G. 'Molecular beacon-functionalized gold nanoparticles as probes in dry-reagent strip biosensor for DNA analysis'. *Chem. Commun. (Camb).* 2009, vol. 7(21), pp. 3065–7.
[86] Elenis D.S., Ioannou P.C., Christopoulos T.K. 'A nanoparticle-based sensor for visual detection of multiple mutations'. *Nanotechnology.* 2011, vol. 22(15), pp. 155501.
[87] Milenia Biotec. *Milenia® QuickLine* [online]. 2015. Available from: http://www.milenia-biotec.de/products/?L=1 [Accessed 19 Dec 2015].
[88] Becton, Dickinson and Company. *BD™ EZ Flu A+B Test* [online]. 2014. Available from: http://www.bd.com/ds/productCenter/256050.asp. [Accessed 12 Jan 2015].
[89] Alexeter Technologies. *RAID* [online]. 2014. Available from: http://www.alexeter.com/biow/Products/products/strips/RAID_DX.asp. [Accessed 12 Jan 2015].
[90] Li J., Macdonald J. 'Multiplex lateral flow detection and binary encoding enables a molecular colorimetric 7-segment display'. *Lab. Chip.* 2015, vol. 16(2), pp. 242–245.
[91] Kalogianni D.P., Litos I.K., Christopoulos T.K., Ioannou P.C. 'Dipstick-type biosensor for visual detection of DNA with oligonucleotide-decorated colored polystyrene microspheres as reporters'. *Biosens. Bioelectron.* 2009, vol. 24(6), pp. 1811–5.

[92] Xia X., Xu Y., Zhao X., Li Q. 'Lateral flow immunoassay using europium chelate-loaded silica nanoparticles as labels'. *Clin. Chem.* 2009, vol. 55(1), pp. 179–82.

[93] Lu B., Smyth M.R., O'Kennedy R. 'Oriented immobilization of antibodies and its applications in immunoassays and immunosensors'. *Analyst.* 1996, vol. 121(3), pp. 29R–32R.

[94] Mashayekhi F., Chiu R.Y., Le A.M., Chao F.C., Wu B.M., Kamei D.T. 'Enhancing the lateral-flow immunoassay for viral detection using an aqueous two-phase micellar system'. *Anal. Bioanal. Chem.* 2010, vol. 398 (7–8), pp. 2955–61.

[95] Qin Z., Chan W.C., Boulware D.R., Akkin T., Butler E.K., Bischof J.C.. 'Significantly improved analytical sensitivity of lateral flow immunoassays by using thermal contrast'. *Angew Chem Int Ed Engl.* 2012, vol. 51(18), pp. 4358–61.

[96] Rivas L., Medina-Sanchez M., de la Escosura-Muniz A., Merkoci A. 'Improving sensitivity of gold nanoparticle-based lateral flow assays by using wax-printed pillars as delay barriers of microfluidics'. *Lab. Chip.* 2014, vol. 14(22), pp. 4406–14.

[97] Parolo C., Medina-Sanchez M., de la Escosura-Muniz A., Merkoci A. 'Simple paper architecture modifications lead to enhanced sensitivity in nanoparticle based lateral flow immunoassays'. *Lab. Chip.* 2013, vol. 13 (3), pp. 386–90.

[98] Parolo C., de la Escosura-Muñiz A., Merkoçi A. 'Enhanced lateral flow immunoassay using gold nanoparticles loaded with enzymes'. *Biosens. Bioelectron.* 2013, vol. 40(1), pp. 412–6.

[99] Gupta S., Huda S., Kilpatrick P.K., Velev O.D. 'Characterization and optimization of gold nanoparticle-based silver-enhanced immunoassays'. *Anal. Chem.* 2007, vol. 79(10), pp. 3810–20.

[100] Abgrall P., Gu´e A-M. 'Lab-on-chip technologies: making a microfluidic network and coupling it into a complete microsystem-a review'. *J. Micromech. Microeng.* 2007, vol. 17(5), pp. 15–49.

[101] Kim T.H., Park J., Kim C.J., Cho Y.K. 'Fully integrated lab-on-a-disc for nucleic acid analysis of food-borne pathogens'. *Anal. Chem.* 2014, vol. 86(8), pp. 3841–8.

[102] Li J., Macdonald J. 'Advances in isothermal amplification: novel strategies inspired by biological processes'. *Biosens. Bioelectron.* 2014, vol. 64C, pp. 196–211.

[103] Hatano B., Maki T., Obara T., *et al.* 'LAMP using a disposable pocket warmer for anthrax detection, a highly mobile and reliable method for anti-bioterrorism'. *Jpn. J. Infect. Dis.* 2010, vol. 63(1), pp. 36–40.

[104] Crannell Z.A., Rohrman B., Richards-Kortum R. 'Equipment-free incubation of recombinase polymerase amplification reactions using body heat'. *PLoS ONE.* 2014, vol. 9(11), pp. e112146.

[105] Martinez A.W., Phillips S.T., Carrilho E., Thomas S.W., Sindi H., Whitesides G.M. 'Simple telemedicine for developing regions: camera

phones and paper-based microfluidic devices for real-time, off-site diagnosis'. *Anal. Chem.* 2008, vol. 80(10), pp. 3699–707.

[106] Feng S., Caire R., Cortazar B., Turan M., Wong A., Ozcan A. 'Immunochromatographic diagnostic test analysis using Google Glass'. *ACS Nano.* 2014, vol. 8(3), pp. 3069–79.

[107] OraSure Technologies Inc. ORAQUICK *In-home HIV Test* [online]. 2014. Available from: http://www.oraquick.com [Accessed 27 Jul 2015].

[108] Sanitoets CC and Sallamander Concepts (Pty) Ltd. *Sanitoest Malaria Home Test Kits* [online]. 2015. Available from: http://www.anytestkits.com/malaria-test-kit.htm. [Accessed 27 Jul 2015].

[109] MIT News Office. *A Paper Diagnostic for Cancer* [online]. 2015. Available from: http://newsoffice.mit.edu/2014/a-paper-diagnostic-for-cancer-0224 [Accessed 27 Jul 2015].

Chapter 14

MicroRNAs and their applications in diagnosis for osteoarthritis

Long Zhang[1], Qian Chen[1,2] and Yupeng Chen[1,2]

14.1 Introduction

Osteoarthritis (OA), age-related loss of the homeostatic balance between cartilage degradation and repair mechanisms primarily involved in articular cartilage is a complex chronic and highly prevalent degenerative joint disease [1]. Large numbers of individuals with OA throughout the world suffer baryodynia most in knees and hips joints [2]. Regardless of the fact that few pathogenesis pathways have been researched and some drugs reduce symptoms and slow the progression of OA, there are still no effective pharmacological methods for prevention and treatment. The difficulties in detecting it at an early stage and lack of effective treatments may be constituted to the lethality of OA. Therefore, there is an urgent need for precious, personalized and predictive markers to diagnose it early and could treat it with the best approach. It is important to further investigate and understand OA pathology to develop effective therapeutic targets to control OA.

Endogenous small noncoding RNAs known as microRNAs (miRNAs), 18–24 nucleotide-long single-stranded RNAs are negatively important regulators of posttranscriptional gene expression in organisms ranging from nematodes to humans [3–5]. MiRNAs are transcribed by RNA polymerase II. A hair pin structure of pri-miRNA ends with single mismatched sequences [6] is established when the RNA polymerase binds to the promoter region of the target DNA sequence. The pri-miRNA will be further processed into pre-miRNA by the RNase III enzyme Drosha and its cofactor DGCR8 [7] in the nucleus. With the help of Exportin-5 [8], pre-miRNA is transported into the cytoplasm for deep processing with the stem loop removed into a double-stranded short RNA duplex [9] by RNase III enzyme Dicer [10]. One strand of the miRNA duplex known as the passenger strand degrade rapidly, and the other strand is selected as the guide miRNA associated

[1]Bone and Joint Research Center, The First Affiliated Hospital and Frontier Institute of Science and Technology, Xi'an JiaoTong University, Xi'an 710061, China

[2]Department of Orthopaedics, Rhode Island Hospital and Warren Alpert Medical School of Brown University, Providence, RI 02903, USA

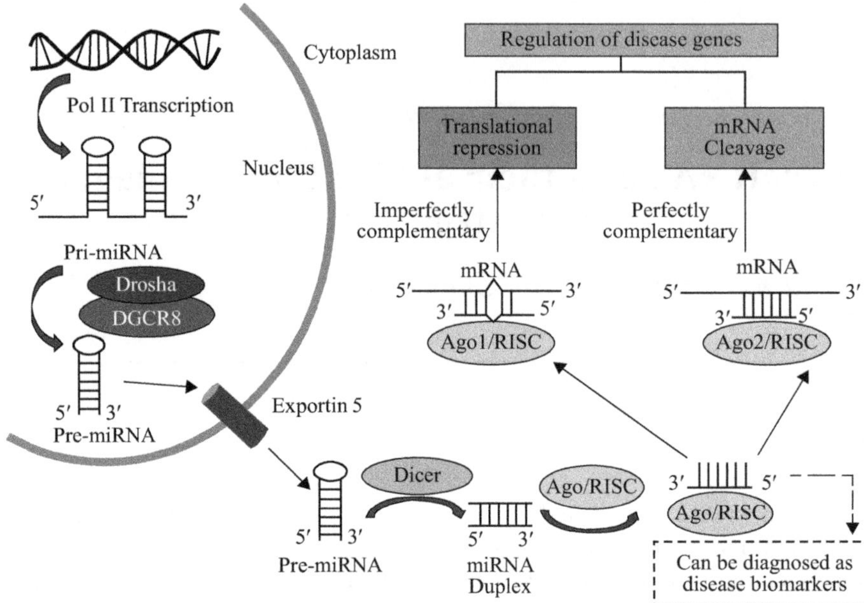

Figure 14.1 Diagrammatical demonstration of the principle of miRNA actions

with Ago protein to form the RISC (RNA induced silencing complex) complex to target specific mRNA [11, 12]. But when miRNA-induced silencing complex (mRISC) acts on mRNA, there are two ways would be occurring. If the miRNA could fully match the mRNA sequence, the mRNA is degraded by the mRISC complex [13]. When the two sequences are imperfectly complementary, the mRNA only be inhibited to translate by mRISC without degradation [12]. The principle of miRNA actions is diagrammatically shown in Figure 14.1.

Numerous studies show that miRNAs are involved in some significant cellular processes like apoptosis [14], differentiation [15], organ development [16], and expected to be diagnostic and prognostic biomarkers of cacoethic tumors [17–21]. Also, miRNA expression was detected both in plasma and synovial fluid from OA patients [22]. A large number of studies show that miRNA plays an important role in regulating the gene expression in OA which is characterized by the progressive destruction of articular cartilage. Therefore, understanding the role of miRNA in OA promises to provide a breakthrough in OA detection and treatment.

14.2 Potential miRNAs as early diagnostic biomarkers for OA

MiRNAs as important molecules in intracellular regulatory processes such as organ development [16] apoptosis [14], cell differentiation [15] and cancer [23], regulate gene expression. Recently, many studies showed that miRNAs could be potentially used as diagnostic markers for many diseases [22], and this could be importantly used in screening asymptomatic patients. MiRNAs are extensively known presenting in plasma, furthermore, miRNAs are existing in dried biological fluids such as semen, vaginal secretions and saliva. This would provide more possibilities for using miRNAs as biomarkers for disease detection and clinical evaluation in the early stage. In the beginning, miRNA-21as biomarker was discovered with a high plasma level in diffuse large B-cell lymphoma patients [24]. Then, diseases detection and prognosis using plasma miRNAs were reported in cancers and other diseases [20, 25]. When studied the miRNA biomarkers for rheumatoid arthritis (RA), Wang *et al.* found that miRNAs showed highly significant differentiation between patients with RA and three groups of patients with other disease like OA, SLE and Graves' disease [26].

OA patients almost suffer baryodynia in knee and hip joints [2]. Though few pathogenesis pathways have been investigated, there are scarcely any drugs could completely cure OA. One reason is that once we discover or feel pain on joints, varying degrees damage occurred. The lethality of OA owes to the difficulties in detecting it at an early stage and lack of effective treatments. At present, detection methods of OA like magnetic resonance imaging (MRI) and X-ray, are not sensitive enough to detect it at the early stages, which will miss the best time of treatment and prevention. Therefore, early diagnostic markers for OA seem to be very necessary. To investigate whether plasma miRNAs can be efficient biomarkers for OA, different miRNAs were studied in OA patients.

14.2.1 miR-146

The biggest annoyance to OA patients is pain produced from onset joints. Light OA conditions would influence the patients' normal movement, and serious illness will cause disability. However, miR-146 is linked to human articular cartilage degeneration and pain-related factors. Studies have shown that chronic pain in OA is caused by Toll-like receptor (TLR) and nuclear factor kappa B (NF-κB) participant inflammatory responses [27, 28], and miR-146 is significantly up-regulated in human peripheral knee OA joint tissues. So, scientific researchers might believe that miR-146 may have a relationship with the inflammatory response. It was confirmed that miR-146 is involved in the inflammatory response [28–31].

Prominent catabolic cytokine IL-1β plays an important role in OA cartilage degeneration. In chondrocytes, IL-1β stimulated OA chondrocytes, 42 miRNAs were up-regulated. On one hand, IL-1β promotes the expression of degenerative enzymes MMPs. On the other hand, it could inhibit chondrocytes synthesis extracellular matrix proteins [32]. And both of them have a relationship with OA occurrence.

Past study has shown that miR-146 is expressed after stimulating the chondrocytes of normal cartilage by IL-1β [33]. There was a significant difference compared with the cells treated without IL-1β. Another factor matrix metalloproteinase-13 (MMP-13), an OA associated enzyme was detected and it was also induced after IL-1β stimulation in the same way as miR-146. In their early studies, miR-146 was highly expressed in early OA cartilage when analyzed using real time PCR. And they revealed that miR-146 is expressed in superficial, middle and deep layers in examining the distribution of miR-146 in OA cartilage by in situ hybridization

(ISH). For further study, they divided OA cartilage into three grades with Mankin score standard. The results showed that acute expression of miR-146 in low grade OA cartilage, and the level of miR-146 expression decreased with the continued degeneration of cartilage. It seemed like that miR-146 was expressed at each stage accompanied by the expression of MMP-13 with a contrary relationship. In late stage, low expression of miR-146 accelerated the degradation of cartilage might be due to loss of miR-146 acting as a repressor of MMP-13. MiR-146 regulates knee joint homeostasis, cartilage degrading proteases and pain-associated inflammatory molecules in particular chondrocytes and synoviocytes. Damaged tissue could be repaired by up-regulation of miR-146 which significantly suppressed the expression of MMP-13 and ADAMTS5.

14.2.2 miR-140

OA as the most common degenerative joint disease accompanied with the degradation of articular cartilage [1, 34]. MicroRNA-140 (miR-140) is almost specially expressed in chondrocytes by the *Mir140* gene [35]. Too many researches about miR-140 have been studied and the results showed that miR-140 was a cartilage-restricted miRNA in zebra fish [36] and mouse embryos [35]. Later, the expression of miR-140 was found in human during chondrogenesis, especially in articular cartilage. MiR-140 expression is highly expressed in normal human cartilage, but significantly decreased in OA cartilage [37–39]. In order to study the potential role of miR-140 in cartilage homeostasis, mice lack of *miR-140* gene was generated by gene targeting. And the *miR140* (-/-) mice could survive but with a defect in the longitudinal growth of the skull and short long bones [40]. Age-related OA-like phenotypes, such as proteoglycan loss and fibrillation of articular cartilage were observed in *miR-140* gene lacking mice. Cartilage damage was protected after over-expression of miR-140 in cartilage [41].

Prominent catabolic cytokine IL-1β one of the critical mediators plays an important role in OA cartilage degeneration. The expression of miR-140 may have relationship with IL-1β. To confirm this, Miyaki *et al.* used IL-1β to stimulate the chondrocytes, and the expression of miR-140 was obviously decreased [38]. To examined whether the expression of OA-related enzymes ADAMTS5 and MMP-13 can be regulated by miR-140. After stimulating the chondrocytes with IL-1β that were transfected with or without miR-140. The result showed that the expression of ADAMTS5 and MMP-13 with the IL-1β stimulation was significantly reduced by miR-140. It has been demonstrated that miR-140 directly up-regulated the expression of cartilage degradation related enzymes MMP-13 and ADAMTS-5, whose over-expression is closely associated with OA [37, 42–44].

All these results indicated that miR-140 is essential for normal endochondral bone development and could regulate cartilage homeostasis to prevent OA occurrence.

14.2.3 miR-22

As we all know, miR-22 is associate with tumorigenesis, because of the expression silencing a family of enzymes called protein TET (ten-eleven-translocation), which play a significant role of tumor suppressor [45, 46]. Moreover, miR-22, whose expression respectively targets PPAR (peroxisome proliferator activated receptor) and BMP-7 (bone morphogenetic protein-7) at the level of mRNA and protein. And inflammatory and catabolic changes were blocked when inhibit the expression of miR-22 in osteoarthritic chondrocytes [39]. Through regulation of overexpression of miR-22, 76% of BMP-7 and 93% of PPAR protein were inhibited in normal chondrocytes. Western blot analysis showed that PPAR and BMP-7 could be regulated both in normal and osteoarthritic chondrocytes. In contrary, when inhibit miR-22 expression in osteoarthritic chondrocytes by antisense miR-22 treatment, 8.35 fold of BMP-7 and 12.55 fold of PPAR were extremely up-regulated and high down-regulation of MMP-13 was observed in Western blot, ELISA and immunofluorescence experiments. This is significant news for OA patients with decreased expression of MMP-13, whose expression is harmful to cartilage by degradation of type II collagen in OA. PPAR is involved in metabolism, but a recent study found that PPAR as a receptor is associate with inflammatory processes through IL-1β and down-regulated in osteoarthritic chondrocytes [39].

IL-1β and MMP-13 protein levels were highly promoted through over-expression of miR-22 or suppression of either BMP-7 or PPAR by RNA interference in normal chondrocytes. The results showed that 5.8 fold of IL-1β and 8.1 fold of MMP-13 expression were up-regulated and 4.9 fold of aggrean expression was down-regulated in normal chondrocytes with over-expression of miR-22. These findings revealed that the expression of miR-22 is related to OA, and down-regulation of miR-22 could be an efficient approach for OA therapy.

14.2.4 miR-27b

There are two *miR-27* genes in the human genome on chromosomes 19 and 9, respectively, *miR-27a* and *miR-27b*, whose products only have one nucleotide difference. For miR-27a, lower expression was showed in OA compared to normal chondrocytes, and it may indirectly regulate MMP-13 expression [37] or not an IL-1β responsive gene [47]. However, miR-27b was found to regulate the expression of MMP-13 in human OA chondrocytes and express lower in OA than that of in normal samples [47]. MiR-27b seed sequence directly binds to the 3′UTR of MMP-13 mRNA and negatively regulates the expression of its target of MMP-13 by modulating NF-κB signal or targeting BMP-7. Over-expression of miR-27b was 0.62 fold of MMP-13 expression on stimulation with IL-1β compared with non-stimulated in OA chondrocytes. And inhibit miR-27b expression in IL-1β stimulated chondrocytes by miR-27b inhibitor resulting in 13% increase in MMP-13 expression compared with control OA chondrocytes. Also, 0.51 fold more MMP-13 was increased in OA chondrocytes transfected with miR-27b inhibitor alone than that of in non-transfected control. Without any further stimulation, miR-27b expression was 67% lower compared with OA and normal samples. Conversely, increased MMP-13 expression could down-regulate miR-27b in IL-1β stimulated chondrocytes [47]. These results suggest that up-regulation of miR-27b in vivo would be a novel therapeutic approach in OA.

Statistical analysis showed that the expression of miRNA-16 in OA patients' plasma was lower than that of in control. The results also showed that the expression of plasma miR-132 in OA patients differed from that of in RA patients, and it could be a potential detection marker for OA and RA [22].

As described earlier, miR-146 intensely expressed in early OA cartilage and the expression decreases with the continued degeneration of cartilage. Comparing with healthy people, lower expression of miR-140, miR-27b and higher expression of miR-22 could be as potential detection markers for OA.

Except for plasma miRNAs studies, synovial fluid miRNAs also be investigated in this study. Through the comparison of miR-16, miR-132, miR-146a and miR-223 from synovial fluid and plasma in OA, lower expression in synovial fluid shows that synovial fluid and plasma miRNAs respectively generate. Synovial fluid miRNAs direct feedback the joint space condition better than plasma miRNAs. Therefore, synovial fluid miRNAs can also be used as detection marker for OA [22].

14.3 MiRNAs biomarker detection technologies

As previously described, circulating miRNAs as biomarkers for various cancers and other disease like OA have been proved. Therefore, high specificity or sensitivity of miRNA detecting methods also play an irreplaceable role in diseases detection and prognosis process. In the past, many methods for miRNAs detection have been developed such as northern blotting [48], microarray [49], ISH [50] and reverse transcription quantitative polymerase chain reaction (RT-qPCR) [51, 52] techniques.

Northern blotting is a common method for miRNA detection, but suffers from low sensitivity and poor quantification of results. Microarray-based method for detecting miRNAs is helpful for large-scale screening without providing quantification of results. ISH as a semi-quantitative method could differentiate single nucleotide differences from miRNA. In miRNAs as biomarkers for diseases detection and prognosis progress, these three methods could only be used for qualitative analysis but not for quantitative analysis. RT-qPCR is one of the most common approaches for sensitive and accurate quantification of miRNA expression. It has been used in identifying miRNAs biomarkers for early detection of numerous diseases [52–55]. Acute expression of miR-146 in low grade OA cartilage, and the level of miR-146 expression decreased with the continued degeneration of cartilage were confirmed by RT-qPCR method in previous study [33]. Although RT-qPCR provides a high quantification and sensitivity of results, it is money-consuming and complex process.

Recently, new methods such as quencher-free fluorescent method [56] and molecular beacon (MB) technology [57] were developed for detection of miRNAs. Researchers developed a quencher-free fluorescent method using the target-triggered recycling signal amplification in combination with a 2-aminopurine probe which is a fluorescent adenine with weak fluorescence in DNA strands but fluorescence enhancement in the free state to detect let-7a miRNA in human non-small-cell lung cancer. This method exhibits high sensitivity that can distinguish the single-base difference between two miRNAs in a limitation quantification of

0.3 fmol. Thus, quencher-free fluorescent approach provides a sensitive miRNA biomarker detection technology. MB technology is a novel DNA and RNA expression detection technology that can be used in living cells. This is a convenient and high sensitively method for miRNA detection because the chitosan (CS)-MB complexes are easily assembled and can be used in other diseases by simply changing the MB of targeted miRNA.

Each of the miRNAs detection technology has its own advantages and disadvantages. The advantages and disadvantages of different miRNAs detection technologies are presented in Table 14.1. Among these approaches, the MB method is noticeable because it could be used not only in vitro [58, 59] but also in vivo [60, 61] with high sensitivity for miRNA detection. MB-based approaches have been used for RNA sensitive detection and distinguish mature and precursor miRNA species without isolation and amplification of RNA [62] or lysis exosomes [58]. Similar to cells, exosomes are small extracellular vesicles that include miRNAs and precious information from their mother cells. Therefore, in vitro detecting miRNAs from exosome for detection of diseases by MB method provides competitive advantages compared with some other methods containing lots of tedious steps such as isolation of the exosomes, exosome lysis, miRNA isolation, cDNA synthesis and real-time PCR analysis. MB of miR-21 was designed and used to detect the expression of miR-21 in the cancer cell-derived exosomes and revealed

Table 14.1 Advantages and disadvantages of different miRNAs detection technologies

	Advantage	**Disadvantage**	**In vivo or vitro**
Northern blotting	Can detect the specific gene expression of cells in the growth and development stage	Low sensitivity and poor quantification of results	In vitro
Microarray	Helpful for large-scale screening	Without providing quantification of results	In vitro
In situ hybridization	Can differentiate single nucleotide differences	Semiquantitative method	In vitro
RT-qPCR	Sensitive and accurate quantification of miRNA expression	Money-consuming and complex process	In vitro
Quencher-free fluorescent	High sensitivity and discriminate single-base difference among miRNAs	Applicable scope have not been widely validated	In vitro
Molecular beacon	Convenient and high sensitively and wide range of application; can be used in vivo; have the potential to assess the expression of multiple miRNAs in a single sample	Over rely on delivery vehicles in vivo study; complex design	In vivo and in vitro

the direct detection technique of exosomal miRNA using MB could be used for diagnose cancer [58]. In addition to the advantages of application in vitro, MB can be used in vivo. However, the discovery of nontoxic, biodegradable and biocompatible MB delivery vehicles limit the application of miRNA detection by MB in vivo. Although, some miRNAs detection with MB based method such as CS [57] and magnetic fluorescence nanoparticles [63] have been developed in vivo, these materials are far from incompetent MB development requirements in vivo delivery. Nontoxic, biodegradable and biocompatible vehicle material will facilitate the development of MB based miRNA detection in vivo.

14.4 Nano-biomaterials for molecular beacon-based miRNA detection

The structure of the conventional MB is similar to pre-miRNA, which both have a loop and a stem. After ripening, the stem part of pre-miRNA usually is selected based on target sequence, but it is the loop of MB to fulfill the similar responsibility. Except for the stem and loop part, there is a fluorophore and a quencher at each end of oligonucleotide hairpin [64, 65]. In the absence of a target, fluorescence is absorbed because fluorescence resonance energy transfer (FRET) between the fluorescent dye and the quencher. However, if the loop part of MB bind the target, the quencher molecule separate from the fluorescent dye and emit fluorescence signals [64, 66] (Figure 14.2). This principle makes MB a suitable probe for miRNA detection in vitro and in situ without lots of tedious steps such as miRNA isolation, cDNA synthesis and real-time PCR analysis, because it has high specificity and low background fluorescence [65].

For specific detection of the target miR-221 in cancer, researcher developed a novel method for aptamer and miR-221 MB–conjugated magnetic fluorescence detection nanoparticles (MFAS) using small oligonucleotides AS1411 aptamer and miR-221 MB, which is complementary to miRNA-221. The AS1411 aptamer with

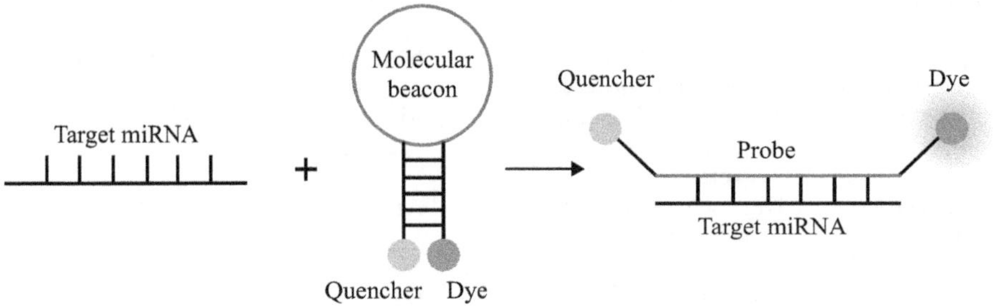

Figure 14.2 Schematic illustration of miRNA detection by molecular beacon. When the loop part of molecular beacon bind the miRNA target, the quencher molecule separate from the fluorescent dye and emit fluorescence signals, otherwise fluorescence is absorbed because FRET between the fluorescent dye and the quencher

favorable pharmacokinetic properties was used for drug delivery into cancer cells and miRNA-221 MB was used to image miR-221. The results showed that MFAS miR-221 MB successfully imaged miR-221 and miRNA MB-based MFAS can be used in many different cancers by detecting other miRNAs in other cancers [63]. Another experiment by co-immobilizing miR-21 MB and AS1411 aptamer on the surface of the fluorescent dye-doped silica nanoparticles into a fluorescent nano-probe (FSiNP-AS/MB) that could specifically and effectively deliver a miR-21 MB into the cancer cells for miR-21 detection. The results showed that FSiNP-AS/MB specifically transferred miR-21 MB into target cells with the binding affinity of AS1411 and produced fluorescence [67].

Too many polymers, such as CS, poly ethylenimine (PEI) and poly(ethylene glycol) (PEG) have been investigated in nucleic acid delivery system. CS is one of the widely studied polymers which are extracted from crustacean shells. It holds the characters of low immunogenicity and minimal toxicity, high biocompatibility and positive charge [57]. Positively charged CS nanoparticles could firmly integrate negatively charged nucleic acid into complex nanoparticles which could be used as plasmid DNA, oligonucleotides and siRNA delivery vehicles [68]. MiR-155 MB probe was self-assembled with low immunogenicity and toxicity CS nanoparticles to study the expression of miR-155 in lung cancer cells [57]. Negatively charged nucleic acid probes could not freely across the cell membrane. When positively charged CS nanoparticles with negatively charged probes steadily combined together, it could be used for delivery vehicle due to the low immunogenicity and high biocompatibility of CS nanoparticles. The result showed that miR-155 MB modified by CS nanoparticles could be effectively delivered and sensitively target the miR-155. PEI is a synthetic positively charged polymer. PEI-based nanocarriers can use PEI alone or be modified with PEG or graphene nanoribbon. For its hydrophilism, PEI could increase the stability of dsRNA and circulation time in serum. Nanoparticles adding PEG could also increase the circulation time in blood and reach the target [69]. PEI-grafted graphene nanoribbon (PEI-g-GNR) could protect locked nucleic acid modified MB (LNA-m-MB) from nuclease digestion with negligible cytotoxicity. The combination of PEI-g-GNR/LNA-m-MB could effectively deliver LNA-m-MB into the cells to recognize the target miRNA [70].

Locked nucleic acid (LNA) is an oligonucleotide derivative of structurally rigid modification that increases the binding affinity [71]. LNA is widely used for protecting the target molecule from cellular nucleases. On the study of quantifying nasopharyngeal carcinoma (NPC) correlative miR-205 in the serum of patients at different NPC stages, a LNA modified MB (LNA/MB) was applied as the detection probe to capture and detect target miR-205 in serum matrix. This method could overcome the background interference and quantified the miR-205 with only 10 μL of serum in 1h with high sensitivity and specificity [72].

Lipid are used as common non-viral gene delivery carriers. Lipid-based cationic liposomes could mix targeting peptides that self-assemble with DNA [73] or siRNA [74] to form LPD or LPR receptor-targeted nanocomplexes (RTNs). This method could enhance the utility of LPD/LPR-RTNs in vivo applications and deliver *BACE1* siRNA into rat brains with significant gene silencing [75]. A thiol-yne click chemistry based synthesis of biomimetic cationic thioether lipid was showed highly efficient siRNA delivery to cells and highly efficient siRNA delivery mouse embryonic stem cells [76]. Even though, it was siRNA or DNA not MB that be delivered, lipid-based cationic liposomes nanocomplexes could give us a feasible formulation for MB-based drug delivery. However, in order to investigate cellular pharmacokinetics of siRNA, cationic lipid nanoparticles were co-encapsulated with MB and fluorescence-labeled siRNA and proved that LNPs could take the target molecules into cells giving function [77].

It has proved that several parts (9–16 amino acids) of proteins have the ability to efficiently pass through biological membranes called protein transduction domains (PTDs) or cell penetrating peptides (CPPs) [78, 79]. This kind of peptide (TAT-1) linking with MB without other delivery reagent could efficiently transfer into living cells for mRNA detection [80] and provide a rapid and sensitive approach for the detection of gene expression.

Those materials used for siRNA or miRNA delivery into living cells could give us a feasible formulation for MB-based drug delivery. Biomaterials modified MBs provides a very promising application for the detection of miRNAs which potentially used as diagnostic markers for many diseases [22, 23, 81, 82] both for the diseases been diagnosed or not.

14.5 Conclusions

MiRNAs play important roles in regulation of posttranscriptional gene expression that involved in some significant cellular processes like apoptosis differentiation and organ development and also be expected as diagnostic and prognostic biomarkers of cacoethic tumors. Many of studies show that OA related cytokines, enzymes or proteins are regulated by miRNAs. Therefore, understanding the role of miRNA in OA promises to provide a breakthrough in OA detection and treatment. To achieve the goal of early detection and treatment OA with effective methods for preventing further deterioration. Finding high reliability diagnosis biomarkers and very sensitive detection technologies for OA seems to be imminent. As mentioned earlier, the occurrence of OA accompanied by changes in the expression of some miRNAs such as miR-146, miR-140, miR-22 and miR-27b. These miRNAs could be potentially used for diagnostic markers for OA detecting at an early stage, which could provide more possibilities for treatment.

To date, as far as we know, methods for miRNAs biomarkers detection in OA mainly use microarray, ISH and RT-Qpcr [33, 39, 55], which are time consuming and could not be used in vivo. Applications of novel miRNAs detection technologies such as quencher-free fluorescent method and MB technology in various cancers also give us great inspiration to take full use of them in OA detection. The most effective and attractive method for miRNA detection is MB-based methods which could be used not only in vitro but also in vivo. However, low immunogenicity, low toxicity, high biocompatibility and high transmission efficiency materials for MB delivery into living cells or in vivo are very vital. In this review, several materials, such as polymers, LNA, lipid and cell penetrating peptide are discussed. Many MB-conjugated materials were successfully used for miRNAs detection on diseases detection. However, the development of simple and high sensitivity methods for OA detection with an efficient material in clinical application still remains a great challenge.

References

[1] Loughlin, J. The genetic epidemiology of human primary osteoarthritis: current status. *Expert Reviews in Molecular Medicine* 7, 1–12 (2005).

[2] Taylor, A. M. Metabolic and endocrine diseases, cartilage calcification and arthritis. *Current Opinion in Rheumatology* 25, 198–203 (2013).

[3] Ambros, V. The functions of animal microRNAs. *Nature* 431, 350–355, doi:10.1038/nature02871 (2004).

[4] Bartel, D. P. MicroRNAs: genomics, biogenesis, mechanism, and function. *Cell* 116, 281–297 (2004).

[5] Farh, K. K., Grimson, A., Jan, C. *et al.* The widespread impact of mammalian MicroRNAs on mRNA repression and evolution. *Science* 310, 1817–1821, doi:10.1126/science.1121158 (2005).

[6] Lee, Y., Jeon, K., Lee, J. T., Kim, S. & Kim, V. N. MicroRNA maturation: stepwise processing and subcellular localization. *The EMBO Journal* 21, 4663–4670 (2002).

[7] Han, J., Lee, Y., Yeom, K. H., Kim, Y. K., Jin, H. & Kim, N. The Drosha-DGCR8 complex in primary microRNA processing. *Genes & Development* 18, 3016–3027, doi:10.1101/gad.1262504 (2004).

[8] Lund, E., Guttinger, S., Calado, A., Dahlberg, J. E. & Kutay, U. Nuclear export of microRNA precursors. *Science* 303, 95–98, doi:10.1126/science.1090599 (2004).

[9] Bossé, G. D. & Simard, M. J. A new twist in the microRNA pathway: not Dicer but Argonaute is required for a microRNA production. *Cell research* 20, 735–737 (2010).

[10] Chendrimada, T. P., Chendrimada, Gregory, R. I. *et al.* TRBP recruits the Dicer complex to Ago2 for microRNA processing and gene silencing. *Nature* 436, 740–744, doi:Doi10.1038/Nature03868 (2005).

[11] Hutvagner, G. & Simard, M. J. Argonaute proteins: key players in RNA silencing. *Nature Reviews Molecular Cell Biology* 9, 22–32, doi: Doi10.1038/Nrm2321 (2008).

[12] Vimalraj, S., Miranda, P., Ramyakrishna, B. & Selvamurugan, N. Regulation of breast cancer and bone metastasis by microRNAs. *Disease Markers* 35, 369–387 (2013).

[13] Brennecke, J., Stark, A., Russell, R. B. & Cohen, S. M. Principles of microRNA–target recognition. *PLoS Biology* 3, e85 (2005).

[14] He, L., He, X., Lowe, S. W. & Hannon, G. J. MicroRNAs join the p53 network—another piece in the tumour-suppression puzzle. *Nature Reviews Cancer* 7, 819–822 (2007).

[15] Chen, C.-Z., Li, L., Lodish, H. F. & Bartel, D. P. MicroRNAs modulate hematopoietic lineage differentiation. *Science* 303, 83–86 (2004).

[16] Callis, T. E., Chen, J.-F. & Wang, D.-Z. MicroRNAs in skeletal and cardiac muscle development. *DNA and Cell Biology* 26, 219–225 (2007).

[17] Mitchell, P. S., Parkin, R. K., Kroh, E. M. *et al.* Circulating microRNAs as stable blood-based markers for cancer detection. *Proceedings of the National Academy of Sciences* 105, 10513–10518 (2008).

[18] Garzon, R., Volinia, S., Liu, C. *et al.* MicroRNA signatures associated with cytogenetics and prognosis in acute myeloid leukemia. *Blood* 111, 3183–3189 (2008).

[19] Zhu, W., Qin, W., Atasoy, U. & Sauter, E. R. Circulating microRNAs in breast cancer and healthy subjects. *BMC Research Notes* 2, 89 (2009).

[20] Heneghan, H., Miller, N., Lowery, A., Sweeney, K. & Kerin, M. MicroRNAs as novel biomarkers for breast cancer. *Journal of Oncology* 2010 (2009).

[21] Schetter, A. J., Leung, S. Y., Sohn, J. J. *et al.* MicroRNA expression profiles associated with prognosis and therapeutic outcome in colon adenocarcinoma. *The Journal of the American Medical Association* 299, 425–436 (2008).

[22] Murata, K., Yoshitomi, H., Tanida, S. *et al.* Research article Plasma and synovial fluid microRNAs as potential biomarkers of rheumatoid arthritis and osteoarthritis. *Arthristis Researh & Therapy* 12, 86–88 (2010).

[23] Kinose, Y., Sawada, K., Nakamura, K. & Kimura, T. The role of microRNAs in ovarian cancer. *BioMed Research International* 2014 (2014).

[24] Lawrie, C. H., Gal, S., Dunlop, H. M. *et al.* Detection of elevated levels of tumour – associated microRNAs in serum of patients with diffuse large B – cell lymphoma. *British Journal of Haematology* 141, 672–675 (2008).

[25] Kosaka, N., Iguchi, H. & Ochiya, T. Circulating microRNA in body fluid: a new potential biomarker for cancer diagnosis and prognosis. *Cancer science* 101, 2087–2092 (2010).

[26] Wang, W., Zhang, Y., Zhu, B. *et al. Plasma microRNA expression profiles in Chinese patients with rheumatoid arthritis. Oncotarget* 6, 42557–42568 (2015).

[27] Liu Bryan, R. & Terkeltaub, R. Chondrocyte innate immune myeloid differentiation factor 88-dependent signaling drives procatabolic effects of the endogenous toll-like receptor 2/toll-like receptor 4 ligands low molecular weight hyaluronan and high mobility group box chromosomal protein 1 in mice. *Arthritis & Rheumatism* 62, 2004–2012 (2010).

[28] Boldin, M. & Chang, K. NF-κB dependent induction of microRNA miR 146. an inhibitor targeted to signaling proteins of innate immune responses. *Proceedings of National Academy of Sciences (USA)* 103, 12481–12486 (2006).

[29] Bhaumik, D., Scott, G. K., Schokrpur, S., Patil, C. K., Campisi, J. & Benz, C. C. Expression of microRNA-146 suppresses NF-κB activity with reduction of metastatic potential in breast cancer cells. *Oncogene* 27, 5643–5647 (2008).

[30] Sonkoly, E., Ståhle, M. & Pivarcsi, A. in *Seminars in cancer biology*. 131–140 (2008).

[31] Nakasa, T., Miyaki, S., Okubo, A. *et al.* Expression of microRNA-146 in rheumatoid arthritis synovial tissue. *Arthritis & Rheumatism* 58, 1284–1292 (2008).

[32] Goldring, M., Birkhead, J., Sandell, L., Kimura, T. & Krane, S. Interleukin 1 suppresses expression of cartilage-specific types II and IX collagens and increases types I and III collagens in human chondrocytes. *Journal of Clinical Investigation* 82, 2026 (1988).

[33] Yamasaki, K., Nakasa, T., Miyaki, S. *et al.* Expression of MicroRNA-146a in osteoarthritis cartilage. *Arthritis & Rheumatism* 60, 1035–1041 (2009).

[34] Feng, S., Jacobsen, S. E. & Reik, W. Epigenetic reprogramming in plant and animal development. *Science* 330, 622–627, doi:10.1126/science.1190614 (2010).

[35] Tuddenham, L., Wheeler, G., Fousara, S. N. *et al.* The cartilage specific microRNA-140 targets histone deacetylase 4 in mouse cells. *FEBS Letters* 580, 4214–4217 (2006).

[36] Wienholds, E., Kloosterman, W., Miska, E. *et al.* MicroRNA expression in zebrafish embryonic development. *Science* 309, 310–311 (2005).

[37] Tardif, G., Hum, D., Pelletier, J.-P., Duval, N. & Martel-Pelletier, J. Regulation of the IGFBP-5 and MMP-13 genes by the microRNAs miR-140 and miR-27a in human osteoarthritic chondrocytes. *BMC Musculoskeletal Disorders* 10, 148 (2009).

[38] Miyaki, S., Nakasa, T., Otsuki, S. *et al.* MicroRNA-140 is expressed in differentiated human articular chondrocytes and modulates interleukin-1 responses. *Arthritis & Rheumatism* 60, 2723–2730 (2009).

[39] Iliopoulos, D., Malizos, K. N., Oikonomou, P. & Tsezou, A. Integrative microRNA and proteomic approaches identify novel osteoarthritis genes and their collaborative metabolic and inflammatory networks. *PLoS ONE* 3, e3740 (2008).

[40] Nakamura, Y., Inloes, J. B., Katagiri, T. & Kobayashi, T. Chondrocyte-specific microRNA-140 regulates endochondral bone development and targets Dnpep to modulate bone morphogenetic protein signaling. *Molecular and cellular biology* 31, 3019–3028 (2011).

[41] Miyaki, S., Sato, T., Inoue, A. *et al.* MicroRNA-140 plays dual roles in both cartilage development and homeostasis. *Genes & Development* 24, 1173–1185 (2010).

[42] Wang, M., Sampson, E. R., Jin, H. *et al.* MMP13 is a critical target gene during the progression of osteoarthritis. *Arthritis Research & Therapy* 15, R5 (2013).

[43] Mitchell, P. G., Magna, H. A., Reeves, L. M. *et al.* Cloning, expression, and type II collagenolytic activity of matrix metalloproteinase-13 from human osteoarthritic cartilage. *Journal of Clinical Investigation* 97, 761 (1996).

[44] Malfait, A.-M., Liu, R.-Q., Ijiri, K., Komiya, S. & Tortorella, M. D. Inhibition of ADAM-TS4 and ADAM-TS5 prevents aggrecan degradation in

osteoarthritic cartilage. *Journal of Biological Chemistry* 277, 22201–22208 (2002).

[45] Song, Su., Ito, K, Ala, U. *et al.* The oncogenic microRNA miR-22 targets the TET2 tumor suppressor to promote hematopoietic stem cell self-renewal and transformation. *Cell Stem Cell* 13, 87–101, doi:http://dx.doi.org/10.1016/j.stem.2013.06.003 (2013).

[46] Song Su., Poliseno, L., Song, M. *et al.* MicroRNA-antagonism regulates breast cancer stemness and metastasis via TET-family-dependent chromatin remodeling. *Cell* 154, 311–324 (2013).

[47] Akhtar, N., Rasheed, Z., Ramamurthy, S., Anbazhagan, A. N., Voss, F. R., & Haqqi, T. M. MicroRNA-27b regulates the expression of matrix metalloproteinase 13 in human osteoarthritis chondrocytes. *Arthritis & Rheumatism* 62, 1361–1371 (2010).

[48] Várallyay, É., Burgyán, J. & Havelda, Z. MicroRNA detection by northern blotting using locked nucleic acid probes. *Nature Protocols* 3, 190–196 (2008).

[49] Thomson, J. M., Parker, J., Perou, C. M. & Hammond, S. M. A custom microarray platform for analysis of microRNA gene expression. *Nature methods* 1, 47–53 (2004).

[50] Nelson, P. T. & Wilfred, B. R. In situ hybridization is a necessary experimental complement to microRNA (miRNA) expression profiling in the human brain. *Neuroscience Letters* 466, 69–72 (2009).

[51] Mocellin, S., Rossi, C. R., Pilati, P., Nitti, D. & Marincola, F. M. Quantitative real-time PCR: a powerful ally in cancer research. *Trends in Molecular Medicine* 9, 189–195 (2003).

[52] Wang, P., Yang, D., Zhang, H. *et al.* Early detection of lung cancer in serum by a panel of microRNA biomarkers. *Clinical Lung Cancer* 16, 313–319 (2014).

[53] Wang, W., Sun, G., Zhang, L., Shi, L. & Zeng, Y. Circulating microRNAs as novel potential biomarkers for early diagnosis of acute stroke in humans. *Journal of Stroke and Cerebrovascular Diseases* 23, 2607–2613 (2014).

[54] Jiang, L., Cheng, Q., Zhang, B.-H. & Zhang, M.-Z. Circulating microRNAs as biomarkers in hepatocellular carcinoma screening: a validation set from China. *Medicine* 94, e603 (2015).

[55] Prado, S. D., Cicione, C., López, E. M. *et al.* Characterization of microRNA expression profiles in normal and osteoarthritic human chondrocytes. *BMC Musculoskeletal Disorders* 13, 144 (2012).

[56] Zhu, G., Liang, L. & Zhang, C. Quencher-free fluorescent method for homogeneously sensitive detection of MicroRNAs in human lung tissues. *Analytical Chemistry* 86, 11410–11416 (2014).

[57] Zhu, H., An, J., Yao, Q. *et al.* Chitosan combined with molecular beacon for Mir-155 detection and imaging in lung cancer. *Molecules* 19, 14710–14722 (2014).

[58] Lee, J. H., Kim, J. A., Kwon, M. H., Kang, J. Y. & Rhee, W. J. In situ single step detection of exosome microRNA using molecular beacon. *Biomaterials* 54, 116–125 (2015).

[59] Baker, M. B., Bao, G. & Searles, C. D. In vitro quantification of specific microRNA using molecular beacons. *Nucleic Acids Research*, gkr1016 (2011).

[60] Yao, Q., Zhang, A., Ma, H. *et al.* Novel molecular beacons to monitor microRNAs in non-small-cell lung cancer. *Molecular and Cellular Probes* 26, 182–187, doi:http://dx.doi.org/10.1016/j.mcp.2012.07.001 (2012).

[61] Kang, W. J., Choa, Y. L., Chae, J. R., Lee, J. D., Choi, K. J. & Kim, S. Molecular beacon-based bioimaging of multiple microRNAs during myogenesis. *Biomaterials* 32, 1915–1922 (2011).

[62] Lin, P., Yu, S. & Yang, P. MicroRNA in lung cancer. *British Journal of Cancer* 103, 1144–1148 (2010).

[63] Kim, J. K., Choi, K.-J., Lee, M., Jo, M.-h. & Kim, S. Molecular imaging of a cancer-targeting theragnostics probe using a nucleolin aptamer-and microRNA-221 molecular beacon-conjugated nanoparticle. *Biomaterials* 33, 207–217 (2012).

[64] Tsourkas, A., Behlke, M. A. & Bao, G. Structure–function relationships of shared-stem and conventional molecular beacons. *Nucleic Acids Research* 30, 4208–4215 (2002).

[65] Nitin, N., Rhee, W. J. & Bao, G. Translation inhibition reveals interaction of 2'-deoxy and 2'-O-methyl molecular beacons with mRNA targets in living cells. *Nucleic Acids Research* 37, 4977–4986 (2009).

[66] Peng, Z., Young, B., Baird, A. E. & Soper, S. A. Single-pair fluorescence resonance energy transfer analysis of mRNA transcripts for highly sensitive gene expression profiling in near real time. *Analytical Chemistry* 85, 7851–7858 (2013).

[67] Li, H., Mu, Y., Qian, S. *et al.* Synthesis of fluorescent dye-doped silica nanoparticles for target-cell-specific delivery and intracellular MicroRNA imaging. *Analyst* 140, 567–573 (2015).

[68] Mao, S., Sun, W. & Kissel, T. Chitosan-based formulations for delivery of DNA and siRNA. *Advanced Drug Delivery Reviews* 62, 12–27 (2010).

[69] Cho, K., Wang, X., Nie, S. & Shin, D. M. Therapeutic nanoparticles for drug delivery in cancer. *Clinical Cancer Research* 14, 1310–1316 (2008).

[70] Dong, H., Ding, L., Yan, F., Ji, H. & Ju, H. The use of polyethylenimine-grafted graphene nanoribbon for cellular delivery of locked nucleic acid modified molecular beacon for recognition of microRNA. *Biomaterials* 32, 3875–3882 (2011).

[71] Campbell, M. A. & Wengel, J. Locked vs. unlocked nucleic acids (LNA vs. UNA): contrasting structures work towards common therapeutic goals. *Chemical Society Reviews* 40, 5680–5689 (2011).

[72] Ho, S.-L., Chan, H.-M., Ha, A. W.-Y., Wong, R. N.-S. & Li, H.-W. Direct quantification of circulating miRNAs in different stages of nasopharyngeal

cancerous serum samples in single molecule level with total internal reflection fluorescence microscopy. *Analytical Chemistry* 86, 9880–9886 (2014).

[73] Du, Z., Munye, M. M., Tagalakis, A. D., Manunta, M. D. & Hart, S. L. The role of the helper lipid on the DNA transfection efficiency of lipopolyplex formulations. *Scientific Reports* 4 (2014).

[74] Tagalakis, A. D., Saraiva, L., McCarthy, D., Gustafsson, K. T. & Hart, S. L. Comparison of nanocomplexes with branched and linear peptides for siRNA delivery. *Biomacromolecules* 14, 761–770 (2013).

[75] Tagalakis, A. D., Castellaro, S., Zhou, H. *et al.* A method for concentrating lipid peptide DNA and sirNa nanocomplexes that retains their structure and transfection efficiency. *International journal of nanomedicine* 10, 2673 (2015).

[76] Li, L., Zahner, D., Su, Y., Gruen, C., Davidson, G. & Levkin, P. A. A biomimetic lipid library for gene delivery through thiol-yne click chemistry. *Biomaterials* 33, 8160–8166 (2012).

[77] Yu, B., Wang, X., Zhou, C. *et al.* Insight into mechanisms of cellular uptake of lipid nanoparticles and intracellular release of small RNAs. *Pharmaceutical Research* 31, 2685–2695 (2014).

[78] Snyder, E. & Dowdy, S. Protein/peptide transduction domains: potential to deliver large DNA molecules into cells. *Current Opinion in Molecular Therapeutics* 3, 147–152 (2001).

[79] Becker-Hapak, M., McAllister, S. S. & Dowdy, S. F. TAT-mediated protein transduction into mammalian cells. *Methods* 24, 247–256 (2001).

[80] Nitin, N., Santangelo, P. J., Kim, G., Nie, S. & Bao, G. Peptide-linked molecular beacons for efficient delivery and rapid mRNA detection in living cells. *Nucleic Acids Research* 32, e58–e58 (2004).

[81] Waldman, S. A. & Terzic, A. MicroRNA signatures as diagnostic and therapeutic targets. *Clinical Chemistry* 54, 943–944 (2008).

[82] Chen, Y., Gao, D.-Y. & Huang, L. In vivo delivery of miRNAs for cancer therapy: challenges and strategies. *Advanced drug delivery reviews* 81, 128–141 (2015).

Chapter 15

Electrochemical capacitive biosensors for point-of-care diagnostics: principles and applications

Paulo R. Bueno[1]

15.1 Introduction

15.1.1 Electrochemistry and biosensors

Electron transfer [1–3] is when the elementary charge, the electron itself, moves from an atom or molecule to another atom or molecule (generally forming atomic or molecular ions) and this phenomenon constitutes the essence of electrochemistry science [4, 5], mechanistically defining the thermodynamic concept of redox par (or reaction), wherein the reduction and oxidation partners change (in a dynamical equilibrium) a certain amount of electrons in between them. Essentially the phenomenon of electron transfer between molecules at interfaces [5] plays a central role not only in living systems (respiration and photosynthetic processes), but also in electrochemistry devices [6] (solar and biofuel cells, batteries, supercapacitors based on pseudocapacitance phenomena and biosensors) in general.

In the development of surface-sensitive devices and techniques, besides involving measurements of potential on the interfaces and current crossing them, the interfacial electrochemistry encompasses double layer interfacial phenomenon [4–6] that essentially is an electrified structure that appears on the surface of an object (herein in a solid phase) when it is exposed to a fluid (herein a liquid electrolyte) and refers to a parallel layers of charge (electrons in the solid phase and ions in the electrolyte phase), as illustrated in Figure 15.1. The first layer of this electrified structure comprises ions (positive or negative) adsorbed onto the solid phase object due to chemical interactions (see Figure 15.1). The second layer is composed of ions attracted to the surface charge via electrostatic (coulomb) forces that electrically screening the first layer. In applying an electric potential in the solid interface, electric current (the amount of electron charge per unit of time) can originate either from electron transfer or double layer charging. These two parallel

[1]Physical Chemistry Department, Institute of Chemistry, Universidade Estadual Paulista (São Paulo State University, UNESP), Nanobionics group, CP 355, 14800-900, Araraquara, São Paulo, Brazil

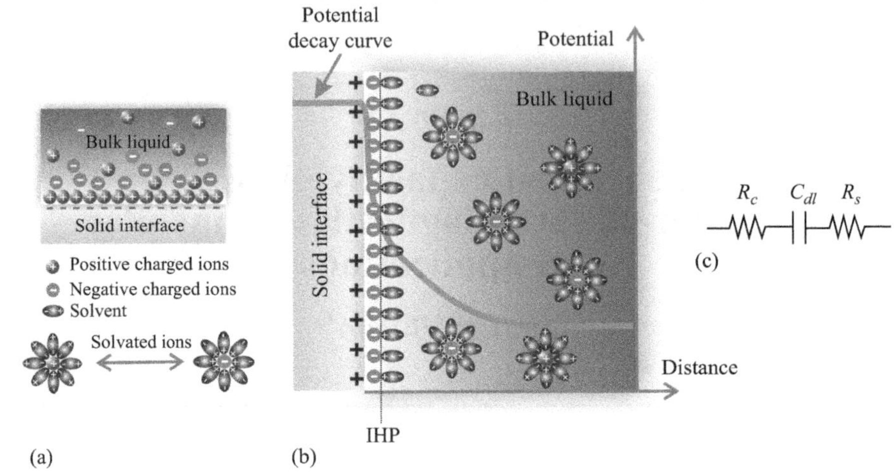

Figure 15.1 Schematic representation (in the absence of faradaic processes) of a junctions constituted of a metallic conductor (solid phase) in contact with an ionic solution (phase) junctions which gives rise to a double layer structure. (a) Double layer structure with negative-charged solid. As shown in (b) depending on the nature of the solid, now positively charged, there is another layer of charges inside the solid. Yet in (b) it is demonstrated an illustration of the potential decay developed from the solid interface up to the bulk of solution crossing the Helmholtz Inner Plane (IHP). The IHP is related with the Helmholtz capacitance in contrast with the Gouy-Chapman capacitance as discussed in the text. (c) The equivalent circuit of the interface represented in (a) and (b) is constituted by a resistance of contact (or metallic plate), R_c, in series with the double-layer capacitance (C_{dl}) and solution (electrolyte) resistance (R_s). Note that in practice $R_c \ll R_s$ and so that the response can be accurately represented only by R_s and C_{dl} equivalent circuit terms

processes, that is, charge transfer and rearrangement of the interfacial charge, are referred as faradaic (involving electron transfer) and non-faradaic (not involving electron transfer, for instance double layer charging), respectively. The faradaic term was coined based on the Faraday constant (96.485 coulombs per mole) which is the number of mole of electrons [4, 5]. Therefore, electro-chemistries generally used this constant to measure the number moles of charge involved in a given redox reaction. Non-faradaic current, therefore, is the measurable electrical current (or fraction of it) that is not involved with electron transfer phenomenon or redox reactions.

For instance and according to the core subject of this chapter, in biosensor devices [7, 8], the interface of the sensor is analytically selective and able to detect any analyte of interest by combining a biological receptor component with a physicochemical transducer concept. Indeed the quantification of biological or biochemical processes is of utmost importance for medical, biological and biotechnological applications [7–9]. Technologically, the conversion of biological information into an electronic signal is challenging due to connecting of an electronic device directly to a biological environment [10, 11]. Electrochemical biosensors provide an attractive means to analyse the content of a biological sample due to the direct conversion of a biological event to an electronic signal. Furthermore, the electron transfer or transport in biological systems is not itself made electronically but essentially and, most importantly, is intrinsically made through electrochemistry reactions.

Therefore, electrochemical biosensors use electrochemical (redox reaction) concepts as transducer signal to convert a biological reaction or a binding event (on the interface) into a measurable and quantifiable electronic signal. The most known electrochemical biosensors (showing successfully commercial applications such as the glucose meter or glucometer as an ultimate example) are based on enzymatic catalysis (the enzymes used in biosensor devices are named redox enzymes), for instance, where the reaction produces or consumes electrons. Furthermore, enzymes can be used as labels bound to antibodies, antigens and oligonucleotides with a specific sequence, thus providing what is known as affinity-based biosensors. As a matter of exemplification, among enzymes used in biotechnology [10] just only a limited number of them are used for monitoring clinically relevant metabolites, and such enzymes are glucose oxidase and glucose dehydrogenase for glucose assays [12, 13] as previously mentioned above, alcohol oxidase for ethanol, NADH-dependent lactate dehydrogenase and lactase, for instance, the cytochrome-*c* with cholesterol esterase for cholesterol, urease for urea and cholesterol oxidase co-immobilized with cholesterol esterase for cholesterol assay from the group of oxidoreductases. Peroxidase and alkaline phosphatase are the most common enzyme labels for electrochemical affinity biosensors [10, 11].

Complementary and concurrently to those above-mentioned enzymatic-based electrochemical devices and assays, there are nowadays other important biological assays and devices such as electrochemical immunosensors [14] which are specifically based on the use of the event of formation of antigen–antibody complex in the sensoring interface to detect and convert, by means of an electrochemical transducer signal, a biological analytical event of interest into a quantifiable electrical signal. The strength of these devices is based on the fact that protein-binding events are one of the most promising classes of tumour marker for earlier cancer diagnostics and therapy monitoring [14, 15]. For example, elevated levels of the serum proteins carcinoembryonic antigen (CEA), carbohydrate antigen (CA) 15-3, CA-19-9 and CA 125 can be associated with several types of cancers [16]. Indeed, the detection and quantification of protein biomarkers in complex biological samples lies central to proteomics and is important in either drug design besides early clinical diagnosis or effective therapeutic application as mentioned earlier. In this latter application the concentration of a protein tumour marker or other large biomolecule in a complex

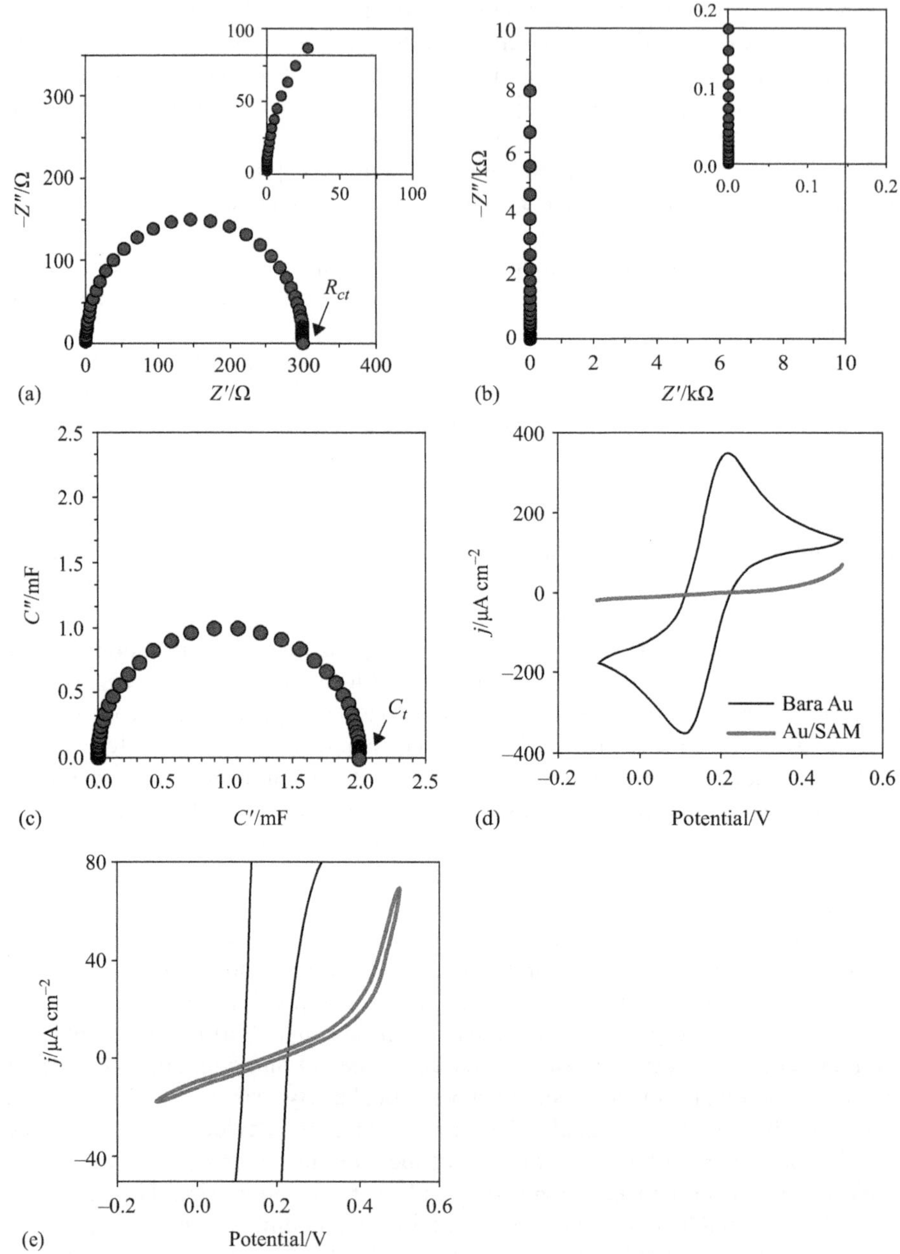

Figure 15.2 (a) Illustration of a Nyquist impedance plot (inset is the high frequency response) for the impedimetric response of a metallic (gold)/solution (electrolyte) interface (with a classical double-layer capacitance existing in parallel to a charge transfer resistance)

biological fluid as blood serum can be measured using traditional immunoassays, which is generally made by through the use of a second, labelled antibody enabling the tumour marker to be quantified, usually by absorbance or other optical measurements, constituting the most common (commercial) immunoassays that use enzyme labels and so that are called enzyme-linked immunosorbent assays (ELISA) [17].

Though sensitive, ELISA approaches [17] are laborious and require a specifically labelled secondary antibody for every antigen of interest. In order to reach higher levels of sensitivity and to move to a detection format which is both potentially cheap, portable and multiplexable, label-free electron chemical and analytical detection methods based on biosensoring interfaces are exceedingly powerful and sensitive.

The (previously) above shortly introduced classes (enzymatic or immunological) of electrochemical biosensors are based on transducer concepts of measuring electrochemical current (amperometric/conductimetric biosensors [18–20], associated with current/conductance of redox reactions), electrochemical potential (potentiometric biosensors [20–23], associated with the change on the redox potential of an electrochemistry reaction) or electron transfer resistance (impedimetric biosensors [24–26]) occurring through the biologically functionalized electrochemical interface, the latter constituting a physical measurement of the easy or difficulty to transfer electrons (by measuring the total resistance of the interface) during the electrochemistry reaction event, as exemplified in Figure 15.2(a). The major goals of this chapter are to make emphasis on another class of biosensors that neither use current, potential or resistance as transducer parameters, but instead it measures and quantifies changes on the energy stored (or its capability of changing/discharging the interface during a biological binding or affinity event) of an

---

containing a redox pair in solution and (ideally) not limited by diffusion. In this situation there is a measurable electron transfer resistance, R_{ct} that can be obtained by the radius of the semicircle as indicated. In (b) it is shown that the same responsive Nyquist impedimetric diagram (inset again is the high-frequency response) after a self-assembly dielectric (non-electroactive) monolayer is formed over the metallic interface, leading to the well-known blocking layer effect. In this case the Nyquist plot does not provide useful information about the capacitive characteristics of the interface. Thus the most useful way to obtain information on processes occurring on this interface is to convert the complex impedance data into complex capacitive data. The Nyquist capacitive plot is shown in (c) where the dominated capacitance, C_t, of the interface can be obtained. (d) Shows the corresponding current–potential response of the interface for bare gold interfacial response before and after dielectric layer is formed over it. It can be observed a huge suppress of the current exchanged between electrode (gold) and the electrolyte containing a redox probe. (e) States for the zoomed current response corresponding to the axis of ordinate in (d)

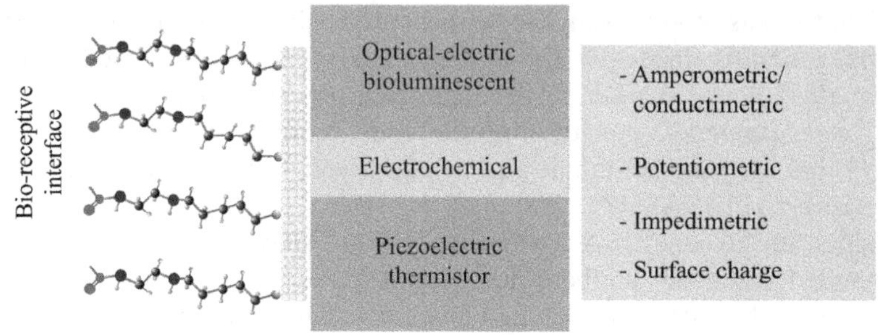

Figure 15.3 In between different types (according to the physical transducer concept) of biosensor (optic-electric, bioluminescent, electrochemical, piezoelectric, thermistors), those devices based on electrochemical transducer concepts are mostly classified in to four different types of sensor devices, i.e. amperometric/conductimetric, potentiometric, impedimetric (associated with the total resistance of the interface) and/or those based on surface charge storage, where capacitive biosensor devices (the main topic of this chapter) are included

electrochemistry interface constituting what we thus will refer to as capacitive biosensor (faradaic or non-faradaic) devices.

Before introducing the concepts involved in using capacitance measurements as an approach to transducer biological event into a measurable electrical signal, through electrochemistry interfaces, we will shortly make reference to the concepts employed on potentiometric including Field Effect Transistor (FET) electrochemical-based methods such as ion-sensitive [27] FETs, amperometric and impedimetric biosensor devices, since they are massively used in electrochemistry biosensor applications as can be observed in specialized literature. This will thus facilitate further comparisons and will help us to classify the electrochemical capacitive biosensors regarding its advantages and/or disadvantages in terms of their potential applications. Finally, we would like to mention that additional measurement techniques, which have been shown useful performance in combination with electrochemical detection, are out of the scope of this chapter, even in terms of conceptual comparisons, such as the electrochemical versions of surface plasmon resonance, optical waveguide light-mode spectroscopy, ellipsometry, quartz crystal microbalance and scanning electrochemical microscopy. Various types of transducers have been shown in Figure 15.3.

15.1.2 Potentiometric, amperometric and impedimetric biosensors

The general performance of electrochemical biosensor devices is often a combination of the surface architectures (that connects the sensing element to the biological sample at the nanometre scale) with the transduction signal used.

In particular it is important to emphasize the importance of the precise control over the delicate interplay between surface nano-architectures, surface functionalization and the chosen sensor transducer principle, as well as the usefulness of complementary characterization tools to interpret and to optimize the sensor's response. In this section we will focus on the transducer principles commonly used in biosensor devices observing that the choice of any of these transducer signals can be optimized according to the chemically projected nano-architecture of the biosensing interface.

15.1.2.1 Potentiometric principles

Biosensors based on potentiometric transducer principle operate through the use of Nernst potential (which, in other words, is the Boltzmann distribution applied to redox-active molecular systems) as derived by Nicolsky-Eisenman (broadly applied in ion-sensitive FET description) or in its simplest common form as presented in (15.1) [4].

$$V = V^0 + \frac{k_B T}{e} \ln \frac{[Ox]}{[Red]} \tag{15.1}$$

where V is the electrode potential measured in the metallic probe (or current collector, the previously mentioned solid phase component of the interface), V^0 is the formal potential of redox probe (pair) in electrolyte solution (or at the electrode's surface) with respect to an appropriate electrochemical potentiostatic reference, k_B is the Boltzmann constant, T is the absolute temperature, e is the elementary charge, $[Ox]/[Red]$ is the ratio between the concentration of oxidized $[Ox]$ and reduced $[Red]$ species in the electrode's surface (current collector). Electrochemical biosensors based on (15.1) monitor changes on V (or $V - V^0$) caused by any biological event occurring on the biosensor's interface that modifies the equilibrium of the redox reaction. Equation (15.1) can easily be restated as a function of variation of the Gibbs free energy of the redox reaction (15.2).

$$\Delta G = e\left(V - V^0\right) = k_B T \ln \frac{[Ox]}{[Red]} \tag{15.2}$$

15.1.2.2 Amperometric principles

Amperometric biosensors are relatively sensitive and operate based on the measurement of the current (i) or current density ($j = i/A$, where A is the geometrical area of the electrode or current collector) associated with an electrochemistry reaction occurring in the biosensor's surface. The simplest form of amperometric detection is through the measurement of a *direct current* (DC) due to the application of an electrochemical potential difference between the current collector and the counter electrode. Although this methodology constitutes an easiest way of monitoring the surface changes of the biological functionalized electrode due to a given biological event, this technique (or transducer approach) has limitations related to the uncompensated resistance that intrinsically exist on this kind of measurement. This effects of uncompensated [28] resistance, R_u, causing an iR_u drop additional to that classically related to the solution resistance, iR_s. The latter series resistance is a sensitive function of the electrochemical cell features and an intrinsic electrolyte resistive term existing on the functionalized surface itself which decrease specificity and selectively of this transducing method especially when high sensitivity is needed at low current density. Together, these both non-faradaic contributions (a parasitic current not associated with the electrochemical reaction itself) [28] can be a limitation in terms of producing visibly non-distorted signal and they are responsible for significant loss of specificity and sometimes sensitivity. This effect may be particularly true within bioelectrochemistry analyses where faradaic current densities can be such (so week) that signal is effectively lost within this (non-faradaic) "noise." The technique nonetheless is strictly good (in batch analysis, for instance) where there is no limitation of using large amount of electroactive material, which can cause, on the other hand, increases on the cost of the device, for instance, especially if a large amount of antibodies/antigens are needed to construct the sensing electrodes. Furthermore, in non-specific and complex biological samples the fouling (of non-specific proteins, for instance) process on the interface can cause high non-faradaic current and noise becomes predominant over the faradaic-specific signal.

15.1.2.3 Impedimetric principles

Impedimetric biosensors are based on the electrochemical impedance measurement which is indeed related to the electrical impedance of the redox reaction to occurs on a specific interface. This can be quantifiable by measuring the electrical impedance of the biosensing interface. The electrical impedance measures the opposition that an electronic circuit presents (in this case those associated with physical chemistry events on the electrochemistry interface) to a current when a small perturbative oscillatory voltage is applied on the electrochemistry interface. Quantitatively it constitutes the mathematical complex ratio between the applied small voltage oscillatory perturbations to the oscillatory current response. We thus specifically define electrochemical impedance $[Z^*(\omega)]$ as a specific form of a transfer function (with a precise mathematical meaning) in the case of voltage and current input/output signals [24, 26]. The asterisk in $Z^*(\omega)$ indicates that the impedance is a complex function. For instance, from a modulated potential (as function of time, t) $V(t) = \overline{V} + \tilde{V}e^{j\omega t}$ input and a sigmoidal output current response $I(t) = \overline{I} + \tilde{I}e^{(j\omega t - \phi)}$ thus $Z^*(\omega) = V(t)/I(t) = Z' + jZ''$, where $j = \sqrt{-1}$ (is the imaginary unit number) and $\omega = 2\pi f$, where f is the linear frequency [24, 26]. ϕ is the phase angle between the perturbation (voltage) and response (current) signals in phasor terminology [24, 26]. Finally, the Z' and Z'' are the real and imaginary terms of the $Z^*(\omega)$ complex function [24, 26].

It is important to note that the impedance $Z^*(\omega)$ is a function of the perturbation frequency, ω. In using different frequencies the technique is known as electrochemical impedance spectroscopy (EIS) because a spectrum of impedances can be constructed as a function of frequency and this approach has been widely used for biomarker determination (or quantification) due to its increased sensitivity, especially through the determination of charge transfer resistance, R_{ct}, as indicated in Figure 15.2. Indeed, the impedance spectrum can be used to obtain intrinsic physical parameters of the interface such as R_{ct} which can be obtained graphically from the impedance diagrams, as shown in Figure 15.2, or by fitting the acquired spectrum to an appropriate equivalent circuit of the biosensing interface.

Furthermore, from the impedance spectrum it is possible to access the faradaic and non-faradaic processes related to the biosensing interface. This means that besides the R_{ct} that is involved exclusively with electron transfer and faradaic events, the double-layer capacitance, C_{dl}, exclusively associated with the charging of double layer through a non-faradaic current, can be equivalently obtained from the impedance spectrum of the interface, even on the parallel occurrence of the charge transfer. Therefore, even on the absence of redox reactions impedance spectroscopy can be obtained and the response (or a particular region of the spectra) can be used as transducer signal. This constitutes what is known as non-faradaic capacitive transducer signal. Therefore, it is possible to divide impedance spectroscopy into faradaic or non-faradaic. The advantage of using impedance is that the electrical impedance of an interface in AC steady state under a constant DC bias is uniquely non-destructive and sensitive to interfacial change which can be either obtained without amplification or labelling of the biological receptor at the biosensing interface.

15.2 Types of capacitance and capacitive phenomena

Before we start to differentiate between what will be referred here as double layer or monolayer (non-faradaic) and electrochemical (faradaic) capacitances and to discuss on how these capacitances can be used in biosensor devices, it is important to state the meaning of capacitance and the physical concept behind its meaning. From undergraduate physics textbooks [29] we know that capacitance is the capability of some chemical (electron gas) system (in an interfacial or bulk form) to store electrical charge per unit of potential difference established within a given reference. Mathematically this physical phenomenon is described by the following expression (15.3).

$$C = \frac{q}{V} \tag{15.3}$$

where C is the capacitance, $q = Ne$ is the amount (N) of unitary charge e (equivalent to 1.6×10^{-19} coulombs) and V is the applied potential with respect to a given reference. C can be equivalently written in differential form as $C = dq/dV$ and so that named differential capacitance. The physical unit of capacitance is faraday (F) which is coulomb per unit of volts. The inverse of capacitance $1/C = V/q$ is directly related to the energy able to be stored in a given chemical system (as we will demonstrate further herein) and physically it is the amount of charge statically stored per difference of potential (or electrical work applied) on the system. It has "similarities" with Ohm's law (or Ohm's phenomenology) where the resistance is defined as $R = V/i$. According to Ohm's law, $i = dq/dt$ is the charge in movement due to a difference of potential applied in the system in opposition to the charge statically stored (q) in a given capacitive system. Therefore, R is related to the energy loss (the amount or fraction of energy lost due to the work done on the system per unit of time when the system is submitted to a difference of potential) in a given scattering process whereas V/q is related (as we will demonstrate below) to the energy statically stored. In other words, in electromagnetic classical theory resistances are associated with dissipative forces whereas capacitances are associated with the conservative forces related to the working done (or energy applied to realize work) on the system. The capability of a chemical system in loss or store energy, therefore, depends on the resistance and capacitance terms obtained or measured in the chemical system.

15.2.1 Electrostatic or geometrical capacitance

If we apply the capacitance concept of (15.3) and use the Gauss's (law) approach to separate charge (under a constant potential difference) between two parallel (and equivalent) conductive plates as shown in Figure 15.4, the calculated capacitance is only a function of the geometry of the system (15.4).

$$C = \varepsilon_r \varepsilon_0 \frac{A}{d} \tag{15.4}$$

where ε_r is the relative static permittivity (sometimes only referred as dielectric constant) of the materials that separate the plates, ε_0 ($\sim 8.85 \times 10^{-12}$ F m^{-1}) is the dielectric constant or dielectric permittivity of the vacuum (or free space), A is the area of the plate and d is the distance between the plates. The same can be applied for a cylindrical, spherical or isolated conductive sphere and we will observe that the calculated capacitance is only a function of geometric characteristic of the system. Because of this particular feature such kind of capacitance is referred as geometrical capacitance. The fact that this capacitance only depends on the geometric characteristic of the system is intrinsically related with coulomb forces where electrons are free to move (from one plate to another) independently of the electronic structure of the chemical system as we will demonstrate later herein. Nonetheless, the capacitance as given in (15.4), since the charge is considered to be statically separated, thus also exemplifies what is known as electrostatic capacitors (devices) or electrostatic capacitance (phenomenon), because it is essentially based only on electrostatic theoretical (Coulomb's law) concepts as the driven forces to separate charges.

15.2.2 Double-layer capacitance

As mentioned earlier the capacitive characteristics of an interface between an electronic conductor (known as current collector) and an electrolyte solution (an ionic conductor) is one of the most important interfacial electrochemical

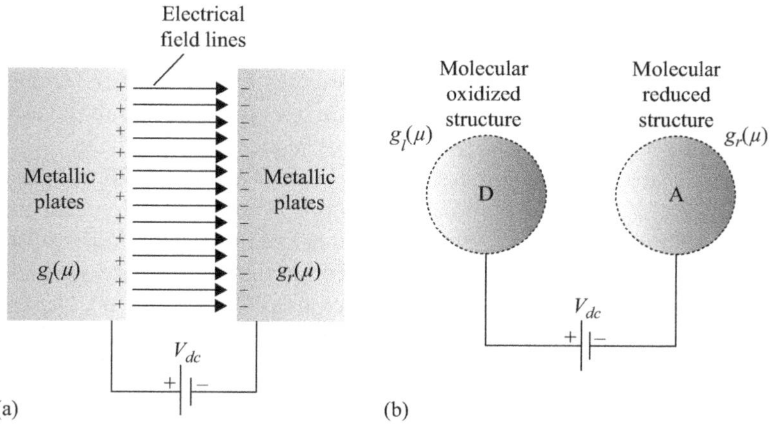

Figure 15.4 The differences existing in separating charges (due to a direct and constant potential difference, V_{dc}) between metallic macroscopic plates and molecular structures depend essentially on the consideration or not of electronic structures. The most general capacitance is the electron chemical capacitance that considers (existing in series) both electrostatic and quantum (electronic structure) contribution terms. (a) As discussed in the text only electrostatic contributions are present in charging macroscopic metallic plates (electronic structures are ignored and chemical structure of the plates does not play any whole on the analysis) and thus the resulting capacitance is the geometrical capacitance. (b) In charging molecular structures (where the molecular scale plays a considerable effect), the quantum capacitance (related with HOMO and LUMO energetic levels) and associated energies cannot be ignored. In (a) and (b) D (oxidized) and A (reduced) refer to electron donor and acceptor molecular structures (redox pair), respectively. Note that there is no quantum capacitive contribution (see (15.9) and (15.10)) for case (a) since both $g_l(\mu)$ and $g_r(\mu)$ are very high. On the other hand, there is significant quantum capacitive contributions in the case of (b) (molecular scale) where $g_l(\mu)$ and $g_r(\mu)$ can be significantly affected by a single electron transfer

phenomenon. This interface is important because it is where electrochemical reactions occur as man-controlled processes driven by galvanostatic or potentiostatic modes. In supposing there is no solvent decomposition or electron transfer during application of a potential in this interface with respect to a given chemical potential reference, a charge storage phenomenon is possible to occur. In such situation the interface is thus referred as ideally polarizable interface, based on thermodynamics reasoning and generally this interface is chargeable since the metallic conductive surface carries an excess of charge, which is balanced by a charge of equal magnitude and opposite sign on the electrolyte (ionic conductor) side of the interface. Although the differences in mobility of the charges existing between the electronic and ionic conductors are greater than the differences in their charge concentrations, it is the lower charge carrier concentration in the electrolyte that contributes to the existence of two charge planes, i.e. the charge of the electrolyte phase extends over a larger region of space, typically 5–20 angstroms. The resulting charge distribution (two narrow regions of equal and opposite charge) is known as *electric double layer*. It can be rationalized as a capacitor similar to that description made in (15.4) with an extremely small effective plate separation, and therefore has a very high capacitance per unit of area ($C/A = \varepsilon_r\varepsilon_0/d$). Depending on the electrolyte concentration and solvent, capacitance measurements of double layer typically have values in between 1 and 40 μF cm^{-2}.

A surprisingly good model for capacitance of these kinds of junctions constituted by the contact of an electronic conductor with an electrolyte (an electronic/ionic interface) is well known as Gouy-Chapman model (or theory) for such an interfacial phenomenon introduced as early as 1910 and is essentially based on combined electrostatics and statistical mechanics [5]. Based on this model the capacitance of the interface is expressed as (15.5) and (15.6).

$$C = \varepsilon_r\varepsilon_0\kappa \tag{15.5}$$

where, κ is the Debye inverse length ($L_D = 1/\kappa$) given by

$$\kappa = \left(\frac{2e^2N_e}{\varepsilon_0\varepsilon_r k_B T}\right)^{1/2} \tag{15.6}$$

where N_e denotes the density of charge (positive or negative) in the bulk of the electrolyte.

At low electrolyte concentration the model of (15.5) is reasonably good but at high electrolyte concentration it fails, where systematic deviation of the model is observed. Indeed, experiments demonstrate that the double-layer capacitance is described by a series combination of the capacitance given by (15.5) that we will now name as C_{GC} and another C_H known as Helmholtz capacitance which is independent of electrolyte concentration. The double-layer capacitance (C_{dl}) is expressed as (15.7) [5]

$$\frac{1}{C_{dl}} = \frac{1}{C_{GC}} + \frac{1}{C_H} \tag{15.7}$$

and constitutes another type of electrostatic capacitive phenomenon in which ions (and not only electrons) are involved and are important entities during the charge mechanisms of this electrochemical interface.

15.2.3 Dipolar capacitance of molecular layers

In biosensor applications it is very important to modify/functionalize the electronic conductive interface (current collector) with a molecular layer or a given electroactive material of interest, which will either serve as biological receptor for the analyte of interest. With this purpose, there are several common surface modification/functionalization techniques. Obviously and additionally with the various electrochemical transduction mechanisms and the choice of the recognition receptor molecules all of them combined will influence the ultimate sensitivity of the sensor. New nanotechnology-based approaches, such as the use of engineered ion-channels in lipid bilayers, the encapsulation of enzymes into vesicles, polymersomes or polyelectrolyte capsules, provide additional possibilities for signal amplification, etc. [10].

The modification of the surface obviously changes the characteristic of the double-layer accordingly to what was demonstrated in the previous section of the double-layer phenomenology and model (for more details see Figures 15.2 and 15.5). A dielectric model for the molecularly modified interface of the current collector was introduced by our research group [30]. The proposed model was based on the formation of a self-assembly molecular layer (an electrically insulator) over a conductive electronic interface (known as dielectric blocking effect) which causes essentially changes on the dielectric characteristics of the interface where ions now have a different dynamics with a dipolar relaxation clearly observed (see Figure 15.5). Therefore, the modification of the simple and classic interfacial model of (15.7) was proposed to occur due to the presence of a dielectric layer on the interface associated with the presence of the monolayer film, spanning between the solid (electronic) and the electrolyte (ionic), as depicted in Figure 15.5. The presence of this intervening hydrated dielectric layer modifies the double-layer capacitance in generating a new resultant term, $\boldsymbol{C_m}$, as expressed in (15.8) [31]

$$\frac{1}{C_m} = \frac{1}{C_b} + \frac{1}{C_{dl}} \tag{15.8}$$

where $\boldsymbol{C_b}$, the bulk capacitance of the monolayer (the expected layer capacitance without ionic ingress), is now the expected capacitance of the layer without electrolyte or proton ions (or cations). The resultant capacitance $\boldsymbol{C_m}$ can be treated as that of the plate (15.4). If $\boldsymbol{C_{dl}} > \boldsymbol{C_b}$, the latter ($\boldsymbol{C_b}$) dominates the interfacial capacitive response and $\boldsymbol{C_b}$ then approaches $\boldsymbol{C_m}$, i.e. $\boldsymbol{C_b} \sim \boldsymbol{C_m}$. Due to the presence of this intervening molecular layer, other relaxations and capacitances can be present due to the entrance and penetration of ions (protons for instance) on the molecular monolayers, which results in a capacitance of this molecular layer within ions on it, named as $\boldsymbol{C_t}$. $\boldsymbol{C_t}$ occurs in parallel to $\boldsymbol{C_m}$ and dominates the capacitive response of the molecular layer. Associated with $\boldsymbol{C_t}$ there is an uncompensated $\boldsymbol{R_t}$ resistance. Both of these resistance and capacitance can be measurable by impedance spectroscopy methods (see Figure 15.5). $\boldsymbol{C_t}$ constitutes essentially a modification of the double-layer capacitance due to the presence of the covalently attached monolayer and embedded ions on it and constitutes another type of electrostatic capacitance that takes into account the dipolar contribution of the monolayer due to the existence of an additional (intrinsically existing) ionic relaxation of the ions inside the molecular layer structure. We refer to this phenomenon (combined series $\boldsymbol{R_t}$ and $\boldsymbol{C_t}$) as an ionic dipolar relaxation process or phenomenon. The associated capacitance ($\boldsymbol{C_t}$) of this process constitutes another type of electrostatic or dielectric capacitance.

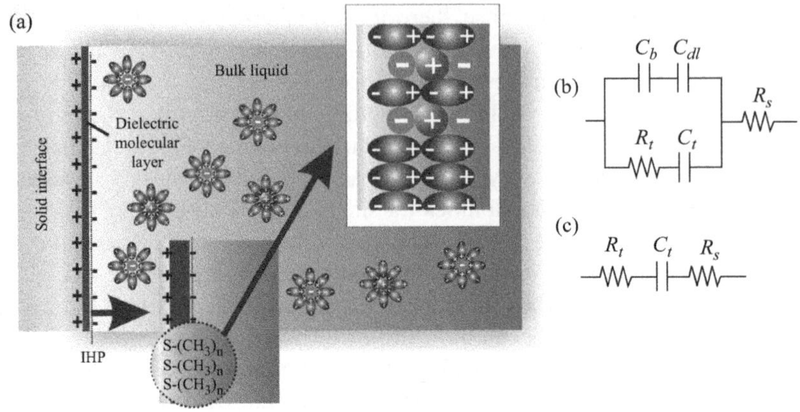

Figure 15.5 In the case of a modification (for instance, functionalization) of the metallic (current collector) electrode with a molecular, for example, with a thiolated (non-redox active) self-assembly monolayer (SAM), the structure of the double layer (as predicted by Helmoltz-Gouy-Chapman combined model) is affected (modified ionic and potential distribution with respect to those shown in Figure 15.1) in a phenomenon which is known as dielectric blocking effect (since this structure contributes to decrease the accessibility of the ions or possible electroactive molecular groups to the current collector), see also Figure 15.2. Once the ions can penetrate into the SAM structure (as exemplified in inset of the present figure), an ionic dipolar relaxation is developed on the blocking molecular layer as a consequence of the restricted movement of the ions inside the modified double-layer structure. Such dipolar relaxation contributes to non-faradaic current which can act as background parasitic signal in faradaic-based biosensors. (b) Is the equivalent circuit where, according to (15.8), the equivalent capacitance between bulk (C_b) of the monolayer and double layer (C_{dl}) is C_m. In situations where ions can penetrate, an additional parallel ionic relaxation phenomenon is introduced (governed by R_t and C_t terms). Because $C_t \gg C_m$, the ultimate equivalent circuit is that shown in (c). Finally observe also that $R_t \gg R_s$ which leads to the blocking dielectric effect as discussed and shown in terms of voltammetric and impedimetric (phenomenological) responses in Figure 15.2

15.2.4 Electrochemical capacitance

As demonstrated above the geometrical, double-layer and dipolar capacitance of molecular layers is of different types (or variations) of a same physical phenomenon known as electrostatic or geometrical capacitance (thus a non-faradaic phenomenon, characterized by the existence of electroactive species, named redox probe). The differences existing between those previously introduced capacitances are due to the absence of ionic species (electrostatic are the only separable charging mechanism) or due to the presence of a given ionic structure on the interface between current collector and electrolyte (non-faradaic electrochemical capacitor). In the absence of an electrolyte there is the pure electrostatic or geometrical capacitance (see (15.4)). In the presence of an electrolyte structure in the interface, Debye length becomes important (see (15.5)) and contributes to the capacitance phenomenology which is introduced as a different way of screening the existing electric field. The electrolyte or ionic structure (including its dynamics) in the interface is, for instance, the only phenomenon that differentiates between pure double-layer and dipolar capacitances (due to the existence of a molecular dielectric blocking layer), see comparatively Figures 15.1 and 15.5.

On the other hand, the electron chemical capacitance [32–35] is the most general capacitive phenomenon existing in physics and also encompasses both electrostatic and chemistry through the knowledge of electronic structure of the atoms and ions that can exist in the interface. In other words, electron chemistry capacitance encompasses electrostatics as well as the electronic structure of the ionic counter-part of a given (electron) chemical structure in contact with current collector or metallic probe. Electrochemistry capacitance, as the name suggests, thus incorporates electron and chemical potential contributions when separating charge between two chemical systems as illustrated in Figure 15.4(b). Therefore, it can be demonstrated from density functional theory concepts (see support information of Reference 33) that this capacitance, referred by us (in an electrochemistry pure context) as redox capacitance (associated with faradaic phenomenon), C_r, is a series combination of the electrostatic (C_e) and quantum capacitances (C_q) (15.9 and 15.10) [32, 33].

$$\frac{1}{C_r} = \frac{1}{C_e} + \frac{1}{C_q} \tag{15.9}$$

where C_e in (15.9) has the same meaning as shown in (15.4) and (15.5), whereas C_q is conceptually given by [33]

$$\frac{1}{C_q} = \frac{1}{e^2}\left[\frac{1}{g_l(\mu)} + \frac{1}{g_r(\mu)}\right] \tag{15.10}$$

where $g_l(\mu)$ and $g_r(\mu)$ are the density of states (states per unit of energy) between two general chemical systems. It can be easily noted that in separating charges by applying a potential difference ($-edV = d\mu$, where μ is the electron chemical potential of the electrons in the metallic conductor or current collector) between two metallic plates as shown in Figure 15.4, the density of states $[g_l(\mu)]$ in both equivalent conductors is huge and C_q is null or neglected [33]. In this case, following (15.9) and (15.10), the measured C_r capacitance reduces to C_e and there is no quantum contribution to the capacitance, as expected.

In the particular situation where a molecule with redox-active centres [so that with a given redox density of states, $g_r(\mu)$, associated with faradaic phenomena] is chemically coupled to a metallic density of states $[g_l(E)]$, as illustrated

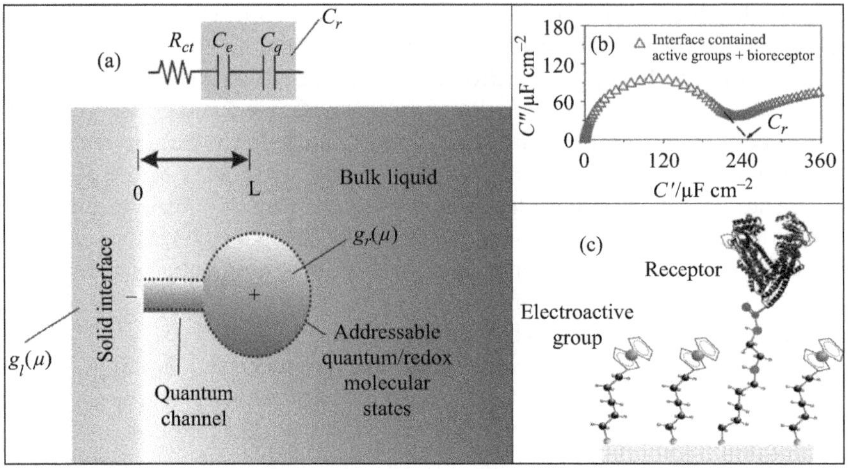

Figure 15.6 When a molecular electroactive (containing redox sites) layer is formed over a current collector (conductive working electrode) electrochemical capacitance, C_r, arises due to the fact that now redox density of states [$g_r(\mu)$] is assessable around redox formal (half-wave) potential. (a) C_r encompasses both (series contributions) electrostatic (C_e) and quantum capacitances (C_q). (b) The value of C_r can be obtained by electrochemistry capacitance spectroscopy (ECS) methods from where a Nyquist capacitive diagram is analysed. C_r value is effectively obtained from the diameter of the semicircle of the Nyquist capacitive diagram. (c) The C_r value obtained from mixed layers containing both redox active and bio-receptive groups (as illustrated in this figure) can be used as highly sensitive transducer signal in biosensors applications

in Figure 15.6(a), thus the metallic density of states is huge comparatively to $g_l(\mu) > g_r(\mu)$ those of molecularly attached redox centres and thus the chemical capacitance (C_q) of the system (15.10) reduces to (15.11) [32, 33]

$$\frac{1}{C_q} = \frac{1}{e^2}\left[\frac{1}{g_r(\mu)}\right] \tag{15.11}$$

or equivalently $C_q = e^2 g_r(\mu)$. In the particular situation where the occupation of C_e or its variation with potential is much lower than C_q for an electrochemical interface containing redox-active states (for instance, a monolayer contained redox centres self-assembled on metallic probe or current collector), the variation or the measurement of C_r as a function of potential follows those of C_q and the density of redox states is clearly accessible in a way that C_r is directly proportional to the redox density of states, $g_r(E)$, of the redox-active monolayer such as (15.12) [32, 33, 36].

$$C_r \propto e^2 g_r(\mu) \tag{15.12}$$

The shape [37] of $g_r(\mu)$ function is of particular importance and follows a Gaussian shape as discussed in Reference [36].

It will be demonstrated in the next section that both electrostatic (non-faradaic as introduced in previous section) and electrochemical capacitances (as introduced in the present section) can be used as transducer signal in engineering biosensors capacitors.

15.3 Capacitive biosensors

Berggren *et al.* [37–39] have pioneered the use of non-faradaic capacitive immunosensors [37, 40, 41]. They applied the concepts for the detection of human chorionic gonadotropin hormone (HCG) and interleukin-2 [39], a microbial infection immune factor, reported more than ten years ago on monoclonal antibody-modified Self-Assembly Modified (SAM) gold electrodes. These assays were reported to be sensitive to targets down to pg mL^{-1} levels [38]. In similar work non-faradaic EIS methods have been reported to detect interferon with an astonishing 8–10 ng mL^{-1} level of sensitivity in buffer at thiolated SAM-Ab interfaces. This is some 10 million times greater sensitivity than typically associated with alternative label-free immunoassays. Rickert and co-workers [42] have reported non-faradaic target detection, based on the immobilization of an antibody on a mixed alkane thiol self-assembly monolayer, by measuring capacitance change. Since then, a large number of non-faradaic EIS assays (including those based on field-effect transistors scheme) have been reported. During the past decade, focus on the ability to reliably assay protein biomarkers has grown and, with this in mind, both faradaic and non-faradaic EIS assays have shown considerable promise.

There are different approaches that have been generally used for non-faradaic capacitance measurements. According to a review on this issue made by Berggren *et al.* [37], either it can be accomplished by measuring the change in the capacitance between two metal conductors in close proximity to each other with the recognition element immobilized between them (interdigitated electrodes), or by measuring the capacitance potentiostatically at an electrode/solution interface with the recognition elements on the surface of the working electrode. In terms of measurement and evaluation of the capacitance values, Berggren *et al.* [37] have emphasized and made focus on impedimetric and transient (step) measurements. Based on classical impedimetric approaches dielectric capacitances can be obtained (or estimated) by fitting impedance spectra to an equivalent circuit (representing the physical chemistry parameters of the system's interface). In using simple RC circuit the capacitance is easily estimated and can be more precisely measured if a Randle's or Randle's-like equivalent circuit is applied, but this latter method obviously demands a time-consuming procedure and can be not suited for real-time measurements if frequency is not optimized. By using transient measurements, non-faradaic capacitances can be measured by perturbing the system with a potential step from where current is measured using (15.13).

$$i(t) = \Delta V/R_s \exp[-t/R_s C_T] \quad (15.13)$$

where $i(t)$ is the measured current response (as a function of time, t) from the potential step perturbation (ΔV, i.e. the pulse potential applied), R_s is the total series resistance and C_T the total capacitance (containing all sort of non-faradaic contributions). Obviously the characteristic time (or the time scale) of the charging process is the product of R_sC_T. In this approach, obviously, the components (different resistive and capacitive terms) of the system cannot be separated. A particular disadvantage of the non-faradaic capacitive methods is those related to selectivity and magnitude of the signal which sometimes can be of the same order of magnitude than those of background.

Accordingly, in trying to optimize the signal and avoid interferences, it is possible to use more sophisticated approaches such as Electrochemical Capacitance Spectroscopy (ECS) from where non-faradaic and faradaic contributions, when existing at the same time, can be elegantly separated [28, 32, 33, 35, 36]. ECS approach is derived from spectroscopic impedance methods and consists in converting complex impedance function, $Z^*(\omega)$, into complex capacitance function, i. e. $C^*(\omega)$. The capacitance analysis is done by obtaining $C^*(\omega)$ by means of impedance $Z^*(\omega)$ using the relationship $C^*(\omega) = 1/i\omega Z^*(\omega)$, in which ω is the angular frequency and $i = \sqrt{-1}$. Practically, the real (C') and imaginary (C'') parts of the complex capacitive function can be directly obtained as a function of real and imaginary terms obtained from the measured complex impedance as $C'(\omega) = Z''\varphi$ and $C''(\omega) = Z'\varphi$, noting that $\varphi = 1/\omega|Z|^2$, where $|Z|$ accounts for the modulus of the impedance function. The applicability of the method is illustrated in Figure 15.7 where it is clearly shown that the response of an electrode which contains both non-faradaic dipolar ionic relaxation and electrochemical (redox) capacitance contributions. The electrochemical signal can be resolved or "purified" from non-faradaic signal [35].

Furthermore, by applying ECS analysis the total capacitance or the redox (electrochemistry) capacitive term can be easily measured/obtained [33, 35, 43], as shown in Figure 15.6(b), as a function of any target or biomarker concentration for a biosensoring interface constituted of a mixed layer containing redox probe attached over the metallic or current collector surface and a receptive layer contained the receptive centres for the biological recognition of the biomarker of interest, see Figure 15.6(c). Therefore, C_r, the redox (electrochemistry) capacitance of the biosensor's molecular receptive layer can be used as a very sensitive (from nano to femto molar) transducer signal [32, 43–46]. The advantage of using this electrochemical signal comparatively to those of non-faradaic is that it can be purified from non-specific binding events which are intrinsically associated with electrostatic interactions [32, 43–46]. In other words, the matrix effect (a well non-specific of the environment that decreases selectivity) can be avoided or be hugely suppressed.

Indeed, it can be observed that by following (15.11) and (15.12) the inverse (this inverse quantity is directly associated with the energy of the interface as will be shown below) of the redox (electrochemical) capacitance, $1/C_r$, can be plotted as a function of biomarker (or analyte) concentration and reports on very sensitive analytical curves (see Figure 15.8(a) and (b)) and equivalently selective (see Figure 15.8(c) and (d)) for important biomarkers [32, 44–46]. The origin of the

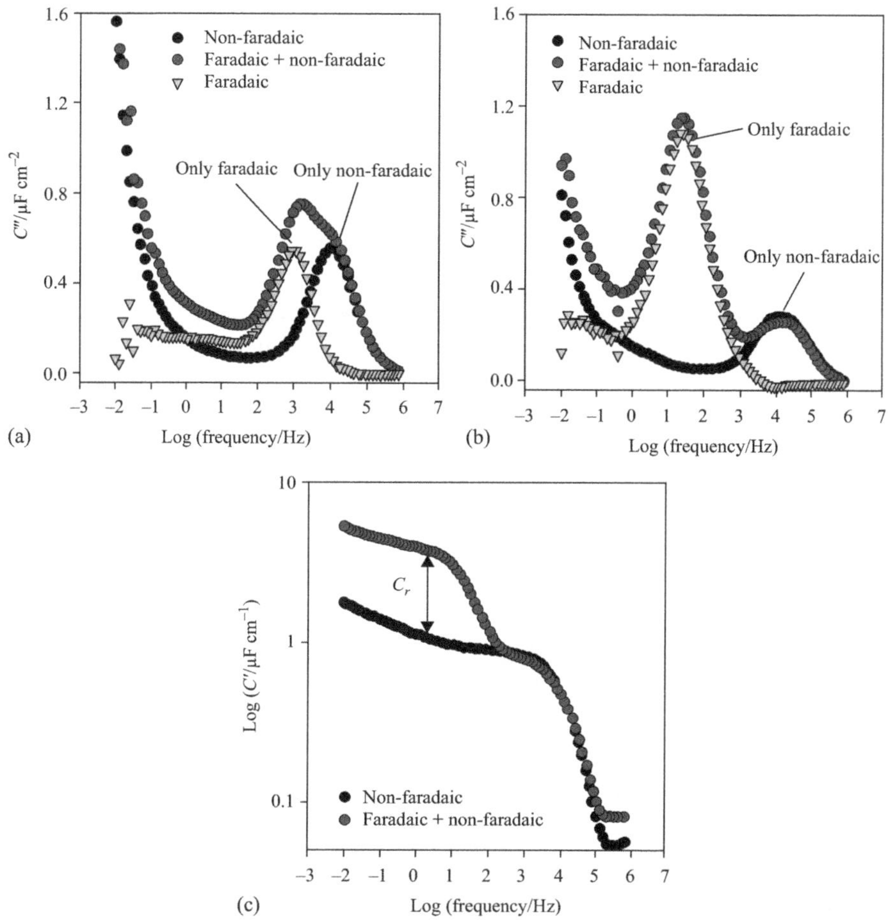

Figure 15.7 *The clear separation of faradaic and non-faradaic capacitive responses can be done by using ECS approach. (a) Non-faradaic contributions (named non-faradaic) are obtained outside of faradaic windows (where obviously only non-faradaic phenomena operate) whereas when the electrochemical potential is poised at faradaic windows (precisely at the formal or half-wave potential) both faradaic and non-faradaic contributions exist (named faradaic + non-faradaic). By using non-faradaic as background signal of this spectroscopic methodology, it is possible to subtract the non-faradaic curve from the back to obtained a "purified" faradaic response (named barely as faradaic). (b) The same as (a) but in this case the processes are separated in time-scale. (c) The additional contribution of faradaic capacitive phenomenon over non-faradaic can be alternatively observed by constructing different Bode diagrams representation. In the present case it is shown the real term of the complex capacitance as a function of frequency (logarithm scale). Reprinted (adapted) with permission from Reference 35. Copyright (2012) American Chemical Society*

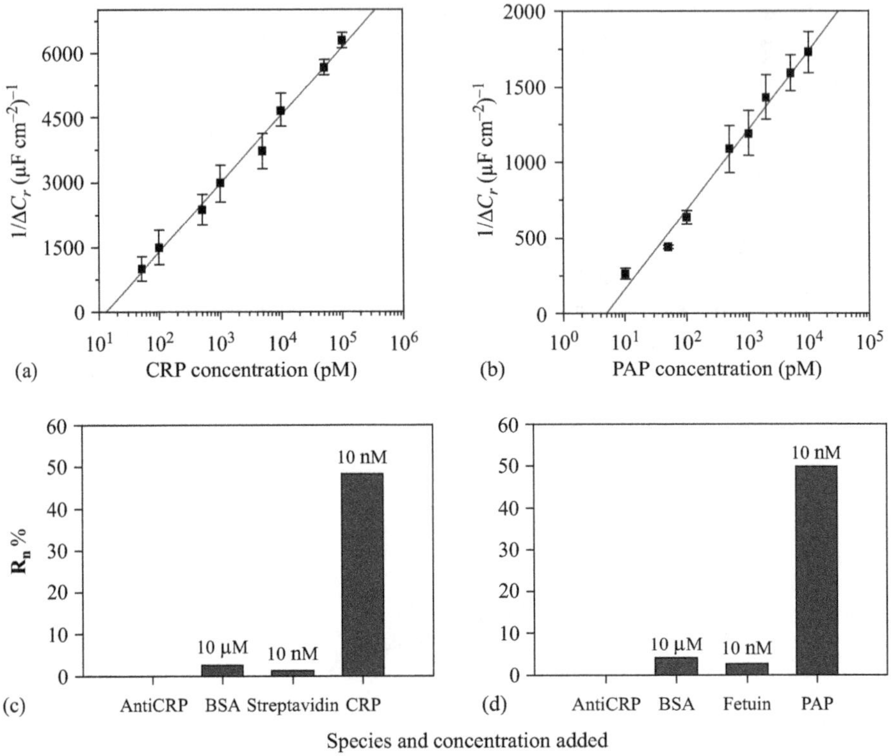

Figure 15.8 Analytic capacitive curves reporting $\boldsymbol{C_r}$ *for (a) CRP to CRP receptive interfaces and (b) PAP to PAP receptive interfaces. Plotted data points represent means and standard deviations across three measured interfaces in each case. Errors reported at 95% confidence.* R^2 *(for CRP) is 0.994 and* R^2 *(for PAP) is 0.990, where* R^2 *is the coefficient of determination. Redox capacitive response of anti-CRP (c) and anti-PAP (d) interfaces in the presence of nonspecific protein as a percentage of the response (*$\boldsymbol{R_n}$*) seen upon selective binding. % response (ordinate axis),* $\boldsymbol{R_n}\% = 100\%\ (\boldsymbol{R_n} - \boldsymbol{R_0})/\boldsymbol{R_0}$*, where calculated with respect to CRP and PAP specific interface response for zeroed target concentration (*$\boldsymbol{R_0}$*). Across both interfaces nonspecific responses were typically less than 4% of* $\boldsymbol{R_0}$ *in contrast to specific responses of 48–50% of* $\boldsymbol{R_0}$*. Reprinted (adapted) with permission from (Joshua Lehr, Flávio C. B. Fernandes, Paulo R. Bueno, Jason J. Davis; Label-free capacitive diagnostics: Exploiting local redox probe state occupancy, Analytical Chemistry). Copyright (2014) American Chemical Society*

high sensitivity of the obtained analytical curves has its origins on the fact that $e^2/C_r = [g_r(\mu)]^{-1} = d\mu/dN_r$, following the theory behind (15.11) and (15.12) paved on conceptual density function theory [33], represents the variation of the electron chemical potential (so that associated with the electrostatic and chemical energy of the interface) of the biosensor's interface with respect to redox state occupations, i.e. the redox density of states function, $g_r(\mu)$, by its definition is given by $g_r(\mu) = dN_r/d\mu$, where N_r is the total density of redox states, i.e. the amount of occupied redox states (reduced or oxidized molecules) existing on the interface. In other words, the electron occupation of the redox molecular layer of a given redox-active biosensing interface is a function of the electron chemical potential of that interface, which ultimately depends on the electrostatic and quantum (electronic) structure of the receptive interface [33]. The redox-active engineering interfaces like those based on redox-active monolayers can be very sensitive to any variation on the molecular electronic or electrostatic structure of such interface as a function of the chemical environment it is exposed to.

Therefore, ultimately, $e^2/C_r = d\mu/dN_r$ is the measurement of the energy (electrostatic and electronically) of the interface. How this energy varies with the change on the electron chemical potential of the interface due to a binding event (that increases as a function of concentration of the target) is shown in Figure 15.8(a) and (b) for two different biomarkers. Indeed, such an increase on the energy of this interface is associated with a decrease on the density of redox states of the interface, N_r, so that there is a decrease on the redox activity of the interface. The mechanistic operation of this kind of biosensing interface has being consistently observed for different structured (or engineering) interfaces, including those based on redox-active peptides [46].

15.4 Summarization and perspectives

In summary, it was possible to classify the electrochemical capacitive biosensor devices based on non-faradaic and faradaic processes. In general, it can be observed that capacitive biosensor are yet in an early stage of development and a long way is thus possible to be walked in terms of interfacial engineering combined with optimization of capacitive transducer signal. The applicability of these kinds of devices is mainly focused in immune sensing applicability aiming, for instance, the development of sensing devices for early diagnostic applications. Nonetheless, other possibilities such as applications focus on virus and air chemical contaminants detection are also open desirable applications to be explored.

The disadvantages of capacitive devices are the needs of a very controllable molecular structured on the surface of the device which is reached with the control of metallic depositions or with mechanical/electrochemical combined polishing. The advantages compared with other electrochemical biosensor devices lay on the point-of-care and bedside applications since there is no need of adding redox probe on the complex biological sample of the patients (obviously in immune sensing applications). Also as an advantage is the multiplex and miniaturization capabilities of these devices, which was practically shown in recent works where these capabilities were incorporated into both the analysis of real patient samples and the simultaneous detection of multiple important markers. We believe that in the future we will observe/access more assay applications built-in up on electrochemical capacitive concepts as useful electroanalytical transducer signal of sensing interfaces and devices.

References

[1] Marcus, R.A., *Electron-transfer reactions in chemistry – theory and experimental (Nobel Lecture)*. Angewandte Chem., 1993. **32**(8): p. 1111–1121.

[2] Marcus, R.A., *Electron-transfer reactions in chemistry – theory and experiment*. Reviews of Modern Physics, 1993. **65**(3): p. 599–610.

[3] Marcus, R.A. and N. Sutin, *Electron transfers in chemistry and biology*. Biochimica et Biophysica Acta, 1985. **811**(3): p. 265–322.

[4] Bard, A.J. and L.R. Faulkner, *Electrochemical Methods Fundamentals and Applications*. 2 ed. 2000, John Wiley & Sons. 850.

[5] Schmickler, W., *Interfacial Electrochemistry*. 1996, Oxford: Oxford University Press.

[6] Bueno, P.R. and C. Gabrielli, *Electrochemistry, Nanomaterials and Nanostructures*. Handbook of Nanostructured Materials for Alternative Energy Device, ed. E.R.L. (Org.). 2008, New York: Springer.

[7] Wang, J., *Electrochemical glucose biosensors*. Chemical Reviews, 2008. **108**(2): p. 814–825.

[8] Patil, A.V., F.B. Fernandes, P.R. Bueno, and J.J. Davis, *Graphene-based protein biomarker detection*. Bioanalysis, 2015. **7**(6): p. 725–742.

[9] Balasubramanian, K. and M. Burghard, *Biosensors based on carbon nanotubes*. Analytical and Bioanalytical Chemistry, 2006. **385**(3): p. 452–468.

[10] Bartlett, P.N., *Bioelectrochemistry: Fundamentals, Experimental Techniques and Applications*. 2008, Chichester: John Wiley & Sons Ltd.

[11] Knopf, G.K. and A.S. Bassi, *Smart Biosensor Technology*. 2007, Rochester, New York: CRC Press.

[12] Wang, J., *Glucose biosensors: 40 years of advances and challenges*. Electroanalysis, 2001. **13**(12): p. 983–988.

[13] Wilson, R. and A.P.F. Turner, *Glucose-oxidase – an ideal enzyme*. Biosensors & Bioelectronics, 1992. **7**(3): p. 165–185.

[14] Wang, J., *Electrochemical biosensors: towards point-of-care cancer diagnostics*. Biosensors & Bioelectronics, 2006. **21**(10): p. 1887–1892.

[15] Luppa, P.B., L.J. Sokoll, and D.W. Chan, *Immunosensors – principles and applications to clinical chemistry*. Clinica Chimica Acta, 2001. **314**(1–2): p. 1–26.

[16] Zhang, M., Cui, F., Lu, S., *et al.*, *Developmental pluripotency-associated 4: a novel predictor for prognosis and a potential therapeutic target for colon cancer*. Journal of Experimental & Clinical Cancer Research. **34**, 2015, doi:10.1186/s13046-015-0176-z.

[17] Lequin, R.M., *Enzyme immunoassay (EIA)/enzyme-linked immunosorbent assay (ELISA)*. Clinical Chemistry, 2005. **51**(12): p. 2415–2418.

[18] Stetter, J.R. and J. Li, *Amperometric gas sensors – a review*. Chemical Reviews, 2008. **108**(2): p. 352–366.

[19] Wang, J., *Amperometric biosensors for clinical and therapeutic drug monitoring: a review*. Journal of Pharmaceutical and Biomedical Analysis, 1999. **19**(1–2): p. 47–53.

[20] Reshetilov, A.N., *Models of biosensors based on principles of potentiometric and amperometric transducers: use in medicine, biotechnology, and environmental monitoring (Review)*. Applied Biochemistry and Microbiology, 1996. **32**(1): p. 72–85.

[21] Bratov, A., N. Abramova, and A. Ipatov, *Recent trends in potentiometric sensor arrays – a review*. Analytica Chimica Acta, 2010. **678**(2): p. 149–159.

[22] Estela, J.M., C. Tomas, A. Cladera, and V. Cerda, *Potentiometric stripping analysis – a review*. Critical Reviews in Analytical Chemistry, 1995. **25**(2): p. 91–141.

[23] Jagner, D., *Potentiometric stripping analysis – a review*. Analyst, 1982. **107**(1275): p. 593–599.

[24] Pejcic, B. and R. De Marco, *Impedance spectroscopy: over 35 years of electrochemical sensor optimization*. Electrochimica Acta, 2006. **51**(28): p. 6217–6229.

[25] Suni, I.I., *Impedance methods for electrochemical sensors using nano-materials*. Trac-Trends in Analytical Chemistry, 2008. **27**(7): p. 604–611.

[26] Patil, A.V., F.C. Bedatty Fernandes, P.R. Bueno, and J.J. Davis, *lmmittance electroanalysis in diagnostics*. Analytical Chemistry, 2015. **87** (2): p. 944–950.

[27] Martinoia, S., G. Massobrio, and L. Lorenzellib, *Modeling ISFET micro-sensor and ISFET-based microsystems: a review*. Sensors and Actuators B-Chemical, 2005. **105**(1): p. 14–27.

[28] Bueno, P.R., F. Fabregat-Santiago, and J.J. Davis, *Elucidating capacitance and resistance terms in confined electroactive molecular layers*. Analytical Chemistry, 2013. **85**(1): p. 411–417.

[29] Griffiths, D.J., *Introduction to Electrodynamics*. 4 ed. 2013, Pearson, Essex, England.

[30] Bakker, E., E. Pretsch, and P. Buhlmann, *Selectivity of potentiometric ion sensors*. Analytical Chemistry, 2000. **72**(6): p. 1127–1133.

[31] Goes, M.S., H. Rahman, J. Ryall, J.J. Davis, and P.R. Bueno, *A dielectric model of self-assembled monolayer interfaces by capacitive spectroscopy*. Langmuir, 2012. **28**(25): p. 9689–9699.

[32] Santos, A., F.C. Carvalho, M.-C. Roque-Barreira, and P.R. Bueno, *Impedance-derived electrochemical capacitance spectroscopy for the evaluation of lectin-glycoprotein binding affinity*. Biosensors & Bioelectronics, 2014. **62**: p. 102–105.

[33] Bueno, P.R., G.T. Feliciano, and J.J. Davis, *Capacitance spectroscopy and density functional theory*. Physical Chemistry Chemical Physics, 2015. **17**(14): p. 9375–9382.

[34] Bueno, P.R., D. Gimenez-Romero, F.F. Ferreira, and G.O. Setti, *Electrochemical capacitance spectroscopy and capacitive relaxation of the change-over process in iron hexacyanoferrate molecular compound.* Electrochimica Acta, 2010. **55**(21): p. 6147–6155.

[35] Bueno, P.R., G. Mizzon, and J.J. Davis, *Capacitance spectroscopy: a versatile approach To resolving the redox density of states and kinetics in redox-active self-assembled monolayers.* Journal of Physical Chemistry B, 2012. **116**(30): p. 8822–8829.

[36] Bueno, P.R. and J.J. Davis, *Elucidating redox level dispersion and local dielectric effects within electroactive molecular films.* Analytical Chemistry, 2014. **86**(4): p. 1977–2004.

[37] Berggren, C., B. Bjarnason, and G. Johansson, *Capacitive biosensors.* Electroanalysis, 2001. **13**(3): p. 173–180.

[38] Berggren, C. and G. Johansson, *Capacitance measurements of antibody-antigen interactions in a flow system.* Analytical Chemistry, 1997. **69**(18): p. 3651–3657.

[39] Berggren, C., B. Bjarnason, and G. Johansson, *Instrumentation for direct capacitive biosensors.* Instrumentation Science & Technology, 1999. **27**(2): p. 131–139.

[40] Mortari, A., Campos-Reales, N., Corda, G., Brown, N.L., and Csöregi, E., *Protein-based capacitive biosensors: a new tool for structure-activity relationship studies.* Electroanalysis, 2008. **20**(24): p. 2677–2684.

[41] Strong, Z.A., A.W. Wang, and C.F. McConaghy, *Hydrogel-actuated capacitive transducer for wireless biosensors.* Biomedical Microdevices, 2002. **4**(2): p. 97–103.

[42] Rickert, J., W. Gopel, W. Beck, G. Jung, and P.A. Heiduschka, *A 'mixed' self-assembled monolayer for an impedimetric immunosensor.* Biosensors & Bioelectronics, 1996. **11**(8): p. 757–768.

[43] Santos, A., J. Davis, and P. Bueno, *Fundamentals and applications of impedimetric and redox capacitive biosensors.* Journal of Analytical and Bioanalytical Techniques S, 2014. **7**: p. 2.

[44] Fernandes, F.C.B., M.S. Goes, J.J. Davis, and P.R. Bueno, *Label free redox capacitive biosensing.* Biosensors & Bioelectronics, 2013. **50**: p. 437–440.

[45] Fernandes, F.C.B., A. Santos, D.C. Martins, M.S. Goes, and P.R. Bueno, *Comparing label free electrochemical impedimetric and capacitive biosensing architectures.* Biosensors & Bioelectronics, 2014. **57**: p. 96–102.

[46] Santos, A., J.P. Piccoli, N.A. Santos-Filho, E.M. Cilli, and P.R. Bueno, *Redox-tagged peptide for capacitive diagnostic assays.* Biosensors & Bioelectronics, 2015. **68**: p. 281–287.

Chapter 16

AC electrokinetics-based capacitive biosensor as a platform technology for on-site detection of biospecific interactions

Jayne Wu[1]

16.1 Introduction

The capability of diagnosing a disease rapidly without the need for a specialized laboratory and personnel is critical to combat diseases and halt epidemics. Current detection methods for proteins and pathogens alike are labor-intensive, lack automation and/or have to be done in central clinical laboratories with trained technicians. In recent years, biosensors have attracted increasingly more research interest because of their potential for low-cost, rapid and portable point-of-care (POC) biomolecule detection and diagnosis [1]. Biosensors can be broadly classified as labeled or label-free detection. Labeled detection methods would require a detectable label and usually complicated procedures to attach labels specifically to the targets. Representative labeled detection methods include fluorescent immunoassay enzyme-linked immunosorbent assay (ELISA). Label-free detection methods do not need the labeling step, usually take few steps to complete and are more suitable for on-site detection/diagnosis [2].

Extensive efforts have been devoted to the development of various label-free bioaffinity sensors to quantify biochemical markers at low abundance, which is critical to many disciplines in life sciences and health care, from disease diagnosis to drug discovery and environment monitoring to bioterrorism [3, 4]. Label-free biosensing strategies are rather diverse, including optical, electrical and mechanical transducers. A few examples are mechanical transducers using acoustic wave resonance, electrical method such as impedance sensing and optical methods such as surface plasmon resonance (SPR) [5]. As arguably the most well-described and widely used version of label-free assays, SPR can provide useful information for the operator, but suffers from serious shortcomings such as high cost and complicated instrumentation, which have prevented the widespread adaptation of this technology [6]. Likewise, less expensive approaches such as acoustic wave sensors

[1]Department of Electrical Engineering and Computer Science, The University of Tennessee, Knoxville, TN 37996, USA

are moderately sensitive but susceptible to interference from environmental factors, limiting their usefulness as well.

Electrical impedance sensors are receiving increasing attention mainly due to its simplicity. These electrical impedance biosensors have been repeatedly shown to provide a robust, economical and easily implemented approach to label-free detection. An advantage of impedance biosensors is that they can be readily reconfigured to detect a variety of target particles, making them readily adaptable for many applications, including detection of gases, DNA, enzymes, proteins and virus. Hardware wise, to re-purpose an impedance sensor, all is needed is to alter the bound probe, with little to no manipulation of the device itself. Further, with impedance sensing, to implement multiplexed assay is relatively straightforward. It can be done by functionalizing different surface regions of the electrode sensor with different probe molecules.

However, two key challenges exist for using biosensors for on-site diagnosis, including impedance biosensors. First, most of the reported molecular assays work well only with purified samples. However, clinical samples very likely have highly complex constitutes, so aggressive processing of practical samples is usually necessary before testing such as extraction, purification and enrichment. To be viable as an on-site diagnostic system, sample preparation must be simple enough to be performed on site. Therefore, it is necessary that the system has the capability to detect a target in a complex solution such as sera or other biological fluid, which, by nature, are enriched with interfering proteins and ionic species. Second, the device must yield test results in a short time with high sensitivity and specificity. Biosensors are efficient in analyzing the fluid in its close vicinity, about 1 pL–nL of sample fluids. So for low abundance analyte, the analyte molecules in the rest of the fluid need to reach the sensor to be detected. If by diffusion alone, the detection may take a long time, from hours to days. Of the detection/diagnostic systems that are currently in use, most still require hours for a single assay (even longer for 'sample to result'), severely limiting their use for the on-site detection of a broad range of biomolecular interactions. Because the slow detection is usually caused by the travel of analyte to the sensor, to reduce the response time, a microscale mechanism is needed to bring the molecules to the sensor. A number of strategies have been investigated to provide sample enrichment, such as membrane pre-concentration, field-amplified sample stacking, isotachophoresis, chromatographic preconcentration, magnetic particles and optical tweezers. However, those methods are either incompatible with protein tests or too complicated to be practical for on-site measurement [7], such as the requirements of special buffer arrangements, reagents, or both. Recent study on alternating current electrokinetics (ACEK) found that electric fields can be used for effective bioparticle enrichment [8–11]. In addition, electrical methods are particularly well suited for miniaturization, because a high field strength can be easily generated with low voltages over a wide range of frequencies.

To achieve real-time, sensitive and label-free detection of binding reactions, we have developed an ACEK capacitive sensing method for use with interdigitated microelectrodes (IDMEs) [12, 13]. Capacitive sensing is a type of non-faradaic impedance sensing. Conventional impedance sensing scans the electrode impedance/capacitance at equilibrium over a range of frequencies at typically 5–10 mV. Here, ACEK capacitive sensing method reads the sensor capacitance continuously at a fixed frequency with a higher voltage level. As such, AC electric fields are strong enough to induce directed transport of biomolecules towards the electrode surfaces. ACEK mechanisms that can be used to enhance biomolecular binding include dielectrophoresis (DEP), AC electro-osmosis (ACEO) and AC electrothermal (ACET) effect. By carefully choosing the detection frequency and optimizing the electrode design, molecular binding at the IDME surface can be directly quantified with high sensitivity, whereas the effects from interfering molecules in the sample will be minimized. The ACEK capacitive sensing system reported here is the first to integrate active guidance of analytes with real-time monitoring of specific biomolecular binding process. This is significant because it allows rapid and easy-to-operate detection of biomolecular binding at low concentrations.

This chapter will demonstrate how ACEK capacitive sensing method is implemented to monitor protein–protein interactions, as well as to detect various bioparticle binding to an electrode [12–15]. It will be shown that it is a rapid, sensitive, quantitative and highly accessible approach to various affinity sensing needs. The development and optimization of the assay will also be given with respect to AC signal and electrode dimensions.

16.2 Mechanisms

16.2.1 Capacitive detection of biomolecular binding on electrode surface

When electrodes are immersed in an electrolyte solution, the electrode surface usually acquires surface charge. To maintain charge neutrality, counter ions will be generated in a very thin layer close to the electrode surface to shield the surface charges, which is commonly known as the electric double layer (EDL). Electrically, the bare electrode surface will yield an interfacial capacitance that can be approximated as $C_{int} = \varepsilon A/\lambda_{edl}$, where C_0 is the interfacial capacitance for a bare electrode, ε is the permittivity of the dielectric layer on electrode surface, A is the surface area exposed in the electrolyte, and λ_{edl} is the thickness of the EDL, i.e. Debye length [16]. In this approximation, C_{int} is regarded as a parallel plate capacitor, with the layer of counter ions as one plate and the electrode surface as the other plate. The separation distance between the two plates is the Debye length of EDL (according to Debye–Huckel Theory). When biomolecules are deposited on the electrode surface, such as the immobilization of probe molecules on an electrode, it is equivalent to increasing the separation between the two electrode plates. The interfacial capacitance then becomes $C_{int} = \varepsilon A/(d_{probe} + \lambda_{edl})$, where d_{probe} is the diameter (size) of the bounded molecular probe. When the target analyte binds specifically to the antigen deposited on the electrodes, the electrode plates of interfacial capacitance are further separated by the diameter of the analyte, $d_{analyte}$.

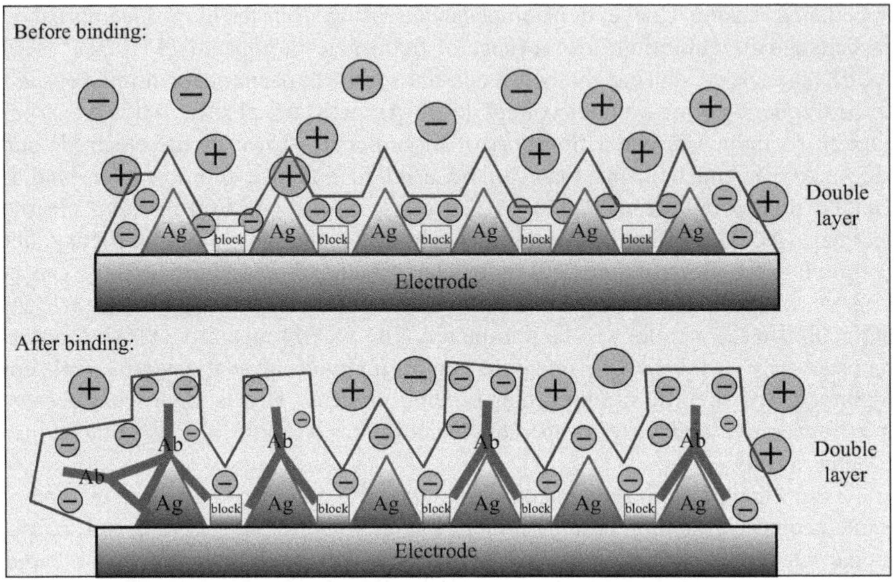

Figure 16.1 Mechanism of capacitive sensing of biomolecular binding at electrode surface, with antibody binding to antigen on the electrode as an example. Top: Before binding, the electrode surface is immobilized with antigen, immersed in an electrolyte. Bottom: Interfacial capacitance C_{int} will decrease after binding, since the separation of counter ions from the electrode surface increases while surface area remains almost the same

Then the interfacial capacitance become $C_{int} = \varepsilon A/(d_{analyte} + d_{probe} + \lambda_{edl})$. Since the interfacial capacitance is sensitive to the dielectric deposition on the electrode, the surface binding can be detected through the relative change in interfacial capacitance with high specificity.

16.2.2 Direct detection of interfacial capacitance

Extensive research has been done on the impedimetric characterization of an electrolyte-electrode system, and many sophisticated equivalent circuits have been developed [17, 18]. Such equivalent circuits usually strive to represent the impedance of the electrolyte-electrode system over a wide range of frequencies. Especially at very low frequency, complicated electrode process and non-ideal electrode surface have been the focus of modeling effort. Our method measures the sensor capacitance at a fixed frequency (usually kHz) to extract the change in the interfacial capacitance, so a simplified equivalent circuit will suffice as it only needs to fit the system impedance over a very narrow frequency range.

A typical equivalent circuit for an electrolyte-electrode system is as shown in Figure 16.2, where R_{ct} and C_{int} account for charge transport at the electrode/electrolyte interface. R_{fluid} is the resistance of the sample fluid, and C_{fluid} is the

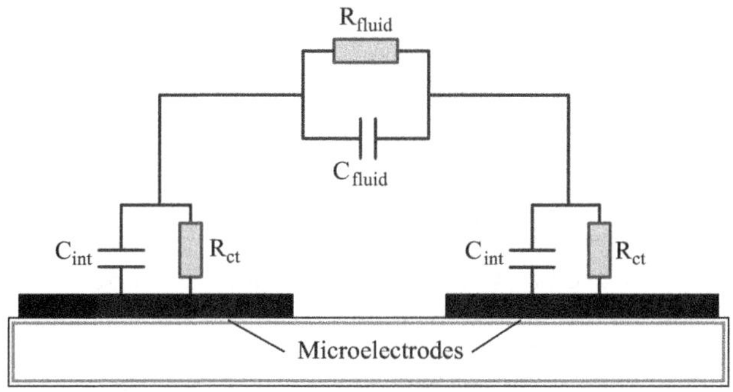

Figure 16.2 A representative equivalent circuit of an 'electrolyte-electrode' system. R_{ct} and C_{int} account for charge transport at the electrode/ electrolyte interface. R_{ct}: charge transfer resistance, C_{int}: interfacial capacitance as illustrated in Figure 16.1. R_{fluid}: electrolyte resistance, C_{fluid}: electrolyte capacitance

capacitance caused by dielectric coupling between the two electrodes with the sample fluid as a medium. At very high frequencies (usually >10 MHz), both C_{fluid} and C_{int} will present much lower impedance than the resistances they are in parallel with, so the sensor impedance will be C_{fluid} and C_{int} in series. At intermediate frequencies (usually 1 kHz to 500 kHz for our sensor), C_{fluid} will present a much larger impedance than R_{fluid}, so electrical current will pass through R_{fluid} instead of C_{fluid}, C_{int} still dominates the charge transfer across the electrode surface. Therefore, the sensor impedance can be approximated as a series connection of R_{fluid} and C_{int}.

Impedance value measured by an impedance analyzer is also in the form of $Z_{meas} = R - jX = R + 1/j\omega C_{meas}$, where R and X are the real part and imaginary part of the measured impedance, respectively. A capacitance value of $C_{meas} = 1/\omega X$, which corresponds approximately to $C_{int}/2$ in Figure 16.2, can be directly found from the imaginary part of measured value. Therefore, the change in C_{meas} can be directly used to indicate the deposition on the electrode surface, which greatly simplifies the process of interpreting experimental data. Our study of the electrode impedance spectra also showed that for the frequency range of interest to biomolecule detection, a serial connection of fluid resistance and interfacial capacitance will suffice to simulate the impedance presented by the electrode/fluid system [12, 13]. Therefore, capacitive sensing at a predetermined frequency provides a straightforward means to detect biomolecular binding on microelectrodes.

16.2.3 ACEK enhancement of affinity sensing

While the concept using impedance sensing for affinity biosensors have been proposed for many years, there have to date been few real-world successes. One major obstacle is long assay time when working with practical concentration of target analytes or the need for preconcentration of analytes. This is mainly due to the fact that the sensors rely on passive diffusion of macro-molecules to the sensor to allow interaction of molecules of interest with the immobilized probes [19]. The diffusion of target analytes to the sensor may take hours even days for the analytes to accumulate to a detectable level. To artificially increase the biomolecular concentration for detection to happen quickly, a significant amount of time, labor and cost is needed to prepare the analyte samples. Further, for binding reaction with fast association, the binding process may very well still be transport-limited. To reduce any adverse effect imposed by transport limitation, ACEK effects are invoked here to accelerate the transport of proteins to the sensor. In our method, a stronger than usual AC signal (typically 5–10 mV in conventional impedance sensing) is used for capacitance interrogation, which will concurrently induce ACEK effects to convect/attract macromolecules to the sensing electrode surface, hence minimizing the effect/limit imposed by mass transport.

The newly emerged ACEK strategy is well suited for lab-on-a-chip based macromolecule enrichment [16, 20]. ACEK methods are implemented by applying non-uniform alternating current electric fields over microelectrodes immersed in electrolyte. Oftentimes planar IDMEs are used, because the electric field distribution around the electrode member is non-uniform and high electrical field strength can be reached easily. Both particle and fluid movement can be induced in the fluid surrounding the microelectrodes, namely microflows by ACEO [21, 22] or ACET effect [23, 24] and particle movement known as DEP [25]. ACEO and ACET effect produce fluid flows that can carry biomolecules from fluid bulk towards the electrodes, while DEP directly exert force on biomolecules through the induced dipole moment. As schematically shown in Figure 16.3, with only an array of microelectrodes, directed fluid/particle movement is induced by AC electric field toward the electrode surface, which is easy to incorporate and simple to operate. Because ACEO requires working fluid of low ionic strength, at which most biomolecules

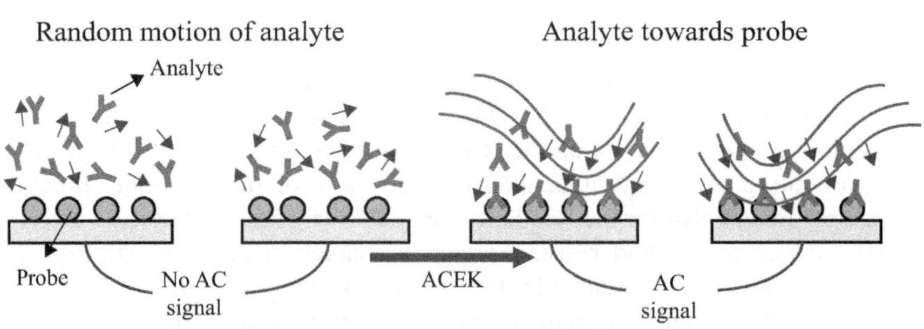

Figure 16.3 Conceptual illustration of biomolecular binding without and with ACEK effects, using antibody–antigen binding as an example. The left shows that binding is achieved through natural diffusion of antibody to meet antigens immobilized on the electrodes. The right shows that antibody is directed toward the electrodes and binds with immobilized antigen, when an AC signal is applied onto the electrodes

will denature, mainly ACET and DEP are of interest to the detection of biomolecular binding in this work.

ACET flows are induced by inhomogeneous electric field and the resultant temperature rise, which further results in localized changes in the electric conductivity and permittivity of the fluid. To maintain electrical neutrality, electrical charges are induced in the fluid, which move under the influence of the electric field to produce microflows. With planar electrodes, ACET effect will induce vortices above each electrode, and the microflows will convect the embedded particles towards the electrode surface [26, 27]. Below a few MHz, ACET effect only depends on AC voltage level. There is no dependence on the size of bioparticles or AC frequency, making ACET effect suitable for enrichment of a broad range of bioparticles. An expression for the ACET force that particles in the fluid would experience is given by (16.1).

$$\langle F_{ET} \rangle = -\frac{1}{2}\left(\frac{\nabla\sigma_m}{\sigma_m} - \frac{\nabla\varepsilon_m}{\varepsilon_m}\right) \cdot \frac{\varepsilon_m |E|^2}{1+(\omega\tau)^2} - \frac{1}{4}\nabla\varepsilon_m |E|^2 \tag{16.1}$$

where σ_m and ε_m are the electrical conductivity and permittivity of the medium, $\tau = \varepsilon_m/\sigma_m$ is its charge relaxation time, and $\omega = 2\pi f$ is radian frequency. E is the electric field strength, T is absolute temperature in K. For aqueous media at 293K, $\frac{\nabla\varepsilon_m}{\varepsilon_m} = \frac{1}{\varepsilon_m}\frac{\partial\varepsilon_m}{\partial T}\nabla T = -0.004\nabla T$, and $\frac{\nabla\sigma_m}{\sigma_m} = \frac{1}{\sigma_m}\frac{\partial\sigma_m}{\partial T}\nabla T = 0.02\nabla T$. At low frequency, $\frac{1}{1+(\omega\tau)^2} \approx 1$. The expression for ACET force (F_{ET}) on fluid can be simplified as [28]:

$$\langle F_{ET} \rangle = -0.011 \cdot \nabla T \cdot \varepsilon_m |E|^2 \approx 0.011 \cdot \frac{\varepsilon_m \sigma_m}{k} \pi \cdot r \cdot |E|^4 \tag{16.2}$$

where k is the thermal conductivity of the fluid and r is half of electrode gap. In the second half of above derivation, order of magnitude estimation is used and the temperature maximum is assumed to locate above the centerline of electrode gap.

Co-existent with ACET effect is DEP force on particles in the fluid. In an electric field, the counterion distribution along bioparticles gives rise to a dipole moment. In the presence of an electric field gradient, the dipole moment experiences a force towards either the high-field intensity region (positive DEP) or the low-field intensity region (negative DEP), depending on factors such as AC frequencies and buffer composition. DEP force on a particle is expressed as (for spherical particle) [28]:

$$\langle F_{DEP} \rangle = \pi a^3 \varepsilon_m \cdot \mathrm{Re}\left[\frac{\tilde{\varepsilon}_p - \tilde{\varepsilon}_m}{\tilde{\varepsilon}_p + 2\tilde{\varepsilon}_m}\right] \nabla |E|^2 \approx 2a^3 \varepsilon_m \cdot \mathrm{Re}\left[\frac{\tilde{\varepsilon}_p - \tilde{\varepsilon}_m}{\tilde{\varepsilon}_p + 2\tilde{\varepsilon}_m}\right] \frac{|E|^2}{r} \tag{16.3}$$

where a is the particle radius; $\tilde{\varepsilon}_p, \tilde{\varepsilon}_m$ are the complex permittivities of the particle and the medium, which are frequency-dependent. $\tilde{\varepsilon}_{p,m} = \varepsilon_{p,m} - i\frac{\sigma_{p,m}}{\omega}$; $\varepsilon_{p,m}$ and $\sigma_{p,m}$ are the permittivities and conductivities of the particles and the medium, respectively. DEP force is dependent on particles size and AC frequency.

In this method, ACET effect will convey bioparticles toward the electrodes from up to microns away. When bioparticles in the fluid come near the electrode surface, they would experience a strong positive-DEP force that would attract them to the surface thus facilitate the binding process. DEP together with ACET effect will have a much larger effective range for bioparticle enrichment.

16.3 Devices and methods

16.3.1 Interdigitated microelectrode sensors

ACEK capacitive sensing adopts planar IDMEs as the sensor, as shown in Figure 16.4. Various electrode materials have been used, including gold, platinum and aluminum. There is no appreciable difference in the sensor performance caused by the electrode materials, other than that the surface chemistry for immobilizing the probe molecules on the electrode metal need to be adjusted.

Different IDME dimensions were tested as well. Main consideration for IDME design is to generate adequate ACEK effect on nanoscale without causing adverse electrode reactions. Since ACEK effects are dependent on electric field strength, which is inversely proportional to the electrode gap, the electrode gap is used as the design metric and IDMEs are denoted by the electrode gap. For example, IDME with electrode width of 2 μm separated by 2 μm gaps is denoted as 2 μm IDME, and electrodes with 5 μm gap is denoted as 5 μm IDME. 2 μm IDME is the most commonly used in our experiments. A scanning electron micrograph of the 2 μm electrode array is shown in Figure 16.4b.

Before being functionalized as affinity sensors, the IDMEs were thoroughly cleaned. First the IDMEs were soaked in acetone for 10 min, then rinsed by isopropyl alcohol for 30 s, deionized water for another 30 s and dried with air gun. A silicone microchamber (2.5 mm in diameter and 0.9 mm in depth, JTR24R, Grace™ Bio-labs) was sealed onto the wafer with IDMEs inside for sample loading, as shown in Figure 16.1. The microchamber is sufficiently high for electric fields and ACEK effects to fully develop in the sample fluid.

IDME sensor preparation includes exposing and cleaning the electrodes, and surface functionalization with probe molecules to achieve specificity. IDMEs were cleaned sequentially with acetone, isopropyl alcohol, de-ionized water and ozone treatment. Then the surface was treated with (3-Aminopropyl) triethoxysilane (APTES) and glutaraldehyde cross linker for reliable immobilization of molecular probes (e.g. antigen). After the probe immobilization, the electrodes were further treated with a blocking agent (SuperBlock, PIERCE).

16.3.2 Sample preparation and electrode functionalization

Sample solutions were prepared using 1 mM phosphate buffer (pH 7.0) containing 15 mM NaCl, referred to as 0.1x phosphate-buffered saline (PBS). 0.1x PBS-T is used for rinsing, which is 0.1x PBS containing 0.05 v/v% Tween 20 (Fisher Scientific, Pittsburgh, PA).

(a)

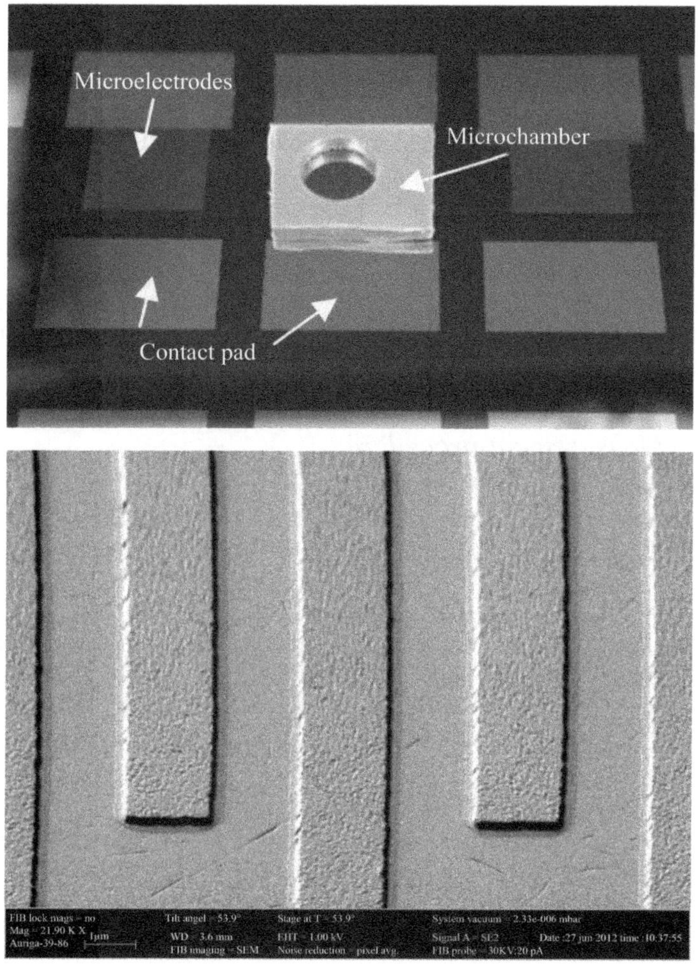

(b)

Figure 16.4 Interdigitated microelectrode (IDME) sensors used for ACEK capacitive sensing. (a) Planar IDME sensor with its microchamber on a silicon wafer. (b) Scanning electron micrograph of the IDME

Before binding assay, the electrode surface is functionalized by immobilizing probe molecules and blocking. For protein detection experiments, the probe molecules were diluted in 0.1x PBS (1 mM phosphate buffer (pH 7.0) containing 15 mM NaCl) at a concentration of 10 μg/mL, which was then loaded into the microchamber and incubated in a humidor at room temperature for 5 h. Afterwards, protein chips were blocked with 0.1x Buffer B, which is 0.1x PBS-T containing 10 v/v% SuperBlock (PIERCE Biotechnology, Rockford, IL). For small molecule detection experiments, aptamer specific to BPA [29] with 5' thiol modifier C6 SH (Sangon Biotech Co., Ltd, Shanghai, China) was immobilized on the electrodes at a concentration of 1 μM, which was also incubated in a humidor at room temperature for 5 h.

Then the aptamer electrodes were blocked with Triton X-100 (0.1 v/v %), which was prepared by adding 10 μL of Triton X-100 solution in 10 mL of distilled water. The quality of the prepared electrodes was evaluated by measuring the interfacial capacitance, as described in Section 16.4.1.

Protein samples were 1:10 serial diluted in 0.1x PBS buffer concentration ranging from 1 pg/mL to 100 ng/mL. For the detection of small molecule, BPA molecule was diluted in 0.1x PBS with concentration ranging from 1 to 1000 fM.

Testing on dummy IDMEs were also conducted to evaluate the specificity of this sensing method. The IDME sensors were prepared by blocking the electrode surfaces without immobilizing probe molecules, known as dummy IDMEs. They were then used against sample solutions as the above.

16.3.3 Measurement procedure

The interfacial capacitance was continuously measured at 100 kHz by an impedance analyzer (Agilent 4294A) for 30 s. We have elected to use an uncommon metric, the normalized capacitance change rate, as the criterion by which we detect binding. Therefore, a fractional change in the measured capacitance is employed to correlate with the deposition on the electrode surface. The percentage change in normalized capacitance is found by normalizing the measured capacitance, then finding the slope of its change versus time (%/min). Normalized capacitance is calculated as Norm $(\mathbf{C_{int,t}}) = \mathbf{C_{int,t}}/\mathbf{C_{int,0}}$, where $\mathbf{C_{int,t}}$ and $\mathbf{C_{int,0}}$ are the measured interfacial capacitances at time t and time zero, respectively. The change rate is found by least square linear fitting method of the Norm $(\mathbf{C_{int,t}})$ versus time curve. Doing so circumvents the need for a reference sensor, minimizes size difference from sensor to senor, further simplifying the detection procedure and instrumentation.

16.4 Experiments

16.4.1 Capacitive sensing for rapid analysis of surface quality control

The quality of electrode surface and its functionalization plays an essential role in the assay reliability and repeatability. As different surface process (e.g. levels of cleanness and surface deposition) correlates strongly with the thickness or topologies of dielectric layers at the electrode surface, the sensor surface will be closely monitored by measuring its C_{int}, the interfacial capacitances. This surface analytical method is simple and quick, and has been validated experimentally [30]. We have developed a set of reference C_{int} values at each step to ensure electrode quality, as shown in Figure 16.5. Electrode preparation includes microfabricating and cleaning the electrodes, and surface functionalization with probe molecules to achieve specificity. Cross linkers (3-Aminopropyl) triethoxysilane (APTES) and glutaraldehyde will be used for reliable probe immobilization.

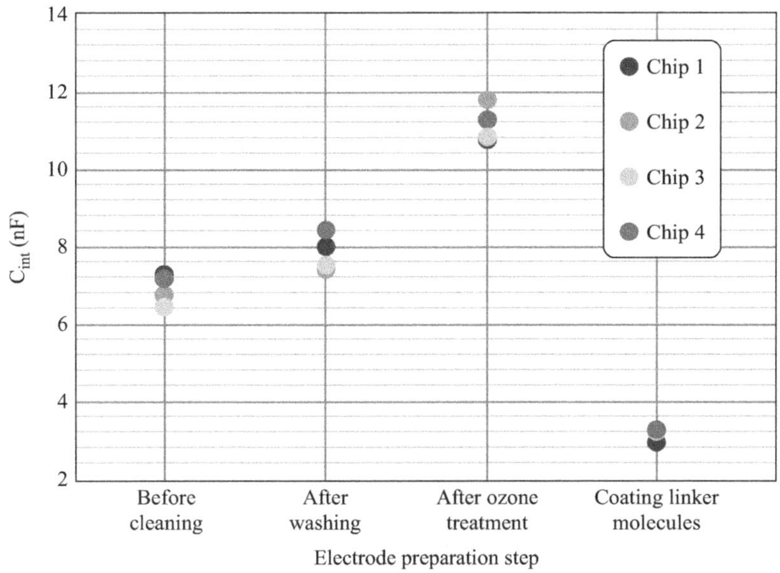

Figure 16.5 Correlation of interfacial capacitance with electrode surface treatment

16.4.2 Capacitance changes due to protein binding and detachment

In the first set of experiments, as a proof of principle, we measured how C_{int} would respond when specific protein was adsorbed onto or desorbed from the functionalized electrode surface. Specific protein–protein interactions of weak affinity, such as between chemotaxis proteins, were tested. Purified untagged bacterial chemotaxis signal transduction proteins from *Azospirillum brasilense*, CheA and CheW, were used as a model system. The interactions between CheA and CheW homologs are expected to yield binding response. When CheW-CheA complex on the electrode surface is exposed to solutions with low level CheA, desorption of CheA will occur because the binding between CheW and CheA is weak. Then a negative response should be detected.

In the preliminary experiments, CheW was immobilized on the electrode surface prior to the tests. Control buffer and CheA samples were added and measured sequentially. The buffer solution was Tris-buffered saline with 50 mM Tris and 150 mM NaCl. 20 μL of CheA protein (average of less than 0.1 mg/mL), purified from *A. brasilense* and in native form, was applied on the electrode sensor, which ran for 5 min using capacitive sensing protocol. The normalized capacitance (C_{int} normalized against its value at time 0) was plotted as a function of time in Figure 16.6. As shown in Figure 16.6, while the capacitance of control sample stayed rather constant during the test, the capacitance decreased monotonically with time due to binding reaction of CheA with CheW. The contrast between binding and no binding is obvious. Desorption was detected when electrode

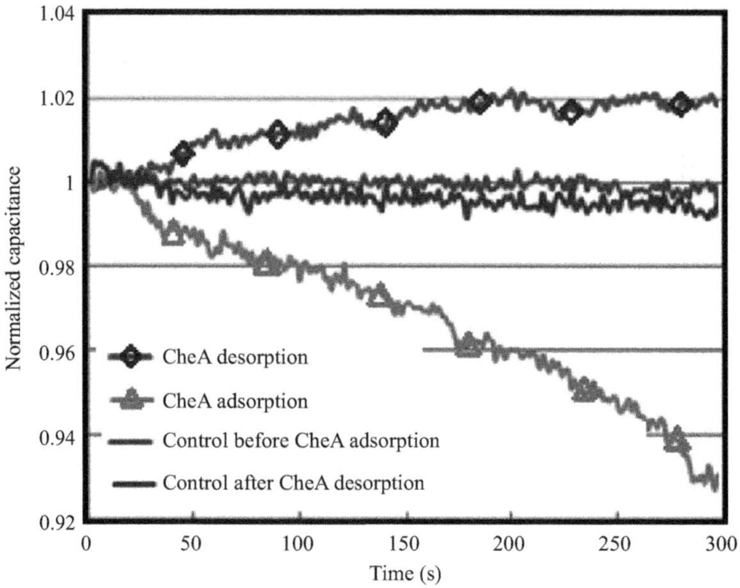

Figure 16.6 Protein adsorption and desorption study by fixed frequency ACEK capacitive sensing method

surfaces were exposed to solutions of low CheA concentration. As expected, the capacitance increased with time and reached its equilibrium as most CheA was released from electrode surface into the solution. Another control experiment was run after CheA desorption experiment, and it also yielded very little capacitance change. The low capacitance change from the control samples indicates that there is good and reliable correlation between specific biomolecular binding and the capacitance change at the electrode surface, and the capacitance changes from the adsorption and desorption tests were not a result of electrochemical reactions and other impedimetric artifacts in the measurements. These preliminary experiments demonstrated that our capacitive sensing method was able to detect expected interactions between CheA and CheR, and it provides a proof of concept for the ability of the technology to detect these interactions quickly and specifically.

16.4.3 Sensitive and quantitative detection

First, quantitative detection of a biomarker protein (D-dimer, marker for pulmonary embolism) was conducted. Pulmonary embolism (PE) is a medical condition that is commonly diagnosed in patients seeking emergency treatment in the United States. Because symptoms of PE are vague and often overlap with other pulmonary conditions, diagnosis may be difficult. By evaluating levels of circulating D-dimer protein (a product of fibrinogen degradation), the physician can eliminate PE as causative factor, given D-dimer levels are normal. Currently, this test is based on the ELISA format, and requires a dedicated laboratory to perform. Clinically, levels of D-dimer protein of less than 250 ng/mL are considered normal.

As shown in Figure 16.7a, human D-dimer protein spiked in PBS solutions was detected by ACEK capacitive sensing method. The electrodes were functionalized with commercial anti-D-dimer antibody and blocking agent Buffer B (PIERCE Biotechnology, IL). Series dilutions of D-dimer spiked in PBS from 100 fg/mL to 10 ng/mL were used, and blank PBS was used as a control sample. After the sample was loaded onto the electrode, its impedance was continuously measured for 1 min using an AC signal of 1 V_{rms} at 100 kHz from a bench-top impedance analyzer (Agilent 4294A). From Figure 16.7a, a clear correlation can be established between the normalized capacitance change rates and the D-dimer concentrations. As D-dimer became more diluted, the capacitance change rate decreased, until it reached 100 fg/mL. Then the change rate became indistinguishable from that of control sample. The limit of detection (LOD) is determined to be the lowest concentration of antibody that could be distinguished from the control sample. So the LOD was found to be around 10 pg/mL, below what is considered as clinically relevant. The results demonstrates that ACEK capacitive sensing is capable of quantitative measurement, is highly sensitive, and is rapid by shortening the assay time from 3 h to <2 min.

For comparison, we have also measured the impedance spectra before and after the 1 min ACEK incubation for various concentrations of D-dimer in the form of Bode plot (Figure 16.7b) and Nyquist plot (Figure 16.7c). Interesting to note, both Bode plot and Nyquist plot cannot indicate obvious impedance changes from 1 pg/mL to 10 ng/mL, while ACEK capacitance measurement method can clearly differentiate D-dimer concentration in the same range. This further demonstrates the advantage of our method – it is more sensitive and reliable since it continuously monitors the dynamic binding process, while other sensors that detect the equilibrium state constantly face the challenges of the time-dependent instability in physiological samples.

16.4.4 Effect of AC frequency

Figure 16.8 shows the sensor capacitances over a wide frequency range, for cases before and after biomolecule deposition on the electrode surface. According to Figure 16.8, the capacitance change is larger at low frequency and diminishes at high frequencies of a few megahertz. This is in agreement with the sensor's equivalent electrical circuit of $R_S - C_{int}$ series connection. The capacitance change becomes smaller with increasing AC frequency, and is unobservable at above 1 MHz. Based on Figure 16.8, it appears that a low frequency will be favored for capacitive measurement since the capacitance difference is larger. This is true for conventional capacitive sensing. However, ACEK capacitive sensing is a kinetic sensing method. It measures the molecular deposition on the electrode surface caused by a specific AC signal. As discussed in the previous section, the AC measuring signal will also induce AC electrokinetic effects to expedite the binding process. The effect on binding by ACEK has been verified using fluorescently labeled antibody in an antigen–antibody binding assay [31].

Our study has shown that two ACEK mechanisms, DEP and ACET effect, are responsible for moving biomolecules toward the electrode surface in biofluids.

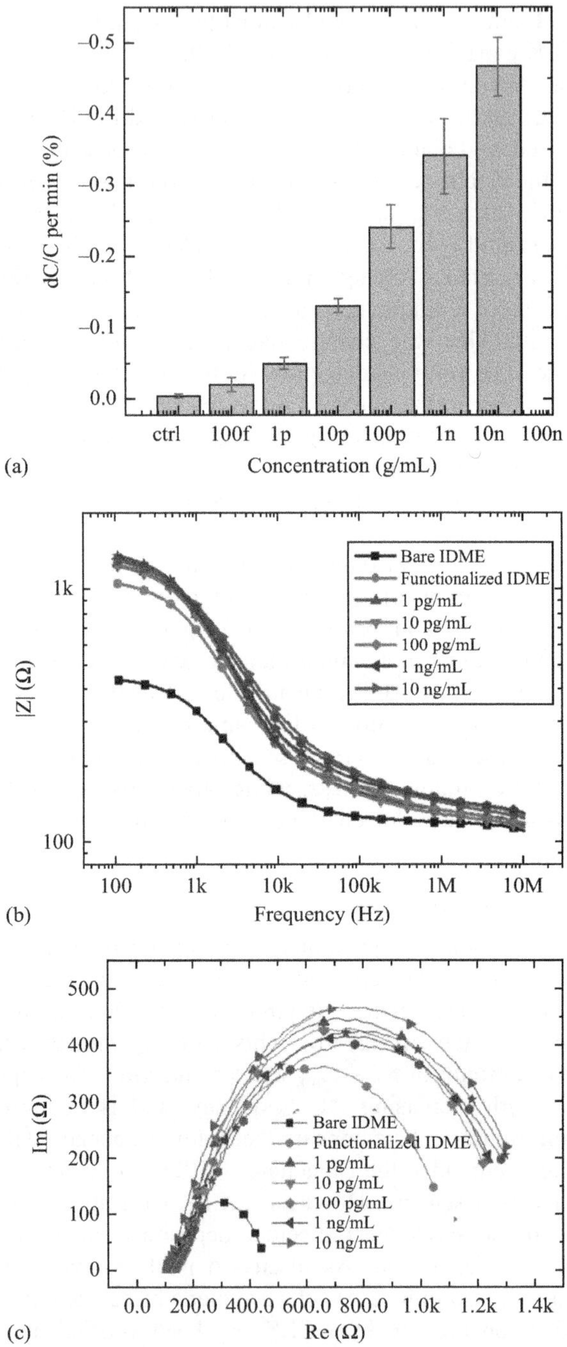

Figure 16.7 Detecting various concentrations of human D-dimer with antibody-functionalized IDME arrays as sensors, using (a) normalized capacitance change rates as the metric, and (b) Bode plots and (c) Nyquist plots of electrode arrays at the end of 1 min ACEK capacitive sensing

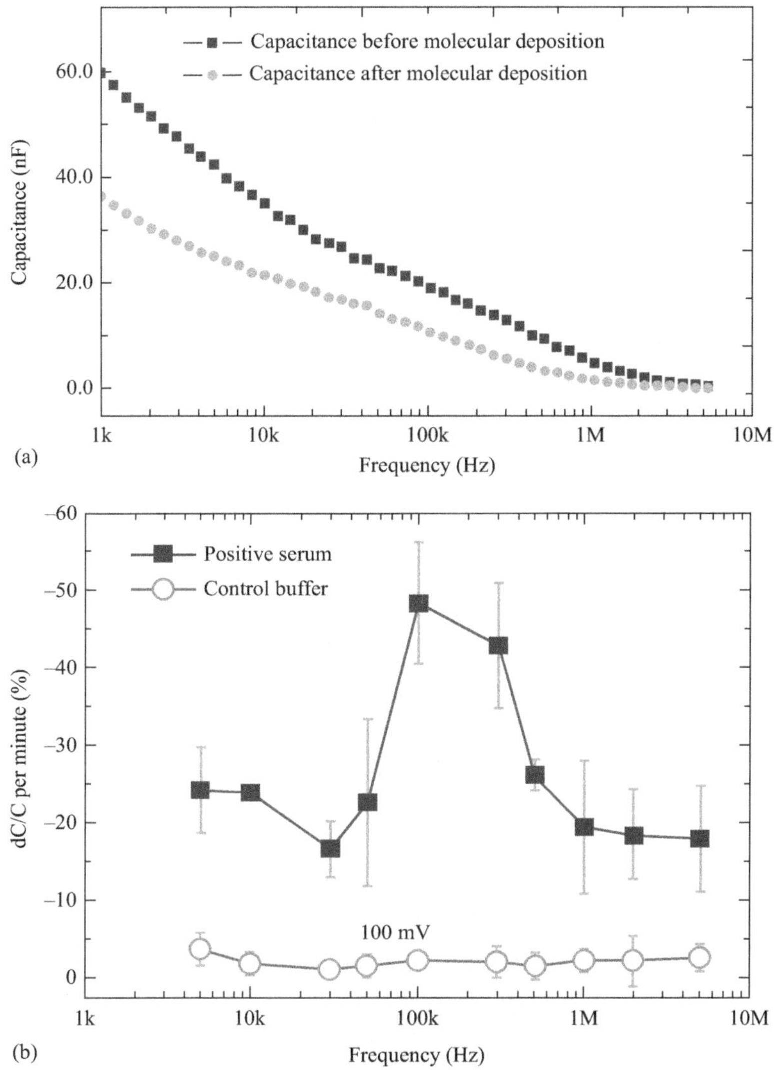

Figure 16.8 (a) Endpoint capacitive sensing of electrode surface, using the capacitances before and after molecular deposition on the electrode surface. The capacitance change is larger at lower frequency. (b) Capacitance change rate due to antigen–antibody binding at various AC frequencies with 100 mV voltage. The change rate reflects the binding process

Between them, DEP is an important, often dominant, mechanism for enhancing biomolecular binding. Since DEP is frequency dependent, the choice of AC frequency should induce positive DEP, which helps attracting biomolecules to the electrode surface for binding and increasing binding events. The frequency dependence of antibody capture by ACEK has been studied by varying the AC frequency used in ACEK capacitive sensing. As shown in Figure 16.8b, a serum sample with target antibody was tested from 5 kHz to 5 MHz at 100 mV_{rms}, and the resultant capacitance change rate showed obvious frequency dependence. The change rate was the largest between 100 and 300 kHz, and quickly dropped when AC frequency deviated from this frequency range. The bell-shaped frequency dependence was clearly indicative of positive DEP effect. When AC frequency was outside the optimal range, the capacitance change rates were still much higher than those of control sample, which indicates enhanced binding by ACET effect. Therefore, for biomolecules of 100 kD or larger, strong DEP enrichment effect is expected, and has been found to be around 100 kHz in our past experiments.

Another consideration of AC frequency is to avoid electrochemical reactions at the electrode surface. Only the electric potential dropping over the fluid/electrode interface could be used to cause electrochemical reactions or other complications such as dissolution/denaturation of our probe/electrode complex, which corresponds to the voltage sustained by the capacitive component in the sensor impedance, referring to the sensor equivalent circuit. As such, most of the AC potential would be applied over the resistive fluid bulk to induce DEP and ACET effect. So, at the chosen frequency, the sensor impedance should be relatively resistive to avoid electrolysis. For example, at 100 kHz, the impedance of our microelectrodes exhibits a phase angle of approximately -5 degrees. As a result, about 8.7% of the potential (8.7 mV_{rms} out of 100 mV_{rms}) would be dropped between the dielectric layer formed by the macromolecules on the electrode surface and the electrolyte, which poses very little risk of electrode fouling. Our preliminary experiments used AC voltage lower than 0.5 V and much lower voltage actually drops over the dielectric layer on the electrodes.

16.4.5 Effect of electrode designs

According to (16.1) and (16.3), DEP and ACET forces are dependent on the electric field strength. To study the effect of AC electric field and IDME dimensions on molecular binding, a range of voltage levels were applied on 2 μm and 5 μm IDMEs to study their detection performance. IgG samples at 10 and 100 ng/mL were tested in the study. The applied voltage on the electrode scales with the electrode gap to obtain the same electric field strength for both types of IDME. The electric field strength is estimated as AC potential/half circle over electrode gap (i.e. π*gap/2) (mV/μm). The sensor responses at different electric field strengths were plotted in Figure 16.9. As shown in Figure 16.9, the capacitance change rates increased rapidly with increasing electric field strength, while the control experiments exhibited consistently low change rates, which distinctly demonstrated the successful detection of specific antibodies. Also, it is noted that at 12.7 mV/μm, the binding responses were relatively small even for 100 ng/mL. This indicates that the voltage level is too low to induce enough ACEK force and flow to effectively enhance the binding performance. As electric field strength intensifies, the sensor responses increases dramatically, due to ACEK effects. Also noted is that 5 μm IDME produces a much larger response than 2 μm IDME, especially at high

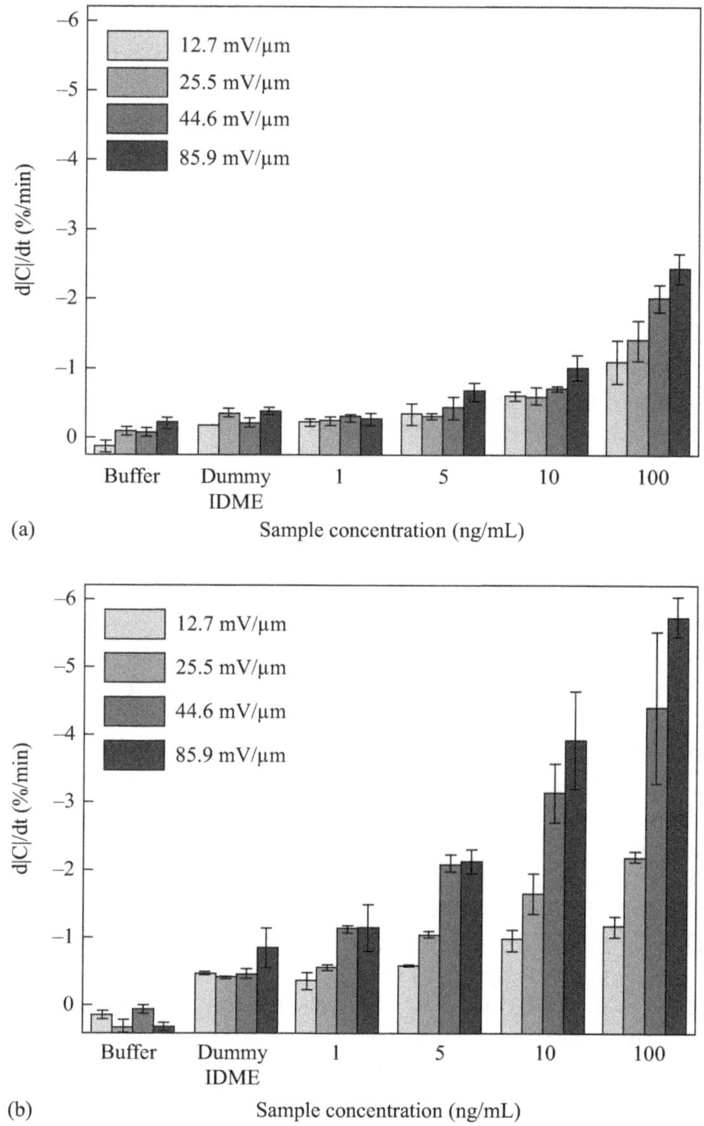

Figure 16.9 ACEK capacitive sensor responses at different electric field strengths. (a) 2 μm electrodes; (b) 5 μm electrodes. Each tested was repeated three times and error bar indicates the standard deviation

electric field strength. For example, at 44.6 mV/μm, the responses of 10 ng/mL from 5 μm IDME is -3.09 ± 0.44 %/min., almost three times higher than that from 2 μm IDME, which is -1.29 ± 0.22 %/min. This indicates that benefit from larger IDME is more obvious at higher electric field strength, which is consistent with (16.2) for ACET force $F_{ACET} \propto r|E|^4$. Based on (16.1) and (16.2), DEP velocity

$u_{DEP} \propto |E_{rms}|^2$ and ACET velocity $u_{ACET} \propto |E_{rms}|^4$, it is reasonable that ACET effect will dominate at higher E field. The difference between 2 and 5 μm IDMEs shown in Figure 16.3 clearly demonstrated the dominating effect of ACET convection at higher electric field.

The LOD can also be found from Figure 16.9. For 2 μm IDME, control buffer shows a capacitance change rate of −0.06 ± 0.06 %/s, tests on dummy IDME shows a change rate of −0.39 ± 0.07 %/s. The change rate of 10 ng/mL reaches −1.29 ± 0.22 %/s, which is more than three standard deviations from that of control tests. 10 ng/mL was thus determined to be the LOD of 2 μm IDME at 85.9 mV/μm. While for 5 μm IDME, an electric field strength of 44.6 mV/μm appears to give better separation for low level of IgG. At 44.6 mV/μm, control buffer and dummy IDME showed change rates of 0.12 ± 0.03 %/s and −0.37 ± 0.28 %/s, respectively. Compared with control tests, 1 ng/mL shows a change rate of −0.81 ± 0.25 %/s, thus was determined to be the LOD of 5 μm IDME at 44.6 mV/μm. The reason that a lower electric field is better for 5 μm IDME is because 5 μm IDME induces stronger ACET effect causing larger non-specific response along with specific binding.

Based on Figure 16.9, it can be concluded that 5 μm IDME is able to generate much stronger ACET convections than 2 μm IDME. Because IgG binding also benefits from DEP attraction [13], Figure 16.9 in fact shows the combined improvement in sensor response from DEP and ACET effects. Since 2 μm IDME produces stronger DEP force field, the actual enhancement in response due to ACET force field is larger than what is exhibited by Figure 16.9.

The benefit of inducing ACET effect can be better illustrated using small molecule detection, because DEP force is size dependent and much weaker on small molecules while ACET effect as a fluidic force is size independent. Figure 16.10a and b show the results of bisphenol A (BPA) detection by 2 μm and 5 μm IDME sensors, respectively. BPA is a small molecule with a molecular weight of only 228 Dalton, while IgG antibody in Figure 16.9 has a molecular weight of 150 kD. Therefore, DEP force is much weaker on BPA than on proteins. In Figure 16.10, the applied electric field strength is 160 mV/μm on 2 μm IDME and 85.9 mV/μm on 5 μm IDME. For both IDMEs, the decrease in capacitance is consistently getting larger with more concentrated BPA samples. However, it can be seen that stronger response was achieved with 5 μm IDME, even though much higher electric field strength is applied on 2 μm IDME. This clearly illustrates the stronger capability of 5 μm IDME in inducing ACET convection. In term of sensor characteristics, 5 μm IDME clearly outperforms 2 μm IDME, with lower LOD (10 fM versus 1 pM) and better specificity.

16.4.6 Selectivity in complex fluids

Experiments were also conducted to demonstrate that ACEK capacitive sensing method is capable of selectively detect target bioparticles from complex clinical matrix. Tests were conducted to detect specific protein from serum [12, 13, 33] and virus particle from nasal swab samples [34]. For serum protein detection, we

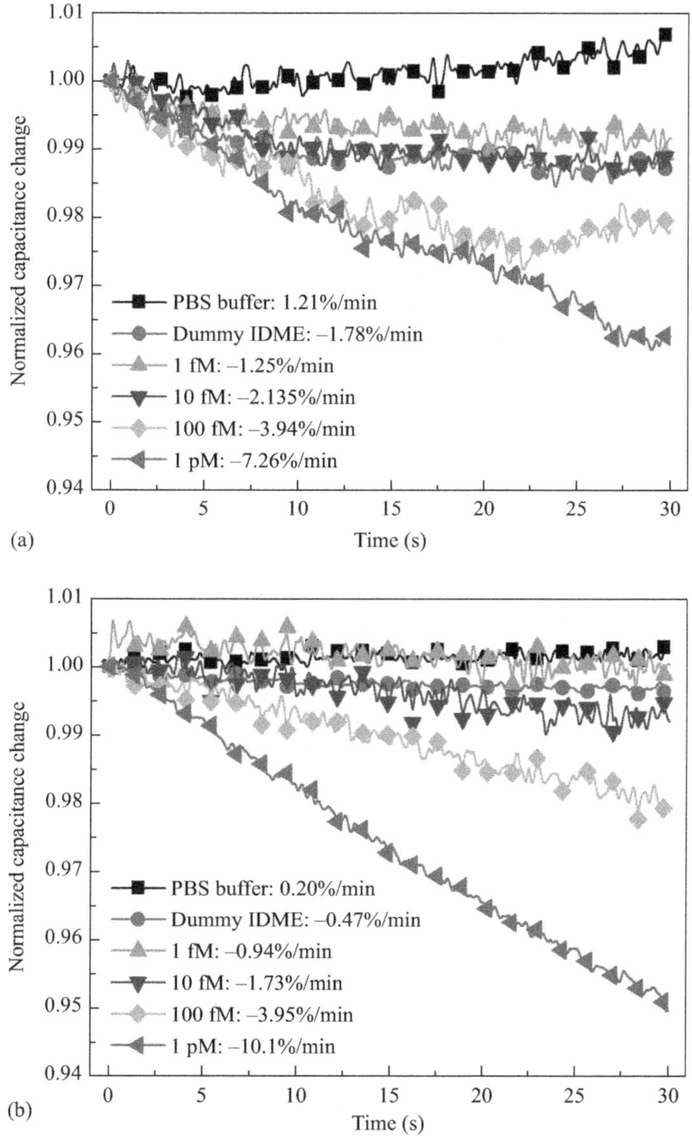

Figure 16.10 BPA detection results on different electrodes. (a) 2 μm IDME at 160 mV/μm, and (b) 5 μm IDME at 86 mV/μm. Each curve is normalized real time capacitance change over 30 s period. Buffer solution is 0.1x PBS on functionalized electrodes, Dummy IDME is 1 pM BPA on dummy electrodes; 1–1000 fM are BPA samples on functionalized electrodes. Each test lasts 30 seconds [32]

successfully demonstrated rapid detection of specific antibodies in three mycobacterial infections (Johne's disease (JD), bovine tuberculosis (TB) and human TB). In Figure 16.11a, raw serum samples from dairy cows tested positive or negative with JD were used as the model complex fluids. Multiple tests were conducted (10 samples, 5 JD-positive and 5 JD-negative). Passive adsorption has been used for IDME functionalization in our experiments, and the serum samples were 1:20 v/v diluted with 0.1x PBS for the tests. The normalized capacitance change rates were given in Figure 16.11. As expected, the capacitances of the JD-negative serum stayed rather constant during the test (little change), while those of JD-positive serum capacitance decreased monotonically with time (negative change) due to binding reaction. The detection results agreed with those by commercially available ELISA tests, and also showed good correction with ELISA response with a Pearson coefficient $R^2 = 0.808$.

For influenza A virus detection, we demonstrated an LOD of 1.5pg/mL. When testing nasal swab samples as shown in the inset of Figure 16.11b, the samples were first diluted with 0.1x PBS at 1:10,000 dilution. In a blind test of 20 clinical swab samples, the results showed a diagnostic sensitivity of 90% and specificity of 70% when benchmarked against an Xpert® Flu by Cepheid (a polymerase chain reaction test). Figure 16.11b demonstrates the specificity of ACEK capacitive sensor for influenza A virus from nasal swabs. Samples in this panel were hand-picked 'weak positives' all undetectable but one by rapid influenza test 'TruFlu', [35] demonstrating high sensitivity of ACEK capacitive sensing. The blind test also correctly identified the influenza B virus sample. This diagnostic method is highly reliable with coefficient of variation around 10%, without much effort spent on surface treatment of the electrodes.

16.5 Conclusions

This chapter presents an 'AC electrokinetic (ACEK) capacitive sensing' technique to monitor and quantitatively characterize protein–protein interactions. 'AC electrokinetic (ACEK) capacitive sensing' is an affinity-sensing platform technology, and was used to conduct a series of proof-of-concept experiments detecting specific antibodies, protein biomarker, virus particles and small molecules. In these experiments, good sensitivity was demonstrated with a response time less than 1 min. Table 16.1 summarizes the analytical performance of this sensing technology.

This work shows high promise in achieving a simple-to-use, sample-in-result-out platform technology that will be considerably more sensitive and significantly faster than traditional immunoassay methods. This sensor enables accurate quantitative measurement of biomarkers in small volumes of blood or other body fluid, and work directly with diluted serum and nasal swab samples. This method can be used to detect a range of diseases and physiological conditions in serum and other bodily fluids. All it needs is to modify the IDMEs for target biomarkers and pathogens. It is expected that this platform technology would be applicable to numerous screening/diagnostic applications at a significantly reduced cost. This technology can also be easily multiplexed for detection of a panel of proteins and pathogens.

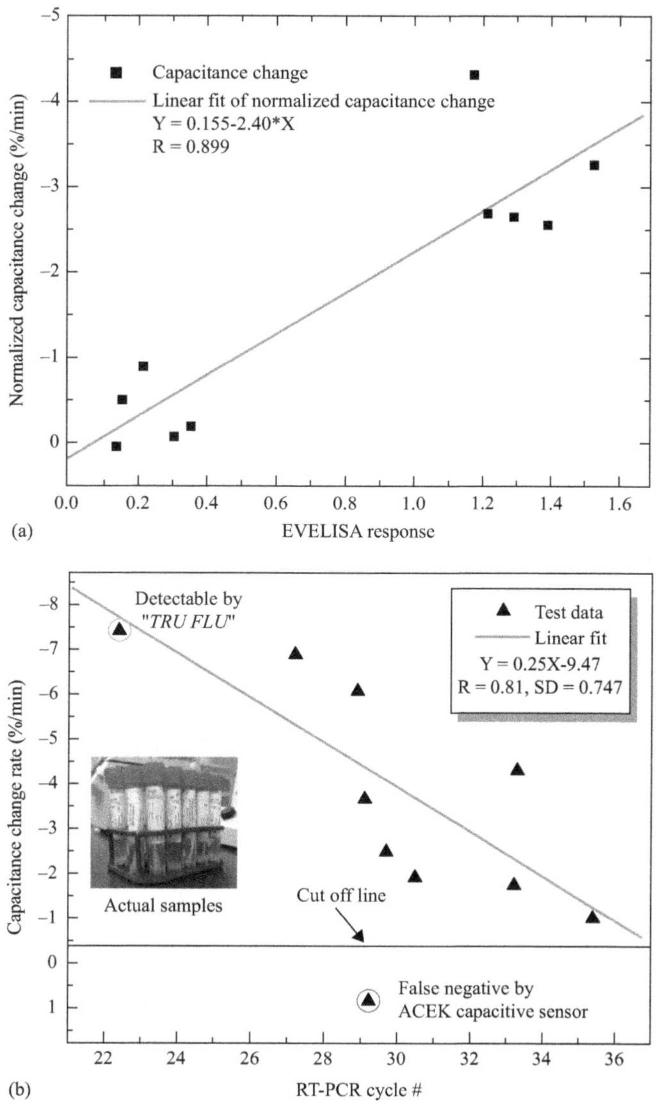

Figure 16.11 *(a) Normalized capacitance changes of IDME arrays functionalized with Johne's Disease (JD)-specific antigen and blocking agent. The samples were JD-positive and negative sera. An AC potential of 500 mV_{rms} at 100 kHz was applied. Correlation of impedance results with animal sera with and without JD infection confirmed by ELISA results. No false positive or negative was found. (b) Comparison of results from ACEK impedance sensor and those from commercial instruments after blind tests of clinical nasal swabs. The strongest positive sample is the upper limit of 'Tru Flu' test by Meridian Biosciences, Inc. The results from ACEK sensor have 90% sensitivity compared with real-time PCR*

Table 16.1 Analytical performance of ACEK capacitive sensor

Type	Detection limit	Sensitivity
Small molecule (aptamer probe)	10 fM	−0.09%/min/log (fM)
Protein (antigen probe)	5 pg/mL (22 fM)	−0.32%/min/pg/mL
Virus particle (antibody probe)	15.25 pg/mL	−1.26%/min/log (pg/mL)

Acknowledgments

The author thanks Profs. Shigetoshi Eda and Gladys Alexandre for their kind collaboration, helpful discussion and sample preparation. She also thanks Mr. Cheng, Dr. Haochen Cui and Dr. Shanshan Li for assistance with experimental data. The work was supported by the University of Tennessee Research Foundation Maturation program.

References

[1] Gruhl, F. J., Rapp, B. E., Länge, K: 'Biosensors for diagnostic applications', *Adv Biochem Eng Biotechnol*. 2013, 133, pp. 115–148.

[2] Daniels, J. S. and Pourmand, N.: 'Label-free impedance biosensors: opportunities and challenges', *Electroanalysis*. 2007, 19(12), pp. 1239–1257.

[3] Nirschl, M., Reuter, F., Voros, J.: 'Review of transducer principles for label-free biomolecular interaction analysis', *Biosensors*. 2011, 1, pp. 70–92.

[4] Ferlay, J., Soerjomataram I., Dikshit R., *et al.*: 'Cancer incidence and mortality worldwide, sources, methods and major patterns in GLOBOCAN 2012', *Int'l J Cancer*. 2015, 136(5), pp. E359–E386.

[5] Guo X.: 'Surface plasmon resonance based biosensor technique: a review', *J Biophotonics*. 5, pp. 483–501.

[6] Gai H., Li Y., Yeung E. S.: 'Optical detection systems on microfluidic chips', *Top Curr Chem*. 304, pp. 171–201.

[7] Weigl, B., Domingo, G., Labarre P., Gerlach, J.: 'Towards non- and minimally instrumented, microfluidics-based diagnostic devices,' *Lab chip*. 2008, 8, pp. 1999–2014.

[8] Wu, J.: 'In situ nanoparticle focusing within microfluidics,' in Kumar C. S. (Ed.), *Microfluidic Devices in Nanotechnology* (John Wiley & Sons, Inc., May 2010), pp. 295–316.

[9] Wu, J.: 'Advances of LOC-based particle manipulation by AC electrical fields', *Recent Patents on Electrical Engineering*. 2008, 1(3), pp. 178–187.

[10] Sin, M. L. Y., Shimabukuro, Y., Wong, P. K.: 'Hybrid electrokinetics for separation, mixing, and concentration of colloidal particles', *Nanotechnology*. 2009, 20, p. 165701.

[11] Yang, K. and Wu, J.: 'Numerical study of in situ preconcentration for rapid and sensitive nanoparticle detection', *Biomicrofluidics*. 2010, 4(3), p. 034106.

[12] Cui, H., Li, S., Yuan, Q., *et al.*: 'An AC electrokinetic impedance immunosensor for rapid detection of tuberculosis', *Analyst*. 2013, 138(23), pp. 7188–7196.

[13] Li, S., Cui, H., Yuan, Q., *et al.*: 'AC electrokinetics-enhanced capacitive immunosensor for point-of-care serodiagnosis of infectious diseases', *Biosens Bioelectron*, 2014, 51, pp. 437–443.

[14] Cui, H., Wu, J., Eda, S., Chen, J., Chen, W., Zheng, L., 'Rapid capacitive detection of femtomolar levels of bisphenol A using an aptamer-modified disposable microelectrode array', *Microchim Acta*, 182(13–14), 2361–2367, 2015.

[15] Li, S., Yuan, Q., Morshed, B., Ke, C., Wu, J.; 'Dielectrophoretic response of DNA and fluorophore in physiological solution by impedimetric characterization', *Biosens Bioelectron*. 2013 41, pp. 649–655.

[16] Morgan, H. and Green, N. G.: *AC Electrokinetics: Colloids and Nanoparticles*' (Research Studies Press, 2003).

[17] Katz, E. and Willner, I.: 'Probing biomolecular interactions at conductive and semiconductive surfaces by impedance spectroscopy: routes to impedimetric immunosensors, DNA-sensors, and enzyme biosensors', *Electroanalysis*. 2003, 15(11), pp. 913–947.

[18] Ohno, R., Ohnuki, H., Wang, H., *et al.*: 'Electrochemical impedance spectroscopy biosensor with interdigitated electrode for detection of human immunoglobulin A', *Biosens. Bioelectron.*, 2013, 40(1), pp. 422–426.

[19] Sheehan, P. E. and Whitman, L. J.: 'Detection limits for nanoscale biosensors', *Nano Lett.* 2005, 5, 803–807.

[20] Wu, J.: 'Interactions of electrical fields with fluids: laboratory-on-a-chip applications', *IET Nanobiotech.*, 2008, 2(1), pp. 14–27.

[21] Green, N. G., Ramos, A., Gonzalez, A., Morgan, H., Castellanos, A.: 'Fluid flow induced by nonuniform AC electric fields in electrolytes on microelectrodes. I. Experimental measurements', *Phys. Rev. E*, 2000, 61(4), p. 4011.

[22] Wu, J., Ben, Y., Battigelli, D., Chang, H.-C. 'Long-range AC electrokinetic trapping and detection of bioparticles', *Industr Eng Chem. Res.* 2005, 44(8), pp. 2815–2822.

[23] Lian, M., Islam, N., Wu, J.: 'AC electrothermal manipulation of conductive fluids and particles for lab-chip applications', *IET Nanobiotech.* 2007, 1(3), pp. 36–43.

[24] Green, N. G., Ramos, A., González, A., Castellanos, A., Morgan, H.: 'Electrothermally induced fluid flow on microelectrodes', *J. Electrostat.*, 2001, 53, 71–87.

[25] Pethig, R.: 'Review article—dielectrophoresis: status of the theory, technology, and applications', *Biomicrofluidics*. 2010, 4, p. 022811.

[26] Yang, C. K., Chang, J. S., Chao, S. D., Wu, K. C.: 'Two dimensional simulation on immunoassay for a biosensor with applying electrothermal effect', *Appl Phys Lett.* 2007, 91(11): p. 113904.
[27] Feldman, H. C., Sigurdson, M., Meinhart, C. D.: 'AC electrothermal enhancement of heterogeneous assays in microfluidics', *Lab. Chip*, 2007, 7, pp. 1553–1559.
[28] Castellanos, A., Ramos, A., Gonzalez, A., Green, N. G., Morgan, H.: 'Electrohydrodynamics and dielectrophoresis in microsystems: scaling laws', *J. Phys. D: Appl. Phys.* 2003, 36, pp. 2584–2597.
[29] Jo, M., Ahn, J. Y., Lee J., *et al.*: 'Development of single-stranded DNA aptamers for specific bisphenol a detection', *Oligonucleotides*. 2011, 21(2), 85–91.
[30] Cui, H., Cheng, C., Wu, J., Eda. S.: 'Rapid detection of progesterone by commercially available microelectrode chips', *Proc. IEEE Sensors.* 2013, pp. 137–140, Nov. 4–6, 2013, Baltimore, MD, USA.
[31] Liu, X., Yang, K., Wadhwa, A., Eda, S., Li, S., Wu, J., 'Development of an AC electrokinetics-based immunoassay system for on-site serodiagnosis of infectious diseases', *Sens Actu A: Physical*. 2011, 171, pp. 406–413.
[32] Cui, H., Cheng, C., Lin, *et al.*: 'Rapid and sensitive detection of small biomolecule by capacitive sensing and low field AC electrothermal effect,' *Sens. Actu. B*. 2016, 226, pp. 245–253.
[33] Li, S., Ren, Y., Cui, H., *et al.*: 'Alternating current electrokinetics enhanced in situ capacitive immunoassay', *Electrophoresis.* 2015, 36, pp. 471–474.
[34] Cheng, C., Cui, H., Yuan, Q., Wu, J., Eda, S., 'Rapid and no-wash detection of avianin fluenza A virus from clinical swab samples', BMES 2014 Annual Meeting, San Antonio, Texas, Oct. 22–25, 2014.
[35] TRU FLU, http://www.meridianbioscience.com/diagnostic-products/respiratory/tru/tru-flu.aspx.

Chapter 17

Fibre optical technology for monitoring and diagnostic applications

Peyman Mirtaheri[1]

17.1 Introduction

Modern sensors have mostly evolved from the tremendous developments in the communication industry, information technology and molecular biology. In particular, the development of optical fibre sensors (OFS) during recent years is related to two of the most important scientific advances of the 1960s, the laser (1960) and modern low-cost optical fibres (1966) [1, 2]. During the early 1980s some of these low-loss optical fibres were used in the development of the first biomedical applied sensors [3].

The great success of optical-fibre sensors is because they can be used to tackle difficult measurement situations where use of conventional sensors is not appropriate. The sensors are usually compact and lightweight, minimally invasive, and can be multiplexed effectively on a single fibre network. They are immune to electromagnetic interference, because there are no electrical currents flowing at the sensing point. Probably the greatest advantage of OFS is still their small size. In most cases, the diameter of bare OFS, usually in the range of 125 to 500 μm, is very appropriate in space-restricted environments such as the instrumented catheters for patients health monitoring or such as thin composite structures. Most frequently, an OFS has an axial geometry suitable also for many applications where this becomes a benefit, such as instrumentation of bolts or similar cylindrical devices. The ability of measuring over distances of several kilometres, without the need for any electrically active component is also an advantage inherited from the fibre optic telecommunication industry. This is an important feature when monitoring large and remote structures such as pipelines or multiple bridges along a single highway.

Biological recognition devices particularly in monitoring and diagnostic applications have attracted extraordinary interest in recent years. This may be because of the key role biosensors play in the development of highly sensitive and

[1]Department of Mechanical, Electronics and Chemical Engineering, Group of Biomedical Engineering, Faculty of Technology, Art and Design, HiOA, Oslo, Norway

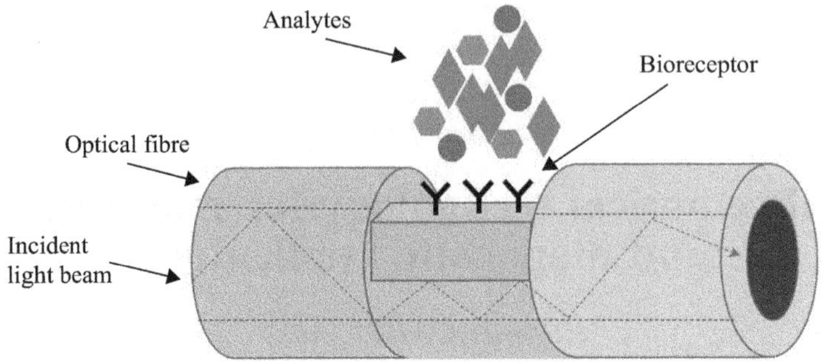

Figure 17.1 Schematic diagram of a typical fibre optical biosensor design

selective chemical analysis, but also in respect with a low-cost production in the recent years.

According to a recently proposed IUPAC definition [4], "*A biosensor is a self-contained integrated device which is capable of providing specific quantitative or semi-quantitative analytical information using a biological recognition element (biochemical receptor) which is in direct spatial contact with a transducer element. A biosensor should be clearly distinguished from a bioanalytical system, which requires additional processing steps, such as reagent addition. Furthermore, a biosensor should be distinguished from a bioprobe which is either disposable after one measurement, i.e. single use, or unable to continuously monitor the analyte concentration.*"

A special type of biosensor that include transducers based on integrated circuit microchips are called as biochips. These type of biosensors are out of the scope of this chapter and will not be further discussed.

Fibre optical biosensors (FOBS), sometimes also called bio-optrodes, are analytical devices incorporating optical fibres and biological recognition molecules [5, 6]. The word "Optrode" is a combination of the words "optical" and "electrode." The term electrode is a misunderstood term normally applied in the field of medicine and sometimes in chemistry, which simply means a sensing part of a device. As illustrated in Figure 17.1 a FOBS is composed of two main components: a bioreceptor and a carrier fibre or waveguide.

17.1.1 Fibre optic technology

Optical fibres are fine strands of glass or plastic, single or bunch of which is used for transmission of light from one compartment to another to large distances. The basic principle of fibre optics, which is based on refractive phenomenon was actually explained by Kepler as early as in 1600s [7]. However, it was not before 1854 that John Tydall demonstrated that light could be conducted through a curved stream of water, providing that a light signal could be bent [8]. As the water has a refractive index that is higher than the air, the light would be trapped and conducted through the water stream.

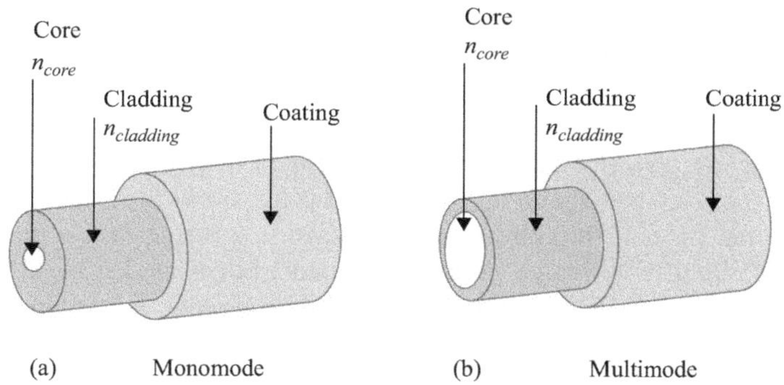

Figure 17.2 Showing the construction of a mono (a) and multimode (b) optical fibres with refractive index for core (n_{core}) and cladding ($n_{cladding}$)

The essential feature for transmission of light with total internal reflection (TIR) in an optical fibre is based on the very same concept, which was demonstrated by Tydall's water experiment. As illustrated in Figure 17.2, an optical fibre has a core with a refractive index n_{core}, and the coating material (cladding) with reflective index $n_{cladding}$ that has to be smaller than n_{core}, i.e. $n_{core} > n_{cladding}$. When a ray of light strikes the boundary interface between these transparent media with different refractive indexes and the angle of incidence is larger than the critical angle, the light would be trapped in the fibre and conducted with small loss. The critical angle can be calculated by the Snell's law [9]:

$$\theta_{critical} = \sin^{-1}\left(\frac{n_{cladding}}{n_{core}}\right) \tag{17.1}$$

Often an optical fibre is described by the numerical aperture (NA) which is a measurement of the ability of an optical fibre to capture light. The higher the value of NA, the more is the light collected for propagation in the fibre:

$$NA = \frac{1}{n_0}\left(n_{core}^2 - n_{cladding}^2\right)^{\frac{1}{2}} \tag{17.2}$$

where n_0 is the refractive index of the medium around the connection of the fibre, which is close to 1 in case of air.

There are two types of optical fibres that are offered, monomode and multimode (see Figure 17.2). Monomode fibres have a narrow core of uniform refractive index profile and transmit only single mode for light of a specific wavelength range and linearly polarized state. On the other hand, multimode fibres have a larger core diameter and can transmit many hundreds light signals.

All optical fibres have a coatings that are applied in concentric layers to prevent damage to the fibre during the drawing application and to maximize fibre strength and micro bend resistance. Unevenly coated fibre will experience non-uniform forces when the coating expands or contracts, and is susceptible to greater signal attenuation. Under proper drawing and coating processes, the coatings are concentric around the fibre, continuous over the length of the application and have constant thickness.

Although the optical fibres were originally designed for light propagation with minimal loss, an optical biosensor requires light to interact with the fibre's surroundings. One way to achieve this interaction is to expose the evanescent field of the transmitted light. If the fibre is tapered down to a diameter less than the core diameter, the light is no longer guided by the core but is guided by the cladding, and the evanescent field will interact with the surrounding environments and its magnitude is enhanced in the tapered region [10, 11].

The penetration depth into the cladding can be calculated by (17.3) [12, 13]:

$$d_p = \frac{\lambda}{2\pi} \cdot \left(n_{core}^2 \sin^2\theta - n_{cladding}^2\right)^{-\frac{1}{2}} \tag{17.3}$$

where λ and θ are the wavelength and angle between core and cladding of the incident light, n_{core} and $a_{cladding}$ are the refractive indexes of the core and cladding. When the fibre is tapered and the fibre is exposed to another surrounding medium, one would change refractive index of the cladding with the refractive index of the substituted medium.

Fibre tapering refers to the process of pulling a fibre while heating, such that the overall diameter of the fibre at the tapered region is less than the original diameter [14]. Currently, two types of tapered fibre geometries in biosensing application are favourable: tapered tips and continuous tapered fibres [15]. In a tapered tip fibre, it consists of an optical fibre which gradually decreases in diameter until it becomes a tiny tip that later becomes the sensing element. On the other hand, a continuous tapered fibre is an optical fibre that is gradually decreasing in diameter (downtaper), which reaches a constant-diameter waist region, and then gradually increases (uptaper) back to the original diameter (see Figure 17.3).

As an example, if an optical fibre is tapered and an aqueous medium in the tapered region is placed. Assuming the wavelength of the incident light is a blue laser (470 nm) which is connected to an optical fibre with a core refractive index of about 1.45 and the incident light angle is about 80°, while the surrounding aqueous

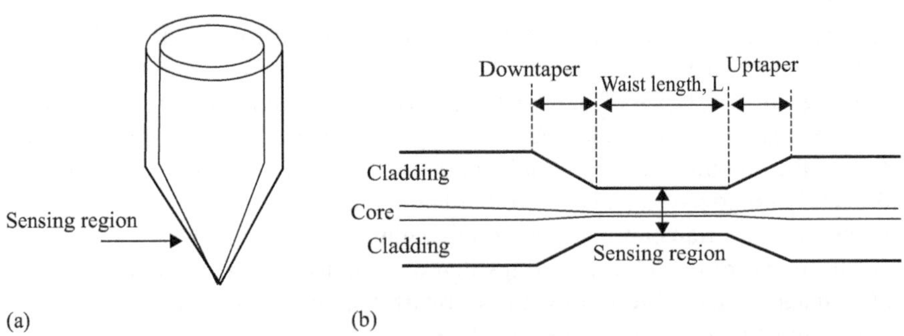

Figure 17.3 Showing the tapering of fibre tip (a) and fibre waist (b)

medium around the fibre has a refractive index between 1.33 and 1.34. The expected penetration depth would be accordingly between 138 and 145 nm.

In general, characteristic dimension of bacterial cells are approximately 1 μm, while that of proteins are on the order of 10 nm. Therefore, depending on the size of the target analyte it may be necessary to increase the penetration depth [16, 17]. The penetration depth is far too small for such sensing purposes [15].

Several investigators have attempted to increase the penetration depth of the evanescent field and facilitate mode coupling by bending [18–22], tapering [23–28], altering the light launching angle [29] and increasing the wavelength [14, 30].

Light propagation through an optical fibre can be described in more detail by the wave theory [16, 31]. The properties of light in the fibre core are determined by the number of modes N that is proportional to the square of the V-number. The V-number of a fibre gives an idea of the number of modes in the fibre and is related to the refractive index difference of the fibre (17.4) [32]:

$$V = (2\pi \cdot R \cdot NA) \cdot \lambda^{-1} \tag{17.4}$$

where R is the radius of the fibre core and NA is the numeric aperture of the fibre. As the refractive index, difference of the fibre core and cladding increases which results in an increase of V-number of the fibre. A single-mode fibre has a V-number that is less than 2.405, while for a multi-mode fibre V-number is greater than 2.405, for most optical wavelengths. In general, one would prefer a fibre with higher V-number which indicates a higher power transmission with less loss.

The losses associated with the V-number mismatching of the fibre arise due to the removal of the cladding and inserting the core of the fibre into an aqueous medium. A minimum value of the taper ratio is needed to avoid large V-number mismatch losses. For a fibre of $NA = 0.2$ (core refractive index 1.46 and cladding 1.45), if the fibre radius is tapered from 100% to 68% of the initial core radius, then the probe will suffer heavily by light attenuation. This has been confirmed experimentally by the group of Golden *et al.* [33]. Thus, in an aqueous medium the minimum radius of the core should be smaller than 68% of the core in order to avoid V-number losses.

17.1.2 Bioreceptors

A bioreceptor is a biologically sensitive element of biosensors, which is responsible for the recognition of an analyte. To a large extend, the choice of the correct bioreceptor decides for the specificity and sensitivity of the final device. There are four main groups of the biological elements [34, 35]:

1. Enzymes, proteins that catalyze specific chemical reactions are also called as biocatalyst. These can be used in a purified form or be present in a micro-organism or in a slice of intact tissue. The mechanisms of operation of these bioreceptors can involve: (1) Conversion of the analyte into a sensor-detectable product, (2) Detection of an analyte that acts as enzyme inhibitor or activator or (3) Evaluation of the modification of enzyme properties upon interaction with the analyte [34].

2. Antibodies and antigens are also called as bioaffinity. An antigen is a molecule that triggers the immune response of an organism to produce an antibody, a glycoprotein produced by lymphocyte B cells which will specifically recognize the antigen that stimulated its production [36].
3. Nucleic acids. The recognition process is based on the complementarity of base pairs (adenine and thymine or cytosine and guanine) of adjacent strands in the double helix of DNA. These sensors are usually known as genosensors. Alternatively, interaction of small pollutants with DNA can generate the recognition signal [37, 38].
4. Receptors, neurotransmitters and hormonal receptors are the body's own biosensors. The binding of a ligand to a receptor triggers an amplified physiological response, such as ion channel opening, secondary messenger system and activation of enzymes [34, 39]. Hence, these biological receptors tend to have an affinity for a range of structurally related compounds or analytes; this topic is interesting for the future generation of biosensors.

17.2 Immobilization

Biosensors work best when the biological and physico-chemical components are kept in close proximity to one another [39]. Their proximity is preserved when the analyte has unlimited access to the biocomponent and when the integrity of the interaction is retained. In general, the biological component has to be properly attached to the optical fibre by immobilization. The immobilization method is determined by the nature of the biocomponent to be immobilized. The type of the optical fibre material and selected measurements technique, and the physical properties of the analyte are important factors that assist in selecting a method. Generally, there are five common methods of immobilization: adsorption, microencapsulation, entrapment, cross linking and covalent binding [40].

17.2.1 Adsorption

It is association of the active component with a film or coating through hydrophobic, hydrophilic and/or ionic interactions [41]. Many substances adsorb enzymes on their surfaces. The adsorption approach itself includes using physical adsorption and chemical adsorption. Physical adsorption is usually weak and involves the formation of van der Waals bonds. Chemical adsorption is much stronger due to the formation of covalent bonds. Advantages are simplicity, absence of a clean-up step and highly reproducible. Drawbacks are susceptible to changes in pH, temperature and ionic strength of the substrate.

17.2.2 Microencapsulation

A semipermeable membrane is used to trap the biomaterial on the optical fibre [42]. This keeps close contact between the biomaterial and the optical fibre. Membrane materials include cellulose acetate [43], polycarbonate [44] or Teflon [45].

It is stable towards changes in temperature, pH, ionic strength and chemical composition [40].

17.2.3 Entrapment

Entrapment immobilization involves the physical trapping of the active biomolecules into a film or coating. In the operation, biomolecules are mixed with a monomer solution. e.g., polymer gel. It is strong, but has a slow diffusion rate of analytes [46].

17.2.4 Cross-linking

It is similar to entrapment, only a polymerization agent (such as glutaraldehyde) is used to provide additional chemical linkages between the active, entrapped component and the film or coating [47]. The biomaterial is chemically bonded to solid supports or to another supporting material such as a gel. It is useful to stabilize adsorbed biomaterials. However, it causes damage to the enzyme, limits the diffusion of the substrate, and there is poor mechanical strength. Finally, we would like to point out that no matter which immobilization method is used, to achieve best performance, the immobilization procedure should be optimized in terms of signal intensity, selectivity and sensitivity by choosing proper materials (e.g., fluorophore) and methods depending on the application [48].

17.2.5 Covalent bonding

Attachment of the active component to the surface of the optical fibre using a chemical reaction. Covalent bonding agent is employed in the biomaterial to support the matrix. e.g., thiol, epoxy, amino, carboxylic. Advantages are stability, avoid problems of leaching. Drawbacks are covalent linkage [49].

17.3 Sensing schemes

The general block diagram of fibre optics sensor system is shown in Figure 17.4. The system generally consists of a light source, optical fibre as transmission channel, sensing element with bioreceptors, optical detector and end processed devices as oscilloscope, optical spectrum analyser and microprocessor-based instrumentation [2]. The light source is usually standard optical components such as light emitting diode [9], lasers and laser diodes but also halogen and xenon lamps are applied. The optical detectors can be photodiodes, Avalanche Photodiode (APD).

Fibre optic biosensors are generally categorized into two groups according to construction that are classified as intrinsic and extrinsic sensors. In an intrinsic sensor is based on evanescent wave. The fibre has two functions: first, the light never leaves the fibre and second, the parameter of interest affects a property of the light propagating through the fibre by acting directly on the fibre itself. The extrinsic sensor or hybrid fibre optic sensor consists of an input and output fibre leading the lights into a "black box," which modulates the light beam upon

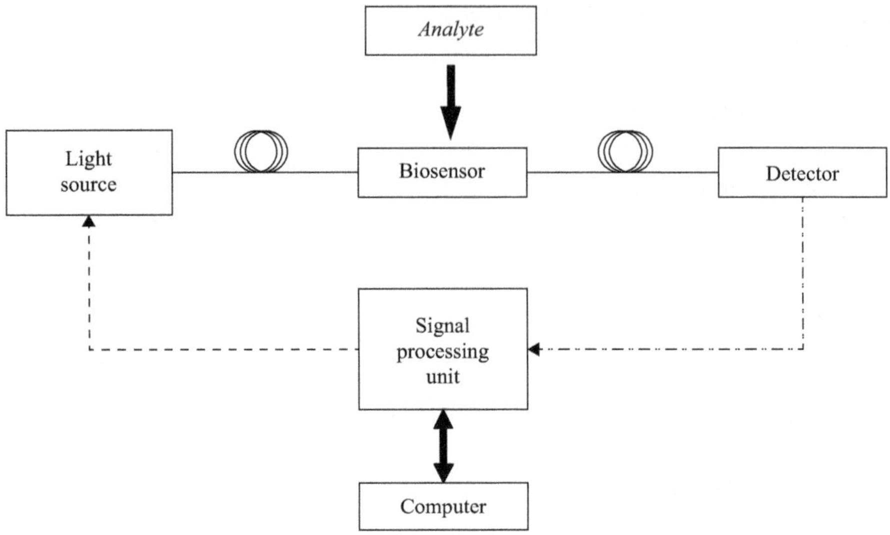

Figure 17.4 Illustrating a general block diagram for an optical biosensing system

activation light and environmental signal. In most cases, the extrinsic sensor may have a linear transfer function as f(x), Which is dependent on the external dye material and its response to the analyte. Normally, there is no way that one could cover a large measuring range, which is described by the limit of detection (LOD).

In most cases, a single fibre is applied as bifurcated fibres that guide incoming and outgoing light. Figure 17.5 illustrates the measurement schematic of the extrinsic and intrinsic sensors.

There are a numerous measurements methods that have been applied for the fibre optical biosensor, however, the most applied measurements methods in regards to the fibre optical biosensors are, absorbance, fluorescence, and inferometeric techniques particularly the surface plasmon resonance (SPR) which has been in a tremendous research focus recently.

17.3.1 Absorbance

The simplest optical-biosensors use absorbance measurements to determine any changes in the concentration of analytes that absorb a given wavelength of light. The biological material is immobilized at the distal end of the optical-fibres and either produces or extracts the analyte that absorbs the light [50]. The system works by transmitting light through an optical fibre to the sample; reflected, scattered or emitted light returns from the sample by a second fibre or by bifurcation of the original fibre. The emitted light signal is interpreted at the detector and is a measure of the concentration of the analyte which is described by the Beer-Lamberts law expressed as:

$$A = \alpha L \eta \tag{17.5}$$

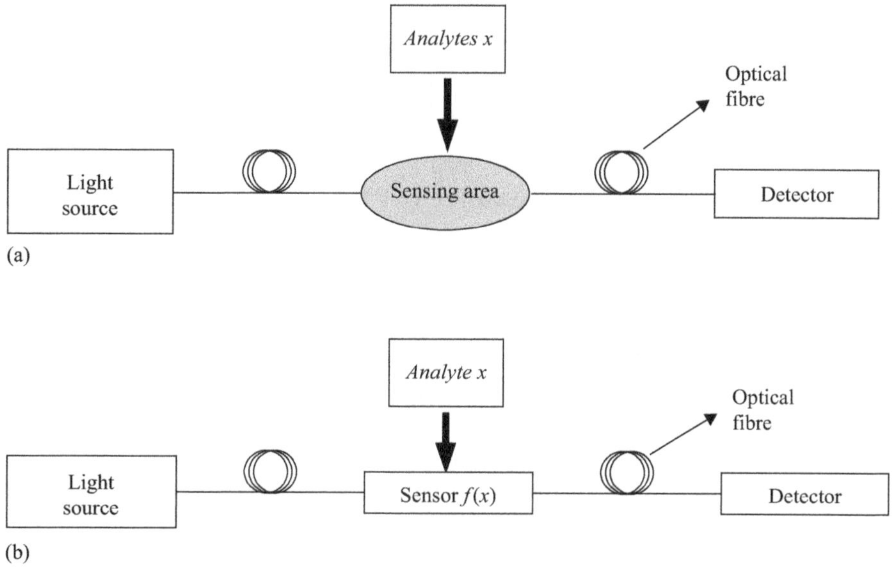

Figure 17.5 Shows the intrinsic (a) and the extrinsic (b) fibre optical sensing (FOS)

where α is absorption coefficient, L is the length of the fibre and η is the fraction of evanescent domain. α is given as:

$$\alpha = \varepsilon[C] \tag{17.6}$$

where ε is molar absorptivity and C is concentration of the analytes to be measured. Sensitivity of de-cladded uniform core fibre is given by [15]:

$$S = \varepsilon L\left(\eta + \frac{d\eta}{dC}\right) \tag{17.7}$$

17.3.2 Fluorescent

A fluorescent measurement is another method used for optical measurements in biosensors. Generally, there are a few analytes that can be directly detected in this manner; otherwise, labels are used. For example, analyte A can react with reagent R to for a product AR. It the measured optical parameter is proportional to the product AR, the response is proportional to A (analyte) at low concentrations. Hence, there is a linear relationship between the ratio of the absorbances at wavelength (AR) and wavelength (R) and the concentration of A. This relationship is independent of R. A competitive binding method is used if neither the analyte nor the reagent shows a spectral change upon binding. In this case, a fluorescent label is used that is similar to the analyte and possesses optical characteristics upon binding [40]. Fluorescence quenching, in which the fluorescence of a compound bounded within the biosensor is affected by the presence of another compound, has been used as another optical transduction method. These sensors are generally used with enzymes, where the production of a product, such as H^+ or O_2, causes quenching of the fluorescence of the bound compound [51, 52].

17.4 Surface plasmon resonance (SPR)

SPR is a unique optical transduction method with numerous applications. SPR is used to probe refractive index changes that occur on the sensor surface. Any physical phenomenon at the surface that alters the refractive surface will trigger a response. Basically, a surface plasmon is an evanescent electromagnetic field generated at the surface of a metal conductor, usually silver or gold, which is excited by incident light of appropriate wavelength. The basic SPR apparatus is referred to as the Kretschman prism arrangement [53].

In a set-up for an OFS, a thin film of metal is coated or deposited on a tapered optical fibre. The metal films form the sensor surface on which the bioreceptor is placed. Light is propagated into the fibre as the TIR occurs, where it is coupled into the plasmon mode of the metal film where it is further measured by an optical photodetector. The changes in the amount of light striking the detection represent the sensor output [39].

Geometric factors which affect the performance of a SPR sensor include the metal thickness, length, waist diameter and launch angle. It was previous stated that the metal coating thickness must be on the order of the wavelength used [54]. In the study done by Sharma *et al.* it was concluded that increasing the length of the sensing region increases the number of reflections, and causes a broader SPR curve with lower SNR [55]. Fabrication and modelling of a uniform-waist single mode SPR sensor was examined by Villatoro *et al.* and it was found that thicker waist diameters resulted in sharper resonance peaks, which increases sensitivity [54].

17.5 Advantageous and disadvantageous of optical fibre biosensors

The incorporation of optical fibre in biosensor which can be used in monitoring and diagnostic application, results in several advantages:

- They have no introduction to electrical hazards close to the patient.
- They are biocompatible to some extent.
- They sometimes do not require contact and therefore the bioreceptor need not to be in direct contact with the optical fibre.
- They can be easily miniaturized at low cost, and therefore attractive for *in vivo* applications.
- They have minimum signal cross talking in a multiple probe.
- They poses less sensitivity with temperature dependency compared to electrochemical methods.

The uncabled fibres are small and flexible making it possible to insert them into tissue by catheters or subcutaneous needles giving advantage of minimally invasive monitoring of most organs. Fibres are non-toxic, chemically inert and intrinsically safe for the patient. In addition, the absence of crosstalk between the fibres allows a multiple sensory measurements in several fibres grouped in a single catheter.

However, at the current time, there are some drawbacks of optical fibre biosensors that can limit their applicability:

- Interference of ambient light and background noise, although it can be avoided by use of suitable light isolation or modulated light detection techniques.
- Possible photobleaching or indicator wash out when indicator phases are employed, and limited stability of the immobilized biological component, although this would also be a drawback for other type of biosensors with different transducer technology.
- Long response times if mass transfer to the reagent phase is needed, although this can be avoided by packing the bioreactor in a well-designed porous media.
- Limited availability of optimized commercial accessories for use with optical fibres.

To handle optical fibre is really more of an art rather than a science. Lining up a fibre to the rest of the measurements system is one of the most physically difficult parts of putting together an optical device.

17.6 Clinical and diagnostic applications

In recent years, the demand has grown in the field of medical diagnostics for simple and disposable devices that also demonstrate fast response times, are user-friendly, cost-efficient and are suitable for mass production. Biosensor technologies offer the potential to fulfil these criteria through an interdisciplinary combination of approaches from nanotechnology, chemistry and medical science.

Clinical diagnostics is a field in which new methods of laboratory analysis for faster, direct, more accurate, more selective, has a high output and less expensive than conventional methods are in high demand.

The ability to assess health status, disease onset and progression, and monitor treatment outcome through a non-invasive method is the main aim to be achieved in health care promotion and delivery and research. There are three prerequisites to reach this goal: specific biomarkers that indicates a healthy or diseased state; a non-invasive approach to detect and monitor the biomarkers; and the technologies to discriminate the biomarkers. The early disease diagnosis is crucial for patient survival and successful prognosis of the disease, so that sensitive and specific methods are required.

Among the numerous humankind diseases, three most relevant cases and the relevant biosensors applied are further discussed. These three cases were chosen because of their worldwide incidence, prevalence, morbidity and mortality, namely, diabetes, cardiovascular diseases (CVD) and cancer.

17.7 Biosensors for diabetes applications

17.7.1 Glucose as diabetes biomarker

About 3% of the population worldwide suffers from diabetes, a leading cause of death, and its incidence is growing fast. Diabetes is a syndrome of disordered metabolism resulting in abnormally high blood sugar levels. Diabetic individuals are at a greater heart disease, stroke, high blood pressure, blindness, kidney failure, neurological disorders risk and other health-related complications without diligent monitoring blood glucose concentrations. Through patient education, regular examinations and tighter blood glucose monitoring, many of these complications can be reduced significantly [56, 57]. Optimal management of diabetes involves patients measuring and recording their own blood glucose levels. Under normal physiological condition, the concentration of fasting plasma glucose is in the range 6.1–6.9 mmol/L, so the variation of the blood glucose level can indicate diabetes mellitus, besides other conditions. Consequently, quantitation of the glucose content is of extreme importance, as it is the main diabetes biomarker. The American Diabetes Association recommends that insulin-dependent type 1 diabetics self-monitor blood glucose 3–4 times daily, while insulin-dependent type 2 diabetics monitor once-daily [58]. However, frequent self-monitoring of glucose concentrations is difficult, given the time, the inconvenience and the discomfort involved with the traditional measurement technique. Several methods for glucose analysis have been reported. However, most of these methods involve complex procedures or are expensive in terms of costs. Although there has been an intense research to develop a simple, sensitive, accurate, micro-volume and low-cost approach for glucose analysis, there is a need for further research before an appropriate device is accepted for rapid field tests and is also effective as an alternative to the existing methods.

17.7.2 Biosensors for glucose measuring

Glucose can be monitored by invasive and non-invasive technologies. Requirements of a sensor for in vivo glucose monitoring include miniaturization of the device, long-term stability, elimination of oxygen dependency, convenience to the user and biocompatibility. Long-term biocompatibility has been the main requirement and has limited the use of in vivo glucose sensors, both subcutaneously and intravascular, to short periods of time. Diffusion of low-molecular-weight substances from the sample across the polyurethane sensor outer membrane results in loss of sensor sensitivity.

One of the solutions to these is enzymatic approach, which used glucose oxidase (GOx) to measure intrinsic fluorescence of GOx [59–62]. In the late 1990s, researchers started to assess a glucose sensor, using the deactivated apo-GOx enzyme, which used the enzyme as a receptor rather than a catalyst [63]. Studies in this area showed that apo-GOx could retain its high specificity, after these investigations, new advances were made in the development of a new biosensor in 2000s [64–66]. One can also mention several receptors including glucose-binding lectins

[67, 68], apo-enzymes [69] and synthetic boronic acid receptors [70] have been employed for glucose detection. Fluorescence-based systems are receiving increasing attention given their high sensitivity. This system causes little or no damage to the host system and enables the measurement of fluorescence intensity as well as fluorescence decay times [71]. To date, there are reports on intrinsic fibre sensors that involve new material and measurements techniques [72, 73]. These are interesting progression towards new measurements devices for glucose measurement devices of the future.

17.8 Biosensors for cardiovascular diseases applications

17.8.1 Cardiovascular disease biomarkers

CVD are highly preventable, yet they are major cause of death of humans over the world. One of the most important reasons of the increasing incidences of CVD and cardiac arrest is hypercholesterolemia, i.e. increased concentration of cholesterol in blood [74, 75]. Hence estimation of cholesterol level in blood is important in clinical applications. The early evaluation of patients with symptoms that indicates an acute coronary syndrome is of great clinical relevance.

Biomarkers have become increasingly important in this setting to supplement electrocardiographic findings and patient history because one or both can be misleading [76–81]. Cardiac troponin is the only marker used routinely nowadays in this setting because it is specific from the myocardial tissue, easily detected and useful for therapeutic decision-making [82]. Determination of the level of other non-myocardial tissue-specific markers might also be helpful, such as myeloperoxidase [83], copeptin [84], growth differentiation factor-15 [85] and C-reactive protein (CRP) [86–88]. The protein CRP, which reflects different aspects of the development of atherosclerosis or acute ischemia, is one of the plasma proteins known as acute-phase proteins and its levels rise dramatically during inflammatory processes occurring in the body. This increment is due to a rise in the plasma concentration of IL-6, which is produced predominantly by macrophages as well as adipocytes. CRP can rise as high as 1000-fold with inflammation. CRP was found to be the only marker of inflammation that independently predicts the risk of a heart attack, however, the detection level are much lower due to the inflammation and thus higher requirement for the sensitivity of the sensor.

17.8.2 Biosensors in cardiovascular disease

Biosensors for cholesterol measurement using fibre optic method was first published in 1990s [89, 90]. Although there is a lot of publication on other technologies rather than the FOBS [91], it is an ongoing research in the field of CVD and fibre optical biosensors [92].

The cardiac markers myoglobin [72] and cardiac troponin I (cTnI) are released from cardiac muscles when they are damaged, and therefore their concentrations can predict the occurrence of myocardial infarction. A fibre-optic SPR sensor to detect markers of MG and cTnI at 3 ng/mL was reported by Masson *et al.* [93]. A direct fluorescence FOBS was also used to detect myoglobin [94]. Cascade Blue-labelled antibody was entrapped in the sensing element. Fluorescence quenching occurred when myoglobin bound to labelled antibody. Using this method, myoglobin was detected at 5 nM. Another study by Tang *et al.* [95] has developed a fibre-optic multi-analyte system which simultaneously quantifies the above two groups of multi-biomarkers related to CVD: anticoagulants (protein C, protein S, antithrombin III and plasminogen) for deficiency diagnosis; and cardiac markers (B-type natriuretic peptide, cardiac troponin I, myoglobin and C-reactive protein) for coronary heart disease diagnosis.

17.9 Biosensors for cancer applications

17.9.1 Cancer biomarkers

Cancer is the leading cause of death in economically developed countries and the second leading cause of death in developing countries. This disease continues to increase globally largely because of the aging and growth of the world population alongside an increasing adoption of cancer-causing behaviours, particularly smoking. Breast cancer is the most frequently diagnosed cancer and the leading cause of cancer death among females and lung cancer is the leading cancer site in males. Breast cancer is now also the leading cause of cancer death among females in economically developing countries, a shift from the previous decade during which the most common cause of cancer death was cervical cancer [96]. Solid cancers are a leading cause of morbidity and mortality worldwide, primarily due to the failure of effective clinical detection and treatment of metastatic disease in distant sites [97, 98]. Cancer can be caused by a range of factors, both genetic and environmental. Chemical, physical and biological factors such as the exposure to carcinogenic chemicals, radiation, bacterial (e.g., stomach cancer), viral infections (e.g., cervical cancer) and toxins (aflatoxin; e.g., liver cancer) can lead to cancer development [99].

As the causes of cancer are so diverse, clinical testing is also very complex. The multi-factorial changes (genetic and epigenetic) can cause the onset of the disease and the formation of cancer cells. However, no single gene is universally altered during this process, but a set of them that brings difficulties to the correct disease diagnosis. All the changes that take place, in the tumours from different locations (organ), as well within tumours from the same location, can be so variable and overlapping that it is difficult to select a specific change or marker for the diagnosis of specific cancers. Therefore, a range of biomarkers can potentially be analysed for disease diagnosis. These biomarkers or molecular signatures can be produced either by the tumour itself or by the body in response to the presence of cancer [100].

The analysis of biomarkers in body fluids such as blood, urine and others is one of the methods applied in the detection of the disease [101]. Multi-marker profiles, both presence and concentration level, can be essential for the diagnosis of early disease onset. These methods should provide information to assist clinicians in making successful treatment decisions and increasing patient survival rate [102]. A range of biomarkers has been identified with different types of cancers. These include DNA modifications, RNA, proteins (enzymes and glycoproteins), hormones and related molecules, molecules of the immune system, oncogenes and other modified molecules [103]. Petricoin *et al.* reported that the blood peptidome provides a higher dimension of information content for cancer biomarker discovery [104]. Several biomarkers are currently being studied; however, few of them can have routine cancer clinical testing importance because of their complexity.

17.9.2 Biosensors in cancer disease

Existing methods of screening for cancer are heavily based on cell morphology using staining and microscopy, which are invasive techniques. Furthermore, tissue removal can miss cancer cells at the early onset of the disease. Biosensor-based detection becomes practical and advantageous for cancer clinical testing, since it is faster, more user-friendly, less expensive and less technically demanding than microarray or proteomic analyses. However, significant technical development is still needed, particularly for protein based biosensors.

Many commercially available platforms use fluorescence labels as the detection system. However, the instruments used for signal readout are usually expensive and are more suitable for laboratory settings. As an example, the Affymetrix gene chip (Affymetrix Inc., Santa Clara, USA) can be used for screening cancer and cancer gene identification. Other biosensor platforms such as grating couplers, resonant mirrors and surface plasmon-based systems have also been used for cancer biomarkers diagnosis. These are classified as label-free and real-time affinity reaction detection systems. Recently, different fibre optical SPR-based biosensors have been developed for cancer markers detection based on the above optical systems [102, 105].

In spite of the achieved development in cancer biosensing, the point-of-care testing is not yet available. In order to achieve this goal challenges must be overcome such as: development of reproducible biomarker assays; improvement in recognition ligands; development of multi-channel biosensors; advances in sample preparation; development of more sensitive transducers; advanced manufacturing techniques; and cost reduction [106].

17.10 Conclusions

Optical fibre biosensors have advanced substantially in recent years. Some fibre-optic biosensors are ready to progress from the research bench to field applications. However, due to the scarcity of commercially available biosensors, overcoming the technical, regulatory and market obstacles is not a trivial matter. Hence, to be successful, all fibre optical biosensor based devices must possess the following characteristics: low detection limits, low cost, simplicity of design and operation, reliability, accuracy, ruggedness, low detection time of analyte, ease of calibration and some degree of reversibility. These devices should be capable of continuous-flow measurements, minimal operator attendance and the determination of multiple analytes. Furthermore, they must compete with other field analytical methods, such as chemical sensors, immunoassays and chemical test kits as well as conventional laboratory techniques. Therefore, fibre optical biosensors should offer new capabilities or significant improvements over existing methods to be successful in an increasingly competitive marketplace. Some of the obstacles common to all field analytical methods include the diversity of compounds and the complexity of matrices in samples, the variability in data quality requirements and the broad range of possible monitoring applications. More specific to optical fibre biosensor technology, the following hurdles have to be tackled in the future: immobilization stability, relatively high development costs for single analyte systems, limited shelf and operational lifetimes for pre-manufactured biorecognition components [107].

There are still more research needed for the development of more robust biomolecules and biomimic receptors that can be used as bioreceptors for sensor design. Validation is still a workhorse in this area and is a crucial issue in development and integration of these devices in monitoring and diagnostic applications.

References

[1] Schaffar BP, Wolfbeis OS. Chemically mediated fiberoptic biosensors. *Bioprocess Technol.* 1991; 15: 163–94.

[2] Grattan KTV, Sun T. Fiber optic sensor technology: an overview. *Sensor Actuat A: Phys.* 2000;82(1–3):40–61.

[3] Peterson JI, Vurek GG. Fiber-optic sensors for biomedical applications. *Science.* 1984;224(4645):123–7.

[4] Thevenot DR, Toth K, Durst RA, Wilson GS. Electrochemical biosensors: recommended definitions and classification – (Technical Report). *Pure Appl Chem.* 1999;71(12):2333–48.

[5] Biran I, Yu X, Walt DR. Optrode-based fiber optic biosensors (bio-optrode). In: Ligler FS, Taitt CR (editors). *Optical Biosensors* (Second Edition). Amsterdam: Elsevier; 2008. p. 3–11.

[6] Griffin GD, Stratis-Cullum DN, McKnight TE. Biosensors. Reference Module in Biomedical Sciences: Elsevier; 2014, ISBN 9780128012383, An update of Griffin GD, Stratis-Cullum DN, Biosensors, Encyclopedia of Microbiology (Third Edition). 2009 (3.ed.). p. 88–103.

[7] Kepler J. Ioannis Kepleri Sae. Cae. Mtis. mathematici Dioptrice seu Demonstratio eorum quae visui & visibilibus propter conspicilla non ita pridem inventa accidunt: praemissae epistolae Galilaei de ijs, quae post editionem Nuncij siderij ope perspicilli, nova & admiranda in coelo deprehensa sunt: examen praefationis Ioannis Penae Galli in Optica Euclidis, de usu optices in philosophia. Augustae Vindelicorum: Typis Davidis Franci; 1611. 4, 28, 80, 4 p. p.

[8] Smith AW. John Tyndall (1820–1893). *The Scientific Monthly* 1920;11(4): 331–340.

[9] Surhone LM, Timpledon MT, Marseken SF. Snell's Law: Optics, Physics, Angle of Incidence, Refraction, Isotropy, Metamaterial, Refractive Index, Willebrord Snellius, Velocity, Ptolemy, Thebaid. Betascript Publishing; 2010.

[10] Yablon AD. Optical Fiber Fusion Splicing: Springer; 2005.

[11] Zhang C, Zhang Z, Song J, Wu C, Song N. Parameter optimization of fusion splicing of photonic crystal fibers and conventional fibers to increase strength. *Opt Fiber Technol.* 2015;22:102–6.

[12] Mendez A, Morse TF. Specialty Optical Fibers Handbook: Elsevier Science; 2011.

[13] Pollock CR. Fundamentals of Optoelectronics: Irwin; 1995.

[14] Villatoro J, Monzón-Hernández D, Mejía E. Fabrication and modeling of uniform-waist single-mode tapered optical fiber sensors. *Appl Opt.* 2003; 42(13):2278–83.

[15] Leung A, Shankar PM, Mutharasan R. A review of fiber-optic biosensors. *Sensor Actuat B: Chem.* 2007;125(2):688–703.

[16] Gannot I, Engineers SoP-oI. Optical Fibers and Sensors for Medical Applications: SPIE; 2005.

[17] Leung A, Rijal K, Shankar PM, Mutharasan R. Effects of geometry on transmission and sensing potential of tapered fiber sensors. *Biosens Bioelectron.* 2006;21(12):2202–9.

[18] Hale ZM, Payne FP, Marks RS, Lowe CR, Levine MM. The single mode tapered optical fibre loop immunosensor. *Biosens Bioelectron.* 1996; 11(1–2):137–48.

[19] Khijwania SK, Gupta BD. Fiber optic evanescent field absorption sensor: effect of fiber parameters and geometry of the probe. *Optic Quant Electron.* 1999;31(8):625–36.

[20] Khijwania SK, Gupta BD. Maximum achievable sensitivity of the fiber optic evanescent field absorption sensor based on the U-shaped probe. *Optic Communicat.* 2000;175(1–3):135–7.

[21] Khijwania SK, Srinivasan KL, Singh JP. An evanescent-wave optical fiber relative humidity sensor with enhanced sensitivity. *Sensor Actuat B: Chem.* 2005;104(2):217–22.

[22] Littlejohn D, Lucas D, Han L. Bent silica fiber evanescent absorption sensors for near-infrared spectroscopy. *Appl Spectrosc.* 1999;53(7):845–9.

[23] Díaz-Herrera N, Navarrete MC, Esteban O, González-Cano A. A fibre-optic temperature sensor based on the deposition of a thermochromic material on an adiabatic taper. *Measure Sci Technol.* 2004;15(2):353.

[24] Grazia A, Riccardo M, Ciaccheri FL. Evanescent wave absorption spectroscopy by means of bi-tapered multimode optical fibers. *Appl Spectrosc.* 1998;52(4):546–51.

[25] Guo S, Albin S. Transmission property and evanescent wave absorption of cladded multimode fiber tapers. *Opt Express.* 2003;11(3):215–23.

[26] Pendock GJ, MacKenzie HS, Payne FP. Dye lasers using tapered optical fibers. *Appl Opt*. 1993;32(27):5236–42.

[27] Villatoro J, Luna-Moreno D, Monzón-Hernández D. Optical fiber hydrogen sensor for concentrations below the lower explosive limit. *Sensor Actuat B: Chem*. 2005;110(1):23–7.

[28] Yang M, Dai J. Fiber optic hydrogen sensors: a review. *Photonic Sens*. 2014;4(4):300–24.

[29] Ahmad M, Hench LL. Effect of taper geometries and launch angle on evanescent wave penetration depth in optical fibers. *Biosens Bioelectron*. 2005;20(7):1312–9.

[30] Moar PN, Huntington ST, Katsifolis J, Cahill LW, Roberts A, Nugent KA. Fabrication, modeling, and direct evanescent field measurement of tapered optical fiber sensors. *J Appl Phys*. 1999;85(7):3395–8.

[31] Messica A, Greenstein A, Katzir A. Theory of fiber-optic, evanescent-wave spectroscopy and sensors. *Appl Opt*. 1996;35(13):2274–84.

[32] Ghatak A, Thyagarajan K. An Introduction to Fiber Optics: Cambridge University Press; 1998.

[33] Golden JP, Anderson GP, Rabbany SY, Ligler FS. An evanescent wave biosensor–Part II: fluorescent signal acquisition from tapered fiber optic probes. *IEEE Trans Biomed Eng*. 1994;41(6):585–91.

[34] Marazuela D, Moreno-Bondi MC. Fiber-optic biosensors–an overview. *Anal Bioanal Chem*. 2002;372(5–6):664–82.

[35] Sassolas A, Blum LJ, Leca-Bouvier BD. Immobilization strategies to develop enzymatic biosensors. *Biotechnol Adv*. 2012;30(3):489–511.

[36] Monk DJ, Walt DR. Optical fiber-based biosensors. *Anal Bioanal Chem*. 2004;379(7–8):931–45.

[37] Aga DS, Thurman E. Environmental immunoassays: alternative techniques for soil and water analysis. *Immun. Tech. for Env. Appl*. 1997;5: 1–20.

[38] Wang J, Rivas G, Cai X, *et al.* DNA electrochemical biosensors for environmental monitoring. A review. *Anal Chim Acta*. 1997;347(1–2):1–8.

[39] Mehrvar M, Bis C, Scharer JM, Young MM, Luong JH. Fiber-optic biosensors-trends and advances. *Anal Sci*. 2000;16(7):677–92.

[40] Eggins BR. Biosensors: An Introduction: Vieweg+Teubner Verlag; 2013.

[41] Masel RI. Principles of Adsorption and Reaction on Solid Surfaces: Wiley; 1996.

[42] Agayn VI, Walt DR (editors). Fiber Optic Sensor Based on Micro-encapsulated Reagents, *Proc. SPIE. Int. Soc. Eng*. 1993; 1797(1):92–5.

[43] Cosnier S, Szunerits S, Marks RS, *et al.* A rapid and easy procedure of biosensor fabrication by micro-encapsulation of enzyme in hydrophilic synthetic latex films. Application to the amperometric determination of glucose. *Electrochem Commun*. 2000;2(12):851–5.

[44] Treloar P, Higson SJ, Desai M, *et al.* Ex-vivo sensors; microencapsulation of enzyme layer in biosensors. In: Guilbault G, Mascini M (editors). *Uses of Immobilized Biological Compounds*. NATO ASI Series. 252. The Netherlands: Springer; 1993. p. 131–40.

[45] Malhotra BD, Chaubey A. Biosensors for clinical diagnostics industry. *Sensor Actuat B: Chem*. 2003;91(1–3):117–27.
[46] Zaitoun MA. Glucose biosensor based on entrapment of glucose oxidase and myoglobin in silica gel by the sol-gel method. *Spectroscopy*. 2005;19(2).
[47] Bidmanova S, Chaloupkova R, Damborsky J, Prokop Z. Development of an enzymatic fiber-optic biosensor for detection of halogenated hydrocarbons. *Anal Bioanal Chem*. 2010;398(5):1891–8.
[48] Sakka S. Sol–Gel Process and Applications. In: Somiya S (editor). *Handbook of Advanced Ceramics* (Second Edition). Oxford: Academic Press; 2013. p. 883–910.
[49] Deshpande DC, Arkansas Uo. Development of a Nanowire Based Titanium Needle Probe Sensor for Glucose Monitoring: University of Arkansas; 2009.
[50] Wise DL. Bioinstrumentation and Biosensors: Taylor & Francis; 1991.
[51] Lakowicz JR. Quenching of Fluorescence. In: Lakowicz J (editor). *Principles of Fluorescence Spectroscopy*. US: Springer; 2006. p. 277–330.
[52] Zhuang X, Ha T, Kim HD, Centner T, Labeit S, Chu S. Fluorescence quenching: a tool for single-molecule protein-folding study. *Proc Nat Acad Sci*. 2000;97(26):14241–4.
[53] Kress-Rogers E. Handbook of Biosensors and Electronic Noses: Medicine, Food, and the Environment: Taylor & Francis; 1996.
[54] Villatoro J, Diez A, Cruz JL, Andres MV. In-line highly sensitive hydrogen sensor based on palladium-coated single-mode tapered fibers. *Sensor J IEEE*. 2003;3(4):533–7.
[55] Sharma AK, Gupta BD. On the sensitivity and signal to noise ratio of a step-index fiber optic surface plasmon resonance sensor with bimetallic layers. *Optic Commun*. 2005;245(1–6):159–69.
[56] Lasker RD. The diabetes control and complications trial. Implications for policy and practice. *N Engl J Med*. 1993;329(14):1035–6.
[57] Turner AP, Pickup JC. Diabetes mellitus: biosensors for research and management. *Biosensors*. 1985;1(1):85–115.
[58] Clark MJ, Jr., Sterrett JJ, Carson DS. Diabetes guidelines: a summary and comparison of the recommendations of the American Diabetes Association, Veterans Health Administration, and American Association of Clinical Endocrinologists. *Clin Ther*. 2000;22(8):899–910; discussion 898.
[59] Li L, Walt DR. Dual-analyte fiber-optic sensor for the simultaneous and continuous measurement of glucose and oxygen. *Anal Chem*. 1995;67(20): 3746–52.
[60] Trettnak W, Leiner MJ, Wolfbeis OS. Optical sensors. Part 34. Fibre optic glucose biosensor with an oxygen optrode as the transducer. *Analyst*. 1988;113(10):1519–23.
[61] Wolfbeis OS. Fiber-optic chemical sensors and biosensors. *Anal Chem*. 2002;74(12):2663–77.

[62] Wolfbeis OS, Durkop A, Wu M, Lin Z. A europium-ion-based luminescent sensing probe for hydrogen peroxide. *Angew Chem Int Ed Engl.* 2002; 41(23):4495–8.
[63] D'Auria S, Herman P, Rossi M, Lakowicz JR. The fluorescence emission of the apo-glucose oxidase from Aspergillus niger as probe to estimate glucose concentrations. *Biochem Biophys Res Commun.* 1999;263(2):550–3.
[64] Chinnayelka S, McShane MJ. Glucose-sensitive nanoassemblies comprising affinity-binding complexes trapped in fuzzy microshells. *J Fluoresc.* 2004;14(5):585–95.
[65] Chinnayelka S, McShane MJ. Microcapsule biosensors using competitive binding resonance energy transfer assays based on apoenzymes. *Anal Chem.* 2005;77(17):5501–11.
[66] Mack AC, Jinshu M, McShane MJ (editors). Transduction of pH and glucose-sensitive hydrogel swelling through fluorescence resonance energy transfer. *Sensors*, 2005 IEEE; 2005 Oct. 30 2005–Nov. 3 2005.
[67] Ballerstadt R, Gowda A, McNichols R. Fluorescence resonance energy transfer-based near-infrared fluorescence sensor for glucose monitoring. *Diabetes Technol Ther.* 2004;6(2):191–200.
[68] Ballerstadt R, Polak A, Beuhler A, Frye J. In vitro long-term performance study of a near-infrared fluorescence affinity sensor for glucose monitoring. *Biosens Bioelectron.* 2004;19(8):905–14.
[69] Chinnayelka S, McShane MJ. RET nanobiosensors using affinity of an apo-enzyme toward its substrate. *Conf Proc IEEE Eng Med Biol Soc.* 2004;4:2599–602.
[70] Moschou E, Sharma B, Deo S, Daunert S. Fluorescence glucose detection: advances toward the ideal in vivo biosensor. *J Fluores.* 2004;14(5): 535–47.
[71] Wolfbeis OS, Klimant I, Werner T, *et al.* Set of luminescence decay time based chemical sensors for clinical applications. *Sensor Actuat B: Chem.* 1998;51(1–3):17–24.
[72] Pahurkar VG, Tamgadge YS, Gambhire AB, Muley GG. Glucose oxidase immobilized PANI cladding modified fiber optic intrinsic biosensor for detection of glucose. *Sensor Actuat B: Chem.* 2015;210:362–8.
[73] Li D, Wu J, Wu P, *et al.* Affinity based glucose measurement using fiber optic surface plasmon resonance sensor with surface modification by borate polymer. *Sensor Actuat B: Chem.* 2015;213:295–304.
[74] Bonow RO. Prevention of cardiovascular disease: challenges and opportunities. *Ital Heart J.* 2004;5 Suppl 6:6S–8S.
[75] Franco M, Cooper RS, Bilal U, Fuster V. Challenges and opportunities for cardiovascular disease prevention. *Am J Med.* 2011;124(2):95–102.
[76] Averna M, Noto D. Clinical utility of novel biomarkers for cardiovascular disease risk stratification. *Intern Emerg Med.* 2012;7 Suppl 3: S263–70.
[77] Ge Y, Wang TJ. Identifying novel biomarkers for cardiovascular disease risk prediction. *J Intern Med.* 2012;272(5):430–9.

[78] Razzouk L, Fusaro M, Esquitin R. Novel biomarkers for risk stratification and identification of life-threatening cardiovascular disease: troponin and beyond. *Curr Cardiol Rev*. 2012;8(2):109–15.

[79] Siasos G. Editorial: Novel inflammatory biomarkers in cardiovascular disease: from molecular mechanisms to therapeutic targets. *Curr Med Chem*. 2015;22(23):2713–5.

[80] Stratz C, Amann M, Berg DD, Morrow DA, Neumann FJ, Hochholzer W. Novel biomarkers in cardiovascular disease: research tools or ready for personalized medicine? *Cardiol Rev*. 2012;20(3):111–17.

[81] Tousoulis D. Novel biomarkers in the prognosis, progression and treatment of cardiovascular disease: the role of microRNAs. *Curr Top Med Chem*. 2013;13(13):1491–2.

[82] Abdolrahim M, Rabiee M, Alhosseini SN, Tahriri M, Yazdanpanah S, Tayebi L. Development of optical biosensor technologies for cardiac troponin recognition. *Anal Biochem*. 2015;485:1–10.

[83] Schindhelm RK, van der Zwan LP, Teerlink T, Scheffer PG. Myeloperoxidase: a useful biomarker for cardiovascular disease risk stratification? *Clin Chem*. 2009;55(8):1462–70.

[84] Giannopoulos G, Deftereos S, Panagopoulou V, *et al.* Copeptin as a biomarker in cardiac disease. *Curr Top Med Chem*. 2013;13(2):231–40.

[85] Kempf T, von Haehling S, Peter T, *et al.* Prognostic utility of growth differentiation factor-15 in patients with chronic heart failure. *J Am Coll Cardiol*. 2007;50(11):1054–60.

[86] Piciu A, Piciu D, Marlowe RJ, Irimie A. Highly-sensitive C-reactive protein, a biomarker of cardiovascular disease risk, in radically-treated differentiated thyroid carcinoma patients after repeated thyroid hormone withholding. *Exp Clin Endocrinol Diabetes*. 2013;121(2):102–8.

[87] Shrestha R, Gyawali P. High sensitivity C-reactive protein: emerging biomarker for primary prevention of cardiovascular disease. *JNMA J Nepal Med Assoc*. 2010;49(179):263.

[88] Willcox BJ, Abbott RD, Yano K, Rodriguez BL, Willcox DC, Curb JD. C-reactive protein, cardiovascular disease and stroke: new roles for an old biomarker. *Expert Rev Neurother*. 2004;4(3):507–18.

[89] Marazuela MD, Cuesta B, Moreno-Bondi MC, Quejido A. Free cholesterol fiber-optic biosensor for serum samples with simplex optimization. *Biosens Bioelectron*. 1997;12(3):233–40.

[90] Trettnak W, Wolfbeis OS. A fiberoptic cholesterol biosensor with an oxygen optrode as the transducer. *Anal Biochem*. 1990;184(1):124–7.

[91] Qureshi A, Gurbuz Y, Niazi JH. Biosensors for cardiac biomarkers detection: a review. *Sensor Actuat B: Chem*. 2012;171–172:62–76.

[92] Wang B, Huang J, Li M, Zhou X (editors). Multifunctional sensing film used for fiber optic cholesterol sensor. 2008;23:72780Q.

[93] Masson JF, Obando L, Beaudoin S, Booksh K. Sensitive and real-time fiber-optic-based surface plasmon resonance sensors for myoglobin and cardiac troponin I. *Talanta*. 2004;62(5):865–70.

[94] Hanbury CM, Miller WG, Harris RB. Fiber-optic immunosensor for measurement of myoglobin. *Clin Chem*. 1997;43(11):2128–36.

[95] Tang L, Ren Y, Hong B, Kang KA. Fluorophore-mediated, fiber-optic, multi-analyte, immunosensing system for rapid diagnosis and prognosis of cardiovascular diseases. *J Biomed Opt*. 2006;11(2):021011.

[96] Jemal A, Bray F, Center MM, Ferlay J, Ward E, Forman D. Global cancer statistics. *CA Cancer J Clin*. 2011;61(2):69–90.

[97] Chambers AF, Groom AC, MacDonald IC. Dissemination and growth of cancer cells in metastatic sites. *Nat Rev Cancer*. 2002;2(8):563–72.

[98] Pantel K, Brakenhoff RH. Dissecting the metastatic cascade. *Nat Rev Cancer*. 2004;4(6):448–56.

[99] Vineis P, Schatzkin A, Potter JD. Models of carcinogenesis: an overview. *Carcinogenesis*. 2010;31(10):1703–9.

[100] Mishra A, Verma M. Cancer biomarkers: are we ready for the prime time? *Cancers*. 2010;2(1):190.

[101] Henry NL, Hayes DF. Cancer biomarkers. *Mol Oncol*. 2012;6(2):140–6.

[102] Tothill IE. Biosensors for cancer markers diagnosis. *Semin Cell Dev Biol*. 2009;20(1):55–62.

[103] Didenko VV. DNA probes using fluorescence resonance energy transfer (FRET): designs and applications. *BioTechniques*. 2001;31(5):1106–21.

[104] Petricoin EF, Belluco C, Araujo RP, Liotta LA. The blood peptidome: a higher dimension of information content for cancer biomarker discovery. *Nat Rev Cancer*. 2006;6(12):961–7.

[105] Francois A, Boehm J, Penno M, Hoffmann P, Monro TM (editors). A novel optical-fiber based surface plasmon resonance sensing architecture and its application to gastric cancer diagnostics. 2011;17:77536Y.

[106] Rasooly A, Jacobson J. Development of biosensors for cancer clinical testing. *Biosens Bioelectron*. 2006;21(10):1851–8.

[107] Gouvêa CMCP. Biosensors for health applications. Biosensors for Health, Environment and Biosecurity, *InTech*. 2011;3:71–86.

Chapter 18

Nanobiosensors for the detection of circulating tumor cells

Na Sun[1] and Renjun Pei[1]

18.1 Introduction

Metastasis is the cause of most cancer mortality. There is tremendous and urgent demand to diagnose cancer at an early stage. Circulating tumor cells (CTCs) are cancer cells shed from primary tumors into blood circulation, which are believed to initiate the spread of cancer [1–3]. Early detection of CTCs and analysis of their cell surface markers will provide critical information for the diagnosis of cancer and personalized therapy, as well as therapeutic efficacy monitoring [4–7]. However, the extremely rare number of CTCs, as few as one single CTC among a few million white blood cells (WBCs) and a few billion red blood cells (RBCs) in 1 mL of patient blood, makes the detection technically challenging. During the past decades, a number of approaches have been developed for CTC detection.

Early technologies developed for CTC detection and enumeration relied on tagging cells with magnetic nanoparticles displaying an antibody specific for the epithelial cell adhesion molecule (EpCAM), which is a marker present on the surfaces of many cancer cells. CellSearch system which uses this approach is the only commercial system approved by the U.S. Food and Drug Administration (FDA) for the detection of CTCs in patients with metastatic breast [8–10], colon [11] and prostate cancers [6]. While the analytical performance of CellSearch as assessed using cell lines is reasonable (with a reported analytical sensitivity of 1 CTC in a 7.5 mL sample), it typically identifies CTCs in the bloodstream for less than 50% of patients with metastatic cancer. As a result, it is primarily used only as a prognostic tool.

A microfluid platform called the "CTC-chip," which consists of an array of anti-EpCAM antibody-coated microposts, was reported to be capable of isolating CTCs with the mean capture yield of 60% as well as the purity of about 50% [12]. Work on advanced CTC capture systems based on microfluid platform or CTC-Chip has received widespread attention. Recently, a microfluidic inertial focusing

[1]Key Laboratory for Nano-Bio Interface, Division of Nanobiomedicine, Suzhou Institute of Nano-Tech and Nano-Bionics, Chinese Academy of Sciences, Suzhou 215123, China

platform, the iCTC chip, was reported with higher sensitivity which combines several types of separation [13]. It depletes smaller red blood cells and platelets in the first microfluidic stage using a mechanical filter. The system then allows CTCs and leukocytes to be sorted using either positive or negative selection via the attachment of magnetic microparticles to the remaining cells, and a magnetic field directs the cells to different isolation chambers. While the integration of microfluidics represents a dramatic change in the CTC detection, allowing for increased capture purity, yield, and sensitivity when compared to the CellSearch system, new techniques with much easier operation, higher efficiency and more affordable cost will be urgently required to further increase these metrics. These techniques can obtain pure and viable CTCs available for further downstream analysis.

With the development of nanotechnology and nanobiomedicine, it is well known that cells could sense and respond to the nanotopography of material. The importance of nanomaterials has been constantly tested with the exploration of the interaction between cells and the nanotopography of material. In the last decade, the nanostructured materials have been incorporated with CTC detecting devices, and the design of nanomaterials becomes the key to overcome current limitations associated with CTC capture and analysis. As there have been some pretty good reviews on nanostructured substrates for guiding cell behaviors [14] or CTC isolation [15, 16], here we will focus on the progress of the design of nanostructured interfaces for CTC biosensors in the past decades, and highlight the new explorations on isolation concepts based on nanostructured interfaces, in an attempt, to achieve available CTCs for accurate downstream detection and analysis.

18.2 Nanostructured interfaces designed for CTC detection

Cells' behaviors on nanostructured surfaces have been extensively explored, including cell adhesion, proliferation and differentiation [17]. Compared to flat surfaces, nanostructured substrates can provide a larger surface area for the immobilization of biomolecules, increasing the binding odds between the ligand and membrane receptor and also total binding force, thus enhancing CTC isolation efficiency. Moreover, the natural extracellular matrix or basement membrane mimicking nanostructured substrates offer a suitable environment for CTC attachment. So far, magnetic nanoparticles [18, 19], silicon nanopillars (NPs)/nanowires [20–24], carbon nanotubes [25], graphene oxide [26], nanoparticle surfaces [27–31], nanofibers [17, 32–34] and nanorough-featured surfaces [35–37] have been used as ultrasensitive platforms in CTC capture and detection.

18.2.1 From micro to nano

For the selection of nanomaterials, silicon nanomaterials are widely used for CTC study due to their silicon NPs biocompatibility and mature fabrication techniques. The effect of silicon NPs geometry of various diameters (120–1100 nm) and spacings (35–800 nm) on CTC-capture yield, cytomorphology and pseudopodia formation was investigated by Yuan Wan *et al.* [38]. The results showed that capture yield was linear to the effective contact area of the NP substrate. Dense NPs with smaller diameter yield a larger effective contact area, and thus were preferred. However, once the spacing between NPs was smaller than the size of a microvillus (<100 nm) or was too large (>800 nm), the cell capture yield and specificity were significantly impaired, respectively. The formation of either lamellipodia or filopodia correlating with adhesion status and elution strength was also confirmed. Specifically, under the same shear stress, lamellipodia were generally formed on NPs with high aspect ratio (>10) where the captured cells were firmly attached; furthermore, significant filopodia formation was observed on NPs with low aspect ratio where captured cells were more prone to detach, indicating filopodia might obtain a newly generated adhesive force to resist shear stress mediated detachment. These findings provide essential guidance in designing NP substrates for more efficient capture of CTCs and manipulation of cytomorphology in future.

Barcode particles, whose encoding information enables simple identification, are another class of attractive nanostructures in the field of multiple bioassays [39]. Zhongze Gu *et al.* [40] presented a new type of barcode particle with the ability to capture, detect and release multiple types of CTCs, as shown in Figure 18.1a. The particles are spherical colloidal crystal clusters decorated with dendrimer-amplified

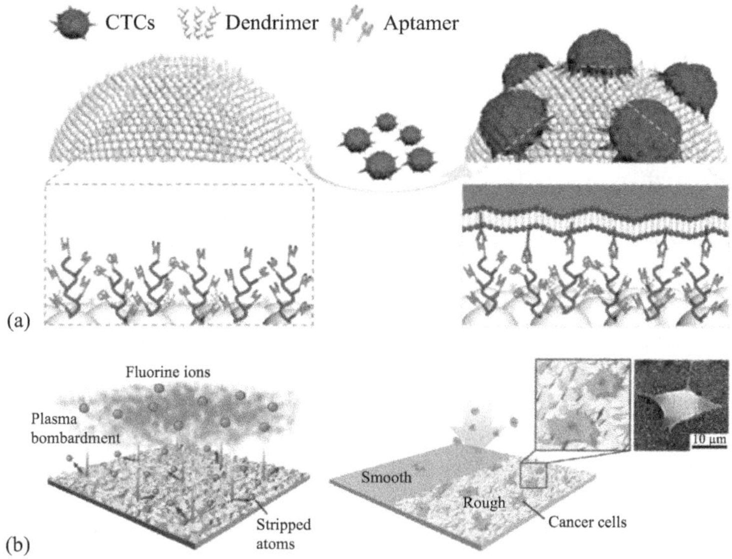

Figure 18.1 (a) Schematic of the barcode particles used for CTC capture; the surface of the barcode particles is decorated with dendrimer and DNA aptamers. Reprinted with permission from Reference 40, © 2014 John Wiley and Sons. (b) Schematic of nanotopography generated by RIE on glass surfaces. Insets show a zoom-in (left) and SEM (right) images of cancer cells captured on nanorough glass surfaces. Reprinted with permission from Reference 35, © 2013 American Chemical Society

aptamer probes. Their size can be adjusted to suit cell dimensions by their microfluidic-droplet templates. Encoding information in the particles is made possible by the characteristic reflection peaks originating from the photonic band gap (PBG) structure of the colloidal crystals, and thus they are very stable. The results showed that the capture specificities for the Ramos and CCRF-CEM cells were 98 ± 1.3% and 97 ± 1.8%, respectively, similar to the levels achieved with microfluidic cell-affinity chromatography devices. It was also demonstrated that the captured CTCs could be sorted accurately.

It is reported that the established interactions between cancer cell surface features and nanoscale structures may provide a possibility of capture without the use of a specific capture moiety. Weiqiang Chen *et al.* [35] exploited the selective adhesion of cancer cells to nanotextured surfaces when compared with blood cells by reactive ion etching (RIE) a glass surface for use in CTC capture. Random nanoroughness on glass surfaces was generated by using RIE, as shown in Figure 18.1b. The RIE-generated nanorough surfaces could efficiently capture different kinds of cancer cells (i.e., MCF-7, MDA-MB-231, Hela, PC3, SUM-149) without using any capture antibody, and the capture yield was increased with increased roughness (Ra, 1–150 nm). Capture yields of 88.7%–95.4% were achieved with nanorough glass surfaces (Ra = 150 nm) for both EpCAM+ MCF-7 and EpCAM- MDA-MB-231 cells, even at low cancer cell concentrations and for both PBMC and lysed blood samples. In spite of the lower capture yield of PBMCs compared to cancer cells by this uncoated nanorough glass surfaces, the purity of target cells was still unsatisfactory. Still, it is a promising strategy to achieve efficient capture at very low cost and is expected to lead to a better isolation and enrichment strategy for live CTCs from cancer patient's blood specimens.

Many nanomaterials, such as graphene, have been extensively employed to fabricate biosensing interfaces. An ultrasensitive and highly specific electrochemical and fluorescent immunosensing method for the detection of CTCs was achieved using a dual signal amplification strategy based on nanobiotechnology by Yuejun Kang *et al.* [30]. The introduction of graphene on the immunosensor surface efficiently accelerated the electron transfer and enhanced the detection signal. The second signal amplification came from the loading of QDs on the silica nanoparticle surface. After immunoreactions, two kinds of tracing tags were co-immobilized on the cell surface that could be conveniently detected by anodic stripping analysis and fluorescence microscopy. In addition, the regeneration of the immunosensor enables the elution and harvesting of the captured CTCs for further molecular analysis. The present immunosensor showed high sensitivity and specificity to detect low-abundance tumor cells with excellent stability, reproducibility and accuracy, indicating its wide potential applications for clinical diagnostics.

18.2.2 From artificial to biomimetic

Structure design is actually the first step to fabricate an ideal nanostructured interface for CTC detection. Experiences indicate that learning from natural biological systems is one of the best ways to design a functional interface. Seeking inspirations from cancer cells themselves as well as biological systems they live in is helpful to create advanced cell-material biointerfaces. Inspired by the topography features and topographical interactions of biological systems, many bio-inspired nanostructures have been created, such as nanofibers and nanofractals.

As the configuration of cell and cell's adhesion, migration, proliferation and differentiation were subject to the ECM, mimicking nanostructure of ECM has attracted great attentions. Inspired by its fiber-like nanostructure, many nanofiber nets have been fabricated for the related cell studies and applications. Considering the geometric orientation of nanostructures embedded in the ECM scaffolds, electrospun TiO_2 nanofibers mimic these horizontally oriented nanostructures that could lead to improved cell/substrate affinity [33]. Nangang Zhang *et al.* fabricated densely packed TiNFs with diameters of 100–300 nm on silicon wafers using electrospinning. The TiNF substrate grafted with anti-EpCAM exhibited more than 18 times of cell-capture yield than the flat Si substrate. On the contrary, relative low ratio of cell-capture yields (between TiNF and flat Si areas) were observed for EpCAM-negative cells (i.e., HeLa and K562), revealing that the horizontally packed TiNFs are sensitive and specific for capturing EpCAM-positive cells.

Shutao Wang's group has carried out plenty of work on fabricating biomimetic materials for CTC detection [24, 41–45]. Many studies have proved that the surface of cancer cells presents fractal morphology. Inspired by this, FAuNSs with controllable fractal dimensions using a one-step electrochemical deposition approach were fabricated by regulating the electrodepositing potential and the concentration of chloride ion [45]. After being coated with EpCAM antibody (anti-EpCAM), the FAuNS interfaces can improve the detection sensitivity by as much as 21 times for an EpCAM-positive cell line compared to the flat Au interface. In the following work, platelet-mimicking microspheres were fabricated by oxidative polymerization of polyaniline (PANi) nanohairs through transverse nano-channels in the shells of hollow polystyrene (PS) microspheres [46]. The micro/nano-hierarchical interface realized highly efficient rare cancer cell isolation from artificial whole blood with extremely low non-specific cell adhesion. This performance is a combination effect of molecule-scaled recognition and structure-scaled topographical interactions between platelet-mimicking microspheres and tumor cells. The high specificity and efficiency of this platelet-inspired multiscaled cytophilic interface can be utilized for the detection of CTCs toward point-of-care cancer diagnosis. Inspired by leukocytes, they have successfully prepared hierarchical biointerfaces for the efficient, specific recognition of cancer cells by the synergistic effect of molecular recognition and hierarchical topographical interaction [43].

In addition to structure mimicking, mimicking soft nature of cancer cells and their microenviroment is an important way to retain the maximum viability of captured CTCs. Therefore, polymer materials have attracted increasing attention which can better match with the soft nature of cells. However, "soft" nanostructures are limited from their fabrication techniques. Still, some polymers have been successfully employed to prepare different nanostructures for CTC detection, including PEDOT nanodots [47], PS nanotubes [41] and PLGA nanofibers [34].

18.2.3 From traditional to smart

Compared to other sensors, there may be one more important functional requirement for CTCs sensors. As the purity as well as viability of obtained CTCs is required for accurate downstream detection and analysis, effective isolation and purification of captured CTCs is one important step.

Special types of polymers called "stimuli-responsive" or "smart" polymers have emerged in recent years. The characteristic feature that makes them smart is their ability to respond to very slight changes in the environment such as temperature, pH, electric field, light or magnetic field.

The nanofiber webs fabricated from stimuli-responsive polymers are of considerable potential for use in filter fabrics, sensors, and electronic devices. The incorporation of stimuli-responsive polymers into nanoscale structures takes advantage of the extremely large surface area and porosity of nanofibers to generate a precise "on-off" switch to control the morphology and function of the nanofiber webs. Extension of these nanoscale effects to the macroscale enables manipulation of the bulk matter and creates the opportunity to develop profitable new applications. Poly(N-isopropylacrylamide) (pNIPAAm) is well known for its sharp conformational transition from expanded coil to compact globule as the temperature is changed around its lower critical solution temperature (LCST). So far, pNIPAAm and its derivatives have been widely used in the fabrication of temperature-responsive surface, films, capsules and hydrogels [48].

Takao Aoyagi *et al.* synthesized the photo-cross-linkable temperature-responsive polymer-based nanofiber webs with reversibly tunable web properties, including swelling/shrinking, mechanical strength, and porosity, as shown in Figure 18.2a [32]. They demonstrated the ability to capture, encapsulate and release cells by transforming the fibrous structure of the nanofiber into hydrogel-like structure by wrapping, swelling and deswelling processes in response to alternations of external temperature. This novel nanofiber enables the facile encapsulation and on-demand release of cells in response to external signals.

Hydrogels have the excellent capabilities of high water retention, tunable mechanical properties and facile exchange of biological metabolites or nutrients, and provide a 3D environment for cell encapsulation. However, the release of cells from hydrogel-based vehicles has mostly been governed by passive mechanisms involving material degradation and cell migration, neither of which allows for the dynamic manipulation of cells. Xiaogang Qu *et al.* developed a novel strategy for reversibly capturing and releasing cells using an NIR responsive graphene oxide-polymer hydrogel [26]. In this work, graphene oxide (GO) was incorporated into pNIPAAm to fabricate 3D NIR-responsive cell vehicles. The pNIPAAm derivative/GO hydrogel was prepared by introducing GO into a monomer solution followed with in situ free radical polymerization. The hydrogel can efficiently capture cells

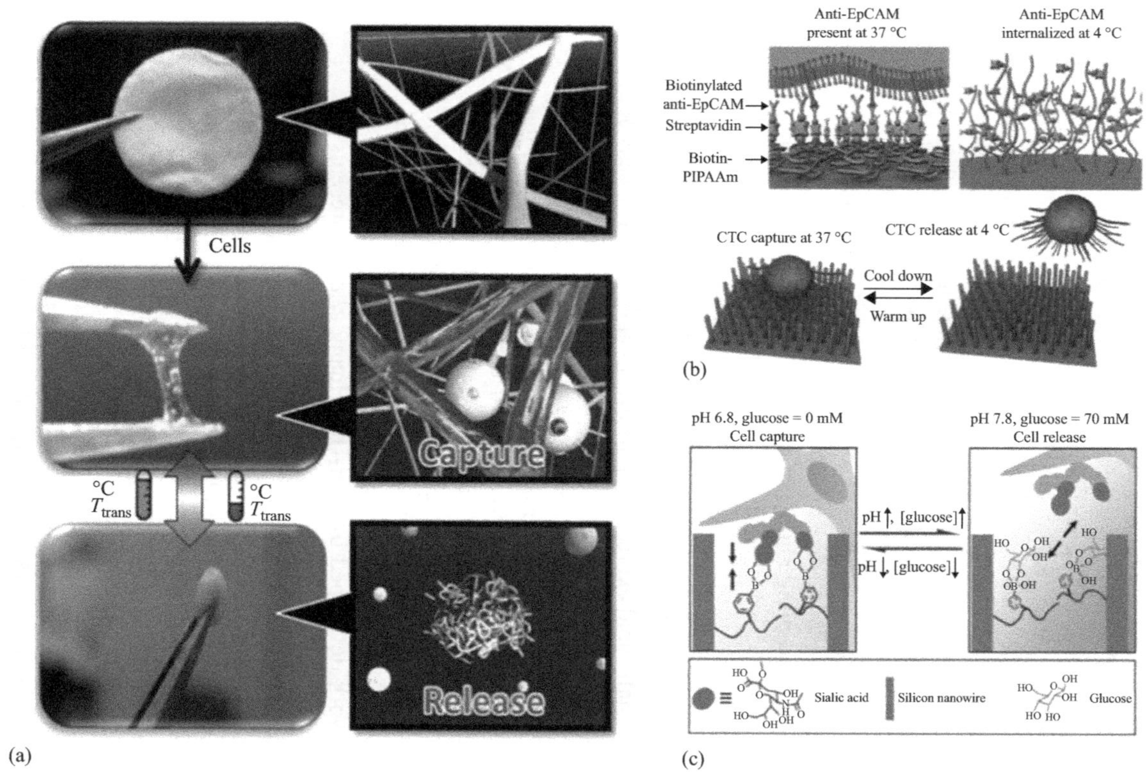

Figure 18.2 *(a) Facile capture and release of cells by using a nanofiber web that transforms from a fibrous to a hydrogel-like structure by wrapping, swelling, and shrinking processes in response to temperature changes. Reprinted with permission from Reference 32, © 2012 John Wiley and Sons. (b) Conceptual illustration of a new-generation nanomaterial-based platform for cell affinity assay capable of not only capturing CTCs with superb efficiency, but also releasing upon stimulating these captured CTCs at a reduced temperature. Reprinted with permission from Reference 50, © 2013 John Wiley and Sons. (c) Cell capture and release induced by pH and glucose. At pH 6.8 in the absence of glucose, the as-prepared surface captures targeted cells due to the specific binding between polyAAPBA brush on the surface and sialic acid existed in the membrane of the cells. By elevating the pH to 7.8 and increasing glucose concentration to 70 mM, competitive binding between tetrahedral anionic polyAAPBA and glucose leads to the release of targeted cells. Reprinted with permission from Reference 52, © 2013 American Chemical Society*

through the bioadhesive ligand RGD, and can also release the cells on demand on application of an NIR light stimulus, which can realize better dynamic control on cells than traditional passive cell depots.

Despite the smart polymers provide a pretty modest environment, the structure fabricating of which remains a challenge for improving capture efficiency of CTCs. Combining the "smart materials" with nanostructures to fabricate some functional biointerfaces is crucial for effective cell detection [49].

Thermo-responsive polymer was then employed to graft on silicon NPs to develop an innovative cell capture and release platform with integrated features of capture-agent directed specific recognition [50, 51]. This platform demonstrates superior performances in capturing cancer cells with high efficiency at 37 °C, and releasing the captured cancer cells with great viability and retained functionality at 4 °C, as shown in Figure 18.2b [50].

Superhydrophilic/superhydrophobic design of surfaces can dominate the effective detection of cancer cells. In Wang's report, superhydrophilic nanoroughness showed selectively absorbing ability to capture CTCs. They reported a pH and glucose dual responsive surface that can efficiently and rapidly switch between capture and release of targeted cancer cells by grafting a poly(acrylamidophenylboronic acid) (polyAAPBA) brush from aligned silicon nanowire (SiNW) array, as shown in Figure 18.2c [52]. PolyAAPBA brush on the SiNW array can form specific binding with sialic acid expressed in the membrane of MCF-7 cells at pH 6.8. With further addition of glucose, a stable complex between tetrahedral anionic polyAAPBA and glucose replaces the polyAAPBA/sialic acid complex, thus releasing the MCF-7 cells. When decreasing PH to 6.8 without glucose, the tetrahedral anionic polyAAPBA is dehydroxylated and can again form specific binding with sialic acid, thereby reversibly capturing targeted MCF-7 cells. In addition, amplified responsiveness and accelerated cell capture/release were observed on polyAAPBA-SiNW, owing to a three-dimensional (3D) contact mode between the SiNW array and the cell protrusions.

Another interesting work developed by Wei-Hua Huang *et al.* represents an additional promising choice for the capture and release of cancer cells [53]. In this work, they fabricated an anti-EpCAM functionalized nanobioprobe (anti-EpCAM-Alg-FMNB), which can be formed and decomposed reversibly to capture and release cancer cells. Ca^{2+}-initiated layer-by-layer (LBL) self-assembly was employed to deposit alginate coating on fluorescent-magnetic nanospheres (FMNS) to fabricate alginate-encapsulated FMNS (Alg-FMNS). The anti-EpCAM-Alg-FMNB can specifically capture EpCAM-positive SK-BR-3 cells but not EpCAM-negative Hela cells and WBCs, and even detect 10^2 spiked SK-BR-3 cells in 1 mL of whole blood with 86% efficiency, demonstrating the novel specificity and sensitivity of this nanobioprobe. Sixty-five percent of captured cells could be released if anti-EpCAM-Alg-FMNB were disintegrated by EDTA treatment. ROS assay, together with annexin V-FITC and PI-based fluorescent assays, showed that ~70% of the released cells maintained their viability and proliferation ability.

18.3 Purification and isolation strategy based on nanostructured interfaces

Nondestructive release of captured cells is now one of important problems urgently to be resolved. Achieving intact CTCs asks for more modest environment for CTC capture and release. Although smart materials that are responsive to light, electricity, compression, temperature and enzymes have been extensively studied to tackle this challenge, it is still challenging to realize highly efficient and specific cell release without sacrificing the structural and functional integrity of the target cells.

It is known that cell responses have been related to both specific (e.g., specific molecules or molecular structures) and nonspecific (e.g., hydrophilicity/hydrophobicity and charge) surface chemical properties. There has been some exploratory but inspiring works attempting to control specific cell release by introducing hydrogels onto the interface to design more modest and effective chemical composition of biointerfaces [54].

Yong Wang's group demonstrated a programmable DNA-responsive hydrogel for cell-type-specific catch and release controlled by nucleic acid hybridization, as shown in Figure 18.3a [55]. Importantly, the entire procedure of regulating the cell-hydrogel interactions does not involve factors destructive to either the cells or the hydrogel. Three single-stranded oligonucleotides are used in this programmable hydrogel-based system, including a primary complementary sequence (CS), a nucleic acid aptamer, and a secondary CS. The primary CS is initially conjugated to the supporting hydrogel through free radical polymerization. It is able to hybridize with the tail of the nucleic acid aptamer and therefore plays the role of a mediator between the hydrogel and the aptamer. An aptamer-functionalized PEG hydrogel was then studied for determining the feasibility of using nucleic acid aptamers to mimic the adhesive binding sites of extracellular matrix [56]. Nucleic acid aptamers can be successfully incorporated into the PEG hydrogel through free radical polymerization. In addition, aptamers can effectively induce cell type-specific adhesion to the PEG hydrogel. The level of cell adhesion can be altered by numerous parameters such as the aptamer concentration, the spacer length and the seeding time. Importantly, CS can block the binding functionality of aptamers in hydrogels and thereby attenuate cell adhesion in physiological conditions. The data presented in this study show that aptamer-functionalized hydrogels are promising biomaterials that can mimic the functions of extracellular matrices (e.g., providing cells with biochemical and biophysical cues).

The proliferation of the rare captured CTCs will be also a significant attempt for further molecular characterization and functional analysis. Nevertheless, few literatures on the culture of the isolated single CTC or rare number CTCs in conventional way have been reported [58–60]. Renjun Pei *et al.* utilized a novel strategy in recent study for further purification and proliferation of the rare number target cells through the following optimized in situ culture of captured cells inspired by "Survival of the fittest," as shown in Figure 18.3b [57]. In this work, a

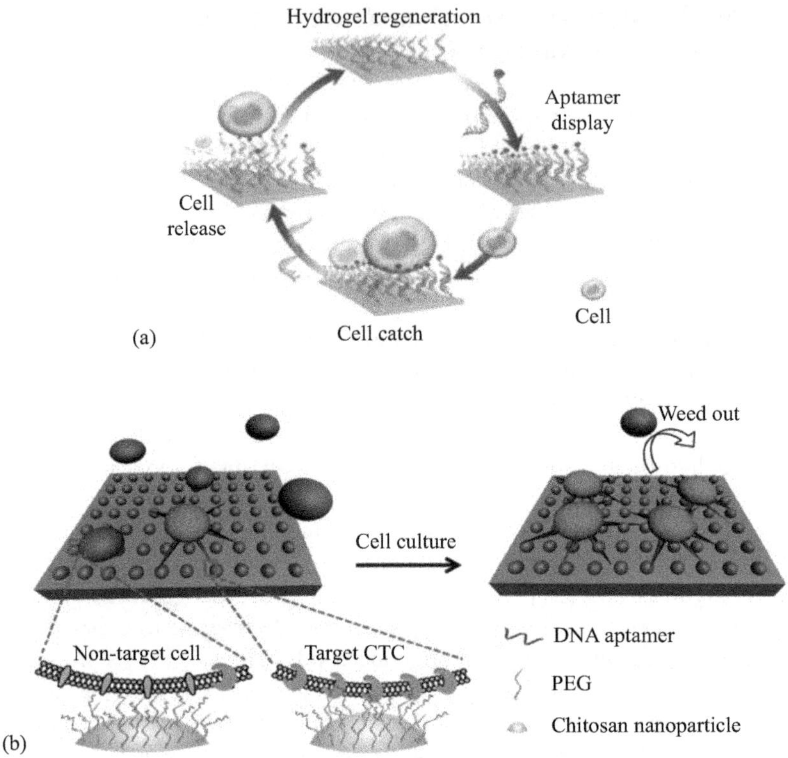

Figure 18.3 *(a) Cell catch and release during the transformation of the aptamer. The hybridization with the primary CS enables the display of the aptamer for cell catch. The secondary CS competes against the primary CS to hybridize and release the aptamer from the hydrogel, resulting in cell release. Reprinted with permission from Reference 55, © 2012 American Chemical Society. (b) Schematic of the chitosan nanoparticle substrate for rare number CTC isolation from non-target cells followed by the optimized in situ culture of captured cells. The in situ culture realized the proliferation of the rare number CTCs and simultaneously weeded out these captured non-target cells (e.g., WBCs) to obtain pure target CTCs for further analysis. Reprinted with permission from Reference 57, © 2015 John Wiley and Sons*

chitosan nanoparticle surface is firstly fabricated by electrospray to provide a cellular compatible interface. A bifunctional PEG employed as "anti-fouling" molecule was then linked onto the chitosan nanoparticle to improve the hydrophilicity of the surface to decrease non-target cell adhesion (e.g., 293T, CCRF-CEM, WBCs). On this basis, the "soft" substrate of chitosan nanoparticles achieved rather high capture efficiency for the isolation of target CTCs (e.g., MCF-7) from the mixed cells when conjugated with cell-specific DNA aptamer. Furthermore, a subsequent in situ culture strategy based on the developed cellular compatible soft interface is introduced for further purification and proliferation of the captured rare number target cells. The WBCs are weeded out after 2 days, and nearly 200 MCF-7 cells are obtained from 7 target cells and more than 90% purity is reached after a 7-day proliferation. This work provides a promising strategy for viable isolation and purification of rare CTCs and it has great potential for achieving clinical validity.

18.4 Conclusions and prospects

In this review, we have summarized the progress of the design of nanostructured interfaces for CTC biosensors in the past decades, and highlighted the new explorations on isolation concepts based on nanostructured interfaces, in an attempt, to achieve available CTCs for accurate downstream detection and analysis. CTC biosensors based on microfluidics have been studied for over several decades, which allow the precise flow control and parameter manipulation to achieve the purity, specificity and high recovery of CTCs from cancer patients. However, these technologies rely on microstructures, trapping arrays or microfilters, limiting further culture and downstream analysis.

Nanostructured substrates have emerged as an ultrasensitive platform in CTC isolation, and various fabrication techniques are now available for preparing different types of nanostructured substrates. The utilization of cell release techniques along with nanostructured substrates would help to enhance cell capture and release technologies. As such, the development of ultrasensitive platforms for CTC isolation based on nanomaterials requires more novel and proper molecular design on the interface to achieve the increased capture efficiency and sensitivity, non-destructive release as well as the culture of CTCs.

On the other hand, nanomaterials can be incorporated into microfluidic platforms, which will provide more room for the improvement of CTC biosensors. Recently, there have been some preliminary attempts to introduce nanomaterials into microfluidics, including magnetic nanoparticles [61–62], graphene oxide [63] and silicon pillars [64, 65]. Although further work is needed to refine the conditions, the extension of these platforms to conventional cell culture and intact cell release will be benefit to the further progress of CTC biosensors.

Acknowledgments

This work was financially supported by the National Natural Science Foundation of China (Nos. 21305154, 21275156), the Natural Science of Foundation of Jiangsu Province (No. BK20130351), the CAS Hundred Talents program and the CAS/SAFEA International Innovation Teams program.

References

[1] Steeg, P. S. Tumor metastasis: mechanistic insights and clinical challenges. *Nat. Med.* **2006**, *12*, 895.

[2] Steeg, P.; Dan Theodorescu, D. Metastasis: a therapeutic target for cancer. *Nat. Clin. Pract. Oncol.* **2008**, *5*, 206.

[3] Williams, S. C. Circulating tumor cells. *Proc. Natl. Acad. Sci.* **2013**, *110*, 4861.

[4] Budd, G. T.; Cristofanilli, M.; Ellis, M. J.; *et al.* Circulating tumor cells versus imaging-predicting overall survival in metastatic breast cancer. *Clin. Cancer Res.* **2006**, *12*, 6403.

[5] Cristofanilli, M.; Budd, G. T.; Ellis, M. J.; *et al.* Circulating tumor cells, disease progression, and survival in metastatic breast cancer. *New Engl. J. Med.* **2004**, *351*, 781.

[6] Olmos, D.; Arkenau, H. T.; Ang, J. E.; *et al.* Circulating tumour cell (CTC) counts as intermediate end points in castration-resistant prostate cancer (CRPC): a single-centre experience. *Ann. Oncol.* **2009**, *20*, 27.

[7] Paterlini-Brechot, P.; Benali, N. L. Circulating tumor cells (CTC) detection: clinical impact and future directions. *Cancer Lett.* **2007**, *253*, 180.

[8] Allard, W. J.; Matera, J.; Miller, M. C. Tumor cells circulate in the peripheral blood of all major carcinomas but not in healthy subjects or patients with nonmalignant diseases. *Clin. Cancer Res.* **2004**, *10*, 6897.

[9] Cristofanilli, M.; Hayes, D. F.; Budd, G. T.; *et al.* Circulating tumor cells: a novel prognostic factor for newly diagnosed metastatic breast cancer. *J. Clin. Oncol.* **2005**, *23*, 1420.

[10] Riethdorf, S.; Fritsche, H.; Muller, V.; *et al.* Detection of circulating tumor cells in peripheral blood of patients with metastatic breast cancer: a validation study of the CellSearch system. *Clin. Cancer Res.* **2007**, *13*, 920.

[11] Cohen, S. J.; Punt, C. J.; Iannotti, N.; *et al.* Prognostic significance of circulating tumor cells in patients with metastatic colorectal cancer. *Ann. Oncol.* **2009**, *20*, 1223.

[12] Nagrath, S.; Sequist, L. V.; Maheswaran, S.; *et al.*. Isolation of rare circulating tumour cells in cancer patients by microchip technology. *Nature* **2007**, *450*, 1235.

[13] Karabacak, N. M.; Spuhler, P. S.; Fachin, F.; *et al.* Microfluidic, marker-free isolation of circulating tumor cells from blood samples. *Nat. Protoc.* **2014**, *9*, 694.

[14] Liu, X.; Wang, S. Three-dimensional nano-biointerface as a new platform for guiding cell fate. *Chem. Soc. Rev.* **2014**, *43*, 2385.

[15] Wang, L.; Asghar, W.; Demirci, U.; Wan, Y. Nanostructured substrates for isolation of circulating tumor cells. *Nano Today.* **2013**, *8*, 374.

[16] Yoon, H.; Kozminsky, M.; Nagrath, S. Emerging role of nanomaterials in circulating tumor cell isolation and analysis. *ACS Nano.* **2014**, *8*, 1995.

[17] Bettinger, C. J.; Langer, R.; Borenstein, J. T. Engineering substrate topography at the micro- and nanoscale to control cell function. *Angewandte Chemie International Edition* **2009**, *48*, 5406.

[18] Wen, C.; Wu, L.; Zhang, Z.; *et al.* Quick-response magnetic nanospheres for rapid, efficient capture and sensitive detection of circulating tumor cells. *ACS Nano.* **2014**, *8*, 941.

[19] Guo, S.; Chen, Y.-Q.; Lu, N.-N.; Wang, X.-Y.; Xie, M.; Sui, W.-P. Ultrasonication-assisted one-step self-assembly preparation of biocompatible fluorescent-magnetic nanobeads for rare cancer cell detection. *Nanotechnology.* **2014**, *25*, 505603.

[20] Lee, S. K.; Kim, D. J.; Lee, G.; Kim, G. S.; Kwak, M.; Fan, R. Specific rare cell capture using micro-patterned silicon nanowire platform. *Biosens. Bioelectron.* **2014**, *54*, 181.

[21] Shen, Q.; Xu, L.; Zhao, L.; *et al.* Specific capture and release of circulating tumor cells using aptamer-modified nanosubstrates. *Adv. Mater.* **2013**, *25*, 2368.

[22] Wang, S.; Wang, H.; Jiao, J.; *et al.* Three-dimensional nanostructured substrates toward efficient capture of circulating tumor cells. *Angew. Chem. Int. Ed.* **2009**, *48*, 8970.

[23] Gach, P. C.; Attayek, P. J.; Whittlesey, R. L.; Yeh, J. J.; Allbritton, N. L. Micropallet arrays for the capture, isolation and culture of circulating tumor cells from whole blood of mice engrafted with primary human pancreatic adenocarcinoma. *Biosens. Bioelectron.* **2014**, *54*, 476.

[24] Lee, S. K.; Kim, G. S.; Wu, Y.; *et al.* Nanowire substrate-based laser scanning cytometry for quantitation of circulating tumor cells. *Nano Lett.* **2012**, *12*, 2697.

[25] Abdolahad, M.; Taghinejad, M.; Taghinejad, H.; Janmaleki, M.; Mohajerzadeh, S. A vertically aligned carbon nanotube-based impedance sensing biosensor for rapid and high sensitive detection of cancer cells. *Lab. Chip.* **2012**, *12*, 1183.

[26] Li, W.; Wang, J.; Ren, J.; Qu, X. 3D graphene oxide-polymer hydrogel: near-infrared light-triggered active scaffold for reversible cell capture and on-demand release. *Adv. Mater.* **2013**, *25*, 6737.

[27] He, R.; Zhao, L.; Liu, Y.; *et al.* Biocompatible TiO_2 nanoparticle-based cell immunoassay for circulating tumor cells capture and identification from cancer patients. *Biomed. Microdevices.* **2013**, *15*, 617.

[28] Huang, C.; Yang, G.; Ha, Q.; Meng, J.; Wang, S. Multifunctional "smart" particles engineered from live immunocytes: toward capture and release of cancer cells. *Adv. Mater.* **2015**, *27*, 310.

[29] Sheng, W.; Chen, T.; Tan, W.; Fan, Z. H. Multivalent DNA nanospheres for enhanced capture of cancer cells in microfluidic devices. *ACS Nano* **2013**, *7*, 7067.

[30] Wu, Y.; Xue, P.; Kang, Y.; Hui, K. M. Highly specific and ultrasensitive graphene-enhanced electrochemical detection of low-abundance tumor cells

using silica nanoparticles coated with antibody-conjugated quantum dots. *Anal. Chem.* **2013**, *85*, 3166.

[31] Jeon, S.; Hong, W.; Lee, E. S.; Cho, Y. High-purity isolation and recovery of circulating tumor cells using conducting polymer-deposited microfluidic device. *Theranostics* **2014**, *4*, 1123.

[32] Kim, Y.-J.; Ebara, M.; Aoyagi, T. A smart nanofiber web that captures and releases cells. *Angew. Chem. Int. Ed.* **2012**, *51*, 10537.

[33] Zhang, N.; Deng, Y.; Tai, Q.; *et al.* Electrospun TiO_2 nanofiber-based cell capture assay for detecting circulating tumor cells from colorectal and gastric cancer patients. *Adv. Mater.* **2012**, *24*, 2756.

[34] Zhao, L.; Lu, Y. T.; Li, F.; *et al.* High-purity prostate circulating tumor cell isolation by a polymer nanofiber-embedded microchip for whole exome sequencing. *Adv. Mater.* **2013**, *25*, 2897.

[35] Chen, W.; Weng, S.; Zhang, F.; *et al.* Nanoroughened surfaces for efficient capture of circulating tumor cells without using capture antibodies. *ACS Nano.* **2013**, *7*, 566.

[36] Wan, Y.; Winter, M.; Delalat, B.; *et al.* Nanostructured polystyrene well plates allow unbiased high-throughput characterization of circulating tumor cells. *ACS Appl. Mater. Interfaces.* **2014**, *6*, 20828.

[37] Chen, W.; Shinuo Weng.; Zhang, F.; *et al.* Nanoroughened Surfaces for Efficient capture of circulating tumor cells without using capture antibodies. *ACS Nano.* **2013**, *7*, 566.

[38] Wang, S.; Wan, Y.; Liu, Y. Effects of nanopillar array diameter and spacing on cancer cell capture and cell *Nanoscale* **2014**, *6*, 12482.

[39] Ye, B.; Ding, H.; Cheng, Y.; *et al.* Photonic crystal microcapsules for label-free multiplex detection. *Adv. Mater.* **2014**, *26*, 3270.

[40] Zheng, F.; Cheng Y.; Wang J.; *et al.* Aptamer-functionalized barcode particles for the capture and detection of multiple types of circulating tumor cells. *Adv. Mater.* **2014**, *26*, 7333.

[41] Liu, X.; Chen, L.; Liu, H.; *et al.* Bio-inspired soft polystyrene nanotube substrate for rapid and highly efficient breast cancer-cell capture. *NPG Asia Mater.* **2013**, 5, e63.

[42] Ma, J.; Wen, L.; Dong, Z.; Zhang, T.; Wang, S.; Jiang, L. Aligned silicon nanowires with fine-tunable tilting angles by metal-assisted chemical etching on off-cut wafers. *physica status solidi (RRL) – Rapid Res. Lett.* **2013**, *7*, 655.

[43] Meng, J.; Liu, H.; Liu, X.; *et al.* Hierarchical biointerfaces assembled by leukocyte-inspired particles for specifically recognizing cancer cells. *Small* **2014**, *10*, 3735.

[44] Zhang, P.; Chen, L.; Xu, T.; *et al.* Programmable fractal nanostructured interfaces for specific recognition and electrochemical release of cancer cells. *Adv. Mater.* **2013**, *25*, 3566.

[45] Zhang, P.; Wang, S. Designing fractal nanostructured biointerfaces for biomedical applications. *Chemphyschem.* **2014**, *15*, 1550.

[46] Liu, X.; Zhang, F.; Wang, Q.; *et al.* Platelet-inspired multiscaled cytophilic interfaces with high specificity and efficiency toward point-of-care cancer diagnosis. *Small.* **2014**, *10*, 4677.

[47] Sekine, J.; Luo, S. C.; Wang, S.; Zhu, B.; Tseng, H. R.; Yu, H. H. Functionalized conducting polymer nanodots for enhanced cell capturing: the synergistic effect of capture agents and nanostructures. *Adv. Mater.* **2011**, *23*, 4788.

[48] Liu, H.; Wang, S. Poly(N-isopropylacrylamide)-based thermo-responsive surfaces with controllable cell adhesion. *Sci. China Chem.* **2014**, *57*, 552.

[49] Ke, Z.; Lin, M.; Chen, J.; *et al.* Programming thermoresponsiveness of NanoVelcro substrates enables effective purification of circulating tumor cells in lung cancer patients. *ACS Nano.* **2015**, *9*, 62.

[50] Hou, S.; Zhao, H.; Zhao, L.; *et al.* Capture and stimulated release of circulating tumor cells on polymer-grafted silicon nanostructures. *Adv. Mater.* **2013**, *25*, 1547.

[51] Liu, H.; Liu, X.; Meng, J.; *et al.* Hydrophobic interaction-mediated capture and release of cancer cells on thermoresponsive nanostructured surfaces. *Adv. Mater.* **2013**, *25*, 922.

[52] Liu, H.; Li, Y.; Sun, K.; *et al.* Dual-responsive surfaces modified with phenylboronic acid-containing polymer brush to reversibly capture and release cancer cells. *J. Am. Chem. Soc.* **2013**, *135*, 7603.

[53] Xie, M.; Lu, N.; Cheng, S.; *et al.* Engineered decomposable multifunctional nanobioprobes for capture and release of rare cancer cells. *Anal. Chem.* **2014**, *86*, 4681.

[54] Li, S.; Chena, N.; Zhang, Z.; Wang, Y. Endonuclease-responsive aptamer-functionalized hydrogel coating for sequential catch and release of cancer cells. *Biomaterials* **2013**, *34*, 460.

[55] Zhang, Z.; Chen, N.; Li, S.; Mark R.. Battig; Wang, Y. Programmable hydrogels for controlled cell catch and release using hybridized aptamers and complementary sequences. *J. Am. Chem. Soc.* **2012**, *134*, 15716.

[56] Chen, N.; Zhang, Z.; Soontornworajit, B.; Zhou, J.; Wang, Y. Cell adhesion on an artificial extracellular matrix using aptamer-functionalized PEG hydrogels. *Biomaterials* **2012**, *33*, 1353.

[57] Su, N.; Wang, J.; Ji, L.; *et al.* A cellular compatible chitosan nanoparticle surface for isolation and in-situ culture of rare number CTCs. *Small.* **2015**, 11, 5444.

[58] Cheng, B.; He, Z.; Zhao, L.; *et al.* Transparent, biocompatible nanostructured surfaces for cancer cell capture and culture. *Int. J. Nanomed.* **2014**, *9*, 2569.

[59] Zhang, Z.; Shiratsuchi, H.; Azizi, E.; *et al.* Expansion of CTCs from early stage lung cancer patients using a microfluidic co-culture modeloncotarget. *Oncotarget.* **2014**, *5*, 12383.

[60] Yu, M.; Bardia, A.; Aceto, N.; *et al.* Cancer therapy. ex vivo culture of circulating breast tumor cells for individualized testing of drug susceptibility. *Science* **2014**, *345*, 216.

[61] Wu, C.; Huang, Y.; Chen, P.; *et al.* Versatile immunomagnetic nanocarrier platform for capturing cancer cells. *ACS Nano* **2013**, *7*, 8816.
[62] Huang, Y. Y.; Hoshino, K.; Chen, P.; *et al.* Immunomagnetic nanoscreening of circulating tumor cells with a motion controlled microfluidic system. *Biomed. Microdevices* **2013**, *15*, 673.
[63] Yoon, H. J.; Kim, T. H.; Zhang, Z.; *et al.* Sensitive capture of circulating tumour cells by functionalized graphene oxide nanosheets. *Nat. Nanotechnol.* **2013**, *8*, 735.
[64] Lin, M.; Chen, J. F.; Lu, Y. T.; *et al.* Nanostructure embedded microchips for detection, isolation, and characterization of circulating tumor cells. *Acc Chem Res* **2014**, *47*, 2941.
[65] Lu, Y. T.; Zhao, L.; Shen, Q.; *et al.* Velcro Chip for CTC enumeration in prostate cancer patients. *Methods* **2013**, *64*, 144.

Chapter 19

Design investigations for robust and continuous online heartbeat monitoring using wearable vs. Doppler-based non-contact vital signs biosensors

V. Das[1,2]*, A. Boothby*[1,3]*, J. Lopez*[1,3] *and D.Y.C. Lie*[1,4]

19.1 Wearable ECG sensors

Vital signs are valuable physiological indicators that can help medical doctors, nurses and healthcare professionals to evaluate and analyze patients' basic health conditions. Conventional vital signs include the body temperature, heart rate, blood pressure, respiratory rate and blood oxygen saturation level (i.e., SpO2, which stands for peripheral capillary oxygen saturation). Continuous monitoring of physiological vital signs is of paramount importance for patients in the Intensive Care Unit (ICU) and Emergency Room (ER). Continuous vital signs monitoring, such as wearing a 24-h Holter monitor, makes it possible to get a much detailed picture of the patient's heart condition with excellent statistics to enable the necessary medical intervention if required. It is also getting more important for medical diagnosis, as well as for telemedicine and wireless-assisted living.

The accurate and robust detection of a person's heart rate is desirable during his/her normal everyday living, as well as under the conditions where uninterrupted clinical observation is required. With the number of individuals succumbing to cardiac disorders, heart rate monitoring and related diagnosis have become more important than ever before. Heart rates are traditionally monitored using the electrical bio-potentials emanating from the heart, which can be tapped either externally at the body-skin surface through transducers, or internally using electrical leads planted inside the ventricular/atrial chamber of the heart. The bio-potential obtained from the body-skin surface is popularly known as Electrocardiogram (ECG) or Elektro-kardiogram (EKG). Similarly the cardiac bio-potential recorded from the ventricular chamber by implants is known as Intracardiac Electrogram or

[1]Department of Electrical and Computer Engineering, Texas Tech University, Lubbock, TX, USA
[2]Texas Instruments, Dallas, TX, USA
[3]Noisefigure Research Inc., Lubbock, TX, USA
[4]Department of Surgery, Texas Tech University Health Science Center, Lubbock, TX, USA

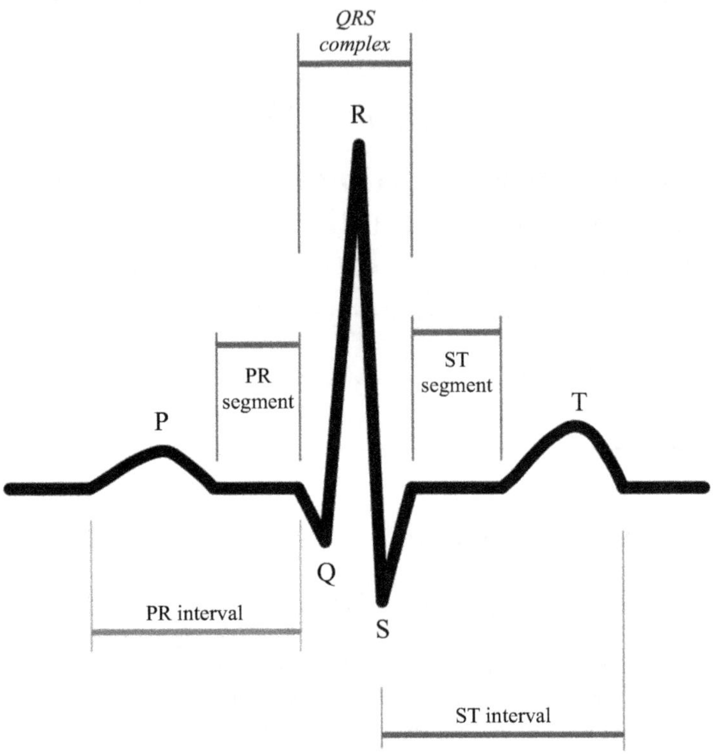

Figure 19.1 Representation of a normal ECG signal [2]

simply Electrogram (EGM). Microwave and Doppler-based techniques have also been explored to estimate heart rates by utilizing the physiological chest-wall displacement corresponding to the periodic cardiac systole-diastole. The concept of *Non-Contact Vital Signs* (NCVS) *Monitoring* using a radio-frequency (RF) Doppler sensor has existed for decades [1].

A normal ECG signal with its components is shown in Figure 19.1 [2]. A typical ECG signal is a surface biopotential from a combination of atrial and ventricular depolarization and repolarization, which translate into electrical events. The atrial depolarization is named as the P-wave, and it signifies the initiation of a cardiac cycle. The QRS complex represents the ventricular depolarization whereas the T-wave represents the ventricular repolarization. The atrial repolarization is overwhelmed by the QRS complex, hence is not noticeable [3].

The intracardiac signals (EGM) can be obtained using bipolar leads placed in the tricuspid valve annulus which lies in the apex region of the right ventricle [3]. Similar to ECG, the EGM is also composed of ventricular events and atrial events. The ventricular events are also termed as "near field" effects whereas the atrial events are known as the "far field" effects. The various components of the EGM signal are also named according to the convention used to describe the components of the ECG waveform. Typically, the analog front end of a wearable ECG sensor or an implantable pacemaker/defibrillator would monitor the cardiac rhythm by recording the periodicity of the ventricular depolarization signal, using the R-wave (or the QRS complex) peaks as they are easier to detect reliably.

Different types of cardiac bio-sensors have evolved over the past few decades, depending upon the type of cardiac signals used to estimate the heart-rate. Wearable cardiac biosensors use ECG as the input for heart-rate detection, whereas Implantable Cardioverter Defibrillator (ICD) uses EGM to monitor heart-rate as well as to provide necessary defibrillation to maintain proper heart rhythm. However, a Doppler-based non-contact vital signs sensor monitors the physiologically modulated cardio-pulmonary *movement* signal to detect the heart rate; more detailed physics of which will be discussed later in this chapter. Next, we will introduce and describe the wearable ECG sensors first, as they are getting smaller and cheaper and more popular on the market today.

Wearable ECG sensors are non-invasive cardiac sensors which use the surface biopotential to record, estimate and monitor the physiological state of the heart. Wearable ECG sensors are available in many varieties, from bulky clinical instrumentation to ambulatory monitoring systems. One of the most popular wearable ECG sensors is the Holter Monitor, where a patient would wear this 5/7 leads wired sensor at the belt to record his/her ECG for 24–72 h continuously and then return to the physicians afterwards for diagnosis and evaluation. When combined with wireless transmission/communications capabilities, the latest wearable ECG sensors can play a very crucial and indispensable role in wireless-assisted living, acute-care centers and for telemetric medicine such that when patients are under constant monitoring for potential medical emergency conditions, they can be attended immediately [4–6].

19.1.1 Components of the wearable ECG sensor system

A typical wearable ECG sensor should include an interface between the skin and the electrical circuitry to tap the cardiac surface biopotentials. Biopotential electrodes in conjunction with special dedicated gels are used for this crucial interface. The electrolytic gels are used to create a conductive layer between the skin and the electrode. Usually silver/silver chloride (Ag/AgCl) electrodes are preferred as they closely resemble the non-polarizable property and are easy to manufacture [3]. The typical body skin-surface electrode and skin interface can be modeled as shown in Figure 19.2. Electrolytic gels when applied on to the skin of the patient for prolonged monitoring may lead to uneasiness as well as skin inflammations due to allergic reactions [7]. We can apply the wearable ECG sensors on a subject by either using wet gel-based electrodes or dry microprobe-based electrodes, depending upon the preferred skin contact. Any type of skin contact can be a cause of irritation and inconvenience in varying degrees, thus hampering the utility and applicability of ECG sensors for long-term mobile monitoring, especially when patients need out-of-hospital monitoring. A non-contact-based ECG sensor completely gets rid of the inconvenience involved in contact-based ECG sensors thus making it more appealing. Capacitive-coupling based non-contact wearable ECG

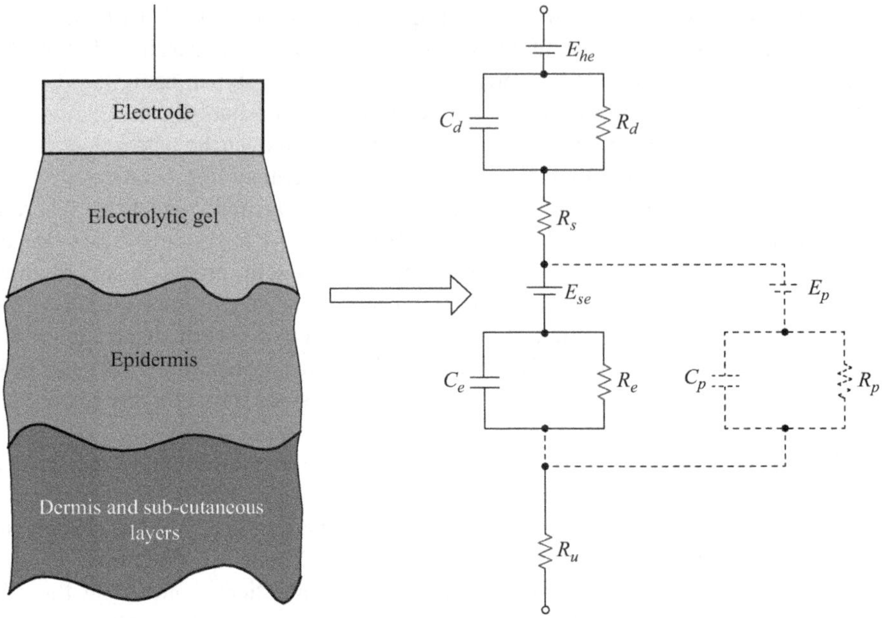

Figure 19.2 Equivalent circuit of an electrode placed on skin [3]

sensors have been recently explored and reported [8], unfortunately they are plagued by degraded ECG signal quality due to much higher impedance presented by the capacitive electrodes and are susceptible to motion artifacts. Latest wearable heart-rate sensors using non-contact optical methods (such as the Apple Watches) have just been launched recently in the second half of 2015. Therefore, even though quite attractive and potentially rather important for mobile heart-rate monitoring, not enough data has been gathered clinically using those devices so they will not be discussed in this chapter.

For a typical wearable ECG sensor, the biopotential electrode is placed next to the Analog Front End (AFE) sensing circuitry. The electrode acts as a transducer between the ionic transport of the nerves on the skin and the electronic transport of the conductive material. This transducer action makes the biopotential electrical ECG signals available (converting from the ionic currents generated by heart movements) for the AFE integrated circuit (IC) to sense. The surface ECG signals from the electrodes are normally weak, having amplitudes in the range from 0.5 mV to 4 mV and containing meaningful information in the frequency range of 0.01–250 Hz [3]. Furthermore, this analog signal has to be made available for digital signal processing in order to show and extract the ECG signal information in a desirable manner. Thus, the AFE circuitry is required to amplify, filter and subsequently digitize the cardiac biopotential signal. Many research groups, however, naturally consider amplification and filtering as the only required functionalities of an AFE circuitry, and treat signal digitization as a separate unit under the analog-to-digital converter (ADC) block [9].

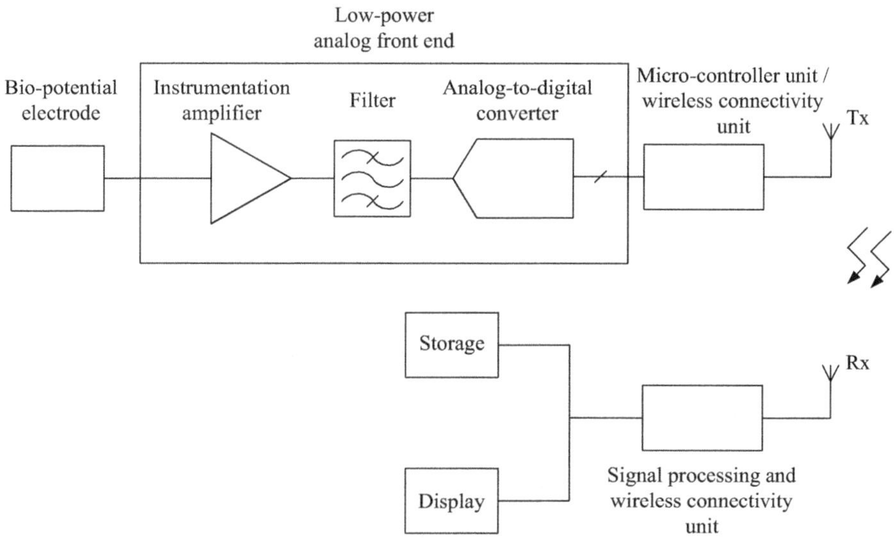

Figure 19.3 A typical wearable ECG sensor system [10]

A typical wearable ECG sensor system consists of the following distinct components, as shown in Figure 19.3 [9,10]:

i. Biopotential Electrode placed at defined points on the human body.
ii. Analog Front End (AFE) Circuitry.
iii. A Microprocessor Unit.
iv. Wireless connectivity.
v. Software designed to monitor and record the physiological data.

In the recent decades the bio-medical community has strived for miniaturization and improvement on the ease of use for the entire ECG recording system to enhance its various performances. Studies on different types of electrodes, circuit topologies and efficient systems implementation, including incorporating wireless connectivity between the ECG sensor and the monitoring computer, have all been reported [4–14]. A key enabler for realizing an efficient, conveniently sized and accurate wearable ECG sensor lies in the AFE circuitry design. To increase the applicability of ECG sensors and to achieve miniature sizes, the power consumption has to be made as small as possible, thus permitting the system to be powered using tiny batteries. Amongst the components of an ECG sensor system, the AFE circuitry plays a pivotal role in deciding the overall power-consumption as it has to be ALWAYS on for continuous monitoring. A low-power high performance monolithic AFE IC, when integrated with the ADC, RF transceivers and microprocessor with memories, can become a completely integrated System-on-Chip (SoC) to help realizing excellent portability, signal integrity, small form factor, and low-power wireless connectivity for robust and continuous ECG monitoring.

The recent advancement in the SoC technologies has made some revolutionary heart-rate monitoring products such as the pacemakers a reality. A more versatile heart-rate monitoring implantable device that can perform both the pacing functionality like a traditional pacemaker, and in addition the ability to do automatic defibrillation will be discussed next: the ICD, which has only become popular in the past couple of decades.

19.2 Implantable cardioverter defibrillator (ICD)

Monitoring of the key cardiac parameters is very important, and if the information obtained from such a monitoring system can be used to provide immediate therapeutic treatment then it can act as a life-saving system. For example, cardiac arrhythmia, which is caused either due to pathological or physiological abnormalities, has been reported to be a prime cause of sudden cardiac death (SCD) [15]. Arrhythmia involves irregular cardiac patterns which lead to cardiac fibrillation, a condition where the cardiac output can be diminishing to even close to zero sometimes, leading to an asystolic state followed by irreparable brain damage and ultimately death [3]. Ventricular fibrillation is the most lethal type of cardiac fibrillation. In the absence of immediate resuscitation, a serious cardiac fibrillation can lead to an instant death. Studies have shown that the chances of survival are strongly dependent on the time delay before which defibrillation was administered [15]. In such a scenario, the availability of an immediate defibrillation using ICDs that can provide successful real-time monitoring and robust detection of lethal arrhythmias can save and have saved numerous lives.

Defibrillation is usually provided using an electric shock to revive the normal cardiac rhythm [3]. If not using an ICD, the external electric shock or "cardioversion" can be provided using electrodes either placed immediately on the myocardium or placed transthoracically. It takes lesser current to provide the required electrical energy when using electrodes placed on the myocardium, but it requires a surgical operation of the heart, so external transthoracic electric shock is often used in cardiac arrhythmias. Arrhythmias may exhibit bradycardia, a condition where the heart rate is way below the normal sinus rhythm; or tachycardia, a condition of faster heart rate that may eventually result in cardiac fibrillation. Defibrillators which are designed such that the defibrillation is synchronized to the R-wave and is administered much ahead of the T-wave are known as cardioverters [3].

Modern ICDs are equipped to provide both defibrillation and pacing, where the high-voltage pulses of about 800 V is used to achieve defibrillation when tachycardia is detected, and a mild electrical pulses of 6–8 V as a part of the pacemaker functionality to stabilize the heart rate in case of bradycardia [13]. Wireless connectivity is also being included in ICDs for enabling medical telemetry and programming for best monitoring of the patients' critical cardiac conditions [17]. A typical modern dual-chamber ICD with the intracardiac transvenous leads inside a human heart is shown in Figure 19.4 as an example.

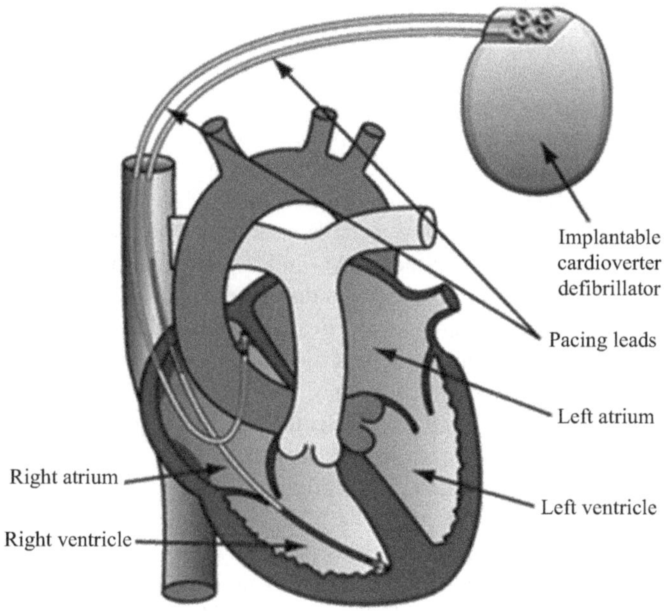

Figure 19.4 An implantable cardioverter defibrillator (ICD) inside a human heart [17]

19.2.1 Components of the ICD system

ICDs are implanted inside human bodies and are expected to last at least for the duration of 5–7 years [15]. The defibrillation and pacemaker functionalities are invoked whenever exigencies like sudden cardiac arrest arise, but the monitoring system is needed to be continually ON for the entire duration of the ICD lifetime. Similar to the wearable ECG sensors, the monitoring/sensing system of ICD comprises the combination of electrodes and analog front end circuits. A modern ICD typically consists of dedicated intracardiac electrodes, AFE circuitry with ADCs, a high-voltage generator, a microprocessor, memories, power-management circuits, large passives (especially the medical-grade capacitors) and sometimes with additional circuitry enabling wireless connectivity [16]. An ICD must have ultralow-power design and aggressive miniaturization, which are made possible by using ICs based SoCs design.

As with the wearable ECG sensors, the electrodes in an ICD system again play a pivotal role in determining the quality and accuracy of intracardiac biopotential signal (EGM) acquisition. Additionally, the leads connecting the ICD device to the electrodes placed in the heart are also a critical part of the entire ICD system. The modern ICD systems use dual-chamber transvenous endocardial leads placed in both the right atrium and the right ventricle. These leads are capable of supporting sensing, pacing, as well as defibrillation of the cardiac rhythms. The transvenous endocardial ICD leads are expected to be good biocompatible electrical conductors, and they also must possess mechanical durability. The leads are exposed to constant and periodic stress due the cardiac contractions, which can result in torsional bending and compression forces being applied on them for almost 37 million times per year [18]. The leads are designed to endure high voltage levels as well as additional thoracic stresses due to the arm and chest movements of the patient. The transvenous leads are also required to have excellent insulation in order to ensure accurate sensing of the intracardiac EGM, and the application of electrical pulses whenever required. The leads have to endure the oxidative stress in chemically hostile environment of the heart [3,18]. Similarly, the ICD electrodes also need to be able to tolerate the mechanical stress due to cardiac activity and must be able to maintain their positions such that they can support the administering of the electrical pulses when required. The electrodes are required not to react and anti-corrosive, as otherwise undesirable irritation to the heart tissues may be experienced, making the implant medically inappropriate. Additionally, interactions/reactions of the electrodes with the heart tissues are to be avoided to prevent an increase in the stimulation threshold (Figure 19.5).

With the recent introduction of a revolutionizing technology called Subcutaneous-ICD systems (S-ICD®, developed by Cameron Health Inc, later acquired by Boston-Scientific Corporation in 2012), the risks and failures related to vascular surgery and prolonged usage of intracardiac transvenous leads can be considerably diminished. These S-ICD® systems use tunneled subcutaneous lead-electrode

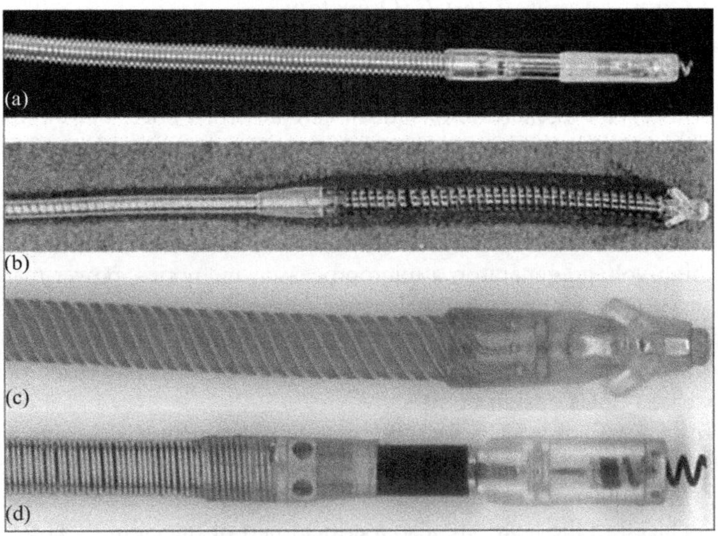

Figure 19.5 Intracardiac transvenous leads: (a) Medtronic Transvene, (b) CPI Endotak, (c) Ventrtex TVL/SPL and (d) St. Jude Medical TVL-ADX 1559 [18]

assembly, placed approximately 1 cm left of the sternum instead of the intracardiac transvenous leads, and are implanted in the small pouch formed under the skin near the sixth rib [20,21]. The S-ICD® systems have obtained FDA approval and are under clinical trials. Preliminary trial results indicate their therapeutic efficiency in tackling ventricular fibrillation, but also reflect inadequacies with respect to ventricular tachycardia due to lack of anti-tachycardia pacing [20]. Furthermore the S-ICD® systems are reported to require higher energy levels to administer the cardiac therapy in comparison with the traditional intracardiac transvenous ICD [19,20]. Additional trials with higher volume of subjects in the age-groups prone to cardiac dysfunction are required to understand and characterize the S-ICD® systems more [20].

The transvenous ICD lead-electrode assembly is followed by its AFE circuitry in an ICD system. Please note that in comparison with the ECG signals, intracardiac EGM signals have stronger amplitudes in the range of 0.1–20 mV [15]. A typical ICD/pacemaker system consists of the following distinct components [17], as shown in Figure 19.6:

1. Intracardiac electrode and transvenous lead assembly.
2. Analog Front End (AFE) Circuits.
3. Bio-Signal Processing Block.
4. System Controller to control the pacing and defibrillation modules.
5. Wireless connectivity.

The wireless connectivity for a modern ICD/pacemaker system depicted in Figure 19.6 is achieved using "Zigbee," which is defined by IEEE 802.15.4 protocol [17]. Zigbee enables data transmission of 40 kbps by utilizing a sub-1 GHz frequency band, making it suitable for low-power implantable implementations like ICD/pacemakers. A low-power high performance completely integrated AFE SoC helps in both longevity and accuracy with digital processing capabilities. We will, therefore, next discuss an indispensable design block of *any* biosensor AFE SoC: the Instrumentation Amplifier (INA). We will show case our novel INA's design and compare our performance vs. those in the literature.

19.3 Biosignal instrumentation amplifier (INA)

The growing needs for important biosensing systems such as the wearable ECG sensors and implantable pacemakers/ICDs have pushed for the continuous improvements in the biosensor design. Some of the most critical requirements for effective biosensor systems are the ultralow-power consumption, the small form factor and the robustness that can still ensure high-quality monitoring for all patients regardless of their sexes, ages, physical conditions, prior medical histories and location (i.e., remote and rural areas). Biosensors are often used for continuous monitoring of biosignals, which are inherently analog in nature and can be electrical signals, Table 19.1. This analog characteristic of the biosignals necessitates the design of analog-front end (AFE) circuitry as the signal sensing block in the

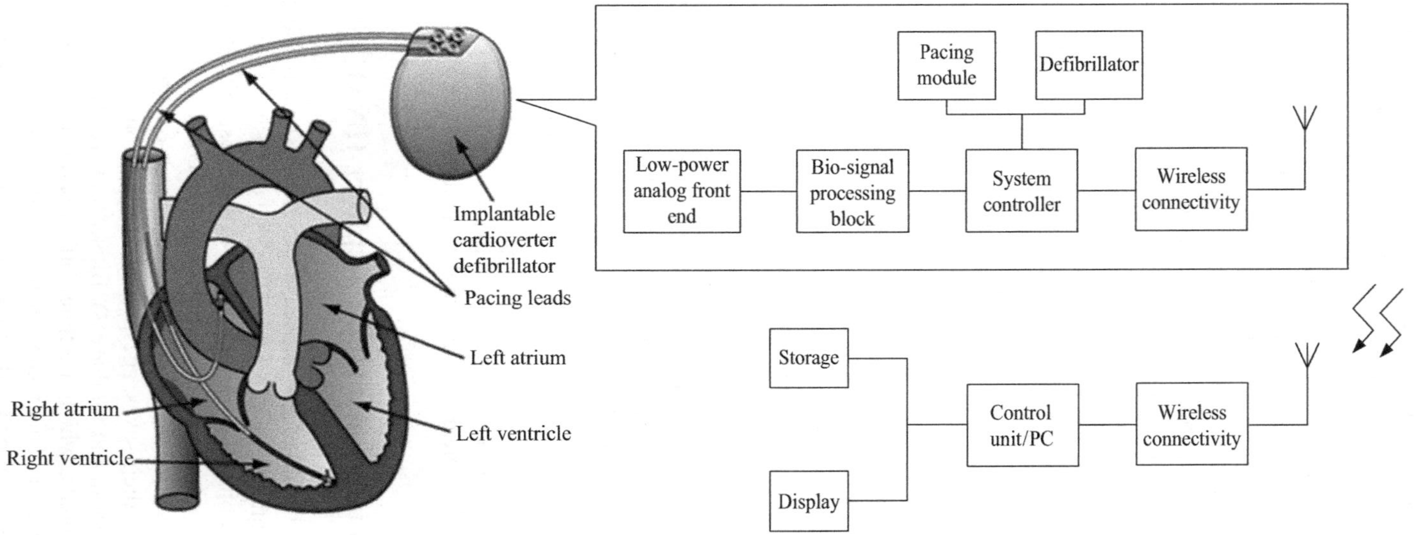

Figure 19.6 A typical modern ICD/pacemaker system [17]

Table 19.1 Biosignal: amplitude and frequency range of ECG vs. EGM [3,15,22]

Bio-signal	Amplitude range	Frequency range
ECG	0.5–4 mV	0.01–250 Hz
EGM	100 μV–20 mV	dc–100 Hz

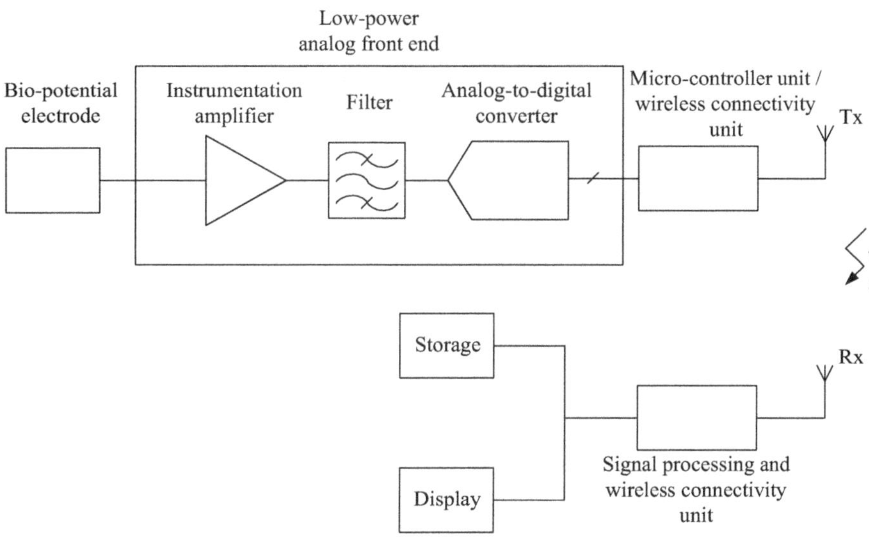

Figure 19.7 A typical wearable ECG sensor showing the AFE circuitry

biosensors. For continuous monitoring, this AFE circuitry needs to be continually operational throughout the life of the biosensor. Thus, if the power consumption of the AFE circuitry can be reduced, then the operational longevity and the effectiveness of the biosensor systems can be improved.

19.3.1 Biosignal Instrumentation Amplifier (INA)

The INA, as shown in Figure 19.7, is the first stage of the AFE circuitry and hence is responsible for defining the overall performance of the biosignal AFE circuitry. The INA interfaces the subsequent AFE circuits and also the electrodes, and hence it has to be designed considering the characters of both. Biosignals are usually associated with electrode dc-offsets, which in the case of ECG arise from the half-cell potentials of the electrode-electrolyte and electrolyte-skin interfaces [3]. Biosignals offer physiological information in the low frequency range (on the order of few Hz), and therefore the in-band noise is often dominated by the $1/f$ noise. Moreover, the presence of the common-mode 60 Hz signal due to mains-power line is always a strong noise source. In view of the above facts, the INA is required to

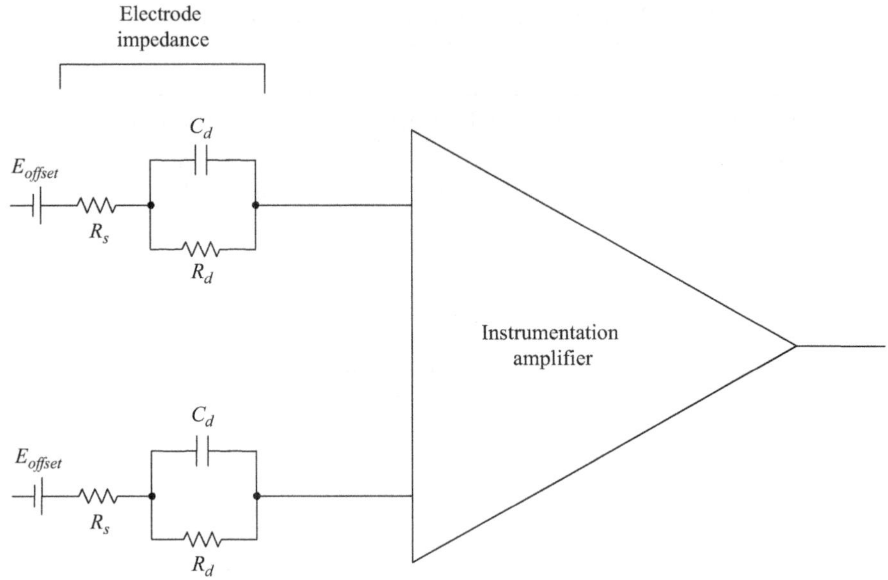

Figure 19.8 Electrode-INA interface, showing the electrode impedance and electrode offsets [3,24,25]

filter the electrode dc-offsets, suppress the in-band $1/f$ noise and reject the common-mode signal to increase the sensitivity to cardiac biosignals [23].

In order to seamlessly interface with the biopotential electrodes, the bio-signal INA needs to be designed to provide high impedance at the amplifier inputs to avoid loading the bio-potential electrodes. A typical electrode-INA interface is shown in Figure 19.8 [3,24,25].

19.3.2 INA design consideration

The noise floor of the INA predominantly decides the sensitivity of the AFE circuitry and therefore, the sensitivity of the biosensor. For example, a noise floor power spectrum density (PSD) of 100 $nV/\sqrt{Hz}$ over a bandwidth of dc to 250 Hz, which is the ECG frequency band, gives an integrated noise value of close to 1.6 μV_{rms} [26]. Commercially available ECG monitoring AFE ICs like ADAS1000 (Analog Devices) and ADS129xR (Texas Instruments) achieve an integrated noise specifications close to 2 μV_{rms} [27,28]. This is the expected noise amplitude in the ECG frequency range, and therefore a biosignal with amplitude *larger* than this noise amplitude can be detected by the amplifier with a noise floor PSD of 100 $nV/\sqrt{Hz}$ or less. The closed-loop dc gain of the INA can be designed in a range of 20 dB to 40 dB depending upon the gain characteristics of the subsequent stages. The common-mode rejection ratio (CMRR) is another important design spec consideration, ideally for battery operated implantable devices a CMRR of greater than

80 dB would be sufficient as it means a suppression of common-mode signal by 10,000 times in comparison with the differential signal [23,26]. However, for wearable biosensors such as ECG sensors, the commercial INAs often need to achieve a very tough CMRR of over 130 dB to effectively remove all the undesired effects due to various sources of mismatches and motion artifacts, etc. [27,28]. The power-supply rejection ratio (PSRR) specification of the amplifier also needs to be carefully considered for a robust design, as any fluctuation on the power-supply needs to be attenuated so as not to influence the amplifier output significantly. PSRR ratings of greater than 60 dB is considered sufficient for battery operated devices [23]. Since the high precision biomedical AFE circuits cater to applications not only limited to battery-operated devices, they often need to achieve a PSRR of 90 dB [28]. In addition, the AFE devices from Analog Devices Inc. and Texas Instruments offer wide range of features such as configurable gain, tunable noise-power performance, thoracic/respiration impedance measurement, just to name a few [27,28]. The operational longevity of wearable ECG sensors or ICD/pacemakers, to a large extent, is determined by the capacities of Li-ion batteries and the current consumption of the AFE circuitry. This operational longevity can be expressed as the equation 19.1:

$$\text{Operational Hours} = \frac{\text{Battery Capacity}}{\text{Current Consumption}} \tag{19.1}$$

According to equation (19.1), a battery capacity of 1.2 Ah and current consumption of 20 μA gives an operational lifetime of close to 7 years; however, this simple calculation does not take into account the deterioration of the battery and potential circuit and component performance over the years. The INA circuit design specifications that we aimed at achieving in this chapter as an example is listed in Table 19.2.

19.3.3 Fully differential folded-cascode based chopper stabilized INA

Considering the above discussed design specs that include a very challenging noise requirement and ultra-lowpower consumption, a chopper-stabilized capacitive feedback fully differential amplifier was design in this work [26,29–32]. Capacitive

Table 19.2 Design specification [26]

Amplifier parameter	Target specification
Supply voltage	<2 V
Supply current	<2 μA
Closed-loop dc-Gain	20–40 dB
Noise [dc–250 Hz]	<2 μV_{rms}
CMRR	>80 dB
PSRR	>60 dB
Bandwidth	>5 kHz

feedback was opted for this design, since realizing accurate capacitor ratios are relatively easier on-chip without trimming. Moreover, using a capacitive feedback enables gain-setting with capacitor ratio, thus reducing errors due to mismatches. The gain of a capacitive feedback amplifier with a finite open-loop gain A is given in (19.2).

$$\frac{V_{out}}{V_{in}} = \frac{C_{in}}{C_{fb} + \dfrac{C_{in} + C_{p,in} + C_{fb}}{A}} \tag{19.2}$$

Here C_{in} is the input capacitor of the feedback network, C_{fb} is the feedback capacitance and $C_{p,in}$ is the parasitic gate capacitance of the input MOSFET device. For the present design two chopper switches were used with one placed at the input and the other placed at the output of the fully differential amplifier. The fully-differential chopper stabilized INA system was designed using the TSMC CMOS 0.18 μm process, and the system-level implementation is shown in the Figure 19.9.

The capacitive feedback system was used for our design shown in Figure 19.9, and was designed to achieve a closed-loop gain of 32 dB. This was realized by using an input capacitor, $C_{in} = 8$ pF and a feedback capacitor $C_{fb} = 0.2$ pF. Higher gain would require a higher input capacitor or a lower feedback capacitor. Higher input capacitance may lower the input impedance of the OTA due to switch-capacitor effect caused by the input chopper [26]. Furthermore, lowering the feedback capacitor may lead to process feasibility issues. Moreover, our biosensor AFE IC would be equipped with variable gain amplifier (VGA), which can boost the signal level when required. To provide the feedback dc-point, a high-resistance ($>10^{12}$ Ω) is required in the feedback path so not to load down the OTA. This high resistance is realized by using MOS-based pseudo-resistors, as shown in Figure 19.9 [26,33,34].

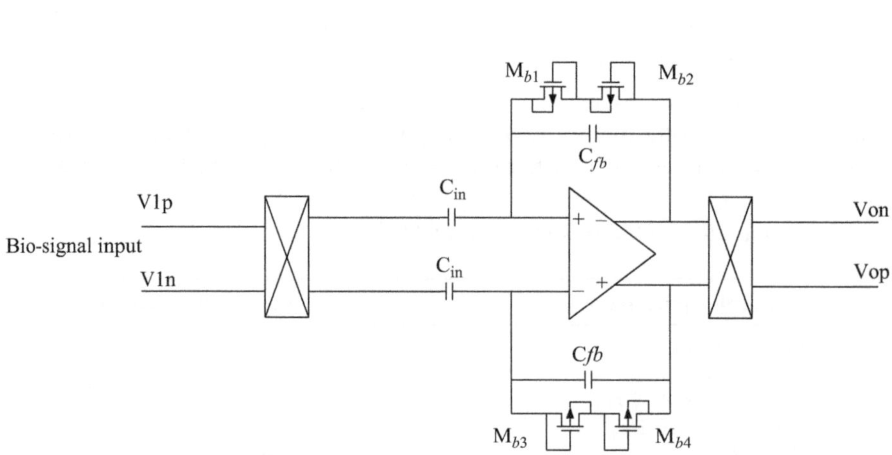

Figure 19.9 Fully-differential capacitive feedback chopper stabilized INA [29,33,34]

In this design, the standard folded-cascode topology with the current scaling technique described in [33] was used to implement the operational transconductance amplifier (OTA). The standard folded-cascode topology aids in the application of current-scaling technique, and also provides adequate gain in a single-stage to implement a feedback network with minimal gain error, thus making the use of a second-stage unnecessary [33,34]. Reduction of an amplification stage also helps the power budget. The current-scaling technique requires the devices in the output (folded) branch of the OTA to be biased such that the quiescent current is a fraction of the quiescent current used to bias the input differential pair. Since the quiescent current in the output branch does not contribute to the overall transconductance, reducing them will not reduce amplifier gain. Application of current scaling reduces the quiescent current in the output branch, which in turn increases the output resistance of each device. This increase in resistance helps in realizing higher gain with just one amplification stage, thus helping a low-power implementation. The noise contributed by the active devices in the output branch is directly proportional to their respective transconductance, hence reducing their quiescent current also helps reducing the noise. The current scaling technique we are using here was similarly proposed in [33,34], which reinforces the low-noise and low-power strategy required to realize a robust and sensitive bio-signal amplifier.

The most important component of the INA circuit design is the folded-cascode OTA, Figure 19.10 depicts its circuit implementation. The designs shown in References 33 and 34 achieved a current ratio of 1:16 between the quiescent current

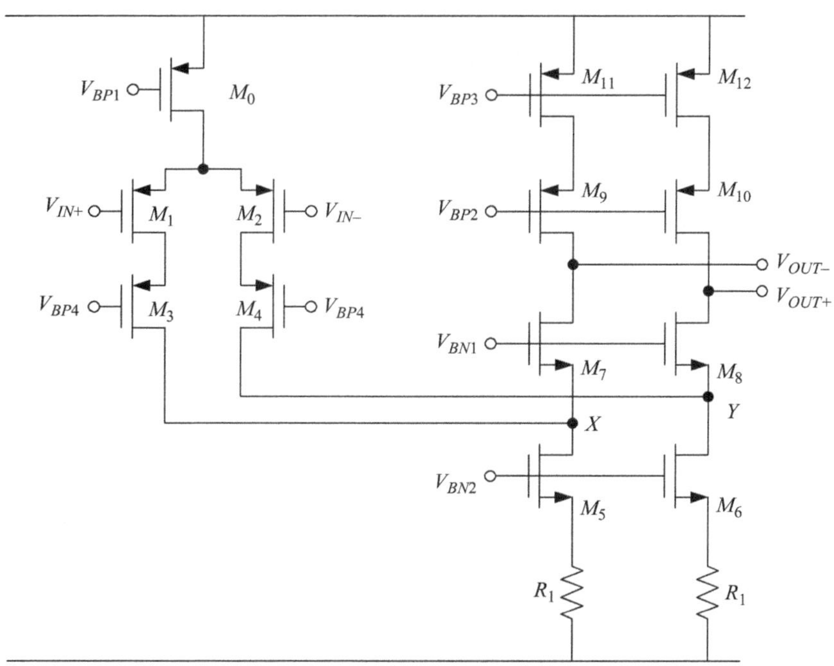

Figure 19.10 Circuit implementation of the folded-cascode OTA [33]

in the output branch vs. the input pair device, but as a conservative approach in our design a current ratio of 1:7 was adopted. Higher ratios can provide better noise performance, but also make the nodes "X" and "Y," (in Figure 19.10) a bit more critical, as the resistance looking into the source of M_7 (M_8) and the drains of M_1 (M_2) (if cascode device M_3 (M_4) is not present) and M_5 (M_6) become comparable, that will inhibit the flow of small signal current to the output branch. Too much reduced flow of small-signal current results in lower effective transconductance (G_m) of the OTA, which can make the design non-functional. This dilemma is overcome by increasing the resistance looking into the drains of input pair by using M_3 and M_4 cascode devices, and increasing the resistance looking into the current sink devices, M_5 and M_6 by using source degeneration resistor R_1. Furthermore, the source degeneration also considerably helps suppressing the transconductance of the noise-contributing M_5 and M_6, resulting in lesser noise.

In order to minimize noise, the other most important requirement is to maximize the effective transconductance (G_m) of the amplifier, which typically is heavily related to the transconductance (g_m) of the input pair. For low-power design, a high transconductance can be achieved by capitalizing on the higher transconductance efficiency of MOS devices in weak-inversion region, as shown in Figure 19.11. Considering the active load devices, there is a trade-off between low-power vs. low-noise implementation, as using devices in sub-threshold region requires less power but it enhances transconductance thus increasing noise. For low-noise strategy, we require a high transconductance (g_m) of the input pair only; thus as a balancing act, the devices M_{11} and M_{12} are operated marginally above threshold region to reduce their noise contribution (Figure 19.12).

The chopper switches were realized using complementary MOS devices. Based on simulation the device sizes of $W/L = 0.5\ \mu m/0.18\ \mu m$ were used. Complementary switching scheme has an inherent advantage with regards to the charge

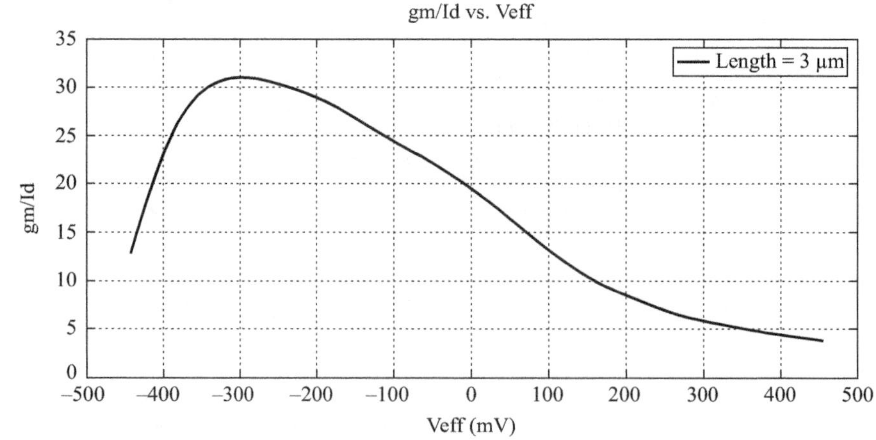

Figure 19.11 Transconductance efficiency for different operating regions of a typical TSMC n-channel MOSFET of length = 3 μm

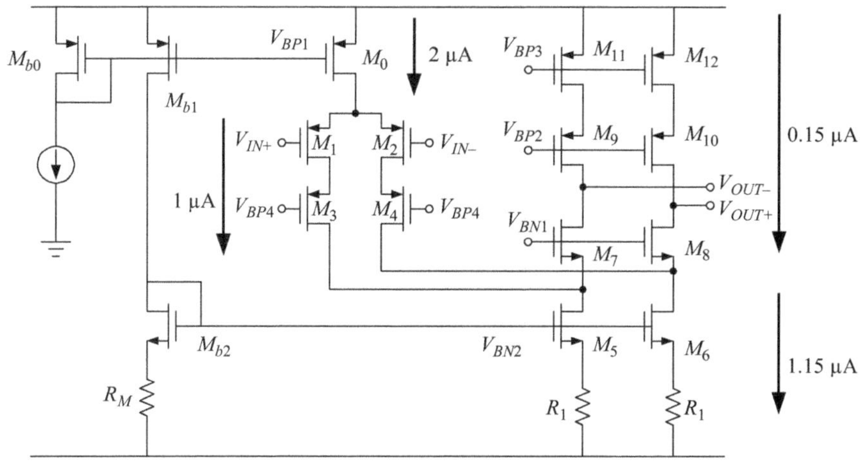

Figure 19.12 The circuit schematic of the OTA with the current-scaling technique

injection and clock feed-through issues [31,35]. The chopper modulation frequency (f_{chop}) of 1 kHz was supplied to a non-overlapping clock generator to generate two clocks, P1 and P2; their complementary clocks, P1′ and P2′ were obtained using subsequent inverter stages.

The chopper modulation frequency of 1 kHz was chosen in agreement with the analysis shown in [31,32] as according to which, a chopper modulation frequency chosen equal to the amplifier corner frequency (f_{corner}) typically provides the best trade-off with respect to the residual noise and spikes observed. Furthermore, the amplifier cut-off ($f_{3\mathrm{dB}}$) and the chopper modulation frequency (f_{chop}) are related asymptotically for values of $f_{3\mathrm{dB}} >> f_{chop}$, and results in the chopper modulated white noise to be almost equal to the original white noise [31]. A higher value of $f_{3\mathrm{dB}}$ vs. f_{chop} also ensures that the amplifier provides stable gain for the signal in the intermediate stage, which as a result of chopping will be at a much higher frequency than the original input signal.

Noise simulation of the INA without the use of chopper stabilization is also shown to highlight the effectiveness of chopper stabilization as an elegant method of noise reduction. The post-layout simulations shown here are only for the case of capacitive (C-only) extraction as a close approximation to the realistic performance of the INA. The noise simulation response of the INA without chopper stabilization has been shown in Figures 19.13 and 19.14, in linear and logarithmic scales, respectively. The logarithmic scale helps in ascertaining the $1/f$ noise corner frequency, which is around 1 kHz for the present design. The periodic noise simulation was used to verify the chopper stabilized INA and the response is shown in Figure 19.15. The $1/f$ noise pole can be seen to be transposed to the chopper frequency, which for the present system is at 1 kHz. The noise response has been summarized in Table 19.3.

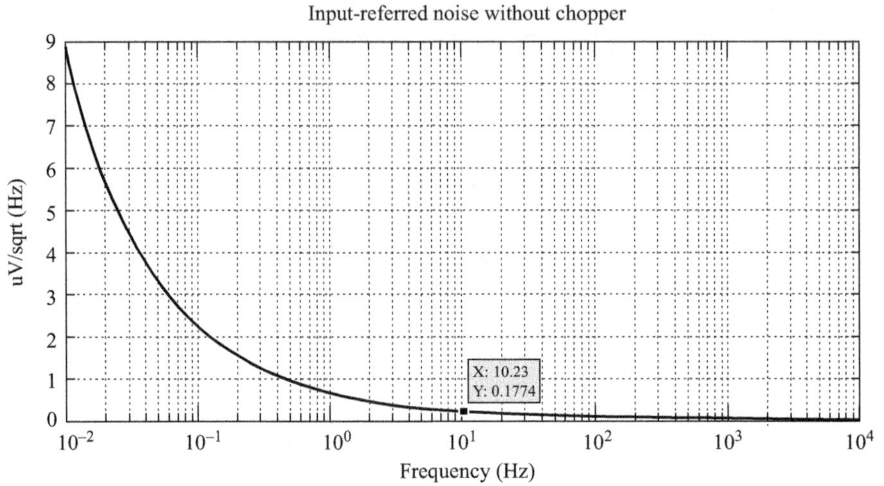

Figure 19.13 Noise simulation response without chopper showing the spot noise at 10 Hz

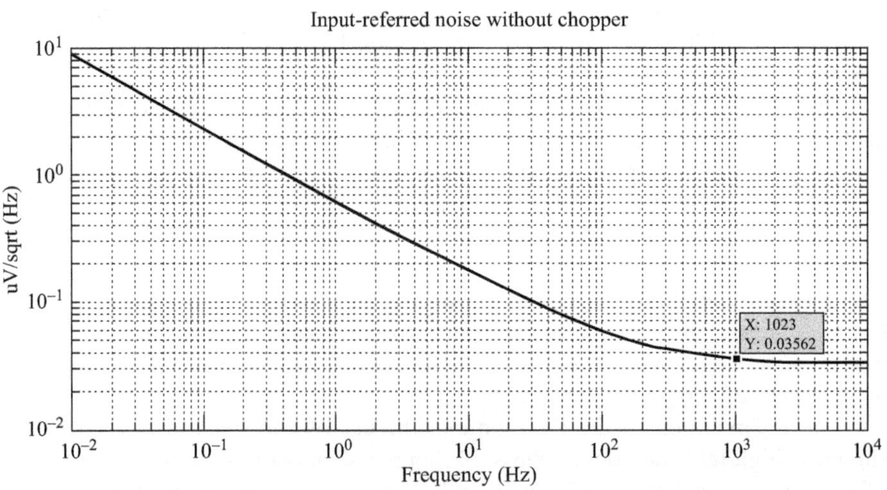

Figure 19.14 Noise simulation response (log) without chopper showing the 1/f noise corner at 1 kHz

The frequency response of the chopper-stabilized INA is shown in Figure 19.16 and a dc-gain of 32.65 dB was achieved. A sudden dip was observed in the vicinity of the chopping frequency of 1 kHz, but this dip will not affect the performance as our range of operation would be from 0.01 to 300 Hz.

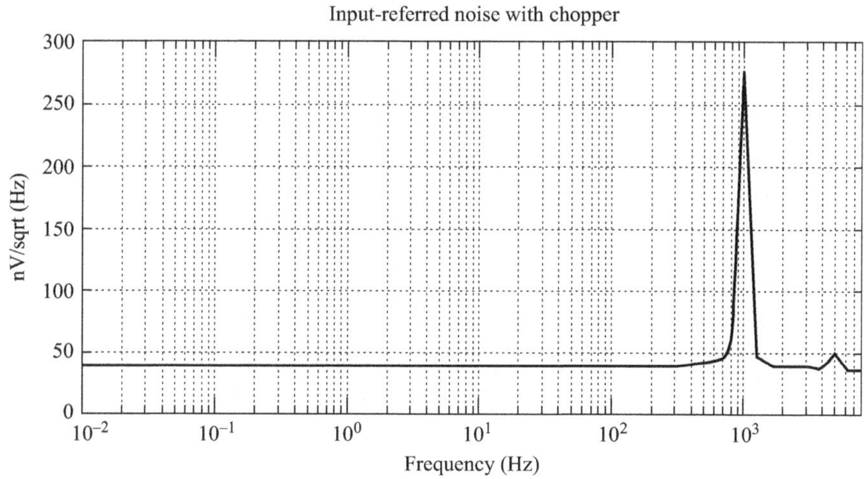

Figure 19.15 Noise simulation response with chopper showing the transposition of the flicker noise pole to 1 kHz

Table 19.3 Noise simulation comparison

Parameter	Without chopper	With chopper
Input-referred noise (0.01–300 Hz)	2.1 μV_{rms}	0.69 μV_{rms}
Spot noise at 10 Hz	180 nV/$\sqrt{}$Hz	39.89 nV/$\sqrt{}$Hz
Corner frequency	1 kHz	$<$10 mHz

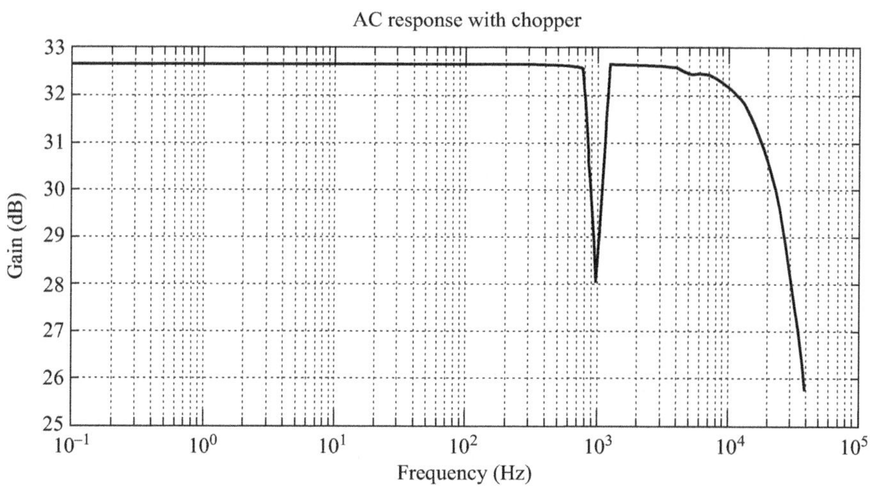

Figure 19.16 Frequency response simulation with chopper

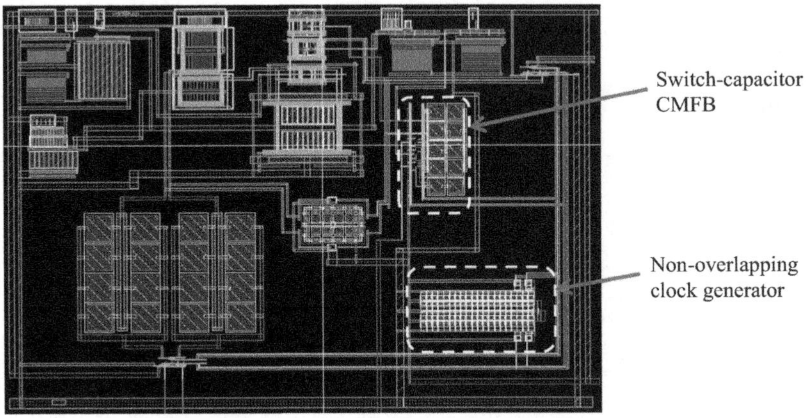

Figure 19.17 Layout of the fully differential capacitive feedback chopper stabilized INA in TSMC CMOS 0.18 μm process

The layout of the fully-differential chopper-stabilized INA with various blocks is shown in Figures 19.17.

19.3.4 State-of-the-art performance comparison

The performance of different low-noise and low-power INA designs applied to different types of bio-signals are compared with the present design, as shown in Table 19.4. One can see our INA design is rather competitive compared with the best in literature.

19.4 Doppler-based non-contact vital signs (NCVS) sensor

It is well-known that using wearable ECG sensors can cause discomforts to the monitored subjects, and the sensors often have to be designed with strict requirements on power consumption and miniature form factor to make them applicable for long term continuous vital signs monitoring. In this context, non-contact vital signs sensing is very attractive, especially for the heart-rate and respiration rate detection based on Doppler radar operating at microwave frequencies that has been reported since 1970s [40,41]. The Doppler-based non-contact vital signs (NCVS) sensor can be used for physiological monitoring of patients with different types of respiration or cardiac complaints without the need of any contact or invasive surgical implants, Figure 19.18. The NCVS sensor uses the external periodic cardiopulmonary movements as the information source to detect the respiration rate and heart rate. The NCVS system can also act as a "life-detection" system when looking for survivors underneath debris and rubbles [42]. In cases of patients with burn injuries or chest wounds, NCVS sensor can be very attractive for the heart-rate monitoring compared with wearable ECG sensors. A robust and advanced NCVS sensor installed on a patient's bed or mounted on the ceiling in hospitals, nursing homes or residential houses can be used for long-term monitoring even without the

Table 19.4 State-of-the-art performance comparison

	Wattanpanitch et al. (2007) [33]	**Qian et al. (2011) [34]**	**Wu et al. (2009) [36]**	**Denison et al. (2007) [26]**	**Fan et al. (2011) [29]**	**Guo et al. (2012) [37]**	**This work (post-layout simulation) [38]**
Current	2.7 μA	0.872 μA	230 μA	1 μA	1 μA	22.4 μA	2 μA
Power	7.6 μW	2.4 μW	1 mW	2 μW	1.8 μW	73.9 μW	4 μW
Gain (dB)	40.85	39.4	40	40	40	26	32.65
Bandwidth	45 Hz–5.32 kHz	0.36 Hz–1.3 kHz	800 kHz	1 kHz	–	30 kHz	25.1 kHz
IRN voltage	3.06 μV_{rms} (10 Hz–98 kHz)	3.07 μV_{rms} (0.5 Hz–30 kHz)	–	1.3 μV_{rms} (0.05 Hz–4 kHz)	6.7 μV_{rms} (0.5 Hz–100 Hz)	0.9 μV_{rms} (1 Hz–200 Hz)	0.69 μV_{rms} (0.05 Hz–300 Hz)
1/*f* noise corner	–	50 Hz	1 mHz	3 Hz	100 mHz	23 Hz	<1 Hz
Noise PSD ($nV/\sqrt{Hz}$)	31	60	15	94	60	32.9	39.89
NEF [39]	2.67	3.09	8.8	4.6	3.3	4.5	2.47
CMRR (dB)	>66	>66	>120	100	134	>110	>66
Chopping frequency (kHz)	–	–	40, 510	4	5	10	1
Process	0.5 μm CMOS	0.6 μm CMOS	0.7 μm CMOS	0.8 μm CMOS	65 nm CMOS	0.35 μm CMOS	0.18 μm CMOS

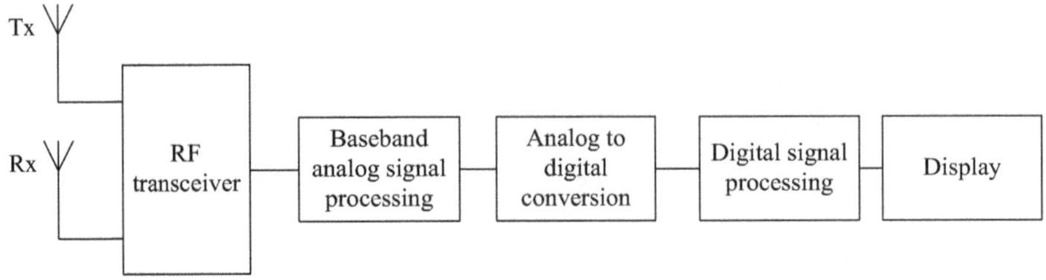

Figure 19.18 A typical Doppler-radar based NCVS sensor [44]

need for the patient's awareness or direct involvement. Since NCVS sensors are usually placed externally at a distance from the patient, they can be powered by mains power from the wall sockets or by rechargeable batteries, thus making them attractive for potential long-term continuous monitoring of heart rate and respiration rate. NCVS sensors can be designed for Industrial, Scientific and Medical (ISM) microwave frequencies, such as 2.4 GHz [43–45] and 5.8 GHz to make them universally acceptable for vital signs monitoring.

According to the Doppler effect theory, a target with a time-varying position and a zero-velocity reflects the incident RF signal with its *phase* modulated signal proportional to the time-varying target movement [43,46]. The NCVS sensor applies this Doppler radar theory by illuminating a stationary patient's chest wall containing periodic movements from both the larger respiration movements of the diaphragm and the smaller heartbeat movements, with a continuous wave (CW) incident wave. The RF transceiver block of the NCVS sensor can act as the CW radar to transmit the signal at an ISM frequency with 0 dBm power, and the phase modulated signal from the physiological movements is reflected from the patient's chest wall, which is then received by the RF transceiver block as well. The reflected signal contains the periodic cardio-pulmonary movement data, and by demodulating the phase of this signal and extracting the time-varying cardio-pulmonary information, we can provide good estimates of the heart rate as well as the respiration rate. The details of this Doppler NCVS principle are explained as followed.

19.4.1 Doppler radar principle for NCVS Sensor

The classic Doppler effect or the Doppler shift in frequency is given as,

$$f_d(t) = \frac{2f}{c}v(t) = 2\frac{v(t)}{\lambda} \tag{19.3}$$

Here $v(t)$ is the velocity of the target, f is the transmitted RF frequency, c is the velocity of propagation and λ is the wavelength of the transmitted signal. Considering the case when the target has a zero net velocity with a periodic cardio-pulmonary movement $x(t)$, the Doppler effect can now be represented as a phase modulation given by [47]:

$$\theta(t) = \frac{2f}{c}(2\pi x(t)) = \frac{4\pi x(t)}{\lambda} \tag{19.4}$$

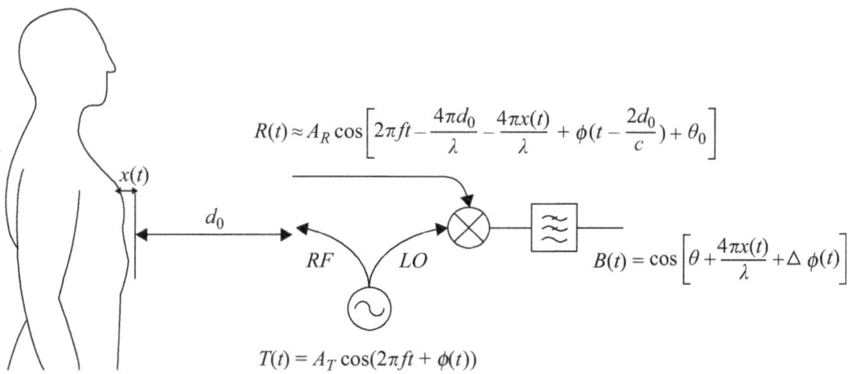

Figure 19.19 Simplified depiction of Doppler-radar principle used for NCVS sensor [48]

The baseband signal obtained after the down-conversion mixing using the CW transmit, $T(t)$ signal shown in Figure 19.19 is given as below (ignoring the amplitudes for simplicity):

$$B(t) = \cos\left[\frac{4\pi d_0}{\lambda} + \frac{4\pi x(t)}{\lambda} + \phi(t) - \phi\left(t - \frac{2d_0}{c}\right) + \theta_0\right] \tag{19.5}$$

On simplification, equation (19.5) can be re-written as,

$$B(t) = \cos\left[\theta + \frac{4\pi x(t)}{\lambda} + \Delta\phi(t)\right] \tag{19.6}$$

Here θ is phase term dependent on the position of the subject with respect to the NCVS sensor, and $\Delta\phi(t)$ is the residual phase noise after range correlation [47]. The "null-point" is seen whenever the LO signal and the incoming RF signal carrying the cardio-pulmonary information are in-phase or 180° out-of-phase, and the optimal sensitivity condition is observed when they are quadrature to each other. As θ is dependent on the distance of the subject from the NCVS sensor, the "null-points" are seen every quarter wavelength ($\lambda/4$). For a 2.4 GHz system, $\lambda/4$ is almost equal to 3 cm, which is a very small distance for optimal adjustments to be done to avoid the "null-points." Considering the above condition, quadrature receivers have been advocated to overcome this problem of the non-quadrature Doppler-based NCVS sensors [46].

19.4.2 Quadrature receiver and arc-tangent demodulation for NCVS sensors

A quadrature receiver is essentially a dual channel receiver where the RF input signal is split in two signal paths (e.g., using a 2-way 0° balun), and each of the RF paths are then down converted using two mixers with quadrature LO inputs to provide image rejection. The mixers' quadrature LO signals can be obtained; for example, from the same LO signal using a 2-way 90° power splitter. Following equation (19.6), the two orthonormal baseband signals obtained after mixing are given as,

$$B_I(t) = \cos\left[\theta + \frac{4\pi x(t)}{\lambda} + \Delta\phi(t)\right] \tag{19.7}$$

and

$$B_Q(t) = \sin\left[\theta + \frac{4\pi x(t)}{\lambda} + \Delta\phi(t)\right] \tag{19.8}$$

Here B_I denotes in-phase baseband signal channel and B_Q denotes the 90° out-of-phase or the quadrature baseband signal channel. When θ is an odd multiple of $\pi/2$, B_I channel experiences a "null-point" whereas B_Q is at its optimum point. Again when θ is an integer multiple of π, B_I channel experiences an optimum point whereas B_Q is at its "null-point." Thus, the mutual orthonormality between the channels ensures that for every $\pi/2$ phase or every $\lambda/4$ distance a simultaneous null-point and an optimum point are observed on either of the channels. Since information on any one of the channel can be used to determine cardio-pulmonary rates, the quadrature receiver, theoretically, can eradicate the problem of null-point for narrow-band signal with perfect I/Q phase and amplitude matching. However, dc-offsets and phase mismatches in the channels usually will degrade the performance of the RADAR system.

Over the years arc-tangent demodulation technique has emerged as a more opted choice due to its simple implementation and reasonably robust performance [44,45,49]. The accuracy of the arc-tangent demodulation technique increases when adequate dc-offset compensation techniques are employed in order to discard the unwanted dc-offset and preserve the dc-information regarding the target position [50,51]. Using equation (19.7) and (19.8) the arc-tangent demodulation can be implemented as represented in equation (19.9) below to obtain the cardio-pulmonary information,

$$\phi_{\text{arc-tangent}}(t) = \arctan\left[\frac{B_Q(t)}{B_I(t)}\right] = \arctan\left[\frac{\sin\left[\theta + \frac{4\pi x(t)}{\lambda} + \Delta\phi(t)\right]}{\cos\left[\theta + \frac{4\pi x(t)}{\lambda} + \Delta\phi(t)\right]}\right]$$

$$= \left[\theta + \frac{4\pi x(t)}{\lambda} + \Delta\phi(t)\right] \tag{19.9}$$

As discussed later, depending upon the range-correlation effect, the residual phase noise term can be considered small enough and the equation (19.9) can be represented as,

$$\phi_{\text{arc-tangent}}(t) \approx \theta + \frac{4\pi x(t)}{\lambda} \tag{19.10}$$

which contains the periodic cardio-pulmonary movement signal we need.

19.4.3 Direct-conversion receiver and range correlation in NCVS sensors

The direct-conversion receivers or zero-IF receivers directly down-convert the RF signal to the baseband for further signal processing, and this reduces the design complexity of the zero-IF receivers when compared to heterodyne receivers. An advantage of using direct-conversion receiver for NCVS sensors is the "range-correlation" effect, which remarkably reduces the noise spectrum at baseband [43,52]. The "range-correlation" effect is applicable in designs where the transceiver uses the same source to generate the transmit signal and the local oscillator (LO) signal for the down-converting mixers. The range-correlation effect in an NCVS is illustrated conceptually in Figure 19.19 [43]. The signal of interest at baseband has the relevant cardio-pulmonary data in the signal range of 0.1–10 Hz where the effect of high phase-noise is detrimental, and this range-correlation effect helps mitigating the VCO phase-noise effect, thus increasing the detection accuracy and robustness. Here in Figure 19.20, $S_\phi(f_0)$ is the phase noise of the signal source used as the LO and the transmit RF signal, $S_{\phi\_delayed}(f_0)$ is the phase noise of the physiological modulated reflected RF signal and $S_{\Delta\phi}(f_0)$ is the residual phase noise seen at baseband after phase noise filter due to the range-correlation effect.

Note the direct-conversion receivers also have their share of disadvantages, where the most important one being the inherent problem of dc-offsets. This dc-offset can be caused when using the same frequency for the mixer LO as the input RF signal. For example, the LO *self-mixing* caused by the LO feedthrough and I/Q mismatches can contribute to inherent dc-offsets. The inherent dc-offset of

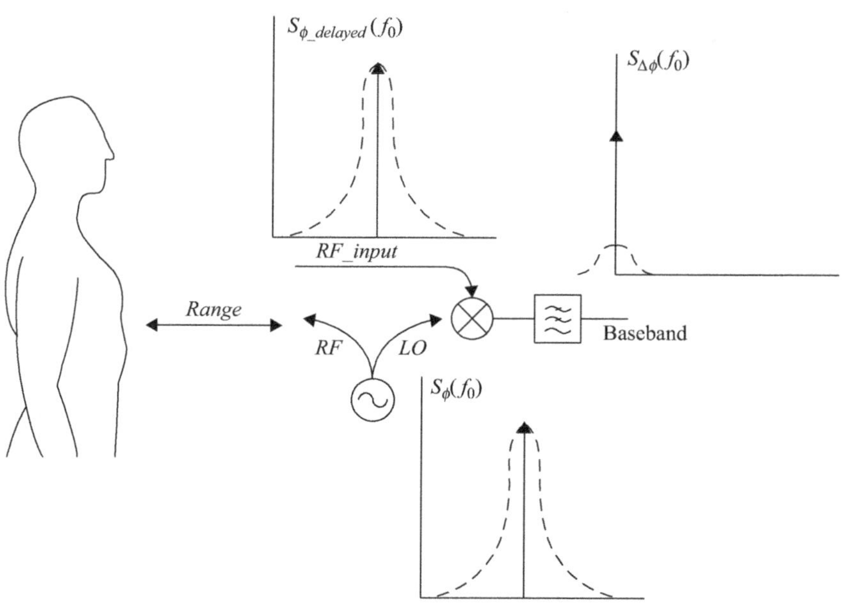

Figure 19.20 Range-correlation effect in a direct-conversion Doppler-based NCVS sensor [43]

the direct-conversion receiver combined with the dc-offset caused by background clutters and the non-cardiopulmonary signals (due to random motions, etc.) can add up to a noticeably large dc-offset, which needs to be filtered or compensated to avoid saturation of the subsequent baseband circuitry. Since the cardio-pulmonary signals are at very low frequencies (close to dc), the issue of dc-offset poses a challenge in accurate detection of the heart rate and respiration rate.

The nature of the antenna such as its gain and directivity also plays an important factor in the sensitivity and robustness of the NCVS sensor system. To minimize the dc-offsets caused by background clutter, experimental data for continuous heart and respiration rate monitoring was recorded in the *anechoic chamber* using the portable fourth-generation NCVS sensor system developed at Dr. Lie's lab. As mentioned before, the NCVS sensor system operates at the 2.4 GHz ISM band using a CW Doppler radar, where periodic chest motions of the monitored subject cause phase modulation that can be demodulated to detect the heart and respiration rates separately [43–45]. The subject is illuminated with separate Tx and Rx antennas to avoid the use of bulky and expensive circulators. The Rx signal which is a phase-modulated and time-delayed version of the Tx signal, is down-converted using the same local oscillator (LO) signal as used for the Tx signal. After down-conversion, full quadrature arctangent demodulation is carried out to extract the time-varying phase information for subsequent cardio-pulmonary rate estimation [44] (Figure 19.21).

Instead of using a stand-alone voltage-controlled oscillator (VCO) for LO frequency generation, the Tx CW signal for this fourth-generation sensor is

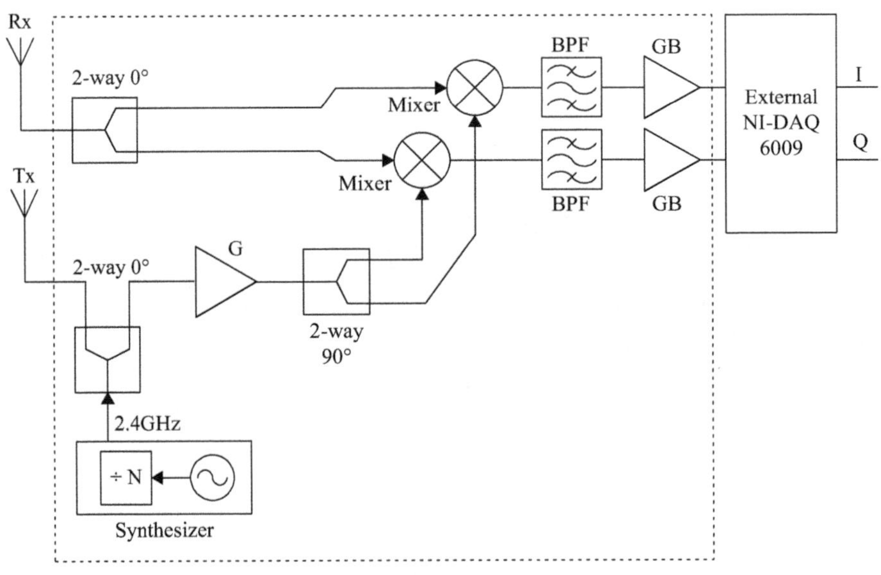

Figure 19.21 Block diagram of our fourth-generation NCVS sensor hardware

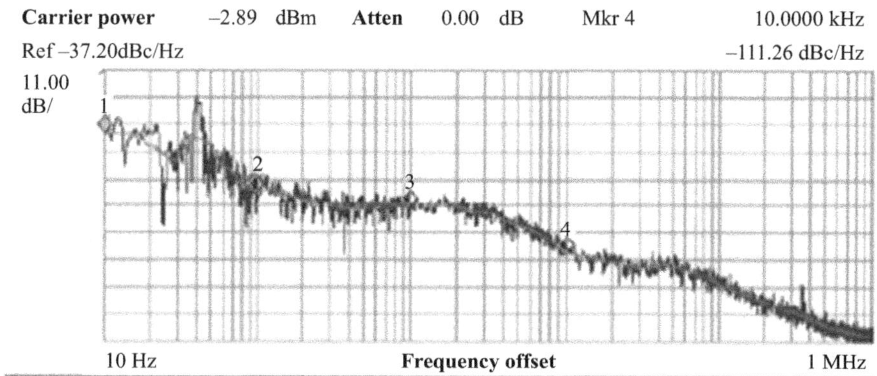

Marker	Trace	Type		X Axis	Value
1	2	Spot	Freq	10 Hz	−62.84 dBo/Hz
2	2	Spot	Freq	100 Hz	−85.83 dBo/Hz
3	2	Spot	Freq	1 kHz	−92.15 dBo/Hz
4	2	Spot	Freq	10 kHz	−111.27 dBo/Hz

Figure 19.22 Measured phase noise (−111 dBc/Hz at 10 kHz offset) of the synthesizer used in our fourth-generation NCVS sensor

generated by a frequency synthesizer with an external Pierce oscillator based 10.24 MHz reference to ensure excellent phase noise and thermal stability (Figure 19.22).

After the I/Q mixers stage, the signal is further conditioned with the Sallen-Key second-order low-pass and high-pass filters with cutoff frequencies at 10 and 0.1 Hz, respectively, using non-inverting op-amps with a voltage gain of 60 dB [47]. This allows us to eliminate a bulky LNA+filter stage used in some other systems [44]. The baseband signal is digitized at a sampling rate of 200 Hz with a National Instruments (NI) USB-6009 Multifunction Data Acquisition Unit (DAQ), which uses a 14-bit ADC with a maximum sampling rate of 48 kS/s, adequate for vital signs detection resolution after baseband filtering [45].

19.4.4 Antenna characterization for NCVS sensor – directivity and radiation patterns

Directivity of an antenna is the ratio of the radiation intensity in a given direction from the antenna to the radiation intensity averaged over all directions [53]. It can also be understood as the power density in a particular direction relative to the total power radiated in all directions [55]. The directivity of antenna is a figure of merit which specifies how focused the antenna is for both transmitting and receiving signals. NCVS sensor systems are required to sense cardio-pulmonary movements, which include heavily attenuated heart movements at the surface of the chest, thereby the directivity of the antenna is a factor in understanding and deciding the performance and sensitivity of the NCVS sensing. We have, therefore, used four different antennas with different characteristics in our NCVS system as shown in

Table 19.5 Basic antenna characteristics based on the radiation patterns

Antenna	Gain (dB)	Frequency (GHz)	E-H plane
Helical	9.8	2.4–2.5	Symmetric
Yagi	7	2.4–2.48	Asymmetric
Log-periodic	7	2.4–2.6	Asymmetric
Patch	7.5	2.4–2.6	Symmetric

Table 19.5 to evaluate their impacts on the overall NCVS system performance. Amongst the four antennas, Yagi, Log-periodic and Patch were commercial-of-the-shelf (COTS) antennas whereas the helical antenna was custom built at Dr. Lie's lab [54] (Figures 19.23–19.26).

Measured 3-dB beam-width or the half-power beamwidth (HPBW) and the side-lobe level (SLL) for the 4 types of antennas used summarized in Table 19.6. It is clear that the custom helical and Yagi antennas are more directional with better side-lobe rejection, and we shall see how their performance impacts the overall NCVS system next.

19.4.5 NCVS system evaluated with several antennas

Each antenna was tested with the sensor system on three different subjects (student volunteers) for 5 readings on each subject, in the anechoic chamber. The experimental setup is shown in Figure 19.27, with the subject sitting 50 cm from the antenna radiation plane. Even though the 50 cm distance was fixed, an I/Q-based CW Doppler NCVS system will still see a nulling issue that occurs periodically every $\lambda/4$ distance (for a 2.4 GHz system is almost equal to 3 cm in free space). This nulling issue happens when the target is placed at 0°, 90°, 180° or 270° from the radiation plane, and results in a large amplitude drop in either the I or Q channel response. Rather than being a problem, this nulling can be considered as a typical characteristic of Doppler-based NCVS systems. As mentioned earlier, the conventional solutions to overcome nulling are to use quadrature receivers with good demodulation algorithms insensitive to nulling, and to improve the system's dc offset and SNR (using good matching with low-noise amplifiers). Since our main goal here is to clearly compare and quantify the antenna performance for optimizing our NCVS sensor system, we have placed the subjects in a non-nulling plane of reference for each antenna for the front vital signs readings only. This allows us to attribute any performance improvements/issues to the antenna selection, rather than the positioning of the subject. Matlab™ and LabVIEW™ were used to process the data for antenna performance analysis.

Different subjects' vital signs were measured from the front, left, right and back sides using our portable NCVS system. The data was taken continuously for 4 min on each subject for each sitting, including a 30 s filter settling time (this long time was because we used large number of taps for the filters to achieve better

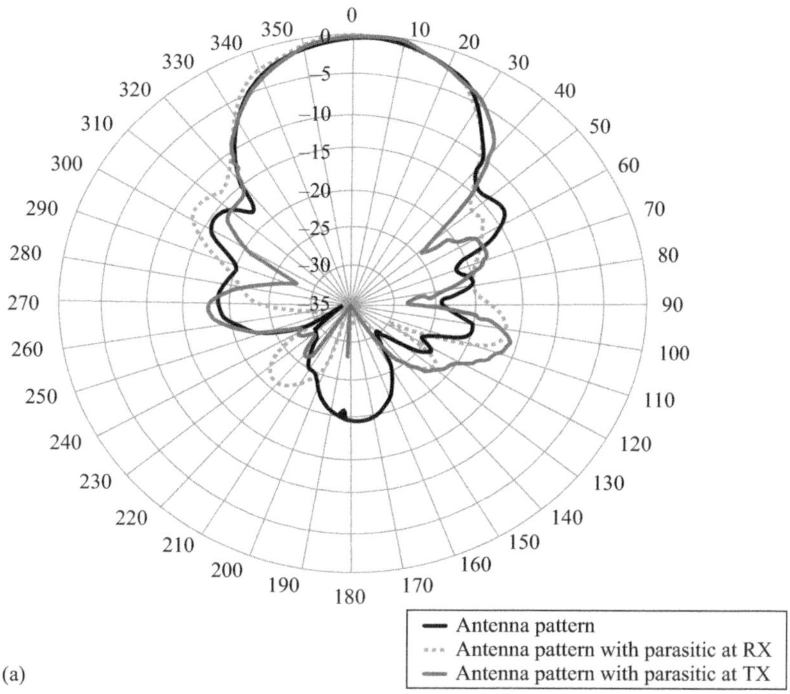

(a)

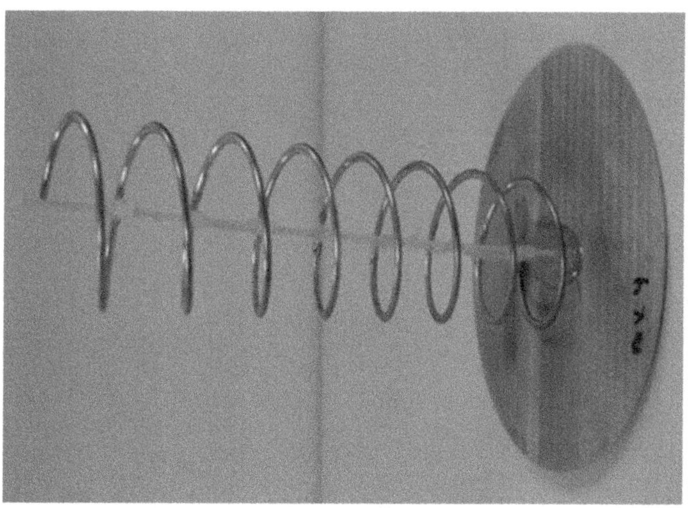

(b)

Figure 19.23 (a) Measured radiation patterns of the custom-built helical antenna. (b) The custom-built helical antenna

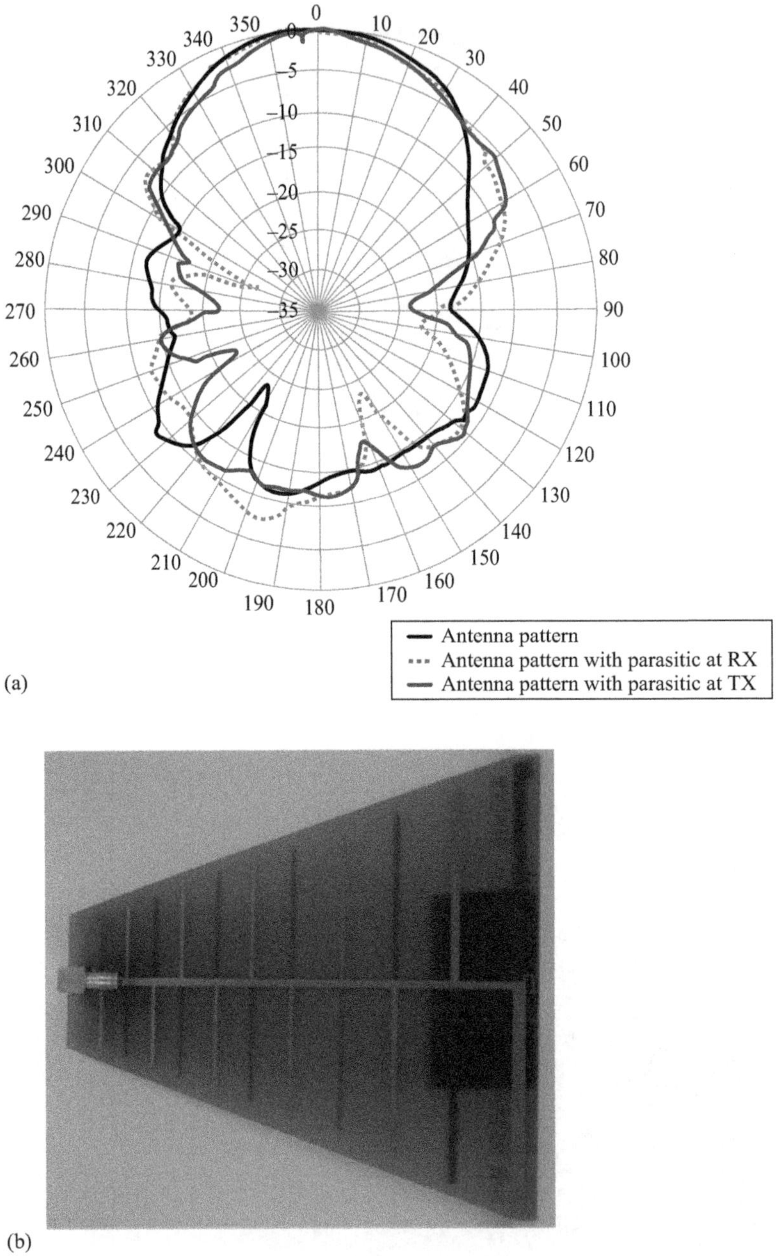

Figure 19.24 (a) Measured radiation patterns of the Log-periodic antenna we used. (b) The Log-periodic antenna

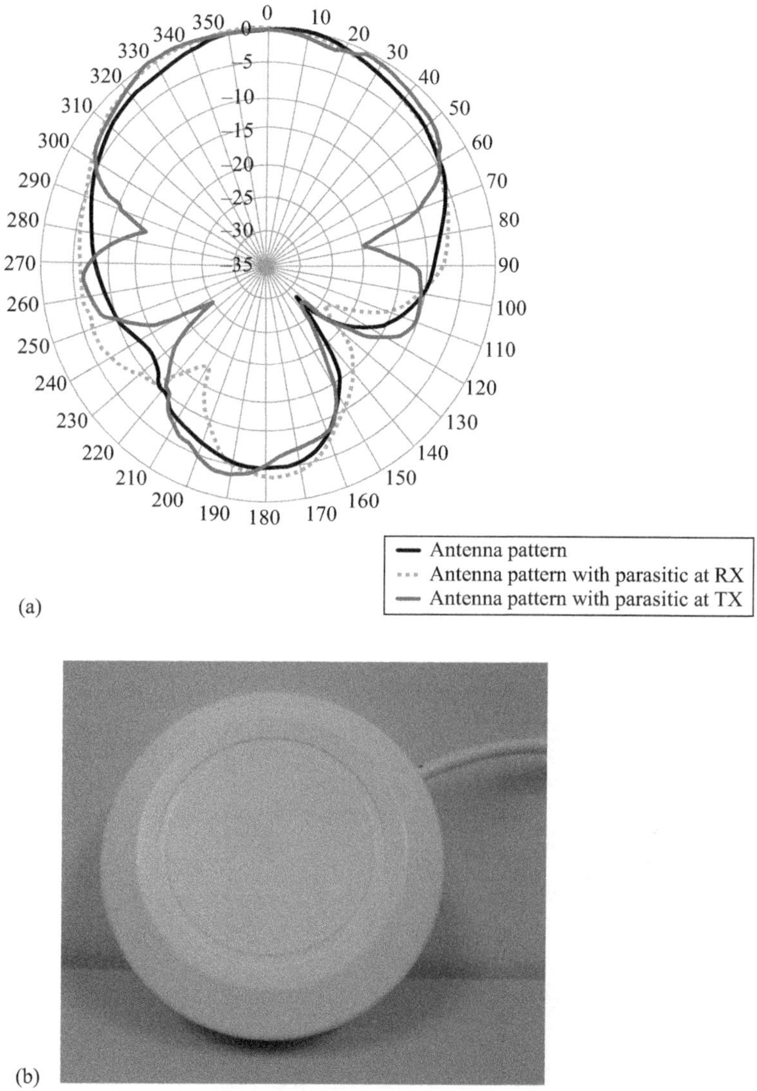

Figure 19.25 (a) Measured radiation patterns of the Patch antenna we used. (b) The Patch antenna

stop-band attenuation). The flow chart for the LabVIEW^{TM} code used in antenna evaluation using our NCVS system is shown in Figure 19.28. The subjects were asked to keep as motionless as possible during the measurement to prevent motion artifacts and to breathe normally.

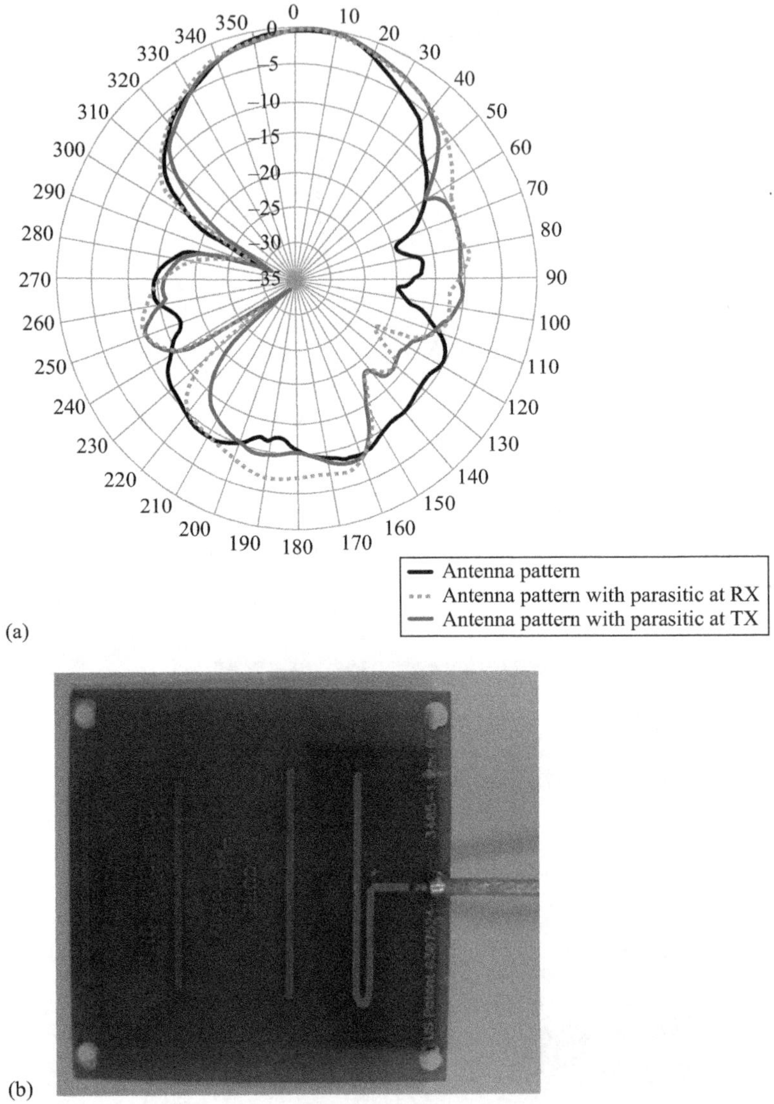

Figure 19.26 (a) Measured radiation patterns of the Yagi antenna we used. (b) The Yagi antenna

Table 19.6 Antenna characteristics based on the radiation patterns

Antenna	Half-power beamwidth (HPBW)	Side-lobe level (SLL)
Helical	44.6°	13.1 dB
Yagi	47°	14.2 dB
Log-periodic	62°	9.4 dB
Patch	92°	5.4 dB

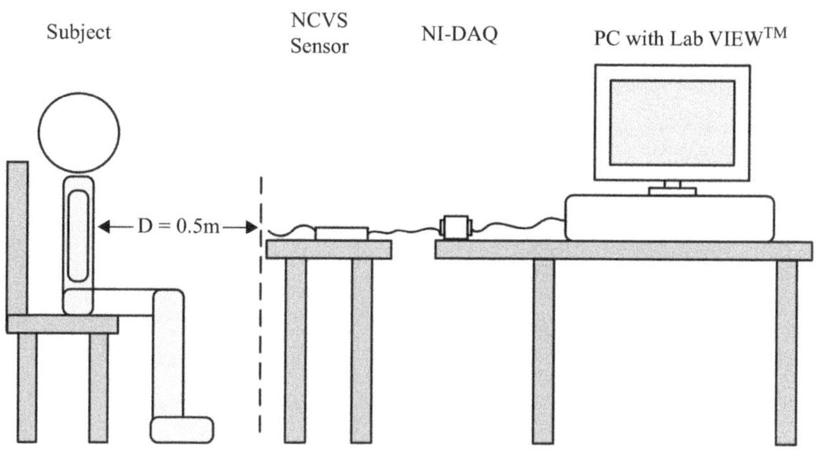

(a)

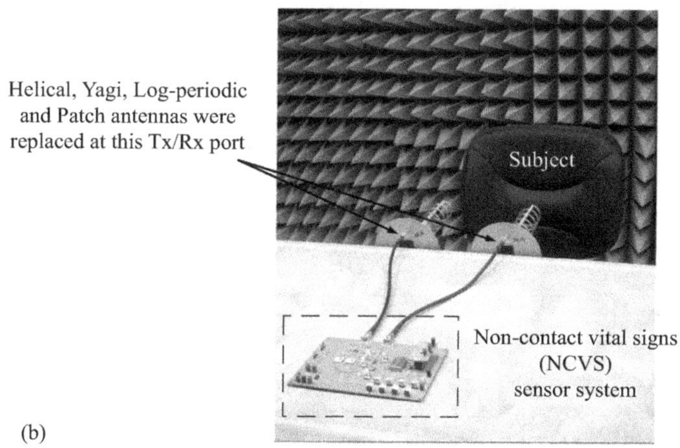

(b)

Figure 19.27 (a) Diagrammatic representation of the NCVS sensor measurement set up; (b) The test setup in the anechoic chamber at Dr Lie's lab

19.4.6 Experimental results and analysis

The helical antenna achieves a tighter error rate than the Yagi, Patch and Log-periodic antennas, as this can be seen in Figure 19.29. The inter-quartile range for the error rates of different antennas is summarized in Table 19.7. The plot shows the values for Rate Error in Beats per Minute (bpm). The data can be best used to directly compare antenna performance when there are negligible nulling effects. The reason for this performance can be directly attributed to the amount of directivity found in the antenna and its symmetry in the magnetic (H) and electric (E) planes. For example, the 3 dB BW of the custom designed helical antenna was measured as 44.6°, versus 62° and 92° for the Log-periodic and Patch antennas,

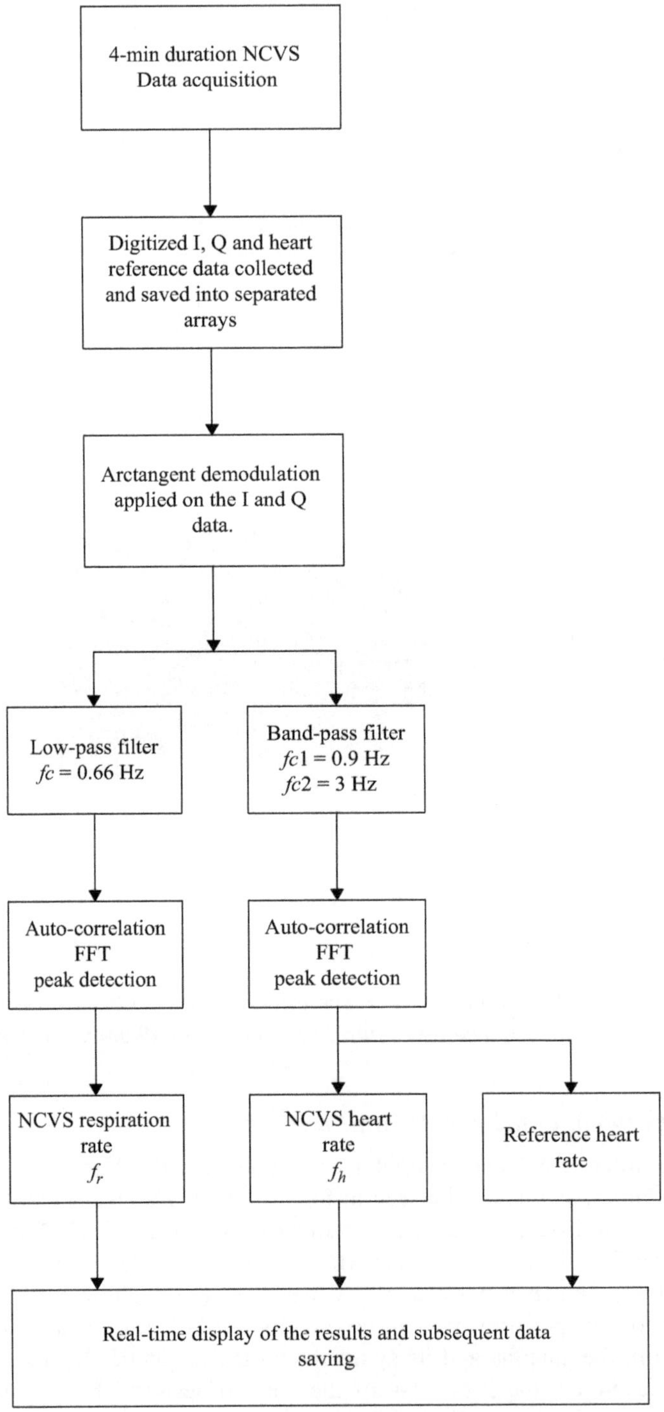

Figure 19.28 The flow chart for the LabVIEW™ code used in antenna evaluation using NCVS system at Dr. Lie's lab

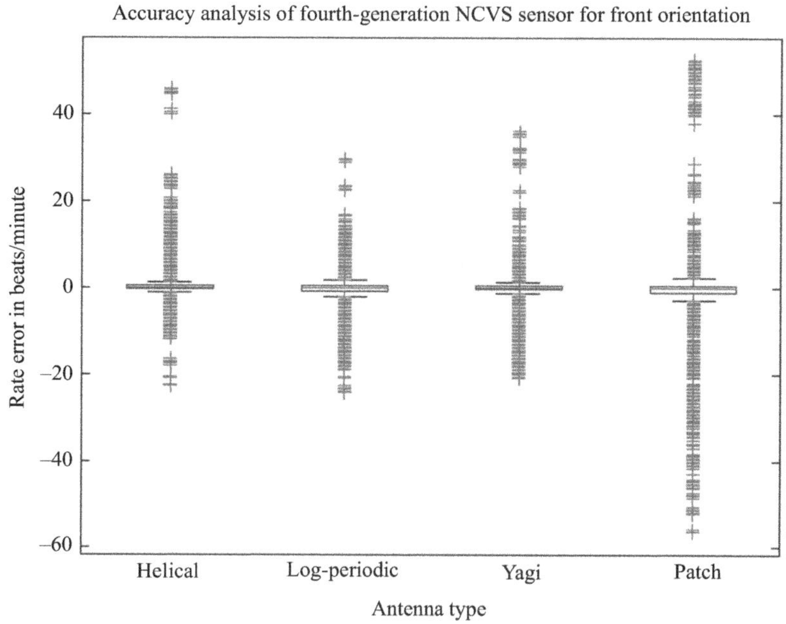

Figure 19.29 Box-Whisker plots for different antennas for subjects' front readings only

Table 19.7 Inter-quartile Range (IQR) for different antennas based on Figure 19.29

Antenna	**Inter-quartile range**
Helical	0.53
Yagi	0.65
Log-periodic	0.98
Patch	1.34

respectively. The Yagi antenna's 3 dB BW is similar to that of the helical antenna, but its pattern is not symmetrical across the E and H planes (about 60° BW in the H plane).

The sensor accuracy and statistics achieved in these experiments for heart rates are summarized in Table 19.8 for front readings of the subjects, which shows that the most directive helical antenna outperforms the rest, while the least directive patch ranks last.

The time-based signal obtained after arctangent demodulation was also extracted from the measurement, as shown in Figure 19.30. The largest detected

Table 19.8 Measured accuracy table for the non-contact vital signs system based on different antennas (for front readings only)

Antenna	Error < 1 bpm	Error < 2 bpm	Error < 5 bpm
Helical	74.53	77.91	84.53
Yagi	70.64	77.25	83.33
Log-periodic	65.04	70.61	76.07
Patch	62.64	67.91	72.73

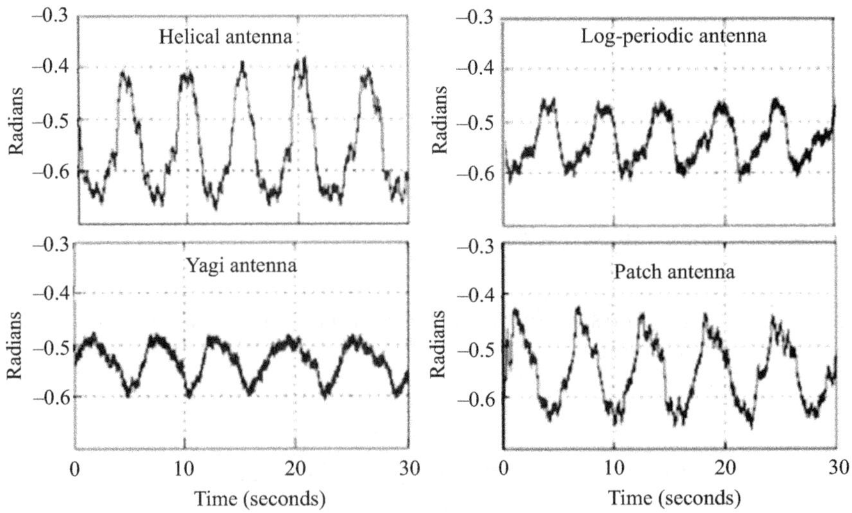

Figure 19.30 Time-based arctangent demodulated signal for heart rate extraction (front readings)

signal was obtained by using the helical antenna, which exceeded those from the Yagi and Log-periodic antennas by close to a factor of 2, indicating a higher gain for the helical antenna as shown in Table 19.5. An additional test was performed with equalized antenna gains for all 4 types of antennas, to verify significance of directivity vis-à-vis gain for sensitive systems like our NCVS sensor, as shown in Table 19.9.

Moreover, respiration rate was also measured during these experiments with excellent ± 1 breaths/min accuracy over 95% of the time. Since the cardiac signal is orders of magnitude smaller than the respiration signal and presents the largest challenges for robust continuous NCVS monitoring, the error of heart rate is expected to be higher compared to the respiration rate [44,56,57]. Thus the heart rate data was used to assess system performance with different antennas. The data shown suggests that the increment in signal radian amplitude strength shown in Figure 19.30, due to the high directivity and symmetric E and H patterns of the

Table 19.9 Measured accuracy table of NCVS system for the gain-equalization experiment (for front readings only)

Antenna	Error < 1 bpm	Error < 2 bpm	Error < 5 bpm
Helical	78.16	81.83	85.59
Yagi	70.64	77.25	83.33
Log-periodic	65.04	70.61	76.07
Patch	62.64	67.91	72.73

helical antenna, can enhance the SNIR of Doppler-based vital signs systems. Further development of the NCVS system includes implementing dc offset error corrections and movement detection algorithms to reduce motion artifacts, allowing improvements in system performance.

19.5 Summary of heart beat sensing techniques

With the various types of heart beat sensing techniques like the wearable ECG sensors, ICD/pacemakers and the Doppler-based non-contact biosensors discussed thus far, it is imperative to investigate the efficient techniques to realize robust and reliable heart rate sensing for a given application. One objective of our research is to understand the system level details and try to derive important design paradigms which would make the existing systems more robust, reliable and power-efficient. A system-level comparison has been shown in Table 19.10, and as can be observed that each of the heart beat sensing technology has its own share of pros and cons. For example, the wearable ECG sensors have better detection accuracy but the use of various electrodes is a cause of discomfort for the monitored patient, thus hampering long-term continuous cardiac monitoring. In the case of pacemakers/ICDs, administering pacing/defibrillation requires a proper knowledge of the instantaneous state of heart deflections, for example if the defibrillation is provided during a T-wave instead of the R-wave it can escalate the fibrillation leading to lethal consequences [3]. Furthermore, defibrillation or pacing is effectively realized only by using the electrode-lead assembly and the sensing-defibrillation module implanted inside the human body. This needs a vascular surgery which is a definite impediment to be used on some patients, even though recently the subcutaneous-ICD (S-ICD®) mentioned earlier may be able to alleviate this serious transvenous surgical pains and electrode-lead failures in the future. On the other hand, the use of NCVS sensor systems for continuous monitoring appears to be attractive for its higher comfort level and relatively relaxed power requirements, but this technology can be plagued with less reliable heart rate detection accuracy due to various artifacts and clutters. The NCVS sensor system records the periodicity of the physical heart movement as rather than the exact heart beat signal, making it impossible to be used for defibrillation; therefore an NCVS sensor system is unlikely to replace the contact-based heart sensing technologies, but will be an excellent complimentary technique to

Table 19.10 Heart beat sensing techniques – a comparison

	Wearable electrocardiogram (ECG) Sensors	**Implantable cardioverter defibrillator (ICD)/pacemaker**	**Doppler-based non-contact vital signs (NCVS) sensor**
Method	Body surface contact	Intracardiac contact	No contact
Signal	ECG	EGM	Reflected phased-modulated signal
Low power consumption	Critical	Extremely critical	Less critical
Power supply	Battery	Li-ion battery	Wall-power or batteries
Position	On the body	Inside the body	Away from the body
Comfort level	Low	Moderate	High
Robustness (detection accuracy)	High	High	Low
Therapy	None	Defibrillation/pacing	None
Miniature form-factor	Recommended	Required	Not critical
Sensing circuit	Analog	Analog	RF-analog
Wireless connectivity	Can be done	Can be done (limited due to power constraints)	Can be done

provide ubiquitous and continuous on-line monitoring, especially for sleep apnea, etc. For each monitoring scenario for a given patient, the optimal choice of one or a combination of the three heart rate sensing techniques requires some good understanding on the limitations and strengths with each technique to realize the best robust and continuous online heartbeat monitoring system.

References

[1] C.G. Caro and J.A. Bloice, "Contactless apnea detector based on radar," *Lancet*, vol. 2, no. 7731, pp. 959–961, Oct. 1971.

[2] National Instruments, "LabVIEW for ECG signal processing," *NI Tutorial 6349*, Aug. 2012.

[3] J.G. Webster, *Medical Instrumentation: Application and Design*, Fourth Edition, John Wiley & Sons, 2009.

[4] R. Fensli, E. Gunnarson and T. Gundersen, "A wearable ECG-recording system for continuous arrhythmia monitoring in a wireless tele-home-care

situation," *Proc. 18th IEEE Symp. Computer-Based Medical Systems*, pp. 407–412, 23–24 Jun. 2005.

[5] J. Welch, F. Guilak and S.D. Baker, "A wireless ECG smart sensor for broad application in life threatening event detection," *Proc. 26th Annu. Int. Conf. IEEE EMBS*, vol. 2, pp. 3447–3449, 1–5 Sept. 2004.

[6] C. Park, P.H. Chou, Ying Bai, R. Matthews and A. Hibbs, "An ultra-wearable, wireless, low power ECG monitoring system," *IEEE Biomed. Circuits Syst.*, pp. 241–244, 29 Nov.–1 Dec. 2006.

[7] C. Assambo and M.J. Burke, "Amplifier input impedance in dry electrode ECG recording," *Annu. Int. Conf. IEEE Eng. Med. Biol. Soc.*, pp. 1774–1777, 3–6 Sept. 2009.

[8] E. Nemati, M.J. Deen and T. Mondal, "A wireless wearable ECG sensor for long-term applications," *IEEE Commun. Mag.*, vol. 50, no. 1, pp. 36–43, Jan. 2012.

[9] L. Fay, V. Misra and R. Sarpeshkar, "A micropower electrocardiogram amplifier," *IEEE Trans. Biomed. Circuits Syst.*, vol. 3, no. 5, pp. 312–320, Oct. 2009.

[10] C.-L. Chang, C.-W. Chang, H.-Y. Huang, *et al.*, "A power-efficient bio-potential acquisition device with DS-MDE sensors for long-term healthcare monitoring applications," *Sensors*, vol. 10, no. 5, pp. 4777–4793, 2010.

[11] F. Pini, C. O'Mahony and K.G. McCarthy, "Electrical characterisation of dry microneedle electrodes for portable bio-potential recording applications," *IEEE Int. Conf. Microelectronics Test Structures (ICMTS)*, pp. 87–90, 19–22 Mar. 2012.

[12] W.H. Ko, M.R. Neuman, R.N. Wolfson and E.T. Yon, "Insulated active electrodes," *IEEE Trans. Ind. Elect. Contr. Instrum.*, vol. IECI-17, pp. 195–198, 1970.

[13] R.M. David and W.M. Portnoy, "Insulated electrogram electrodes," *Med. Biol. Eng.*, vol. 10, pp. 742–751, 1972.

[14] H. Gray, *Anatomy of the Human Body*, 20th ed., Philadelphia: Lea & Febiger, 1918.

[15] J.A. Warren, R.D. Drehe, R.V. Jaworski and J.J. Putzke, "Implantable cardioverter defibrillators," *Proc. IEEE*, vol. 84, no. 3, pp. 468–479, Mar. 1996.

[16] W. Hu, Y.-T. Liu, T. Nguyen, B. Dsouza and D.Y.C. Lie, "Ultralow-power analog front-end IC design for an implantable cardioverter defibrillator (ICD)," *2011 IEEE 9th Int. Conf. ASIC (ASICON)*, pp. 1018–1021, 25–28 Oct. 2011.

[17] U. Cho, Y. Jung, S. Lim and J. Kim, "Implantable bio-medical SoC for ICD with wireless communication system," *IEEE 59th Electron. Compon. Technol. Conf.*, pp. 1086–1091, 26–29 May 2009.

[18] H.M. Haqqani and H.G. Mond, "The implantable cardioverter-defibrillator lead: principles, progress, and promises," *Pacing Clin. Electrophsiol.*, vol. 32, pp. 1336–1353, 2009.

[19] A. Gupta, A. Al-Ahmad and P.J. Wang, "Subcutaneous implantable cardioverter-defibrillator technology," *Cardiac Electrophysiology Clinics,* vol. 1, no. 1, pp. 147–154, Dec. 2009.

[20] G.H. Brady, W.M. Smith, M.A. Hood, *et al.*, "An entirely subcutaneous implantable cardioverter defibrillator," *New Eng. J. Med.,* vol. 363, pp. 36–44, 2010.

[21] R. Capatto, W.M. Smith, M.A. Hood, *et al.*, "Subcutaneous chronic implantable defibrillation system in humans," *J. Interv. Card. Electrophysiol.*, vol. 34, no. 3, pp. 325–32, Sept. 2012.

[22] A.E. Zadeh, "Nano-power switched-capacitor bandpass filters for medical implantable pacemakers and defibrillators," *51st Midwest Symp. Circuits Syst.*, pp. 29–32, 10–13 Aug. 2008.

[23] R.F. Yazicioglu, P. Merken, R. Puers and C.V. Hoof, "A 60 μW 60 nV/$\sqrt{}$Hz readout front-end for portable biopotential acuqisition systems," *IEEE J. Solid-State Circuits,* vol. 42, no. 5, pp. 1100–1109, May 2007.

[24] N. Verma, A. Shoeb, J. Bohorquez, J. Dawson, J. Guttag and A. Chandrakasan, "A 60 μW 60 nV/$\sqrt{}$Hz readout front-end for portable biopotential acquisition systems," *IEEE J. Solid-State Circuits,* vol. 45, no. 4, pp. 804–816, Apr. 2010.

[25] C. Assambo and M.J. Burke, "Amplifier input impedance in dry electrode ECG recording," *Annu. Int. Conf. IEEE Eng. Med. Biol. Soc. (EMBC),* pp. 1774–1777, 3–6 Sept. 2009

[26] T. Denison, K. Consoer, W. Santa, A. Avestruz, J. Cooley and A. Kelly, "A 2 μW 100 nV/$\sqrt{}$Hz chopper-stabilized instrumentation amplifier for chronic measurement of neural field potentials," *IEEE J. Solid State Circuits*, vol. 42, no. 12, pp. 2934–2945, Dec. 2007.

[27] Analog Devices Inc., "ADAS1000 – low-power, five electrode electrocardiogram (ECG) analog front end," *ADAS1000 Data Sheet, Rev.,* Aug. 2012.

[28] Texas Instruments, "ADS1292R – low-power, 2-channel, 24-bit analog front End FOR biopotentials measurements," *ADS1292R Data Sheet, Rev. B*, Sept. 2012.

[29] Q. Fan, F. Sebastiano, J.H. Huijsing and K.A.A. Makinwa, "A 1.8 μW 60 nV/$\sqrt{}$Hz capacitively-coupled chopper instrumentation amplifier in 65 nm CMOS for wireless sensor nodes," *IEEE J. Solid State Circuits*, vol. 46, no. 7, pp. 1534–1543, Jul. 2011.

[30] P.K. Chan, K.A. Ng and X.L. Zhang, "A CMOS Chopper-Stabilized Differential Difference Amplifier for Biomedical Integrated Circuits", *47th IEEE Intl. Midwest Symp. Circuits Systems*, vol. III, pp. 33–36, 2004.

[31] C. Enz and G. Temes, "Circuit Techniques for Reducing the Effects of Op-Amp Imperfections: Autozeroing, Correlated Double Sampling and Chopper Stabilization", *Invited Paper, Proc. IEEE*, vol. 84, No. 11, pp. 1584–1612, Nov. 1996.

[32] C. Enz, E.A. Vittoz and F. Krummenacher, "A CMOS chopper amplifier," *Invited Paper, IEEE J. Solid-State Circuits,* vol. SC-22, no. 3, pp. 335–342, Jun. 1987.

[33] W. Wattanpanitch, M. Fee and R. Sarpeshkar, "An energy efficient micropower neural recording amplifier 60 μW 60 nV/$\sqrt{}$Hz readout front-end for portable biopotential acquisition systems," *IEEE Trans. Biomed. Circuits Syst.*, vol. 1, pp. 136–147, Jun. 2007.

[34] C. Qian, J. Parramon and E. Sánchez-Sinencio, "A micropower low-noise neural recording front-end circuit for epileptic seizure detection," *IEEE J. Solid-State Circuits*, vol. 46, no. 6, pp. 1392–1405, Jun. 2011.

[35] P.E. Allen and D.R. Holberg, *CMOS Analog Circuit Design*, 2nd ed. New York: Oxford University Press, 2003.

[36] R. Wu, K.A.A. Makinwa and J.H. Huijsing, "A chopper current feedback instrumentation amplifier with 1 mHz 1/*f* noise corner and an AC-coupled ripple reduction loop," *IEEE J. Solid-State Circuits,* vol. 44, no. 12, Dec. 2009.

[37] J. Guo, J. Yuan, J. Huang, J.K.-Y. Law, C.-K. Yeung and M. Chan, "32.9 nV/rt Hz -60.6 dB THD dual-band micro-electrode array signal acquisition IC", *IEEE J. Solid State Circuits*, vol. 47, no. 5, pp. 1209–1220, May 2012.

[38] V. Das, D.Y.C Lie and T. Nguyen, "A fully integrated low noise CMOS instrumentation amplifier design for low power biosensors," *IEEE Midwest Symp. on Circuits and Systems (MWSCAS)*, pp. 535–538, 3–6 Aug. 2014.

[39] R.R. Harrison and C. Charles, "A low-power low-noise CMOS amplifier for neural recording applications," *IEEE J. Solid-State Circuits,* vol. 38, no. 6, pp. 958–965, June, 2003.

[40] C.I. Franks, B.H. Brown and D.M. Johnston, "Contactless respiration monitoring of infants," *Med. Biol. Eng.*, vol. 14, no. 3, pp. 306–312, May 1976.

[41] J.C. Lin, J. Kiernicki, M. Kiernicki and P.B. Wollschlaeger, "Microwave apexcardiography," *IEEE Tran. Microw. Theory and Tech.*, vol. 27, pp. 618–620, 1979.

[42] K.M. Chen, Y. Huang, J. Zhang and A. Norman, "Microwave life-detection systems for searching human subjects under earthquake rubble and behind barrier," *IEEE Trans. Biomed. Eng.*, vol. 27, pp. 105–114, Jan. 2000.

[43] A.D. Droitcour, "Non-contact measurement of heart and respiration rates with a single chip microwave Doppler radar", *Doctoral Thesis, Stanford University, CA,* 2006.

[44] B.K. Park, O. Boric-Lubecke and V. Lubecke, "Arctangent demodulation with DC offset compensation in quadrature doppler radar receiver systems," *IEEE Trans. Microw. Theory Tech.*, vol. 55, no. 5, pp. 1073–1079, 2007.

[45] R. Ichapurapu, S. Jain, M.U. Kakade, D.Y.C. Lie and R.E. Bannister, "A 2.4 GHz non-contact biosensor system for continuous vital-signs monitoring on a single PCB," *Proc. IEEE ASICON*, pp. 925–928, 2009.

[46] B.K. Park, S. Yamada, O. Boric-Lubecke and V. Lubecke, "Single-channel receiver limitations in Doppler radar measurements of periodic motion," *IEEE Radio Wireless Symp.*, pp. 99–102, 17–19 Jan. 2006.

[47] R. Ichapurapu, "A 2.4 GHz non-contact biosensor system for continuous vital-signs monitoring," *Master Thesis, Texas Tech, TX,* 2010.

[48] A.D. Droitcour, O. Boric-Lubecke, V. Lubecke, J. Lin and G.T.A. Kovacs, "Range correlation and I/Q performance benefits in single chip silicon Doppler radars for non-contact cardiopulmonary monitoring," *IEEE Trans. Microw. Theory Tech.,* vol. 52, no. 3, pp. 838–848, Mar. 2004.

[49] V. Das, A. Boothby, R. Hwang, T. Nguyen, J. Lopez and D.Y.C. Lie, "Antenna evaluation of a non-contact vital signs sensor for continuous heart and respiration rate monitoring," *IEEE Topical Conf. Biomed. Wireless Technol., Netw. Sens. Syst. (BioWireleSS)*, pp. 13–16, 15–18 Jan. 2012.

[50] M. Valkama, M. Renfors and V. Koivunen, "Advanced methods for I/Q imbalance compensation in communication receivers," *IEEE Trans. Signal. Process.,* vol. 49, no. 10, pp. 2335–2344, Oct. 2001.

[51] B.K. Park, V. Lubecke, O. Boric-Lubecke and A. Host-Madsen, "Center tracking quadrature demodulation for a doppler radar motion detector," *Microw. Symp. IEEE/MTT-S Int.*, pp. 1323–1326, 3–8 Jun. 2007.

[52] M.C. Budge Jr. and M.P. Burt, "Range correlation effects on phase and amplitude noise", *Proc. IEEE Southeastcon, Charlotte, NC*, pp. 5–9, 1993.

[53] C.A. Balanis, *Antenna Theory: Analysis and Design*, 2nd edition, John Wiley Sons, 1997.

[54] A. Boothby, R. Hwang, V. Das, J. Lopez and D.Y.C. Lie, "Design of axial-mode helical antennas for Doppler-based continuous non-contact vital signs monitoring sensors, *IEEE Radio Wireless Symp. (RWS*), pp. 87–90, 15–18 Jan. 2012.

[55] W.L. Stutzman., "Estimating directivity and gain of antennas," *IEEE Antennas Propag. Mag.*, vol. 40, no. 4, pp. 7–11, Aug. 1998.

[56] D.R. Morgan and M.G. Zierdt, "Novel signal processing techniques for Doppler radar cardiopulmonary sensing," *Signal Process.,* vol. 89, no. 1, pp. 45–66, Jan. 2009.

[57] B.-J. Jang, S.-H. Wi, J.-G. Yook, M.-Q. Lee and K.-J. Lee, "Wireless bio-radar sensor for heartbeat and respiration detection," *Prog. Electromag. Res. C.* vol. 5, 149–168, 2008.

Chapter 20

Lab on a chip for point-of-care analysis of drugs in body fluids

Feng Li[1,2], Rosanne M. Guijt[2] and Michael C. Breadmore[1]

20.1 Introduction

Lab-on-chip systems, also known as micro total analysis systems (μTASs), can be defined as integrated microfluidic systems that can perform all of the stages of biological and chemical laboratory processes. Microfluidics is the study and use of fluids at the sub-millimeter length scale. At this scale, only small volumes are required and diffusion is fast, and owing to the unique fluidic behavior at this length scale, complex laboratory tasks can be miniaturized and integrated into a small device. The portability, compactness, high levels of integration, automation and parallelization features in lab-on-a-chip technology is an emerging trend in point-of-care diagnostics [1].

Analytical drug tests are usually performed in a central laboratory by trained laboratory technicians, and in the case of therapeutic drug monitoring the patient typically has to wait for several hours to days to receive the test results before treatment can be adjusted. This is a problem for some acute diseases that need rapid and immediate intervention, such as the treatment of sepsis in an intensive care unit. It is also impedes the workflow for law enforcement officers trying to determine if a suspect has been using drugs of abuse.

Point-of-collection testing (POCT) systems are instruments that do not need special laboratory workers or huge machines, and can provide rapid in vitro testing at the point of collection: a patients' bed-site in hospital or institution, a doctor's office, the ambulance or at home. The obtained information can be directly applied to manage health care by evaluating the therapeutic efficiency, or for the analysis of drug of abuse at the roadside, a crime scene or the workplace [2]. The benefit of a rapid outcome is that it allows for action to be taken immediately, improving health outcomes for the patient and their quality of life, and the more widespread

[1]Australian Centre for Research on Separation Science, School of Chemistry, University of Tasmania, Private Bag 75, Hobart, Tasmania 7001, Australia
[2]School of Medicine and Australian Centre for Research on Separation Science, University of Tasmania, Private Bag 26, Hobart, Tasmania 7001, Australia

screening for drugs of abuse that will make society a safer environment to live and work. In this chapter, we will first discuss some basics about POCT, then lab-on-chip systems for POCT will be presented, including materials and fabrication, detection and applications to drug analysis in body fluids.

20.2 Point-of-collection testing (POCT)

Therapeutic drug monitoring (TDM) makes it possible for a health care practitioner to assess the efficacy of pharmacotherapy and adjust the administrated dose to the optimal level. Typically, dosage is determined by a clinical practitioner based on best practice guidelines, with perhaps some consideration of individual traits such as sex, weight and age, often ignoring the inter-individual differences between patients with regard to their genetic, environmental and lifestyle factors. Depending on the therapeutic index, the ratio of the drug level that causes significant adverse effects divided by drug level required for the desired therapeutic effect, this approach may result in some patients experiencing the desirable therapeutic effects, while others do not have the effect and/or may suffer from toxic effects. Dosage adjustment only based on clinical symptoms is not recommended, hence the importance of TDM for narrow therapeutic index compounds and in situations where patient characteristics do not resemble a healthy individual.

There is also a need for rapid and accurate analysis of drug of abuse. Drug of abuse can be classified as depressants such as barbiturates and benzodiazepines, stimulants such as amphetamines and cocaine, analgesics such as opioids and psychotomimetics such as marijuana based on their pharmacological effect [3]. Drug of abuse can be found in competitive sports, crime scenes, driving, or within the workplace, which may cause serious social problems or affect the ability to control machinery or vehicles.

Currently, testing for drugs is typically performed in a centralized laboratory, although there are a few exceptions like qualitative lateral flow tests used in roadside drug testing. There is an obvious delay and significant expense associated with this as samples must be collected, preserved during transport to the laboratory, prepared and treated for analysis by a trained laboratory technician, the interpreted results returned to inform any possible action that may occur as a result of the test. This process compromises the quality of care, and delays medical or legal intervention.

POCT systems are fully automated instruments that do not require special laboratory workers or large instruments, and can provide rapid in vitro testing results at the site where the sample is collected, or digitally transmit this information to a healthcare provider [2]. Usually little, or ultimately no, prior sample pre-treatment is needed such that the POCT device is 'sample-in/answer-out'. Currently POCT systems are rarely as good as central laboratory testing in terms of the precision and accuracy, and regular confirmatory central laboratory testing is often required. Compared with central laboratory testing, POCT enables faster response times owing to the alleviation of sample transport and communication issues, which is important for acute disease diagnosis and for samples that are unstable over time. Ideally POCT is easy to use and can be operated by non-expert without user interventions [4].

An effective POCT system needs to meet a number of requirements: affordable, sensitive, specific, user-friendly, rapid and robust, preferably equipment-free, deliverable, which is abbreviated as 'ASSURED' [5]. Affordability is very important, especially for widespread implementation and in the developing world. Accuracy (sensitivity and specificity) of the result and robustness relate to the reliability of the POCT. Ease-of-use is a primary requirement because POCT should be designed to be used onsite by persons with little training. The testing should be rapid with minimal manual sample handling. Recognizing some equipment will be required when going beyond colorimetric lateral flow assays, the POCT should be small, portable, preferable battery operated such that it can be transported and used easily.

The most widespread POCT system is the blood glucose meter used by diabetic patients, which has developed over 30 years into a sophisticated and reliable test that provides analytical data that is as good as what can be obtained in a centralized laboratory. Regular A1c testing in a laboratory facility, however, is still required to confirm blood glucose levels are managed appropriately. The glucose test is the very forefront in the field of POCT, but there are very few other examples that provide high accuracy quantitative data.

20.3 Lab-on-chip system for POCT

Lab-on-a-chip systems, which are also known as micro total analysis systems (μTAS), miniaturize, integrate and automate all of the steps necessary for a complete sample analysis. The portability, compactness, and automation of processes and parallelization features of lab-on-a-chip devices make it an ideal platform for the development of POCT [4]. In this section, the instrument aspects of lab-on-chip systems including materials and fabrication and detection will be discussed firstly, after which the application of the lab-on-chip systems will be explored with a focus on the application in POCT.

20.3.1 Materials and fabrication

Fabrication of microfluidic devices is the first step in making a μTAS device. A wide variety of materials has been used to fabricate microfluidic devices, and can be classified as inorganic materials (silicon, glass, etc.), elastomers and plastics (PDMS, PMMA, PC, etc.) and paper. Very simple methods using dry film photoresists and overhead transparencies printed with toner have also been used for research purposes.

The first generation of microfluidic devices were made in silicon and glass [6], arising from their widespread use in microelectronics. Highly precise micro- and nano-structures can be realized using a process typically including photolithography followed by wet or dry etching. While glass and silicon have many excellent properties, their material and processing costs are relatively high. For example, hydrofluoric acid used for wet etching is hazardous and special facilities are required for its handling and disposal. RIE for dry etching requires expensive instrumentation and the gases used are also quite expensive. Furthermore, bonding or sealing of glass and silicon is quite demanding and requires special conditions (high temperature, pressure and a relatively clean environment). Even though some low temperature bonding strategies have been developed, like calcium-assisted glass-to-glass bonding [7], bonding continues to be a significant challenge.

Microchips based on polymers were introduced in the 1990s. Polymers are available with an increasing variety of properties, allowing scientists to select the material most suitable for their purpose. Polymers can be inexpensive, and their fabrication is simpler than that for glass and silicon, and up-scaling is well established in the plastic manufacturing industry. An especially popular material is polydimethylsiloxane (PDMS), an insulating elastomer with good optical transparency over a wide range of wavelengths. Introduced by Effenhauser *et al.* and further developed by the Whitesides group, the process of casting PDMS structures form a microstructured template is called soft lithography. The mixture of liquid PDMS precursor and curing agent is poured onto a template and cured (typically done in an oven to accelerate the cross linking reaction). The patterned PDMS substrate can be easily peeled off from the template because of the low surface tension of PDMS, and can then be reversibly or irreversibly bonded to another PDMS slab, glass or other substrate. This simple process does not require a clean room, making PDMS a very popular material in many research laboratories. In practice, however, PDMS has some disadvantages: the hydrophobicity and structure of PDMS facilitates the adsorption and absorption of hydrophobic analytes [8], and PDMS is incompatible with many organic solvents. Also, its low stiffness limits the aspect ratios that can be realized because of collapsing and self-adhesion, an issue that becomes particularly significant when moving to nanofluidics. Balancing the advantages and disadvantages, PDMS is more suitable for research laboratories than for mass-produced products.

Harder thermoplastics like polymethylmethacrylate (PMMA), polycarbonate (PC) and cyclic olefin copolymer (COC) can be used for the production of polymer microchips using mass-production compatible processes like micro-embossing and injection molding. Their higher stiffness reduces the sagging issue plaguing PDMS structures and microdevices in thermoplastics can be produced at low cost with a very high production rate. However, the high setup costs for embossing and injection molding due to the expense of the fabrication of a high resolution mould makes it more attractive for commercial production than for research and development laboratories.

Paper has become the most popular alternative microfluidic material because of its very low cost. It is made of cellulose which is highly porous and has excellent fluid wicking properties. While paper chromatography has benefited from this for many decades, Whitesides's group demonstrated simple microfluidic capability directing fluid by patterning the paper with a hydrophobic material in 2007 [9]. Structuring paper-based microfluidic devices has been done through wax printing, inkjet printing, standard photolithography, laser cutting and other methods [10]. There are several advantages utilizing paper to fabricate microchips, as it is cheap, fabrication is easy and simple, it can be easily disposed of by burning, which is particularly important for bioassays which may contain biofluids and biohazardous reagents. Significant for POCT is that fluidic transport is driven by capillary forces, hence power-free. There are some drawbacks for the applicability in paper-based microfluidic devices, as there is only a limited range of detection methods compatible with sensitive detection in paper (colorimetry, luminescence and electrochemical detection) as the detection sensitivity is limited by the channel fabric material [11]. Many laboratory processes cannot be replicated in paper, with chromatographic separations for example showing inferior performance.

Toner is a complex powder composite used in laser printers to form an image on polyester film or wax paper [12]. During the process, the powder becomes a fluid which forms a solid structure attached to the transparency sheet or to the wax paper surface. Toner based microfluidic devices can be fabricated through direct laser printing on a polyester film, or by the transfer of a toner layer from wax paper to a higher affinity surface like glass or PDMS. Toner has the potential to become a powerful approach for rapid prototyping and low-cost mass production of microfluidic devices because, unlike photolithography, no mask, sophisticated instrumentation or clean room facilities are needed. However, the channel size is highly dependent on the resolution of the printer, and the channel edges are not sharp, and further research into the use of high-resolution laser printers and/or other materials to realize narrower and better-defined microchannels is required to improve the analytical performance of such devices.

Dry film photoresist (acrylate-based photopolymers) was originally developed for printed circuit board (PCB) fabrication, and introduced to fabricate microfluidic structures by Vulto *et al.* [13]. Dry film photoresist has many advantages over liquid resists, including good conformability, excellent adhesion to other substrates, uniform height distribution, simple and reliable processing, low exposure energy, and short processing time. In addition, channels with specified depth can be achieved because commercial dry film resist has uniform thickness [14].

The selection of the most appropriate material and fabrication method remains complex. Firstly the requirements for laboratory research and commercialization are different, for laboratory research, ease in prototyping to optimize performance of device come first, while for commercial purpose, the production cost and reliability are the most important [15].

20.3.2 Detection

The ability to identify and quantify the target analytes, detection is the final step in the analytical process. A wide range of detectors have been applied in microfluidics, with optical, electrochemical and mass spectrometry dominating the field. Examples relevant to POC analysis are discussed below.

20.3.2.1 Optical detection

The most common detection method in lab-on-a-chip systems is fluorescence due to its high sensitivity and ease of integration. The excitation light source may be a laser or increasingly frequently, a light-emitting diode (LED), with the emitted light collected with a photomultiplier tube (PMT) or a charged couple device (CCD). This setup with an argon ion laser was used for the determination of ephedrine and acebutolol in urine [16, 17] with detection limits as low as 500–1000 ng/L. However, a drawback of this method is a lengthy derivatization process required prior to analysis, explaining the interest in the development of label-free detection methods for POC analysis.

Absorbance detection mainly includes ultraviolet (UV) and infrared (IR) detection. Micellar electrokinetic chromatography (MEKC) in a quartz/poly (methyl methacrylate) microfluidic device coupled with a home-made ultraviolet (UV) detector was used for the separation and detection of amphetamine and seven other illicit drugs within 240 s [18]. The device consisted of a PMMA holder positioned on top of a PCB. A fused silica capillary could be placed in the PMMA holder, connecting the buffer reservoirs. A crack in the capillary at the location of the sample reservoir enabled for electrokinetic injection of the sample. A detection reservoir enabled the focusing of the UV light onto the capillary and photodiode. The position of the capillary in the detection reservoir could be adjusted to optimize alignment. After passing through the channel, the light beam was focused onto the photodiode *via* a lens to collect the signal (Figure 20.1). A similar device was used to detect barbiturates and benzodiazepines in plasma. Under optimal conditions, barbiturates and benzodiazepines could be baseline separated within 200 s with separation efficiency up to 380,000 plates m^{-1}, and the limit of detection was down to 27 ng mL^{-1} for phenobarbital spiked in plasma. While interesting, this device is not a real sample-in/answer-out system, because solid-phase extraction was conducted off-chip to remove interferences [19].

Infrared spectroscopy integrated in a microfluidic device has been used for detection of cocaine in saliva. In this method, the saliva sample was treated using a syringe filter to remove debris and mucins that may clog the channels or cause surface adhesion. Two flows containing saliva and tetrachloroethylene,

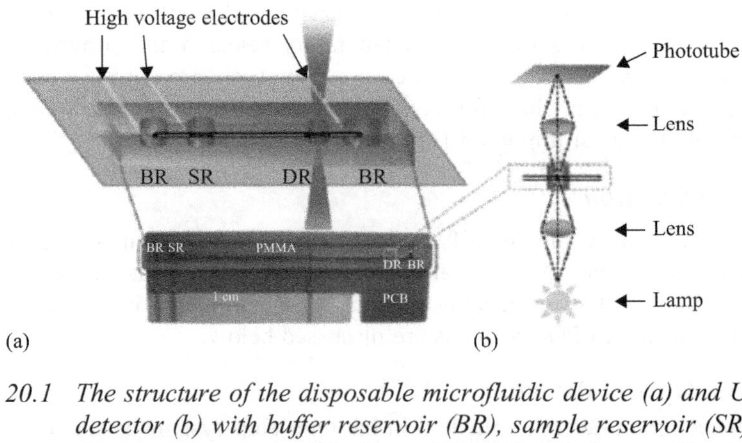

Figure 20.1 The structure of the disposable microfluidic device (a) and UV detector (b) with buffer reservoir (BR), sample reservoir (SR) and detection reservoir (DR). Reproduced from Reference 18 with permission from Royal Society of Chemistry

respectively, merged to generate oil-in-water droplets for the extraction of cocaine from saliva. The IR absorbing cocaine was detected against the IR transparent tetrachloroethylene background, using the integrated sensing device at a wavelength of 5.71 μm (wavenumber 1750 cm^{-1}) indicative of the absorption peak of cocaine [20]. Absorbance detection is less commonly used when compared with fluorescence detection because its sensitivity is limited by the optical path length, which is typically short in microfluidic devices [21]. Furthermore absorbance detection requires specific functional groups, for example conjugated double bond and the microchip material must be transparent in the UV or IR region or the chip material needs to be replaced by a second, transparent material at the detection spot.

Chemiluminescence detection is attractive because it has similar sensitivity to fluorescence and does not requiring a light source. This detection approach relies on the chemical reaction of analytes with reagent to produce light which can directly be detected with a PMT or CCD. Electrochemiluminescence (ECL) detection is a variant in which the active reagent is generated at the surface of an electrode. An electrochemical analyzer was used to perform cyclic voltammetry and provide potentials for the oxidation of Ru $(bpy)_3{}^{2+}$ to Ru $(bpy)_3{}^{3+}$. ECL signals were monitored by a multifunctional chemi- and bio-luminescent analytical system for microchip electrophoresis. The μM LOD of this method was equivalent to previous reports, but the separation time was reduced and the separation efficiency was improved. Heroin and codeine in urine were detected within 100 s [22].

20.3.2.2 Electrochemical detection

Electrochemical detection is a well suited for POCT as the detection signal is only mass dependant, not pathlength dependant thus it does not loose sensitivity as rapidly as optical methods when miniaturized. Further, the chemical signal can be directly transferred to an electronic read-out from the electrodes, so the instrument tends to be more compact and easier to miniaturize [21]. Analytes do not need chromophores, but amperometric detection need electrochemically active groups. Conductometry, in contrast, is a universal technique and widely used in chip-based electrophoretic systems. For example, a PMMA microchip was used for on-line coupling of isotachophoresis (ITP) with zone electrophoresis (ZE) and in-line conductivity detection to determine valproate in serum. The sample was filtered using a 0.45 μm filter before analysis. ITP is useful for biological samples as it separates analytes from matrix components while allowing trace analytes to be concentrated into a narrow band. This helps to disrupt the drug-protein equilibrium, increasing the free drug fraction. Valproate could be quantified within less than 10 min with a limit of detection (LOD) (1–2 μmol/L) well below the therapeutic range (0.35–0.69 mmol/L) [23].

Amperometric detection is based on measuring the oxidation or reduction currents of analytes. This provides excellent sensitivity, but is restricted to electroactive species. Amperometric detection was coupled with an enzymatic conversion following the electrophoretic separation of glucose, ascorbic acid, acetaminophen and uric acid [24]. Glucose is oxidized to gluconic acid and hydrogen peroxide by the enzyme, with the hydrogen peroxide detected by amperometry with the signal directly proportional to the amount of glucose. The device is a simple T-cross design with reservoirs for sample, buffer-enzyme, and buffer. Sample is first injected followed by application of a potential to the buffer-enzyme reservoir to accomplish the enzymatic reaction during the separation step. The enzymatically liberated neutral peroxide is electrophoretically resolved from electroactive interferences ascorbic acid and uric acid during the separation. The peroxide arising from the glucose oxidation is detected within 100 s, and analysis of all electroactive constituents is completed within 4 min. The co-migration of acetaminophen with hydrogen peroxide (both are neutral electroactive species) could be resolved by performing two successive assays: one in the presence of glucose oxidase to determine the signal arising from glucose and acetaminophen, the second in absence of the enzyme to determine only acetaminophen. This device improved the investigation of the effect of ascorbic and uric acid in diabetic patients.

20.3.2.3 Mass spectrometry

Mass spectrometry is a powerful technique because it has the ability to detect and identify. This ensures more accurate quantitation as it reduces inaccuracies arising from overlapping compounds. Miniaturized ultrafiltration of a phenobarbital antibody and barbiturates, including the sequential loading, washing, and dissociation steps were performed in a PDMS microchip followed by the ESI-MS. The affinity capture of phenobarbital allowed it to be concentrated 50 times before identification using the MS [25]. The main disadvantage of MS is that its size is not compact enough for portable use like optical and electrochemical detection. Recently a miniaturized mass spectrometer has been coupled with digital microfluidics (DMF) for the detection of cocaine, benzoylecgonine and codeine in dried urine samples [26], the schematic of selective extraction of drug from dried urine and devices setup is shown in Figure 20.2. The DMF devices assembled with a urine-spotted ITO-glass top plate and a patterned chromium-glass bottom plate, the urine samples were extracted by methanol through DMF devices, and then the extracted samples containing drugs were sprayed into the MS detector for detection. Four analytes were quantified within 15 min and the LOD can be as low as 40 ng/mL. Even though this was a miniaturized MS, the instrument was 25 kg and thus is not yet ideally suited for POCT unless it was housed in a central facility. A hand-held ion trap MS has been developed for defense applications and it is likely that as the cost of this type of MS decreases, that its use for POCT will become more viable.

20.3.3 POCT drug analysis in body fluids with lab-on-chip systems

20.3.3.1 Analysis of drugs in urine

Urine is a body fluid commonly used for drug analysis as it is non-invasive, simple, fast and low-cost. With the drug concentration in urine varying with the urine production, it is more frequently used for qualitative assays, for example for testing for suspected drug abuse in the forensic analysis, but qualitative assays correcting for the urine production are also feasible.

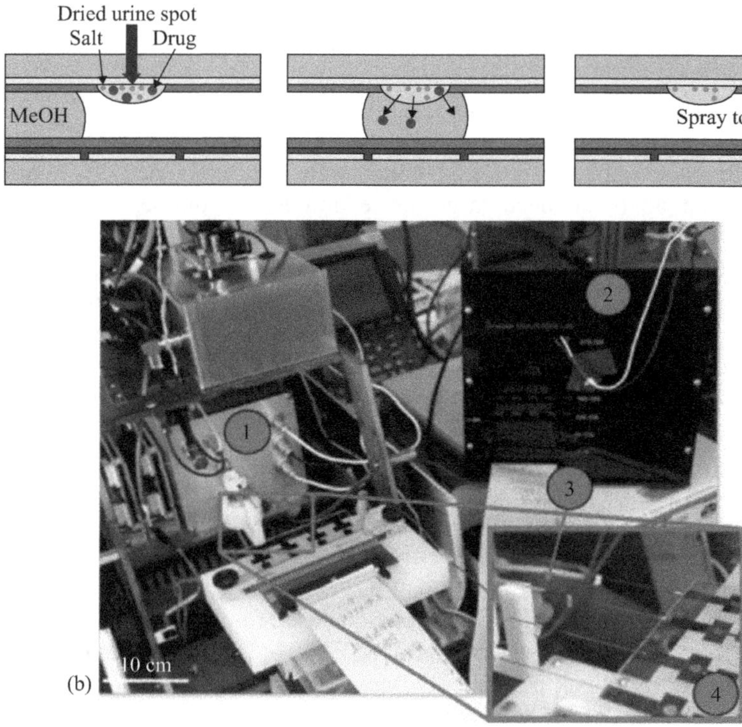

(a)

(b)

Figure 20.2 *(a) Side-view scheme (left-to-right) illustrating the selective extraction of drug from dried urine. (b) Picture of setup, with numbers indicating (1) Mini-12 miniature mass spectrometer. (2) Digital microfluidic 'DropBot' automation system, (3) MS interface, and (4) DMF device. Reproduced from Reference 26 with permission from the American Chemical Society*

20.3.3.1.1 Therapeutical drugs analysis

Urine is relatively clean, hence chemical analysis only requires limited sample treatment, and a number of lab-on-a-chip devices have been developed for the analysis of prescription drugs in urine. Kriikku *et al.* performed ITP-ZE in a PMMA microchip for the determination of β-blocker drugs, atenolol, oxprenolol and acebutolol in urine [16]. Solid-phase extraction (SPE) was conducted to remove the water-soluble hydrophilic matrix compounds, and then followed by ITP-ZE for concentration and analysis. Even though a single PMMA device could be used for over 200 analyses, the detection of β-blockers in real samples was not possible because of the co-migration of analytes and interferences. The sensitivity of the device compared poorly with capillary CE, reporting a higher detection limit in the chip than in a capillary. Detlev combined microchip electrophoresis to simultaneously detect the natively fluorescent diuretics, amiloride, triamterene, bendroflumethiazide and bumetanide. An HeCd laser was used for excitation and all the investigated diuretic drugs could be detected simultaneously and sensitively without interference of endogenous compounds in urine [27].

20.3.3.1.2 Illicit drugs analysis

Liquid–liquid extraction (LLE) as sample treatment technique is an alternative to SPE to eliminate matrix effect and concentrate the analytes [28]. While the benchtop-based approach need large space and large volumes of sample and solvent and associated with a significant risk of contamination due to the manual handling, LLE has also been down-scaled to microfluidic devices to reduce sample, solvent and chemical consumption, and increase portability. For example, an LLE microchip was used for sample pretreatment combined with gas chromatography (GC) for the analysis of amphetamine-like stimulants in urine [29]. In this method, 1-chlorobutane was used to extract drugs from urine following alkalization to neutralize the basic stimulants. Microchannels were partially modified with capillarity restricted modification (CARM) method to stabilize the interface between 1-chlorobutane and alkalized urine. After extraction, the treated urine samples were collected for GC analysis. Similar results were obtained for the on-chip and off-chip extraction of methoxyphenamine from urine, indicating the potential of this approach.

Another example of an extraction technique used for the analysis of drugs from urine is electro membrane extraction (EME). The microfluidic EME device consisted of a 25 μm thick porous polypropylene membrane bonded between two polymethyl methacrylate (PMMA) substrates with channel structures orientated toward the membrane [30, 31]. The supported liquid membrane (SLM) was created by locally filling the pores of the membrane with 2-nitrophenyl octyl ether (NPOE). The sample solution, containing five basic model analytes (pethidine, nortriptyline, methadone, haloperidol, and loperamide) in 10 mM HCl, or acidified urine was pumped through the 50 μm deep donor channel on one side of the membrane. When a voltage was applied across the membrane, the protonated basic drugs migrated toward the cathode and were hence selectively extracted from the sample flow through the organic phase held in the membrane into the 7 μL of acceptor solution (10 mM HCl). In conventional LLE, analyte extraction is based on passive diffusion and controlled by the partition coefficients, while in the EME system analytes were transported electrokinetically across the SLM, reducing the extraction time [30]. The acceptor solution was stagnant, and when the extraction was finished, it was removed using a pipette and analyzed offline by CE. To realize on-line analysis, a flow of acceptor solution was introduced, allowing the detection of analytes in the acceptor solution using an online UV detector or a mass spectrometer [31]. Using the setup shown in Figure 20.3 various biological fluids including urine and whole blood could be analyzed. The SLM composition and analytes properties strongly affect the extraction selectivity and efficiency, and hence careful optimization is necessary for each analyte set.

Detection of the drugs in abuse in urine is very important in forensic analysis and a number of microfluidic devices have been developed for this application. Qiang *et al.* performed micellar electrokinetic chromatography (MEKC) in a

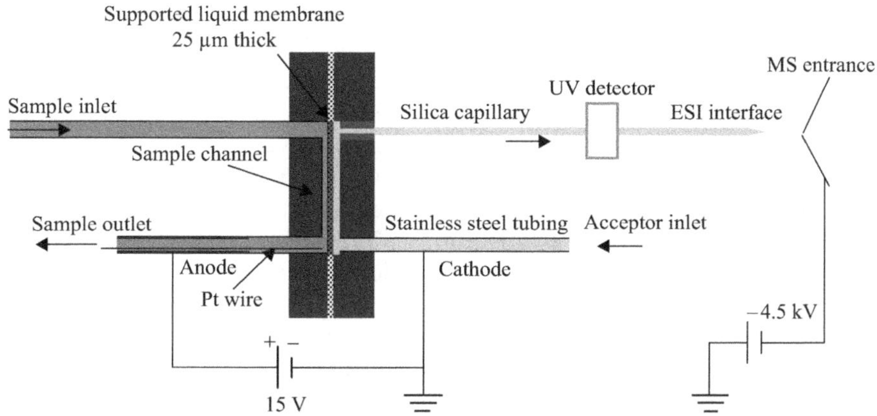

Figure 20.3 Schematic illustration of on-chip electro membrane system. Reproduced from Reference 31 with permission from the American Chemical Society

quartz/poly(methyl methacrylate) microfluidic device using ultraviolet (UV) detector for the detection of amphetamine and seven other illicit drugs. Prior to analysis, the urine samples were extracted with organic solvents to exclude the interference of salts in the samples. All eight drugs could be baseline separated with 240 s and the efficiency is good with the separation efficiency up to 600,000 plates m^{-1}. With a LOD about 5 times below previously reported immunoassays, this assay could be useful in the screening for illicit drugs because of the lower rate of false negative results [18]. Hamid developed a competitive enzyme-linked immunosorbent assay (ELISA) on a disposable plastic microchip to detect amphetamine in plasma and urine without any need for sample clean-up. Compared to the conventional ELISA, the microchip approach was more rapid because the incubation time can be reduced to 10 min instead of a few hours as in standard microtiter plate assays [32].

Narcotics including heroin, codeine and morphine were also determined in urine using microfluidic technology [18, 22, 26, 33, 34]. Qian-Li Zhang combined microchip-based CE with electrochemical detector (ECD) to simultaneously determine morphine and codeine. These two drugs were successfully separated within 140 s and then quantified. In order to improve the resolution, β-CD and acetonitrile were added to the buffer [33]. Microchip MEKC with ECL detection for heroin and codeine was presented by Du and Wang. In this paper, a novel electrolyte system including hydrophilic ionic liquids $BMIMBF_4$ and sodium dodecyl sulfate (SDS) was used to lower the electrophoresis current, and accordingly less Joule heating then better separation performance [22]. Prior to analysis, urine samples were filtered through 0.22 μm membranes and then diluted by 100-fold to decrease the effect of interferences and the ionic strength of the sample matrix. The separation was achieved in 20 mM $BMIMBF_4$ SDS and detection conditions involved 5 mM $Ru(bpy)_3^{2+}$ in 50 mM phosphate buffer (pH 8.5).

Kirby *et al.* coupled a digital microfluidic (DMF) system and a miniature mass spectrometer (MS) for the quantitation of cocaine and codeine in dried urine samples. The dried urine samples were extracted by methanol using DMF devices fabricated with a urine-spotted ITO-glass top plate and a patterned chromium-glass bottom plate. The extracted samples containing drugs were introduced to nanoESI capillaries and sprayed into the MS detector. The LOD of this method was in the ng/mL range and also benefited from portable, quantitative, on-site analysis and maybe useful in a wide range of applications. The efficacy of the DMF extraction method was evaluated by comparing the conductivity of samples before and after extraction, it showed a nearly 70% reduction of the conductivity presenting a good efficacy. However, they found that the salt in the extracts was not zero, which can be troublesome for ESI MS analysis [26]. Ephedrine and pseudoephedrine in urine were also quantified with good sensitivity using microchip based CE with argon ion LIF detection [17].

20.3.3.2 Analysis of drugs in blood

The most common approach in medical diagnostics is a blood test, as blood contains abundant information about the health status of the individual. Plasma is the colorless watery fluid of the blood and lymph that contains no red blood cells, but in which other blood cells (erythrocytes, leukocytes and thrombocytes) are suspended, and serum plasma where the blood clotting factors (fibrinogen) have been removed [35]. Plasma and serum and even whole blood have been used for the detection of drugs. Therapeutic drugs can be tested to evaluate their efficacy and also guide a patient's treatment to adjust the administrated dose to the optimal level for effective therapeutic dose with minimal side effects. Addictive drugs such as codeine can be monitored to detect and prevent drug abuse and illicit trafficking.

20.3.3.2.1 Therapeutical drugs analysis

Theophylline in serum has been determined by immunoassay-capillary electrophoresis (IA-CE) and fluorescence polarization immunoassay (FPIA) [36, 37]. Chiem and co-workers integrated reagent mixing, immune reaction and CE separation on one microfluidic device for competitive immunoassay of serum theophylline. Electroosmotic pumping was used to mix the diluted serum sample and labeled theophylline in a 1:1 ratio, which was then reacted with theophylline antibody. After on-chip reaction, the mixture was injected into the separation channel for analysis [36]. FPIA is a commercial method to quantify some drugs with narrow therapeutic range such as theophylline, vancomicin, cyclosporin. A microchip-based FPIA was developed to determine the theophylline in serum, accelerating the conventional FPIA, which needs 10 min, by almost a factor 10 as only 65 s is required to complete the analysis [37].

Determination of valproate from serum has been achieved by PMMA microchip-based ZE coupled on-line with ITP sample pretreatment and in-line conductivity detection. The serum sample was first diluted with water and filtered before being injected into the system. The drugs in serum could be quantified within 10 min and the limit of detection (LOD) (1–2 μmol/L) was far below the therapeutic range

(0.35–0.69 mmol/L) [23]. ImmunoChip using a cloned enzyme donor immunoassay (CEDIA) and a Beta-Glo assay system was applied to simultaneously determine three kinds of antiepileptic drugs, carbamazepine, phenytoin and valproic acid in serum. This platform provides a precise and relatively fast technique for detection antiepileptic drugs without separation steps, and the total analysis time was less than 6 min, which is much more rapid than the conventional immunoassay methods. Furthermore, the linear range covered the therapeutic range: 0–20, 0–30, and 0–150 μg/mL, respectively. However, the cross reaction of active metabolites with antibodies may cause positive bias, especially when the concentration of metabolites was high. So further comparison of this method and other conventional methods like HPLC-MS was needed to evaluate its accuracy and specificity [38].

When serum is used as test sample, serum needs to be obtained from whole blood prior to analysis, which is not convenient for integration and automation. When whole blood itself can be used, realizing a sample-in/answer-out system is more straight-forward. Lithium is used as a mood stabilizer to treat bipolar mood disorders, and it has been researched as a possible treatment for cluster headaches [39]. The narrow therapeutic range of lithium (0.4–1.2 mmol/L) necessitates frequent TDM to avoid adverse effects. Vrouwe and co-workers combined microchip capillary electrophoresis with conductivity detection to measure lithium in whole blood. Lithium was separated from other inorganic cations like sodium and potassium by CE and a detection limit for lithium of 0.15 mmol/L was realized, which is below the therapeutic range. This method allows point-of-care measurements from a drop of whole blood [40, 41], with the system shown in Figure 20.4. The blood is placed on the device and a filter integrated in the device removes blood cells and platelets. Channels are coated with polyacrylamide to reduce non-specific binding of proteins to the microchannel surfaces thereby improving the quality and accuracy of the result.

A microfluidic diffusion immunoassay (DIA) was used for analysis of phenytoin from whole blood with fluorescence detection [42] as shown in Figure 20.5. The mixing of the reagents in this method is mainly through diffusion. A T-sensor allows diffusion of side-by-side streams, one containing both labeled and sample analyte and the other containing antigen-specific antibody (polyclonal). Binding of analyte to antibody slows their diffusion, and then the concentration of analyte can be calculated based on the diffusion change before and after binding. Iophenoxate was used to decrease interferences from phenytoin binding to albumin. The linear range was 0–400 μmol/L and the limit of detection (LOD) was 8.1 nmol/L. The assay is useful for TDM in blood (therapeutic range in plasma is 40–80 μmol/L) in less than 1 min. Direct analysis of diluted blood samples was achieved without removal of blood cells from blood samples, and the assay compared favorably with FPIA measurements.

Shallan *et al.* developed a sample-in/answer-out device combing the extraction, separation and detection of quinine sulfate spiked in whole blood [43]. Nanochannels were fabricated using dielectric breakdown in PDMS integrated with microchannels for separation. Tuning the size of the nanochannels was achieved by

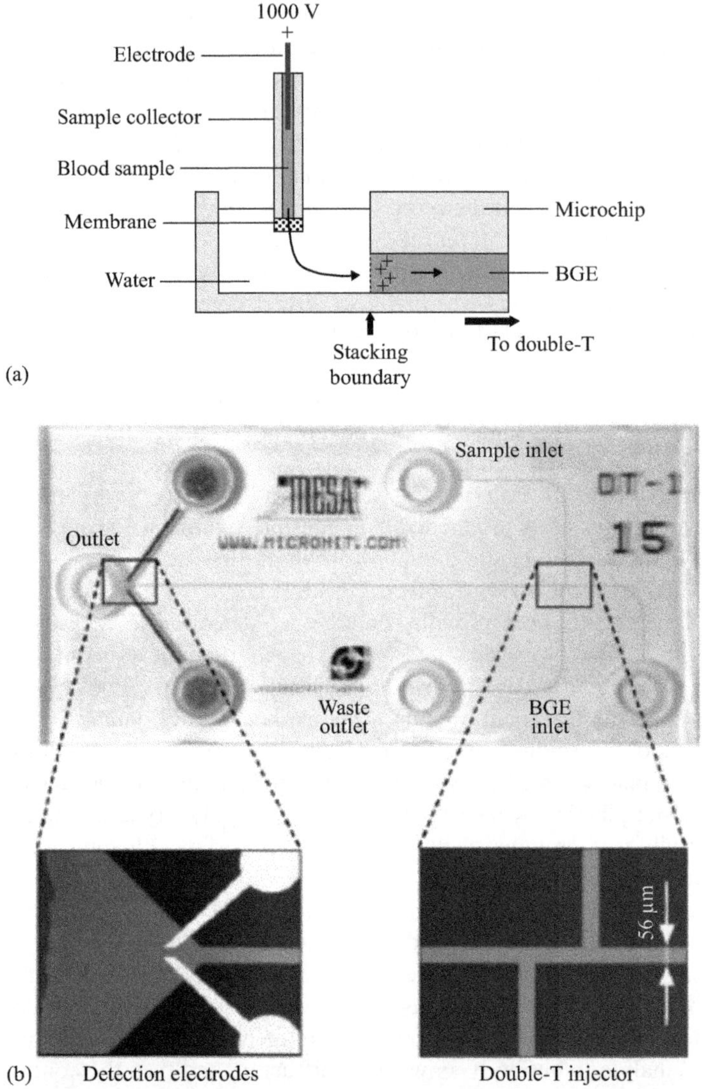

Figure 20.4 *(a) schematic representation of the sample-to chip interface. (b) Photograph of the Double-T microchip with dimensions of 30 × 15 mm^2. Insets show the position of the electrodes used for the conductivity detection and the channel intersection defining the sample volume. Reproduced from References 40 and 41 with permission from the American Association for Clinical Chemistry and the Wiley-VCH Verlag GmbH and Co. KGaA, Weinheim*

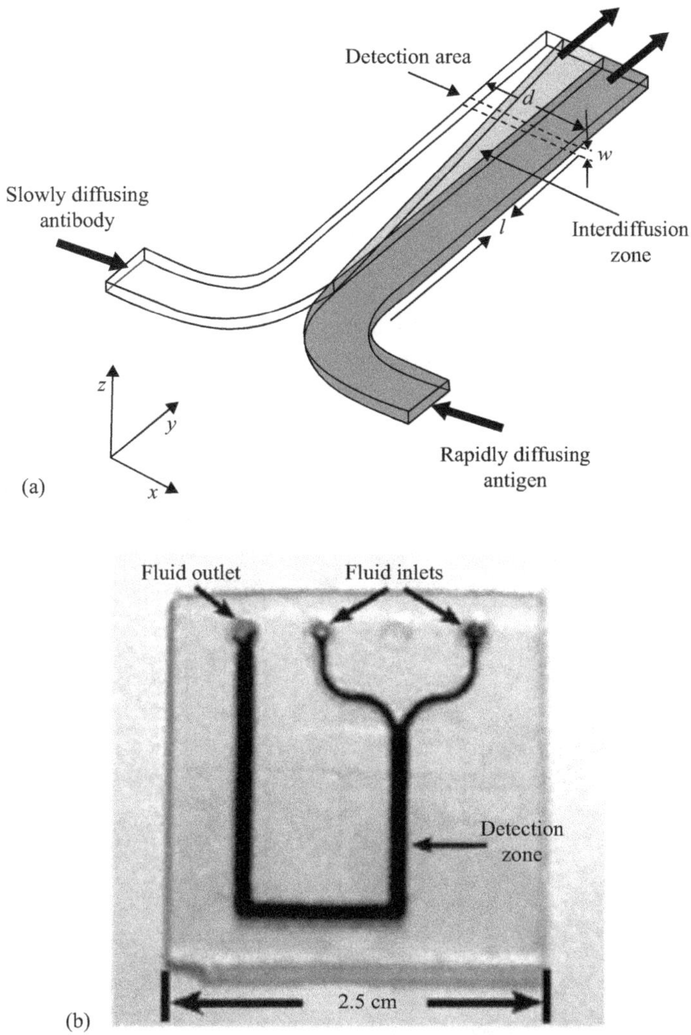

Figure 20.5 *Diffusion immunoassay in a T-sensor. (a) Schematic of a diffusion immunoassay (DIA) implemented in the simplest possible T-sensor. Reagents are pumped separately through device inlets and meet at the junction. At this point, under laminar flow conditions, reagents flow side by side and mix only by diffusion. For a competitive binding assay, sample containing antigen to be measured spiked with a fixed concentration of labeled antigen is pumped through one inlet and a fixed concentration of antibody (Ab) through the other. Assay measurement is made at one location (l) downstream where reagents have had sufficient time to interdiffuse and react. Diffusive transport of analyte is measured across the d dimension. The diffusive transport of antigen is altered depending on the fraction that binds to Ab and is the basis for determination of sample antigen concentration.*
(b) Photograph of a microfluidic device used for testing. The flow channel is filled with dye for visualization. Reproduced from Reference 42 with permission from 2001 Nature Publishing Group

setting a different threshold current during breakdown. This provides control of the permeability to different size molecules, as shown in Figure 20.6. The target drug, quinine, can be extracted from whole blood without any other sample preparation. ITP was performed after extraction to selectively concentrate quinine for detection. The same authors presented a second micro/nanofluidic devices with two nanojunctions of different pore size to create an electrokinetic size and mobility trap which was then coupled with electrophoresis to determine ampicillin in whole blood [44]. This method performed the desalting of the analytes in the smaller nanojunction, which improves the purity of the analytes and had a better performance, reaching therapeutic detection limits within 5 min.

Dried blood spots (DBS) have gained more attention in recent years as a diagnostic sample. The blood is stored on filter paper without other treatment, which is very convenient and easy to handle. Other advantages include the small sample

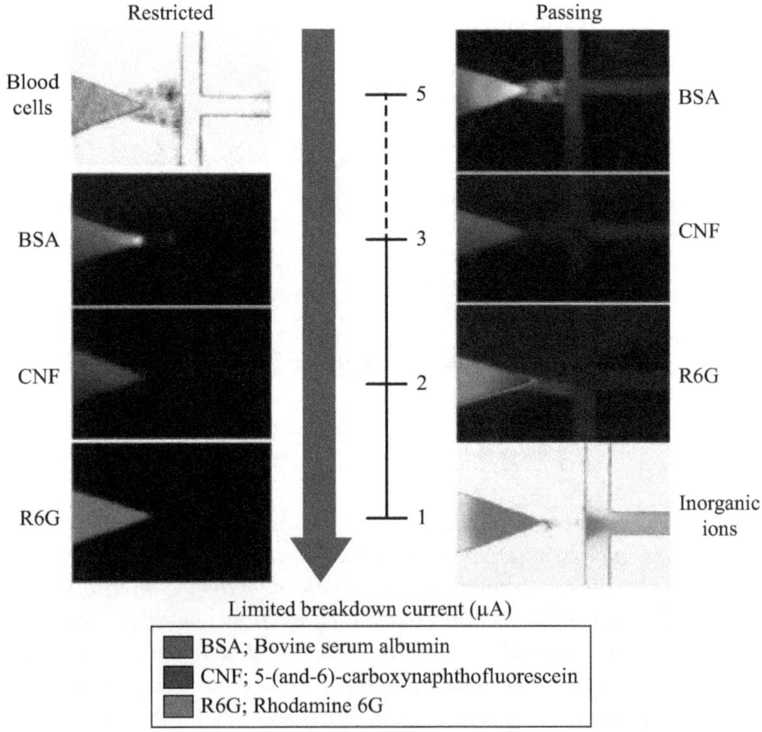

Figure 20.6 Screen shots showing the permeability of nanochannels created with decreasing current limits for red blood cells, labeled BSA, CNF, R6G and the inorganic ions, iron(III) and thiocyanate. Images on the left show blocked transport while those on the right show permeability. In each image, sample compartment is on the left and separation channel on the right. Reproduced from [43] with permission from Royal Society of Chemistry

volume, the enhanced stability without need to cool/freeze and hence easy transportation [45]. A wide variety of techniques to analyze DBS have emerged, including microfluidics ones. Succinylacetone, a marker for hepatorenal tyrosinemia in DBS samples has been quantified using digital microfluidics (DMF) coupled with nano-electrospray ionization mass spectrometry (nESI-MS), moreover this system also included a feedback control system that enhance the fidelity droplet manipulation across DBS samples without manual intervention. The LOD of Succinylacetone was 4.95 μM which was below the monitoring concentration range of 16–150 μM making the microfluidic method suitable for screening purposes. Comparison to gold-standard methods like MS/MS was conducted to prove its reliability [46].

20.3.3.2.2 Illicit drugs analysis

Psychotropic drugs including barbiturates and benzodiazepines in plasma were analyzed using microfluidic devices [19, 47, 48]. Jin Sheng and coworkers combined microfluidic MEKC with UV detection and solid-phase extraction to detect barbiturates and benzodiazepines in plasma. The device used compromised one fused-silica capillary for separation and detection, a poly (methyl methacrylate) board with four reservoirs as support substrate, and a printed circuit board to apply high voltages. Under optimal conditions, barbiturates and benzodiazepines could be baseline separated within 200 s with separation efficiency up to 380,000 plates m^{-1}, and an LOD of 27 ng/mL^{-1} was obtained for phenobarbital spiked in plasma [19]. Competitive immunoassay was conducted in a microfluidic device to determine the content of phenobarbital in plasma. The detection was based on the competitive immunoreaction between phenobarbital and fluorescein isothiocyanate (FITC)-labeled phenobarbital. The concentration of phenobarbital in the sample is directly proportional to that of free FITC-labeled phenobarbital, but inversely proportional to that of immune complex [47, 48]. Serum could also be used directly without any other sample treatment.

The illicit drug cocaine, has been detected in serum using a Microfluidic Electrochemical Aptamer-based Sensor (MECAS) chip which integrated cocaine-specific DNA aptamer with electrochemical detection system. Low concentration of cocaine can be detected directly in unprocessed serum sample continuously and real-time. But the same as other heterogeneous immunoassay, this system also needs the immobilization of the aptamer probe which is tedious and time-consuming [49].

20.3.3.3 Analysis of drugs in saliva and other subtracts

Saliva offers several advantages over blood for analysis, its collection is non-invasive to patients, and comparative easier to obtain by unskilled people. However, the high viscosity and inhomogeneous amalgam create major difficulties in using saliva as sample fluid [50].

20.3.3.3.1 Therapeutic drugs analysis

In order to detect phenytoin in saliva samples, sample pretreatment is used to decrease surface fouling interferences from mucin and other large particles. A filter membrane was used to deplete the cells, debris, and mucins, and then an H-filter was used to extract the analyte from the remaining large molecular weight species in the filtered saliva sample through separating solutes from mixed samples based on their diffusion in laminar flow. 3.6 times less fouling than untreated saliva method before was achieved, with 97% and 92% reduction in glycoproteins and proteins, respectively. However, this method diluted the original analytes concentration by 80% which posed a significant problem for detection [51].

20.3.3.3.2 Illicit drugs analysis in saliva

Saliva is the preferred biological fluid for forensic analysis of drug abuse taken by mouth. Methamphetamine in saliva was determined using a microfluidic device with surface-enhanced Raman spectroscopy (SERS), and a limit of qualification of 10 nM was obtained [52]. Cocaine in saliva was also quantified using infrared detection [20, 53, 54]. Wägli *et al.* used a microfluidic drop-based liquid-liquid extraction and infrared spectroscopy to detect of cocaine in saliva. Saliva was first filtered using a syringe filter to remove debris and mucins, and mixed with tetrachloroethylene (IR transparent) to generate oil-in-water droplets with the cocaine in tetrachloroethylene determined by IR with integrated sensing devices and an optical waveguide [20]. Microfluidic-based extraction combined with Fourier-Transform Infrared (FTIR) attenuated total reflection (ATR) spectroscopy was developed to determine cocaine and street cocaine in saliva. The drawback of this method is limited to laboratories due to its large device size, which is not suitable for portable analysis [54]. Integration of microfluidic devices with a mid-IR Ge waveguide has been applied to detect cocaine in saliva, while the detection limit of this method was not competitive compared to other optical methods, it does have the advantage of compact size of mid-IR Ge waveguide which allows the design of portable systems [54].

20.4 Conclusions and future directions

Microfluidic lab-on-a-chip technology is ideally suited for POCT when all of the necessary functional processes have been integrated to create a sample-in/answer-out device and thus is particularly attractive for the detection of drugs in body fluids. There have been various demonstrations of lab-on-a-chip devices to detect both therapeutic and illicit drugs, which have the potential to simplify the diagnostic step and relieve the central laboratory workers' burden. However, currently very few devices have real sample-in/answer-out POCT capability, because of the challenge in dealing with biological fluids and the reliance on extensive sample preparation to remove interferences from the biological matrix. This ultimately remains the main challenge in this area although it is questionable whether the best approach is simply to miniaturized and integrate existing laboratory approaches for sample treatment. Recent progress using unique nanofluidic phenomena for sample treatment has been shown as a simple approach to make sample-in/answer-out systems for drugs in biological fluids. Continued work in this area, and others unique to the microfluidic platform, will see the development of simple, functional and reliable lab-on-a-chip systems suitable for POCT of drugs in body fluids.

References

[1] Whitesides, G.M. 'The origins and the future of microfluidics'. *Nature.* 2006; **442**(7101): 368–373.

[2] Gubala V., Harris L.F., Ricco A.J., Tan M.X., Williams D.E. 'Point of care diagnostics: status and future'. *Anal. Chem.* 2012; **84**(2): 487–515.

[3] Lledo-Fernandez C., Banks C.E. 'An overview of quantifying and screening drugs of abuse in biological samples: past and present'. *Anal. Methods.* 2011; **3**(6): 1227–1245.

[4] Jung W., Han J., Choi J.W., Ahn C.H. 'Point-of-care testing (POCT) diagnostic systems using microfluidic lab-on-a-chip technologies'. *Microelectron. Eng.* 2015; **132**: 46–57.

[5] Urdea M., Penny L.A., Olmsted S.S., *et al.* 'Requirements for high impact-diagnostics in the developing world'. *Nature.* 2006; **444**(Suppl 1): 73–79.

[6] Reyes D.R., Iossifidis D., Auroux P.A., Manz A. 'Micro total analysis systems. 1. introduction, theory, and technology'. *Anal. Chem.* 2002; **74**(12): 2623–2636.

[7] Allen P.B., Chiu D.T. 'Calcium-assisted glass-to-glass bonding for fabrication of glass microfluidic devices'. *Anal. Chem.* 2008; **80**(18): 7153–7157.

[8] Ocvirk G., Munroe M., Tang T., Oleschuk R., Westra K., Harrison D.J. 'Electrokinetic control of fluid flow in native poly(dimethylsiloxane) capillaryelectrophoresis devices'. *Electrophoresis.* 2000; **21**(1): 107–115.

[9] Martinez, A.W.; Phillips, S.T.; Butte, M.J.; Whitesides, G.M. 'Patterned paper as a platform for inexpensive, low-volume, portable bioassays'. *Angew. Chem. Int. Ed.* 2007; **46**(8): 1318−1320.

[10] Cate D.M., Adkins J.A., Mettakoonpitak J., Henry C.S. 'Recent developments in paper-based microfluidic devices'. *Anal. Chem.* 2015; **87**(1): 19–41.

[11] Li, X., Ballerini, D.R., Shen, W. 'A perspective on paper-based microfluidics: current status and future trends'. *Biomicrofluidics.* 2012; **6**(1): 11301.

[12] Coltro, W.K.T., Carrilho, E., in: Landers, J.P. (Ed.) *Handbook of Capillary and Microchip Electrophoresis and Associated Microtechniques*, 3rd Edn, CRC Press, New York 2007, pp. 1169–1184.

[13] Vulto P., Glade N., Altomare L., *et al.* 'Microfluidic channel fabrication in dry film resist for production and prototyping of hybrid chips'. *Lab. Chip.* 2005; **5**(2): 158–162.

[14] Tsai Y.C., Jen H.P., Lin K.W., Hsieh Y.Z. 'Fabrication of microfluidic devices using dry film photoresist for microchip capillary electrophoresis'. *J Chromatogr A.* 2006; **1111**(2): 267–271.

[15] Ren K., Zhou J., Wu H. 'Materials for microfluidic chip fabrication'. *Acc. Chem. Res.* 2013; **46**(11): 2396–2406.

[16] Kriikku P., Graß B., Hokkanen A., Stuns I., Sirén H. 'Isotachophoresis of β-blockers in a capillary and on a poly (methyl methacrylate) chip'. *Electrophoresis.* 2004; **25**(10–11): 1687–1694.

[17] Belder D., Tolba K., Nagl S. 'Rapid quantitative determination of ephedra alkaloids in tablet formulations and human urine by microchip electrophoresis'. *Electrophoresis*. 2011; **32**(3–4): 440–447.
[18] Qiang W., Zhai C., Lei J., *et al.* 'Disposable microfluidic device with ultraviolet detection for highly resolved screening of illicit drugs'. *Analyst*. 2009; **134**(9): 1834–1839.
[19] Sheng J., Lei J., Ju H., Song C., Zhang D. Rapid ultraviolet monitoring of multiple psychotropic drugs with a renewable microfluidic device. *Anal. Chim. Acta*. 2010; **679**(1–2): 1–6.
[20] Wägli P., Chang Y.C., Hans K., *et al.* 'Microfluidic droplet-based liquid–liquid extraction and on-chip IR spectroscopy detection of cocaine in human saliva'. *Anal. Chem.* 2013; **85**(15): 7558–7565.
[21] Schwarz M.A., Hauser P.C. 'Recent developments in detection methods for microfabricated analytical devices'. *Lab. Chip*. 2001; **1**(1): 1–6.
[22] Du Y., Wang E. 'Separation and detection of narcotic drugs on a microchip using micellar electrokinetic chromatography and electrochemiluminescence'. *Electroanalysis* 2008; **20**(6): 643–647.
[23] Ölvecká E., Koníková M., Grobuschek N., Kaniansky D., Stanislawski B. 'Direct determination of valproate in serum by zone electrophoresis–isotachophoresis on a column-coupling chip'. *J. Sep. Sci.* 2003; **26**(8): 693–700.
[24] Wang J., Chatrathi M.P., Tian B., Polsky R. 'Microfabricated electrophoresis chips for simultaneous bioassays of glucose, uric acid, ascorbic acid, and acetaminophen'. *Anal. Chem.* 2000; **72**(11): 2514–2518.
[25] Jiang Y., Wang P.C., Locascio L.E., Lee C.S. 'Integrated plastic microfluidic devices with ESI-MS for drug screening and residue analysis'. *Anal. Chem.* 2001; **73**(9): 2048–2053.
[26] Kirby A.E., Lafrenière N.M., Seale B., Hendricks P.I., Cooks R.G., Wheeler A.R. 'Analysis on the go: quantitation of drugs of abuse in dried urine with digital microfluidics and miniature mass spectrometry'. *Anal. Chem.* 2014; **86**(12): 6121–6129.
[27] Tolba K.; Belder D. 'Fast quantitative determination of diuretic drugs in tablets and human urine by microchip electrophoresis with native fluorescence detection'. *Electrophoresis*. 2007; **28**(16): 2934–2941.
[28] Bayne S., Carlin M. *Forensic Applications of High Performance Liquid Chromatography (Analytical Concepts in Forensic Chemistry)* CRC Press, Boca Raton, FL 2010.
[29] Miyaguchi H., Tokeshi M., Kikutani Y., Hibara A., Inoue H. and Kitamori T. 'Microchip-based liquid–liquid extraction for gas-chromatography analysis of amphetamine-type stimulants in urine'. *J. Chromatogr. A*. 2006; **1129**(1): 105–110.
[30] Petersen N.J., Jensen H., Hansen S.H., Foss, S.T., Snakenborg D., Pedersen-Bjergaard S. 'On-chip electro membrane extraction'. *Microfluid. Nanofluid.* 2010; **9**(4–5): 881–888.

[31] Petersen N.J., Foss, S.T., Jensen, H., *et al.* 'On-chip electro membrane extraction with online ultraviolet and mass spectrometric detection'. *Anal. Chem.* 2011; **83**(1): 44–51.

[32] Far H.R.M., Torabi F., Danielsson B., Khayyami M. 'ELISA on a microchip with a photodiode for detection of amphetamine in plasma and urine'. *J. Anal. Toxicol.* 2005; **29**(8): 790–793.

[33] Zhang Q.L., Xu J.J., Li X.Y., Lian H.Z., Chen H.Y. 'Determination of morphine and codeine in urine using poly (dimethylsiloxane) microchip electrophoresis with electrochemical detection'. *J. Pharmaceut. Biomed. Anal.* 2007; **43**(1): 237–242.

[34] Sheng J., Ping Q., Lei, J., Ju, H. Song, C., Zhang D. 'Fast and high-performance screening of narcotic drugs on a microfluidic device by micellar electrokinetic capillary chromatography'. *Analyt. Lett.* 2012; **45**(7): 652–664.

[35] Song Y., Huang Y.Y., Liu X., Zhang X., Ferrari M., Qin L. 'Point-of-care technologies for molecular diagnostics using a drop of blood'. *Trends Biotechnol.* 2014; **32**(3): 132–139.

[36] Chen W., Peng C., Jin Z., *et al.* 'Ultrasensitive immunoassay of 7-amino-clonazepam in human urine based on CdTe nanoparticle bioconjugations by fabricated microfluidic chip'. *Biosens. Bioelectron.* 2009; **24**(7): 2051–2056.

[37] Jiang Y., Wang P.-C, Locascio L.E., Lee C.S. 'Integrated plastic microfluidic devices with ESI-MS for drug screening and residue analysis'. *Anal. Chem.* 2001; **73**(9): 2048–2053.

[38] Yang X., Janatova J., Juenke J.M., McMillin G.A., Andrade J.D. 'An ImmunoChip prototype for simultaneous detection of antiepileptic drugs using an enhanced one-step homogeneous immunoassay'. *Anal. Biochem.* 2007; **365**(2): 222–229.

[39] Lieb J., Zeff A. 'Lithium treatment of chronic cluster headaches'. *Br. J. Psychiatry.* 1978; **133**: 556–558.

[40] Vrouwe E.X., Luttge R., Vermes I., Van Den Berg A. 'Microchip capillary electrophoresis for point-of-care analysis of lithium'. *Clin. Chem.* 2007; **53**(1): 117–123.

[41] Vrouwe E.X., Lüttge R., Olthuis W., van den Berg A. 'Microchip analysis of lithium in blood using moving boundary electrophoresis and zone electrophoresis'. *Electrophoresis* 2005; **26**(15): 3032–3042.

[42] Hatch, A., Kamholz, A., Hawkins, K., *et al.* 'A rapid diffusion immunoassay in a T-sensor'. *Nat. Biotech.* 2001; **19**(5): 461–465.

[43] Shallan A.I., Gaudry A.J., Guijt R.M., Breadmore M.C. 'Tuneable nanochannel formation for sample-in/answer-out devices'. *Chem Commun (Camb).* 2013; **49**(27): 2816–2818.

[44] Shallan A.I., Gaudry A.J., Guijt R.M., Breadmore M.C. 'Electrokinetic size and mobility traps for on-site therapeutic drug monitoring'. 2015; doi: 10.1002/anie.201501794.

[45] Meyer M.R. 'Trends in analyzing emerging drugs of abuse – from seized samples to body samples'. *Anal. Bioanal. Chem.* 2014; **406**(25): 6105–6110.

[46] Shih S.C., Yang H., Jebrail M.J., Fobel R., McIntosh N., Al-Dirbashi O.Y. 'Dried blood spot analysis by digital microfluidics coupled to nano-electrospray ionization mass spectrometry'. *Anal. Chem.* 2012; **84**(8): 3731–3738.

[47] Huang Y., Zhao S., Shi M., Liu J., Liang H. 'Competitive immunoassay of phenobarbital by microchip electrophoresis with laser induced fluorescence detection'. *Anal. Chim. Acta* 2011; **694**(1–2): 162–166.

[48] Huang Y., Zhao S., Shi M., Liang H. 'One-way multiplexed immunoassay strategy for simultaneous determination of multi-analytes by microchip electrophoresis'. *Analyst* 2011; **136**(10): 2119–2124.

[49] Swensen J.S., Xiao Y., Ferguson B.S., *et al.* 'Continuous, real-time monitoring of cocaine in undiluted blood serum via a microfluidic, electrochemical aptamer-based sensor'. *J. Am. Chem. Soc.* 2009; **131**(12): 4262–6426.

[50] de Almeida Pdel V., Grégio A.M., Machado M.A., de Lima A.A., Azevedo L.R. 'Saliva composition and functions: a comprehensive review'. *J. Contemp. Dent. Pract.* 2008; **9**(3): 72–80.

[51] Helton K.L., Nelson K.E., Fu E., Yager, P. 'Conditioning saliva for use in a microfluidic biosensor'. *Lab Chip* 2008; **8**(11): 1847–1851.

[52] Andreou C., Hoonejani M.R., Barmi M.R., Moskovits M., Meinhart C.D. 'Rapid detection of drugs of abuse in saliva using surface enhanced raman spectroscopy and microfluidics'. *ACS Nano.* 2013; **7**(8): 7157–7164.

[53] Hans K.M.C., Müller M., Petrosyan T., Sigrist M.W. 'Infrared detection of cocaine and street cocaine in saliva with a one-step extraction'. 2014; **6**(3), 666–673.

[54] Chang Y.C., Wägli P., Paeder V., *et al.* 'Cocaine detection by a mid-infrared waveguide integrated with a microfluidic chip'. *Lab Chip.* 2012; **12**(17): 3020–3023.

Chapter 21

Hydrogel-based biosensors: fundamentals and applications

Gargi Ghosh[1], *Saurav Datta*[2] *and Anju Kumari*[2]

21.1 Introduction

A biosensor is an analytical tool that combines a biological (detection/recognition) element with a physicochemical element in addition to the signal processors. History of biosensor dates back to 1962 when Clark and Lyons developed glucose sensor by embedding glucose oxidase in a dialysis membrane [1]. The early studies spurred slew of other studies which integrated different biorecognition elements including enzymes, antibodies, nucleic acids, and cells onto physicochemical transducers to fabricate biosensors for applications in diverse areas including clinical diagnosis, food technology, military, industrial, and environmental monitoring [2]. Due to the perennial need of biosensors for monitoring blood glucose, analyzing whole blood, point-of-care markets, and for applications in drug discovery and drug screening, health care applications continue to dominate the market of biosensors globally. The exponential rise in the R&D activities worldwide coupled with the rise in incidence of diabetes and chronic diseases including cancer, heart disease, stroke, and tuberculosis have propelled the market growth of biosensors in medical diagnostics. The market for biosensors is on the rise with Transparency Market Research (http://www.transparencymarketresearch.com/biosensors-market.html) projections showing an increase in the global market for biosensors from US $12.46 billion in 2013 to US $21.64 in 2020.

One of the most important aspects in the successful development of biosensors involves immobilization/binding of the biomolecules. The simplest way to attach biomolecules to the surface involves adsorption of the molecules from the solution. However, weak interactions between the surface and the biomolecules as well as changes in the conformation of the molecules often reduce the sensitivity of the biosensors. Apart from physical adsorption, the biomolecules can be chemically conjugated to the surfaces via utilization of various functional groups including

[1]Bioengineering Program, Department of Mechanical Engineering, University of Michigan-Dearborn, MI 48128, USA
[2]Department of Biotechnology, Indian Institute of Technology, Roorkee 247667, Uttarkhand, India

epoxy, amino, thiol, and silane. However, the strategy involving the direct immobilization of functional molecules on to the surface of the electrodes/solid substrates via chemical conjugation is limited by low binding capacities. This challenge can be addressed by introduction of an integrated matrix which not only protects the biomolecules from self-aggregation and provides an aqueous environment to prevent their dehydration but also interfaces them with the devices. Hydrogels have emerged as a preferred matrix.

Hydrogels are three dimensional polymeric networks which are able to absorb aqueous solution. The hydrated environment within the hydrogels permits the immobilized biomolecules to retain their structure and activity. Due to their favorable mass transfer and interfacial properties, immobilized or entrapped biomolecules remain accessible and can interact with the analytes. In addition, the hydrogel-based biosensors also leverage the hydrogel specific properties including swelling, phase transitions, and optical transparency to enhance the signal/noise ratio for sensing. Furthermore, by virtue of good biocompatibility and ability to protect the biorecognition elements from bio-fouling, the hydrogel matrices also improve the sensitivity of the implantable biosensors.

21.2 General properties of hydrogel

21.2.1 Equilibrium swelling

Equilibrium swelling refers to the steady state when the volume change of hydrogel has occurred on being placed in contact with a thermodynamically compatible solvent. The equilibrium swelling of hydrogel depends on the polymer concentration as well as on crosslinking and the charge densities of the polymeric network. The change in volume of the hydrogels results in deformation of the polymeric chains and, therefore, in their thermodynamic properties. It was proposed that the free enthalpy change [3–5] involved in the swelling are:

1. Free enthalpy of mixing due to the mixing of the polymer with the solvent molecules, ΔG_m
2. Free enthalpy of the elastic deformation, ΔG_{el}

$$\Delta G = \Delta G_m + \Delta G_{el} \tag{21.1}$$

$$\text{or,}\quad \Delta\mu = \Delta\mu_m + \Delta\mu_{el} \tag{21.2}$$

The difference in chemical potential can be related to the osmotic pressure of the gel. Flory has drawn the analogy between swelling equilibrium and osmotic equilibrium [3–5]. The swelling pressure or total osmotic pressure (Π) is given by the difference between the osmotic pressure (Π_m) due polymer-solvent mixing and the elastic response (Π_{el}) of the polymeric networks of the swollen hydrogel. At the equilibrium swelling state of the hydrogel, the swelling pressure or total osmotic pressure is zero.

$$\Pi = \Pi_m + \Pi_{el} = 0 \tag{21.3}$$

Flory and Huggins established that for a polymer solution, the chemical potential of mixing can be expressed as:

$$\Delta\mu_m = RT\left[\ln(1-\varphi_2) + \varphi_2\left(1 - \frac{1}{x}\right) + \chi\varphi_2^2\right] \tag{21.4}$$

where, φ_2 is the polymer volume fraction, χ is Flory-Huggins interaction parameter which takes into consideration the energy of interdispersing polymer and solvent molecules and x is the ratio of molar volume of polymer to that of the solvent.

Considering a polymeric network to be one molecule of infinite molecular weight, $1/x = 0$,

The swelling pressure of the network is given by (21.5):

$$\Pi = \frac{RT}{V_1}\left(\ln\varphi_1 + \varphi_2 + \chi\varphi_2^2\right) + \frac{\upsilon\mathrm{RT}}{V_0}\left[\frac{\varphi_2}{2\varphi_{2,0}} - \left(\frac{\varphi_2}{\varphi_{2,0}}\right)^{1/3}\right] \tag{21.5}$$

where, φ_1 is the solvent volume fraction, V_1 is the molar volume of the solvent, V_0 is the gel volume for the reference state, υ = the molar volume of elastic active polymer chains in the gel at the reference volume fraction, $\varphi_{2,0}$.

Polyelectrolyte hydrogels are comprised of weak acid or basic groups which can easily get protonated/deprotonated depending on the surrounding aqueous solution. This ionization process leads to a change in charge density within the polymeric network as well as the concentrations of mobile ions inside and outside the gels which in turn results in swelling or shrinking of the gel. In case of polyelectrolyte hydrogels, the contribution of the electrostatic interaction (Π_{ion}) needs to be considered. Therefore, (21.3) is rewritten as:

$$\Pi = \Pi_m + \Pi_{el} + \Pi_{ion} = 0 \tag{21.6}$$

$$\Pi = \frac{RT}{V_1}\left(\ln\varphi_1 + \varphi_2 + \chi\varphi_2^2\right) + \frac{\upsilon\mathrm{RT}}{V_0}\left[\frac{\varphi_2}{2\varphi_{2,0}} - \left(\frac{\varphi_2}{\varphi_{2,0}}\right)^{1/3}\right] + \mathrm{RT}\Delta C_{tot} \tag{21.7}$$

where ΔC_{tot} is total difference in molar concentration of mobile ions between the gel and the surrounding aqueous solution and is given by Donnan equilibrium.

The hydrogel swelling characteristics has been exploited for various biosensing applications. For example, boronic acid derivative containing hydrogel has been synthesized which swells reversibly in presence of glucose [6, 7]. The swelling characteristics of these glucose sensitive hydrogel have been found to directly correlate with the physiological glucose concentrations. The change in hydrogel volume can also alter the apparent diffraction spectrum of the embedded photonic crystals which in turn can be detected via reflectance spectroscopy. Coupling the volume change of the hydrogel with the molecular recognition of target analyte leads to the development of label free sensor platform. Such optically diffracting hydrogels have been utilized for screening the kinase activity in vitro and in cellular extracts [8]. In addition, biosensors coupling pH-sensitive hydrogels with proton-generating enzymatic reactions have been developed. For example, glucose biosensor can be developed by immobilizing glucose oxidase within the pH sensitive hydrogels. In response to glucose concentration, the pH value is lowered when gluconic acid is produced via the glucose oxidase enzymatic reaction. Hydrogels with basic amine side groups get protonated leading to electrostatic repulsion and swelling of the hydrogel. Moreover, glucose oxidase conjugated polystyrene nanospheres have been incorporated within pH-sensitive hydrogel matrices. Swelling of hydrogel in presence of glucose resulted in enhanced distance between the nanospheres which led to a shift of diffracted wavelength [9]. This sensor can be implanted into the contact lenses to detect changes in glucose level in the tear fluid. Using an adaptable MEMS fabrication platform poly HEMA-based biosensor was developed with capacitive pressure sensing as the transducing principles. The change in hydrogel volume in response to the analyte concentration exerted contact pressure on a deformable conducting diaphragm resulting in a capacitance change [10].

21.2.2 Swelling kinetics

The swelling and shrinking of hydrogels requires the time-dependent transport of the swelling agent. To initiate the swelling, the swelling agents (solvents or ions) need to diffuse into the polymeric network. The penetration of these agents results in reorientation of the polymeric chains. The relation between the diffusion of the swelling agents and the relaxation of the polymer chains can be utilized to distinguish different modes of diffusion.

I. Case I or Fickian diffusion: In this case, the polymeric chains have high mobility and the solvents can easily penetrate the rubbery network. Therefore, the solvent diffusion rate (R_{diff}) is significantly slower than the rate of relaxation (R_{relax}) of the polymer chains ($R_{diff} << R_{relax}$). The swelling of the hydrogel is determined by the diffusion of the swelling agent. The mass uptake is proportional to the square root of diffusion time, $Q \sim t^{1/2}$.
II. Non-Fickian diffusion: The polymeric chains are not mobile enough to permit easy penetration of the solvents. Depending on the relative rates of chain relaxation and diffusion, Non-Fickian diffusion can be categorized into two subsections: Case II diffusion and Case III or anomalous diffusion.
   a. Case II diffusion: In this case, the rate of penetration is higher than the rate of relaxation of the polymer chains ($R_{diff} >> R_{relax}$). Case II diffusion is characterized by a mass uptake that is proportional to time, $Q \sim t$.
   b. Case III or anomalous diffusion: Both rates are comparable ($R_{diff} \sim R_{relax}$). The mass uptake, $Q \sim t^{a}$.

Several mathematical models have been developed to describe the swelling kinetics of the hydrogels. The Fickian diffusion models apply Fick's law to the distribution of the solvent within the polymeric networks. The "collective" or "cooperative" diffusion models, developed by Tanaka and Fillmore, take into account both the solvent diffusion and net chain motion. The collective diffusion coefficient is given by:

$$D = \left(K + \frac{4}{3}G\right)f \tag{21.8}$$

where, f is the friction coefficient between the network and the solvent, K and G are the bulk and shear moduli.

The cooperative diffusion coefficient can also be determined by measuring the swelling of a gel of given geometry as a function of time. For a spherical gel, this theory correlates the change of radius due to swelling with time as follows:

$$\frac{r(t=\infty) - r(t)}{r(t=\infty) - r(t=0)} = \frac{\Delta r(t)}{\Delta r_0} = \frac{6}{\pi^2}\sum_{n=1}^{\infty} n^{-2}\exp\left(-n^2\frac{t}{\tau}\right) \tag{21.9}$$

where $r(t=\infty)$, $r(t=0)$, and $r(t)$ are the radius of the gel at equilibrium, initially, and at any time t, τ is the relaxation time of the polymer. For $t/\tau > 0.25$, τ can be obtained from the slope of the plot of ln $(\Delta r(t)/\Delta r_0)$ versus time. The cooperative diffusion coefficient can then be calculated according to:

$$D_{coop} = \frac{r(t \to \infty)^2}{\pi^2 \tau} \tag{21.10}$$

Typically, the cooperative diffusion coefficient is in the order 10^{-7} cm^2/s.

21.2.3 Pore size/porosity of the gels

The response time (τ) of the smart hydrogels depends on the cooperative diffusion coefficient (D_{coop}) and the square of the characteristic length, l.

$$\tau \sim \frac{l^2}{D_{coop}} \tag{21.11}$$

The response time can be effectively reduced by synthesizing macroporous gels. Porosity of the hydrogels can be altered by varying the crosslinking density which in turn can be achieved by altering the concentration of crosslinking agent, monomer concentration, crosslinking time, as well as by varying the chain length of the monomer. In addition, porosity can be induced in the hydrogels via utilization of porogens, foaming agent, freeze-drying, and phase separation. Porogens, such as salts, organic solvents, and inert materials including glucose, sucrose, polyethylene glycol (PEG), exclude growing polymer chains from regions within the hydrogel matrix and following polymerization leave behind a network of interconnected pores [11]. In our earlier studies we have demonstrated that tuning the porosity of the gel can improve the assay sensitivity. A detection limit of 10 pg/ml was achieved for detection of vascular endothelial growth factor (VEGF) using anti-VEGF-antibody immobilized non-porous hydrogel microparticles. However, tuning the porosity using PEG porogen yielded a detection limit of 2.5 pg/ml indicating the sensitivity of the assay exceeds that of the conventional technologies [11]. This improved sensitivity can be attributed to the enhanced porous architecture of the gels which permitted increased penetration of the target analytes within the 3D polymeric networks and thereby improved the accessibility of the immobilized antibodies.

21.3 Immobilization of biomolecules and applications as biosensors

Various strategies are employed for incorporating the recognition element within the hydrogel matrix as depicted in Figure 21.1. Among these, covalent immobilization, entrapment, and physical deposition (followed by cross-linking) are the most commonly used techniques. Electrostatic immobilization is emerging as another potential technique for incorporating the charged recognition elements onto the hydrogel matrix. For site-directed attachment of the recognition elements, affinity-based immobilization of biomolecules is performed. At times, supplemental functionalities, such as nanoparticles, are introduced to enhance the performance of the recognition

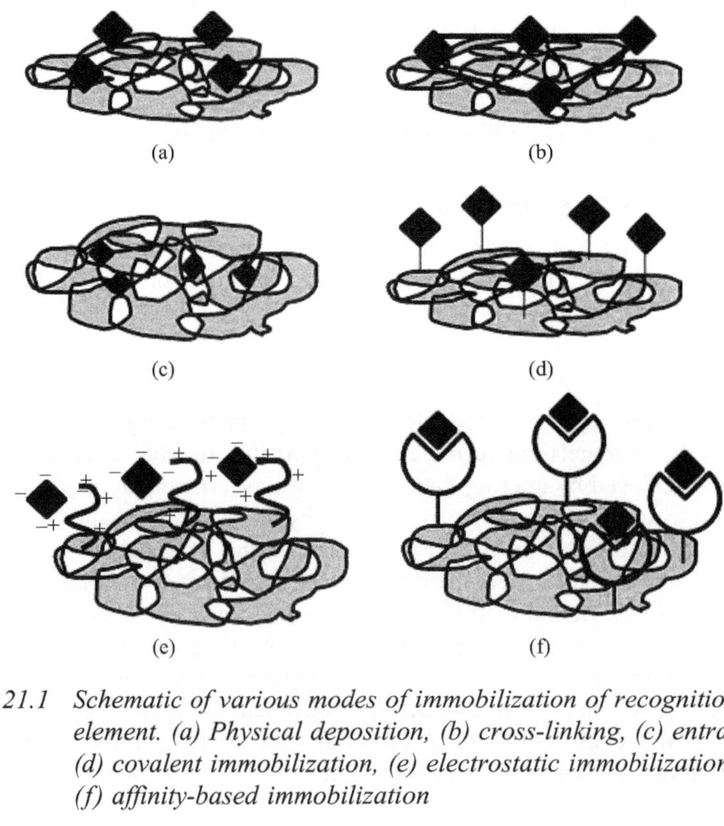

Figure 21.1 Schematic of various modes of immobilization of recognition element. (a) Physical deposition, (b) cross-linking, (c) entrapment, (d) covalent immobilization, (e) electrostatic immobilization, and (f) affinity-based immobilization

element. Here, we briefly describe the basic principles of various immobilization techniques for incorporating recognition elements, such as enzymes, nucleic acids, proteins/peptides, and whole cells, within hydrogel matrix followed by few applications of the same.

21.3.1 Physical deposition and cross-linking

Physical deposition is the simplest form of immobilization of biomolecules, where the recognition element is loosely adhered to the hydrogel matrix primarily by van der Waals or hydrophobic interactions (Figure 21.1 (a)). Advantage of physical deposition is simplicity and cost effectiveness, however, lack of stability is a major disadvantage associated with it. To overcome the disadvantage of poor stability in physical deposition, often it is followed by cross-linking of the biomolecules by suitable cross-linker (Figure 21.1 (b)). Cross-linking could lead to loss of activity of the immobilized biomolecules. Hence, choice of appropriate cross-linker and method of cross-linking are critical. Molecules with reactive groups on terminal positions are typically used as cross-linker.

Glutaraldehyde [$CH_2(CH_2CHO)_2$], with two terminal aldehyde groups, is one of the widely used cross-linkers. Glutaraldehyde was used for cross-linking of glucose oxidase (GOX) enzyme on Pt-nanoparticles (PtNPs)-polyaniline (PANI) hydrogel coated electrode [12]. Another approach of cross-linking was demonstrated by the development of quantum-dot-tagged, DNA-responsive hydrogel photonic beads capable of label-free DNA detection in multiplexing mode [13]. DNA-responsive hydrogel photonic beads were fabricated using a pre-gel solution consisting of acrylamide (2 M), N,N′-methylenebisacrylamide (10 mM), 5′- and 3′-acryloyl-modified ssDNA (10 mM) and a photoinitiator (1.5% v/v). Label-free detection of DNA was achieved by specific hybridization of target DNA and the cross-linked single stranded DNA in the hydrogel that resulted in hydrogel shrinking, which was detected for quantification of the target DNA. Peptide-based supramolecular hydrogel is another group of important biomaterials, which favorably utilizes the cross-linking mode of immobilization. Generally, peptide-based hydrogels are mechanically weak with storage moduli in the range of 10–1000 Pa. Introduction of 3,4-dihydroxyphenylalanine cross-linking into the hydrogel significantly enhanced the mechanical strength (storage moduli of more than 0.2 MPa) [14].

21.3.2 Entrapment

In entrapment, the recognition element is physically enclosed within the hydrogel matrix (Figure 21.1 (c)). Like physical deposition, no chemical bond formation is involved in entrapment as well. However, due to the physical encapsulation within a structured network, it offers a more stable form of immobilization compared to physical deposition. Overall, entrapment provides a simple, cost effective, and efficient mode of immobilization. Reduced accessibility of the recognition element by the target molecules (due to the physical barrier of the enclosing network) could be a challenge for entrapment. Polymers of ethylene glycol- and acrylic-derivatives are frequently used to create the network for entrapping the recognition elements in biosensors.

Poly(ethylene glycol) (PEG)-based hydrogel was used for entrapment of glucose oxidase (GOX) and lactate oxidase (LOX) on gold electrode [15]. GOX/LOX were mixed with poly(ethylene glycol) diacrylate (PEGDA) and other reagents and exposed to unfiltered UV light to form cross-linked hydrogel (photopolymerization) with entrapped GOX and LOX molecules. Apart from that acrylamide, crosslinked with N,N′-methylenebisacrylamide (BIS, non-degradable), and PEGDA (degradable) were utilized to entrap β-galactosidase (lactase) enzyme [16]. Besides, poly-N-isopropylacrylamide (PNIPAAM), silk fibroin and cellulose nanocrystals (CNC)-based hydrogels were also used for entrapment of alcohol oxidase (AOx) onto a nanoplatinum–graphene modified electrode [17].

Entrapment is also used as preferred method of immobilization for biosensors involving aptamers. Aptamers are single-stranded DNA or RNA (ssDNA or ssRNA) molecules that are used as recognition elements in biosensors and bind to analytes, such as proteins and peptides, with high affinity and specificity. A colorimetric agent-caging hydrogel as a platform that relies on DNA base-pair recognition and aptamer–target interactions was utilized for simple and rapid target detection with the naked eye [18]. Two DNA strands, which have complementary adjacent area of a DNA aptamer sequence, were used along with the aptamer to form the hydrogel and enzyme was kept entrapped inside the hydrogel network.

In molecular imprinting, a template molecule is physically entrapped within the voids of the cross-linked polymer. Removal of the template molecule creates molecularly selective sites that are highly selective for the rebinding of the molecules of similar shape and size as the template molecules. Biomolecules, such as proteins, cannot withstand the operating conditions typically used for MIP. Hydrogel-based molecularly imprinted polymers (HydroMIPs) was developed with high selectivity for template proteins [19]. Acrylamide polymer-based HydroMIP with bovine hemoglobin and trypsin as template molecules was found to be a simple diagnostic system for the detection of proteins in disease diagnostics.

Whole cells are also entrapped within hydrogel matrix for detection of analytes. Hydrogel-entrapped *Escherichia coli* sensor was developed for detecting organophosphates (OPs), which are used as pesticides, insecticides and warfare reagents [20]. Organophosphate hydrolase (OPH) enzyme can detect OPs, however, immobilized OPH enzyme demonstrates significantly reduced activity and stability after immobilization. As an alternative, genetically engineered *E. coli* was immobilized within the hydrogel beads. Similarly, a hydrogel patterning and transferring (HPT) method was described that facilitates the quantitative analysis of synthetically engineered genetic circuits within bacterial cells [21]. In HPT method, bacterial cells were encapsulated in the alginate hydrogel-patterns by using polydimethylsiloxane (PDMS) template.

21.3.3 Covalent immobilization

In this technique, biomolecules are covalently attached with the active groups, such as carboxylic acid, amine, and aldehyde, that are previously introduced within the hydrogel matrix (Figure 21.1 (d)). Covalent immobilization enables a stable attachment of the biomolecules, thereby, eliminating the possibility of leakage during the process. However, the major disadvantages are the random covalent attachment that leads to loss of active sites and proximity to the solid polymeric support that leads to denaturation of biomolecules. Various important strategies for covalent immobilization of recognition elements in biosensor are briefly described below.

Via imidazole-intermediate: 1,1′-carbonyldiimidazole (CDI) is used as a precursor for covalent immobilization via imidazole-intermediate within the hydrogels containing hydroxyl (–OH) or amine groups (–NH_2). CDI contains two terminal imidazole groups, which are favorable "leaving groups," and therefore, readily participate in substitution reaction. CDI reacts in succession with the –OH/–NH_2 group of the hydrogel (release of the first imidazole group) and –NH_2 group of the recognition element (e.g. enzyme) (release of the second imidazole group).

Via aldehyde-intermediate: Amine containing hydrogel reacts with glutaraldehyde to form an aldehyde-intermediate via Schiff's base reaction with one aldehyde group of glutaraldehyde. The aldehyde-intermediate containing the second aldehyde group then reacts with the amine group of the recognition element (e.g. enzyme) to covalently immobilize it via Schiff's base reaction.

Via carbodiimide-intermediate: One of the most frequently used strategies for the immobilization of recognition element is the formation of peptide bonds (amide) between the biomolecules (e.g. enzymes) and the functional groups present in the hydrogel. Reaction between carboxylic acid and amine groups (peptide bond formation) is not favorable under normal conditions; hence carbodiimide chemistry is employed to form peptide bond between an enzyme and the hydrogel matrix for covalent attachment. In this approach, the peptide bond formation occurs via formation of a carbodiimide-intermediate using N-hydroxy succinimide (NHS) and a carbodiimide compound (e.g. 1-ethyl-3,3-(dimethylaminopropyl) carbodiimide or EDC) under normal operating conditions.

Development of electrochemical biosensors using GOX or horseradish peroxidase (HRP) along with gold nanoparticles (AuNPs)-containing hydrogel was reported [22]. Mercapto-carboxylic acid (MCA)-modified Au-NPs were prepared by ligand exchange between MCA and citrate-stabilized AuNPs. GOX or HRP molecules were then immobilized onto the MCA-AuNPs using standard EDC/NHS carbodiimide conjugation chemistry between the carboxylic acid groups of MCA and amine groups of the enzyme. After conjugation, the Au-NPs along with the enzyme were dispersed in the prepolymer solution of PEGDA, which was photolithographically patterned in alignment with an array of Au-electrodes fabricated on glass. This led into functionalization of Au-electrode arrays resulting AuNP/GOX or AuNP/HRP carrying hydrogel microstructures, which exhibited improved conductivity and high sensitivity.

In another approach, glucose biosensor was developed based on glucose oxidase (GOX) enzyme and polyaniline (PANI), and chitosan (CS)-coupled carbon nanotubes (CS-CNTs) as signal amplifiers [23]. Covalent immobilization of GOX with the hydrogel matrix was conducted by attaching the amine groups of GOX with the amine groups of CS using carbonyl-di-imidazole (CDI) as described above. GOX was also covalently immobilized onto CS hydrogel matrix (incorporated with multiwalled carbon nanotubes) using glutaraldehyde as the bridging agent [24]. Aldehyde group of glutaraldehyde reacts with the amine group of CS, thereby activating CS for further attachment of GOX by Schiff's reaction between the other aldehyde group of CS-GA and amine group of GOX.

Highly sensitive colorimetric DNA-detecting biosensor was prepared using DNA-functionalized monolithic hydrogels and AuNPs with the aid of covalent bonding [25]. Two kinds of probe DNA molecules were used. One was modified with an acrydite on the 5′ end to achieve covalent attachment to the polyacrylamide hydrogel matrix. The other DNA contained a 3′-thiol modification for attachment to AuNPs. In the presence of the target DNA, the AuNPs were linked to the hydrogel for colorimetric detection. Covalent immobilization of acrydite-modified DNA (thymine rich) on positive (allylamine), neutral (polyacrylamide) and negative (2-acrylamido-2-methyl-1-propanesulfonic acid or AMPS) hydrogels for Hg^{2+} detection has also been reported [26].

21.3.4 Electrostatic immobilization

Reversible attachment via electrostatic interactions has enabled a paradigm shift in immobilization of biomolecules. Biomolecules, such as enzymes/proteins, contain net positive charge at a pH below its isoelectric point (p_I) and net negative charge at a pH above its p_I. In this mode of attachment, hydrogel matrix composed of charged groups are synthesized. Then, operating conditions are adjusted based on p_I to obtain opposite charge on the recognition element, which attaches to the hydrogel matrix by electrostatic interaction between the oppositely charged groups (Figure 21.1 (e)). Electrostatically immobilized biomolecules offer improved activity compared to the covalently immobilized biomolecules. In addition, they also provide improved stability compared to the free biomolecules. It also enables reusability of the hydrogel matrix due to reversible mode of attachment, i.e. an enzyme can be detached by nullifying the electrostatic interaction and new enzyme can be loaded on the same hydrogel matrix. DEAE-Sepharose positively charged anion exchange beads were used for immobilizing negatively charged choline oxidase (ChOX). ChOX-immobilized beads were then entrapped within either calcium alginate or tetramethoxy silane (TMOS) gels for choline detection [27]. A DNA-based biosensor was reported for detection of Hg^{2+}. In the absence of Hg^{2+}; the unfolded anionic DNA interacted with positively charged SYBR Green I (SG) to give strong yellow background fluorescence, while in the presence of Hg^{2+}, DNA became folded and interacted with cationic SG I to emit a green fluorescence.

Unfolded DNA (anionic) + SG I (cationic) = yellow fluorescence
Folded DNA (anionic) + SG I (cationic) + Hg^{2+} = green fluorescence

21.3.5 Affinity-based immobilization

The most sophisticated technique for attachment of recognition element is affinity-based immobilization, where a highly selective biological interaction between a ligand in the hydrogel and a tag in the recognition element is utilized for the immobilization (Figure 21.1 (f)). Antigen-antibody, strept(avidin)-biotin, Ni-histidine are few examples of the affinity couples employed for immobilization in biosensors. Affinity-based immobilization technique enables benefits of both native and immobilized forms of biomolecules, i.e. it retains the activity of the biomolecules in native state along with the higher stability of the traditional covalent bonding. Although, this technique possesses high selectivity and provides high activity and stability, it offers challenges in the form of complex and expensive synthesis steps.

Electrochemical immune-sensors that are prepared based on the specific interaction between antibody and antigen have found wide applications in clinical diagnosis for the detection of different kinds of protein biomarkers. Antibody of the target protein biomarker is immobilized into the porous structure of hydrogel that responses in the presence of the target antigen from a mixture of other biomolecules. Multiple biomarkers are detected by immobilizing the corresponding antibodies of the target biomarkers [28]. The hydrogels prepared from self-assembly of amino acids are of special interest because of its biocompatibility and the facile self-assemble process. In addition, the functional groups on the amino acid molecules enable chemical and biological modifications of the hydrogels. This strategy was employed to prepare a novel supramolecular hydrogel containing ferrocene (Fc)-modified phenylalanine (F) and GOX for the detection of human IgG [29]. Furthermore, rapid protein profiling is possible using antibody microarray as demonstrated with beads-in-gel microarrays by developing a 3D antibody microarray based on the entrapment of antibody-coated micro beads within alginate droplets [30].

For biosensors based on proteins/peptide-based hydrogels, often biotin-(strept) avidin interaction is used. Biotin-(strept) avidin is the strongest known non-covalent interaction. The target protein is biotin-tagged by genetic modification, whereas the hydrogel is functionalized with strept(avidin) to interact with the biotin-tagged protein or vice-versa. Hydrogel microlenses were prepared using poly (N-isopropylacrylamide-co-acrylic acid) microgels and were functionalized with biotin via EDC coupling. It was then used to detect multivalent binding of both avidin and polyclonal anti-biotin [31].

21.4 Multi-analyte detecting system

The biochip- or bio-microarray based-technologies have been developed to permit large scale genomic, proteomic, and functional genomic analyses. High-throughput and high content biomarker detection due to advantages such as fast analysis, low sample consumption, effective cost, and portability underscore the application of these arrays in biomedical fields including diagnostics, drug development, and toxicology studies. Currently, protein arrays can be classified as antibody array (array of polyclonal or monoclonal antibodies for detection/quantification of proteins in biological samples), antigen or reverse array (antigens arrayed to detect antibodies), functional array (array of purified proteins for characterizing protein–protein or protein–small molecule interactions), capture array (array of non-protein molecules such as aptamers or molecular imprinted polymers), and suspension array (coded microparticles in solution for detection of biomarkers in biofluids).

Hydrogel-based microchips were successfully adapted by Rubina *et al.* for quantitative detection of a series of plant (ricin and viscumin) and bacterial (staphylococcal enterotoxin B, tetanus and diphtheria toxins, and lethal factor of anthrax) toxins [32]. The study demonstrated that different types of immunoassays (direct, competitive, and sandwich type) could be successfully carried out on hydrogel-based planar arrays. Yang *et al.* utilized chitosan hydrogels on etched glass slides for detection of cancer biomarkers [33]. The study revealed that the optimal immobilization conditions vary for different antibodies. Under optimized conditions, the detection limit for tumor antigen could be as low as 10 pM [33]. Frequent abnormal amplification or activation of kinases has been implicated in the cause and progression of many cancers. The studies using polyacrylamide- or polyacrylic acid-based planar array had demonstrated specific detection of epidermal growth factor receptor (EGFR) or MET tyrosine kinase activity in cancer cell lysates [34–36]. Furthermore, these studies had also established the potential of the protein-acrylamide copolymer hydrogel arrays to screen for the most effective small molecule kinase inhibitors for the treatment of individual patients.

However, fixed design and low flexibility limit their applications in the clinical setting. Recent years have witnessed a change in paradigm from conventional planar microarrays to novel suspension arrays for multiplexed detection of proteins, nucleic acid, and other biomarkers. Compared with the planar arrays, the suspension arrays offer the advantages of (i) higher flexibility by facilitating modification of the probe-set, (ii) enhanced reaction kinetics due to radial diffusion of analytes/targets, (iii) shorter incubation times, (iv) consumption of less samples, and (v) lower cost. Unlike spatial coding of planar arrays, suspension arrays mostly involve encoded microparticles which are utilized in combination with flow cytometry for detection of biomolecules. Careful manipulation of the intrinsic optical properties enable multiplexed detection of target analytes from a single sample solution. However, these systems suffer from several limitations involving spectral overlap between encoding and reporting fluorophores and higher costs for manufacture and detection. Recent efforts have been directed toward generating hydrogel microparticles that will permit using single fluorophore and eliminating spectral overlap or crosstalk often encountered in color-coded microparticles during multiplexed analysis. One approach toward this has been fabrication of chemically and geometrically complex microparticles via flow lithography [37–39]. Multifunctional particles with distinct regions were synthesized with high degree of reproducibility by polymerizing across laminar co-flowing streams of monomer. Separate "code" and "probe" regions enable identification of the particle and simultaneous detection of multiple analytes present in single solution. Another approach has been fabricating shape-coded particles [40–42]. De-coding the shape-coded particles is easier since shapes of the particles are related to the identity of the target molecules and therefore can be utilized for point-of-care applications. In addition, the spatial coding of planar array was leveraged with the operational efficiencies of suspension array, to generate on-chip microgel droplets within an integrated serpentine trapper array [43]. This convergence of tunable porous hydrogel with efficient microfluidics enhanced the penetration of the target analytes within the trapped microgels and thereby improved the detection sensitivity.

21.5 Summary

While significant advancements have been made in the field of biosensors, a major challenge that needs to be addressed involves development of sensors for point-of-care applications or applications in resource limited settings. Achieving such innovations will require (i) long-term stability and sensitivity of the sensor, (ii) user-friendly data acquisition and read-out, and (iii) portability of the sensor. Integration of hydrogel matrices can address the stability and sensitivity issue of the sensor by enhancing the immobilization of various biomolecules.

References

[1] Clark L.C., Lyons C. "Electrode systems for continuous monitoring in cardiovascular surgery." *Annals of the New York Academy of Sciences*. 1962; 102: 29–45.

[2] Kirsch J., Siltanen C., Zhou Q., Revzin A., Simonia A. "Biosensor technology: recent advances in threat agent detection and medicine." *Chemical Society Reviews*. 2013; 42 (22): 8733–8768.

[3] Flory P.J. "Network structure and elastic properties of vulcanized rubber." *Chemical Reviews*. 1944; 35: 51–75.

[4] Flory P.J., Rehner J. Jr. "Statistical mechanics of cross-linked polymer networks I rubber like elasticity." *Journal of Chemical Physics*. 1943; 11: 512–520.

[5] Flory P.J., Rehner J. Jr. "Statistical mechanics of cross-linked polymer networks II swelling." *Journal of Chemical Physics*. 1943; 11: 521–526.

[6] Beiber B., Musick K., Matsumoto A., Panitch A., Nauman E., Irazoqui P. "Toward a continuous intravascular glucose monitoring system." *Sensors (Basel)*. 2011; 11(1): 409–424.

[7] Mesch M., Zhang C., Braun P.V., Giessen, H. "Functionalized hydrogel on plasmonic nanoantennas for noninvasive glucose sensing." *ACS Photonics*. 2015; 2(4): 475–480.

[8] MacConaghy K.I., Chadly D.M., Stoykovisch M.P., Kaar, J.L. "Optically diffracting hydrogels for screening kinase activity in vitro and in cell lysate:

impact of material and solution properties". *Analytical Chemistry*. 2015; 87 (6): 3467–3475.

[9] Holtz J.H., Asher S.A. "Polymerized colloidal crystal hydrogel films as intelligent chemical sensing materials." *Nature*. 1997; 389: 829–832.

[10] Strong Z.A., Wang A.W., McConaghy C.F. "Hydrogel actuated capacitive transducer for wireless biosensors." *Biomedical Microdevices*. 2002; 4: 97–103.

[11] Al Ameen M.A., Li J., Beer D.G., Ghosh G. "Sensitive, quantitative, and high-throughput detection of angiogenic markers using shape-coded hydrogel microparticles." *Analyst*. 2015; 140: 4530–4539.

[12] Zhai D., Liu B., Shi Y., *et al.* "Highly sensitive glucose sensor based on Pt nanoparticle/polyaniline hydrogel heterostructures." *ACS Nano*. 2013; 7: 3540–3546.

[13] Zhao Y., Zhao X., Tang B., *et al.* "Quantum-dot-tagged bioresponsive hydrogel suspension array for multiplex label-free DNA detection." *Advanced Functional Materials*. 2010; 20: 976–982.

[14] Li Y., Ding Y., Qin M., Cao Y., Wang W. "An enzyme-assisted nanoparticle crosslinking approach to enhance the mechanical strength of peptide-based supramolecular hydrogels." *Chemical Communications*. 2013; 49: 8653–8655.

[15] Yan J., Pedrosa V.A., Simonian A.L., Revzin A. "Immobilizing enzymes onto electrode arrays by hydrogel photolithography to fabricate multi-analyte electrochemical biosensors." *Applied Materials and Interfaces*. 2010; 2: 748–755.

[16] Mariani A.M., Natoli M.E., Kofinas P. "Enzymatic activity preservation and protection through entrapment within degradable hydrogels." *Biotechnology and Bioengineering*. 2013; 9999: 1–9.

[17] Burrs S.L., Vanegas D.C., Bhargava M., *et al.* "A comparative study of graphene–hydrogel hybrid bionanocomposites for biosensing." *Analyst*. 2015; 140: 1466.

[18] Zhu Z., Wu C., Liu H., *et al.* "An aptamer cross-linked hydrogel as a colorimetric platform for visual detection." *Angewandte Chemie* 2010; 122: 1070–1074.

[19] Reddy S.M., Phan Q.T., El-Sharif H., Govada L., Stevenson D., Chayen N.E. "Protein crystallization and biosensor applications of hydrogel-based molecularly imprinted polymers." *Biomacromolecules*. 2012; 13: 3959–3965.

[20] Fleischauer V., Heo J. "An organophosphate sensor based on photo-crosslinked hydrogel-entrapped *E. coli*." *Analytical Sciences*. 2014; 30: 937–942.

[21] Choi S.W., Kim M., Park S., Lee S.K., Kim T. "Patterning and transferring hydrogel-encapsulated bacterial cells for quantitative analysis of synthetically engineered genetic circuits." *Biomaterials*. 2012, 33: 624–633.

[22] Pedrosa V.A., Yan J., Simonian A.L., Revzin A. "Micropatterned nanocomposite hydrogels for biosensing applications." *Electroanalysis*. 2011; 23: 1142–1149.

[23] Wan D., Yuan S., Li G.L., Neoh K.G., Kang E.T. "Glucose biosensor from covalent immobilization of chitosan-coupled carbon nanotubes on polyaniline-modified gold electrode." *Applied Materials and Interfaces*. 2010, 11: 3083–3091.

[24] Fatoni A., Numnuam A. "A highly stable oxygen-independent glucose biosensor based on a chitosan-albumin cryogel incorporated with carbon nanotubes and ferrocene." *Sensors and Actuators B*. 2013; 185: 725–734.

[25] Baeissa A., Dave N., Smith B.D., Liu J. "DNA-functionalized monolithic hydrogels and gold nanoparticles for colorimetric DNA detection." *Applied Materials and Interfaces*. 2010; 2: 3594–3600.

[26] Joseph K.A., Dave N., Liu J. "Electrostatically directed visual fluorescence response of DNA-functionalized monolithic hydrogels for highly sensitive $Hg2^{+}$ detection." *Applied Materials Interfaces*. 2011; 3: 733–739.

[27] Leca-Bouvier B.D., Sassolas A., Blum L.J. "Polyluminol/hydrogel composites as new electrochemiluminescent-active sensing layers." *Analytical and Bioanalytical Chemistry*. 2014; 406: 5657–5667.

[28] Luk Y., Weldon M., Shetye G., Basner S.A., Simon S.A., Burton E. "Woven hydrogel based biosensor." US Patent number US2013/0196309. 2013.

[29] Zhou M., Sun Z., Shen C., Li Z., Zhang Y., Yang M. "Application of hydrogel prepared from ferrocene functionalized amino acid in the design of novel electrochemical immunosensing platform." *Biosensors and Bioelectronics*. 2013; 49: 243–248.

[30] Li H., Leulmi R.F., Juncker D. "Hydrogel droplet microarrays with trapped antibody-functionalized beads for multiplexed protein analysis." *Lab on a Chip*. 2011; 11: 528–534.

[31] Kim J., Nayak S., Lyon L.A. "Bioresponsive hydrogel microlenses." *Journal of American Chemical Society*. 2005; 127: 9588–9592.

[32] Rubina A.Y., Dyukova V.I., Dementieva E.I., *et al.* "Quantitative immunoassay of biotoxins on hydrogel-based protein microchips." *Analytical Biochemistry*. 2005; 340(2): 317–329.

[33] Yang Z., Chevolot Y., Ataman-Onal Y., Choquet-Kastylevsky, G., Souteyrand E., Laurenceau E. "Cancer biomarkers detection using 3D microstructured protein chip: implementation of customized multiplex immunoassay." *Sensors and Actuators B: Chemical*. 2012; 175: 22–28.

[34] Ghosh G., Lee A.G., Palecek S.P. "Hydrogel based protein array for quantifying epidermal growth factor receptor activity in cell lysates." *Analytical Biochemistry*. 2009; 393 (2): 205–214.

[35] Ghosh G., Yan, X., Lee A.G., Palecek S.P. "Quantifying the sensitivities of EGF receptor (EGFR) tyrosine kinase inhibitors in drug resistant non-small cell lung cancer (NSCLC) cells using hydrogel-based peptide array." *Biosensors and Bioelectronics*. 2010; 26(2): 424–431.

[36] Powers A.D., Liu B., Lee A.G., Palecek S.P. "Macroporous hydrogel micropillars for quantifying Met kinase activity in cancer cell lysates." *Analyst*. 2012; 137(17):4052–4061.

[37] Srinivas R.L., Chapin S.C., Doyle P.S. Aptamer-functionalized microgel particles for protein detection. *Analytical Chemistry*. 2011; 83: 9138–9145.

[38] Chapin S.C., Appleyard D.C., Pregibon D.C., Doyle P.S. "Rapid microRNA profiling on encoded gel micropartilces." *Angewandte Chemie*. 2011; 50: 2289–2293.

[39] Choi N.W., Kim J., Chapin S.C., *et al.* "Multiplexed detection of mRNA using porosity tuned hydrogel microparticles." *Analytical Chemistry*. 2012; 84: 9370–9378.

[40] Al Ameen M.A., Ghosh G. "Sensitive quantification of vascular endothelial growth factor (VEGF) using porosity induced hydrogel microspheres." *Biosensors and Bioelectronics*. 2013; 49: 105–110.

[41] Jang E., Koh W.-G. "Multiplexed enzyme-based bioassay within microfluidic devices using shape-coded hydrogel microparticles." *Sensors and Actuators B: Chemical*. 2010; 143(2): 681–688.

[42] Park S., Lee H.J., Koh W.-G. "Multiplex immunoassay platforms based on shape-coded poly (ethylene glycol) hydrogel microparticles incorporating acrylic acid." *Sensors*. 2012; 12(6): 8426–8436.

[43] Zhao Z., Al-Ameen M.A., Duan K., Ghosh G., Lo J.F. "On-chop porous microgel generation for microfluidic enhanced VEGF detection." *Biosensors and Bioelectronics*. 2015; 74: 305–312.

Chapter 22

Applications of graphene microelectrodes in clinical analysis

Georgia-Paraskevi Nikoleli[1], Dimitrios P. Nikolelis[2], Theodoros Varzakas[3], Spyridoula Bratakou[2], Vasillios N. Psychoyios[1] and Stephanos Karapetis[1]

22.1 Biosensors based on nanostructured materials

Biosensors have become important practical tools in the field of healthcare, chemical and biological analysis, environmental monitoring, food safety control, and homeland security. The performance of biosensors depends on their components, among which the matrix material, i.e., the layer between the biorecognition layer and the transducer, plays a crucial role in defining the stability, sensitivity and shelf life of a biosensor [1]. Electrochemical biosensors are of particular interest due to their several advantages such as low detection limits, short response times, long-term stability, power requirements, low cost, ease of operation and miniaturization capability. A current goal for these types of biosensors is the construction of *point-of-care* diagnostic devices.

Nanoscale structures like graphene nanowires, nanotubes, nanowalls and nanorods offer many unique features and show great promise for faster response and higher sensitivity at the device interface. Their nanometer dimensions show an increased sensing surface to volume and strong binding properties, thus allowing a higher sensitivity. Because of the graphene interesting advantages among other nanomaterials, this chapter is devoted to the increasing applications of this material for the fabrication of highly sensitive and selective electrochemical biosensors. This chapter will focus only on applications of this nanomaterial as surface modifier. Some examples of the most interesting capabilities provided by graphene-based (bio) electrodes to the electrochemical detection of analytes and to other

[1]Laboratory of Inorganic & Analytical Chemistry, School of Chemical Engineering, Department of Chemical Sciences, National Technical University of Athens, 9 Iroon Polytechniou St., Athens 157 80, Greece
[2]Laboratory of Environmental Chemistry, Department of Chemistry, University of Athens, Panepistimioupolis-Kouponia, G-15771 Athens, Greece
[3]Technological Educational Institute of Peloponnese, Department of Food Technology, Kalamata, Greece

bioelectronic affinity assays (e.g., DNA hybridization and immuno-assays) will be discussed along with future prospects and challenges.

22.2 Graphene nanomaterials used in electrochemical biosensors fabrication

Graphene nanomaterials (graphene nanowires, nanotubes, nanowalls, and nanorods) have become popular materials for fabricating electrode matrices for electrochemical sensing and biosensin. Graphene is the mother of all graphitic forms including zero-dimensional fullerenes, one-dimensional carbon nanotubes, and three-dimensional graphite [2].

Graphene, defined as a single-layer two-dimensional sp^2-hybridized carbon, is currently the most intensively studied material. This single-atom-thick sheet of carbon atoms arrayed in a honeycomb pattern is the world's thinnest, strongest, and stiffest material, as well as being an excellent conductor of both heat and electricity [3]. Graphene is attractive for electrochemistry because it is a conductive yet transparent material with a low cost and low environmental impact, a wide electrochemical potential window, low electrical resistance in comparison to glassy carbon (GC), atomic thickness and well-defined redox peaks. Peak-to-peak values under cyclic voltammetry (CV) are low, suggesting rapid electron transfer kinetics, and its apparent electron transfer rate is orders of magnitude higher than that of GC. Moreover, the rate of electron transfer has shown to be surface dependent and increased significantly by the introduction of a high density of edge-plane defect sites on graphene surface which provides multiple electrochemically active sites [4]. Its entire volume is exposed to the surrounding due to its 2D structure, making it very efficient in detecting adsorbed molecules. Graphene-based devices possess also the required biocompatibility to be amenable for in situ biosensing. It has also been reported that the edges of graphene sheets possess a variety of oxygenated species that can support efficient electrical wiring of the redox centers of several heme-containing metalloproteins to the electrode and also enhance the adsorption and desorption of molecules [4, 5].

Graphene-based nanomaterials can be classified in relation to the method of production. They can be produced by chemical vapor deposition (CVD) growth, by mechanical exfoliation of graphite, or by exfoliation of graphite oxide. Neither CVD-produced graphene nor mechanically exfoliated graphene contains large quantities of defects or functionalities. Bulk quantities of graphene-based nanomaterials are typically prepared by different methods, such as the thermal exfoliation of graphite oxide which leads to a material called thermally reduced graphene (TRGO) or, for example, sono-assisted exfoliation of graphite oxide to graphene oxide (GO), which can be further reduced chemically or electrochemically. The products are typically referred to as chemically reduced GO (CRGO) or electrochemically reduced GO (ERGO). TRGO contains large amounts of defects and significantly differs from pristine graphene, which has a perfect honeycomb lattice structure. GO has a structure that is not fully planar because the

sp^2 carbon network is heavily damaged. It contains large amounts of oxygen-containing groups, which can be beneficial to the functionalization through the action of the biomolecules for biorecognition events during biosensing. Reduced forms of GO have a partly restored sp^2 lattice but still hold some fraction of oxygen-containing groups [6]. Therefore, one could have a large graphene "tool-box" to choose the right type of graphene for the right application and transduction mechanism [7]. Most of graphene used in electrochemistry is graphene produced from GO chemical/thermal reduction, which is also called functionalized graphene sheets or chemically reduced GO, and usually has abundant structural defects and functional groups which are advantageous for electrochemical applications. It has been demonstrated that ERGO exhibits much better performance for electrochemical applications than CRGO. Moreover, Chua *et al.* [8] demonstrated that not all graphene materials are beneficial for the detection at lab-on-chip devices. Their findings could provide valuable insights into the future applicability of graphene materials towards practical applications.

22.3 Miniaturized graphene electrochemical biosensors for health monitoring

Taking advantage of the relative simplicity, easy miniaturization, possibility of in situ measurements, low-cost and high sensitivity and selectivity of electroanalytical techniques, different graphene-based electrochemical biosensors have been developed for the detection of target analytes. Besides graphene is an excellent conductor of electrical charge with high surface area which facilitates large amounts of defects and thus, electroactive sites [9]. Heterogeneous electron transfer (the transfer of electrons between graphene and the molecule in the solution necessary for the oxidation/reduction of the electroactive specie) occurs at its edges or at defects in the basal plane.

An exhaustive revision of the literature regarding the applicability of graphene nanostructures in electrochemical biosensing demonstrated their use in the implementation of enzymatic, immune- and DNA-sensing platforms. Some relevant examples about these three types of bioplatforms will be briefly discussed in the following sections.

22.3.1 Enzymatic biosensors

Given the tremendous market and investment in sensing glucose for diabetic patients, a wide number of graphene-based electrochemical biosensors have been employed for the determination of this target analyte. In these biosensors the biorecognition element used is glucose oxidase (GOx) which oxidizes glucose to gluconic acid and shuffles electrons into the oxygen which is dissolved in the solution, and then reduced to hydrogen peroxide, which is typically detected electrochemically.

However, in several examples, direct electron transfer (DET) from the enzyme (without the need of O_2 as an electron acceptor) has been demonstrated [10].

A novel and highly sensitive electroanalytical sensing nanocomposite material based on the use of exfoliated graphite nanoplatelets (xGnP) was reported for the development of a glucose biosensor [11]. The glucose biosensing interface, prepared by casting GOx and xGnP in a Nafion water–isopropyl-alcohol solution, showed rapid response time (5 s), high sensitivity (14.17 μA $mM^{-1}\cdot cm^{-2}$ and LOD of 10 μM), good selectivity and long-term stability.

Wang *et al.* [12] reported a facile strategy to prepare N-doped graphene by using nitrogen plasma treatment of graphene synthesized *via* a chemical method. Moreover, the as-prepared N-doped graphene has displayed high electrocatalytic activity for reduction of hydrogen peroxide and fast Direct Electron Transfer (DET) kinetics for GOx able to detect as low as 0.01 mM glucose in the presence of interferences.

The direct electrochemistry of GOx immobilized in a modified electrode based on a composite film of exfoliated graphite nanosheets (GNSs) and Nafion was achieved with a fast electron transfer rate (12.6 s^{-1}) by Fu *et al.* [13]. The resulting biosensors exhibited higher sensitivity (3.4 μA mM^{-1}), compared advantageously in terms of cost and ease of preparation with the carbon nanotubes (CNTs)-based modified electrodes and should have wide applications in third-generation biosensors, bioelectronics and electrocatalysis.

DET of GOx was achieved also using polyvinylpyrrolidone-protected graphene/polyethylenimine-functionalized ionic liquid (PFIL)/GOx electrochemical biosensors [14] and GOx immobilized into thin films of chitosan containing nanocomposites of graphene and gold nanoparticles (AuNPs) at gold electrodes [15]. Both platforms showed obvious electrocatalysis toward O_2 and H_2O_2 reduction and excellent performance for electrochemical biosensing of glucose.

A novel, highly efficient needle-type glucose sensor based was developed by GOx immobilization through the direct interaction between carboxyl acid groups of the RGO and amines of GOx together with the electrostatic interactions existing between the positively charged polymeric ionic liquid (PIL) and GOx [6]. This combined system can provide a favorable microenvironment for the GOx to retain its good bioactivity. The enzyme-coated graphene biosensor exhibited glucose-dependent electrochemical measurements against an Ag/AgCl reference electrode. The excellent performance of the resulting electrochemical biosensor which exhibits a broad linear range up to 100 mM glucose concentration, a sensitivity of 5.59 μA/decade and a stable output response, paves the way to its potential applications in clinical diagnosis.

Electrochemical (bio) sensors based on graphene nanostructures have been developed for the detection of other relevant analytes such as H_2O_2, cholesterol, NADH, ethanol and urea.

Studies performed by Zhou *et al.* [16] demonstrated also a greatly enhanced electrochemical reactivity of H_2O_2 and NADH at a CRGO-modified GC electrodes and a better analytical performance at the CRGO/GC-based bioelectrodes (in connection with GOx and alcohol dehydrogenase (ADH)) for the detection of glucose and ethanol compared with graphite/GC- or GC-based bioelectrodes. These results revealed that CRGO with the nature of a single sheet showed favorable electrochemical activity demonstrating to be a highly promising robust and advanced carbon electrode material which may hold great promise for electrochemical sensors and biosensors design.

Other interesting biosensing platforms based on DET were reported for the detection of H_2O_2 with a single-layer graphene nanoplatelet-horseradish peroxidase (HRP) composite film [17] or using hemoglobin immobilized on a composite film of graphene and chitosan [18].

A novel H_2O_2 biosensor based on a biphenyldimethanethiol BPT/AuNPs/graphene/HRP composite was developed [19]. The resulting biosensor showed an excellent electrocatalytic performance with high sensitivity (LOD of 1.5×10^{-6} M) and fast response to H_2O_2.

A hierarchical enzyme–graphene nanocomposite for H_2O_2 amperometric detection has been fabricated through electrostatic self-assembly of HRP and sodium dodecyl benzene sulfonate (SDBS) functionalized GSs [20]. The SDBS-functionalized GSs can not only provide large, open and accessible two-dimensional surfaces for tethering of the enzymes, but also 'flexible distance' and restack by adapting to the dimensions of the biomolecules through electrostatic self-assembly, attribute of great importance for retaining the native conformations of the guest enzymes. The HRP–GSs composites display excellent electrocatalytic performance toward the reduction of H_2O_2 with fast response, wide linear range, high sensitivity, low LOD and a two-month storage stability. These desirable electrochemical performances are attributed to an excellent biocompatibility and superb electron transport efficiency of GSs, as well as to a high HRP loading and synergistic catalytic effect of the HRP–GSs bionanocomposites toward H_2O_2. As graphene can be readily non-covalently functionalized by "designer" aromatic molecules with different electrostatic properties, the proposed self-assembly strategy was described as affording a facile and effective platform for the assembly of various biomolecules into hierarchically ordered bionanocomposites in biosensing and biocatalytic applications.

Dey *et al.* described the development of a highly sensitive amperometric biosensor for the sensing of H_2O_2 and cholesterol by immobilization of cholesterol oxidase (ChOx) and cholesterol esterase on the surface of Pt nanoparticle decorated chemically synthesized graphene (GNS-nPt) [21]. This sensing platform demonstrated a sensitive detection of H_2O_2 with an LOD of 0.5 nM in the absence of any redox mediator or enzyme at a >100 mV less positive potential with respect to the bulk Pt electrode. The bienzyme integrated nanostructured platform showed a high selective and sensitivity detection of cholesterol ((2.07 ± 0.1) $\mu A\ \mu M^{-1} cm^{-2}$), an LOD of 0.2 μM, high stability and fast response time. These results demonstrated that the Pt nanoparticle decorated graphene is a promising and biocompatible material for the electroanalysis of biologically important analytes in real sample analysis.

Another amperometric layer-by-layer biosensor for cholesterol based on an electrochemical microelectrode with graphene films synthesized by thermal CVD method coated on Fe_3O_4-doped polyaniline (PANi) films and immobilization of ChOx onto the working electrode with glutaraldehyde agent was also developed [22].

These layer-by-layer fabricated bioelectrode exhibited excellent analytical quantification in the wide cholesterol concentration range from 2 to 20 mM with high sensitivity (74 μA $mM^{-1}cm^{-2}$) and fast response time (<5 s).

Shan *et al.* achieved low-potential β-nicotinamide adenine dinucleotide (NADH) detection and biosensing for ethanol by immobilization of an ionic liquid-functionalized graphene (IL-graphene) and the enzyme alcohol dehydrogenase (ADH) on chitosan-modified GC electrode [23]. The IL-graphene/chitosan-modified GC electrode showed a more stable and low-potential amperometric detection of NADH when compared with the bare electrode, eliminated surface fouling effects and exhibited a good linearity (0.25–2 mM) and a high sensitivity of 37.43 μA mM^{-1} cm^{-2}, resulting a novel and promising biocompatible platform for the development of dehydrogenase-based amperometric biosensors. Using ADH as a model enzyme, a rapid and highly sensitive amperometric biosensor for ethanol, with a low LOD (5 μM), was constructed by immobilizing ADH on the IL-graphene/chitosan-modified GC electrode. Moreover, the proposed biosensor was used to determine ethanol in real samples with results in good agreement with those certified by the supplier, thus demonstrating that such IL-functionalized graphene nanocomposite provided a biocompatible platform for the development of electrochemical biosensors with low cost, convenient preparation and very good analytical performance with great potential for practical applications.

GSs modified GC electrodes (GSs/GC electrodes) have been presented and applied for the electrochemical bio-sensing of NADH and ethanol (after ADH immobilization) displaying a more desirable analytical performance in the amperometric detection of ethanol, compared with the conventional graphite functionalized and bare GC-based bio-electrodes [24]. GSs/GC electrodes exhibited good performance with fast, high selective and sensitive response, a wide linear range and low LOD and accurate determination of ethanol in real samples.

A potentiometric and miniaturized cholesterol biosensor based on physical adsorption of ChOx onto exfoliated GSs onto a thin copper wire has been described by Israr *et al.* [25]. This potentiometric biosensor revealed excellent stability, reusability, selectivity and sensitivity (~82 mV/decade) for the detection of cholesterol biomolecules in the 1×10^{-6} M to 1×10^{-3} M logarithmic range, a quick output response (~4 s) and a good shelf life while storing in appropriate environmental conditions, ideal for practical applications.

A miniaturized potentiometric urea lipid film based biosensor with great analytical performance has been developed by Nikoleli *et al.* [26] using GSs successfully exfoliated onto a thin copper wire (Figure 22.1).

A novel potentiometric cholesterol biosensor has been fabricated through the immobilization of the stabilized polymeric lipid membrane onto graphene electrode [27]. The stabilized polymeric lipid membrane is composed of cholesterol oxidase enzyme and polymerization mixture; which holds paramount influence on the properties of cholesterol biosensor (Figure 22.2). The presented biosensor reveals an appreciable reproducibility, good selectivity and high sensing capability with linear slope curve of ~64 mV/decade. The strong biocompatibility among the

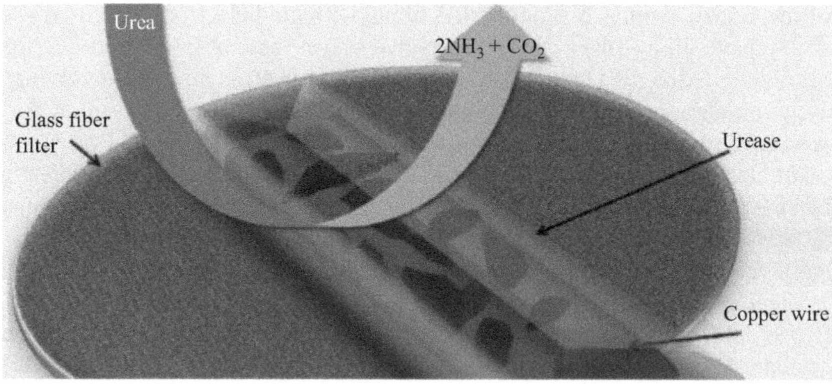

Figure 22.1 Schematic image of the urea biosensor. Reprinted from Reference 26 with permission. Copyright 2013, Electroanalysis, Wiley VCH

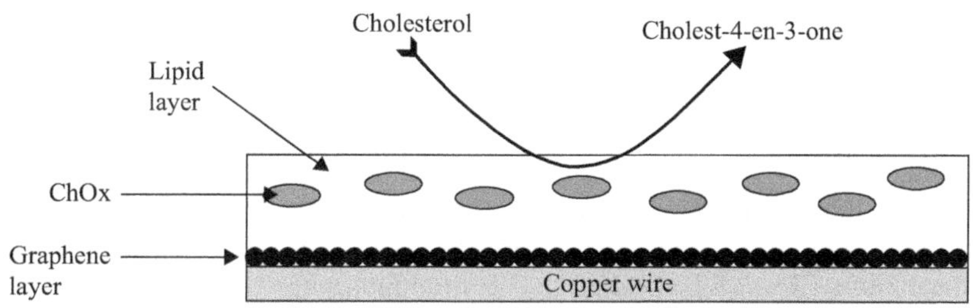

Figure 22.2 Scheme of the biosensor design. Reprinted from Reference 27 with permission. Copyright 2013, Centr. Eur. J. Chem, Springer

stabilized polymeric lipid membrane and human biofluids provides the possibility to use for the real blood samples/practical applications.

22.3.2 Immunosensors

Graphene-based bioplatforms has demonstrated also to be interesting for electrochemical immunosensing. In immunosensing, the direct electrochemical detection of antibody-antigen recognition is usually not possible and electrochemically active labels must typically be used. There are two main strategies in which graphene can be used in electrochemical immunosensors: graphene nanostructures can be used as carrier labels or as modifiers of electrochemical transducers.

Although substantial improvements in the performance of electrochemical immunosensors have been achieved by using graphene nanomaterials for tagging [7, 28, 29] in this chapter, we will describe in more detail only those approaches which exploit its use as electrochemical transducers modifier.

Examples of the use of graphene nanostructured transducer surfaces include the development of very sensitive CEA immunosensors based on gold nanoflower-labeled anti-CEA antibodies along with gold electrode modified with a DNA-graphene film followed by a layer-by-layer assembly of anti-CEA/gold nanoflower/thionine [30] or using a new dual-amplification strategy involving the catalytic recycling of the product by glucose oxidase-conjugated gold-silver hollow microspheres (used as signal tags) coupled with an artificial catalase, Prussian blue nanoparticles, on a graphene-based immunosensing platform [31]. Similarly, graphene sheets sensor platforms in connection with inorganic or organic nanomaterials as advanced labels were used to develop high sensitive immunosensors for the detection of prostate specific antigen (PSA) [32–35] and breast cancer susceptibility gene (BRCA1) [35]. As an example, poly (ethylene glycol) epoly (lactic acid) (PEGePLA) polymeric vesicles were prepared and used to simultaneously encapsulate Fe_3O_4 NPs and immobilize secondary antibody (Ab2) for the fabrication of an electrochemical immunosensor for PSA by primary antibody (Ab1) immobilization onto a GS surface [34].

Hybrid nanoarchitectures, consisting of carbon and inorganic nanomaterials, have shown extremely useful for immobilizing the antibody receptor with high stability and bioactivity [3]. Several studies described also the use of graphene/AuNPs hybrid architectures for enhancing electrode transducers for electrochemical immunosensing [30, 36–39].

A miniaturized potentiometric D-dimer biosensor on graphene nanosheets with incorporated lipid films was recently developed [40]. The graphene electrode was used for the development of a very selective and sensitive immunosensor for the detection of D-dimer by immobilizing the mouse anti human D-dimer antibody on stabilized lipid films (Figure 22.3). The immunosensor responded for the wide

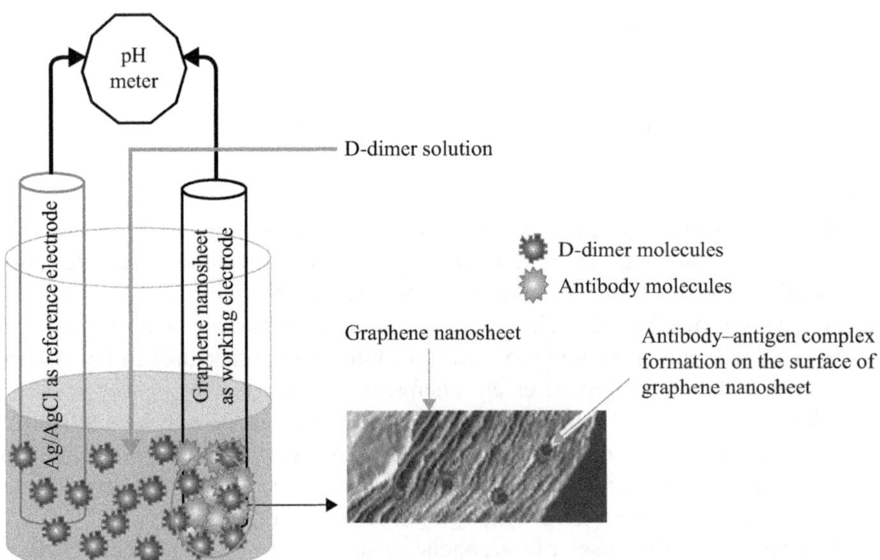

Figure 22.3 Setup of potentiometric D-dimer experiments

range of D-dimer concentrations with fast response time of ca. 15 s. The presented potentiometric D-dimer biosensor is easy to construct and exhibits good reproducibility, reusability, selectivity, rapid response times, long shelf life and high sensitivity of ca. 59 mV/decade over the D-dimer logarithmic concentration range from 10^{-6} mg/L to 10^{-3}mg/L.

22.3.3 DNA sensors

Graphene-based biosensors have found another large field of application in electrochemical DNA sensing. For the electrochemical detection of nucleic acids reagent-less or reagent-based approaches have been reported. In the first group the direct or catalyzed oxidation of DNA bases, as well as charge transport reactions mediated by the π-stacked base pairs are included. Reagent-based methods are usually based on the redox reactions of reporter molecules which bind specifically to either single-stranded or double-stranded DNA or enzymes recruited to the electrode surface by specific probe-target interactions [41, 42]. Although reagent-less methods avoid the need of introducing a reagent during the protocol, and then washing the reagent out and consequently are easier to automate than reagent-based methods which may be time-consuming or more expensive they usually offer poorer sensitivity. Additionally, although on traditional carbon materials, such as glassy carbon and graphite, the adenine (A) and guanine (G) bases give analytically useful signals but cytosine (C) and thymine (T) do not [7]. However, Zhou *et al.* [16] demonstrated that a CRGO-modified GC electrode (CRGO/GC electrode) provides well-resolved signals of all free bases of DNA (G, A, T and C) and showed more favorable electron transfer kinetics than graphite-modified GC and GC electrodes. This greatly enhanced electrochemical reactivity of the four free bases of DNA at the CRGO/GC electrode makes this electrode a better choice for the electrochemical biosensing of four DNA bases in both the single-stranded DNA (ssDNA) and double-stranded DNA (dsDNA) at physiological pH without a prehydrolysis step. The applicability of this promising CRGO/GC electrode was demonstrated for the label-free detection of a SNP site in short oligomers with a particular sequence without any hybridization or labeling processes, suggesting the potential applications of CRGO in the label-free electrochemical detection of DNA hybridization or DNA damage for further research.

Lim *et al.* [43] found that anodized epitaxial graphene (EG), high edge plane defects, was a good choice biosensing platform for the detection of nucleic acids, dopamine and uric and ascorbic acids. In these electrodes the graphene was grown on a substrate where the basal plane is exposed to the solution like in basal plane pyrolytic graphite but with a smaller number of graphene layers. These anodized EG voltammetric sensors allowed to resolve as individual peaks mixtures of nucleic acids (A, T, C, G) or biomolecules (AA, UA, DA) using differential pulse voltammetry (DPV), to realize the simultaneous detection of all four DNA bases in double stranded DNA (dsDNA) without a prehydrolysis step, and also to differentiate single stranded DNA from dsDNA. Their results demonstrated that the electrochemical oxidation of pristine epitaxially grown graphene introduced a high number of edge plane defects on its surface (similarly to what it was previously described multiwalled carbon nanotubes (MWCNTs) [44]) providing a platform with significantly increased and better resolved responses, ideal for high-resolution electrochemical sensing.

Stacked graphene nanofibers (SGNFs) demonstrated also superior electrochemical performance for oxidation of DNA bases over CNTs (two to four times higher currents) due to an exceptionally high number of accessible graphene sheet edges on the surface of the nanofibers when compared to carbon nanotubes [45]. These SGNFs, which are the direct opposites of carbon nanotubes because they consist of perpendicularly stacked graphene sheets along the c-axis, exhibiting exclusively electrochemically active edges (with the exception of terminal basal planes), provided also higher sensitivity than edge-plane pyrolytic graphite (EPPG), GC, or graphite microparticle-based electrodes (GMPs). These authors demonstrated the sensitive oxidation of influenza A (H1N1)-related strands on these SGNF-based electrodes, which could therefore be applied to label-free DNA analysis.

A GO modified light addressable potentiometric sensor (GO-LAPS) modified with an ssDNA probe has been developed to the detection of complementary ssDNA sequences of different length (30, 21, and 14 base pairs) [46]. This GO-LAPS-based platform which demonstrated to be sensitive for short-chain ssDNA detection (the target DNA could be determined in the concentration range from 1 pM to 10 nM) could also be applied to other kinds of biological detection, such as DNA-targeted drugs, tumor markers or single cells.

22.4 Conclusions and future prospects

As a result of the unique physical and chemical properties of graphene nanostructures, in the past few years the literature has experienced an explosive growth of the research works in this topic, especially in the area of electrochemical (bio) sensing.

This chapter has selectively summarized recent approaches (particularly from the last decade) in the rapidly developing area of electrochemical sensors and biosensors based on graphene nanostructures for the detection of clinically and environmentally relevant analytes. The advances discussed clearly demonstrated the considerable growth experienced by electrochemical biosensors technology in terms of applicability and complexity of devices due to the utilization of electrodes-modified with graphene in order to increase the power detection of specific molecules and the development of new methodologies for biomolecules immobilization. A great number of the highlighted applications on the enzyme-based graphene nanobiosensors have focused on glucose sensing using GOx, due to the importance of diagnosing and managing diabetes. The most common issue associated with glucose sensors is slow electron transfer to the electrode after glucose oxidation due to inhibition of flavin adenine dinucleotide (FAD) cofactors, which form the redox center of GOx, by the protective glycoprotein shell. However, graphene-based composites, because of their good electronic properties and biocompatibility, have demonstrated to achieve the DET of this redox enzyme and maintain its bioactivity well, obviating the need for co-substrates or mediators, and their eco-friendliness could pave the way for the development of superior reagentless biosensing devices, nontoxic, bio-safe, and biocompatible, which could then be employed for developing implantable biosensors. The advantages of rapid response and the potential for miniaturization demonstrated also by these graphene nanostructured-based sensor platforms toward glucose detection have proved to be extrapolated for the detection of other biomedically important analytes (glutamate, ethanol, cholesterol, urea, NADH, H_2O_2, etc.) by functionalization with the appropriate enzyme/s. Although it is still a challenge, enzyme-based bioassays on these nanobioplatforms are also expected to be useful for multianalyte detection, opening up the possibility of fabricating innovative biosensor arrays with desired properties for health care.

Apart from enzymes graphene nanostructures-based platforms have been employed as immobilization matrixes for other attractive bioreceptors (such as DNA, aptamers, and antibodies) to implement other types of bioaffinity sensors with great analytical performance for the electrochemical detection of other biomolecules of interest such as protein and genetic biomarkers involved in important diseases such as cancer.

These novel bioplatforms have demonstrated to develop many new signal transduction technologies in biosensors, arising from the sub-micrometer dimensions that can be utilized for simple and rapid in vivo analysis, providing a new horizon for novel functions with a variety of important applications in medical diagnostics, such as the possibility to perform biologically relevant measurements inside living cells.

Future efforts will aim also at guiding and tailoring the synthesis of novel materials for meeting specific electrochemical biosensing applications and needs. These newly developed bioconjugated nanoarchitectures are expected to display even better properties than current nanobiointerfaces and hence to impart excellent performance onto electrochemical biosensors and to further expand the realm of graphene-based electrochemical (bio) sensors.

Acknowledgments

The authors express their acknowledgments for the financial help of the Greek Ministry of Development, General Secretariat of Research and Technology and the European Commission (in particular the European Regional Development fund and National Resources) which co-funded the present research project in the framework of Greece-Slovakia bilateral projects (Contract 12SLO_ET30_1036).

References

[1] Arya S. K., Saha S., Ramirez-Vick J. E., Gupta V., Bhansali S., Singh S. P. "Recent advances in ZnO nanostructures and thin films for biosensor applications: review." *Anal. Chim. Acta* 2012, vol. 737, pp. 1–21.

[2] Rao C. N. R., Biswas K., Subrahmanyam K. S., Govindaraj A. "Graphene, the new nanocarbon." *J. Mater. Chem.* 2009, vol. 19, pp. 2457–69.

[3] Georgakilas V., Otyepka M., Bourlinos A. B., *et al.* "Functionalization of graphene: covalent and non-covalent approaches, derivatives and applications." *Chem. Rev.* 2012, vol. 112, pp. 6156–214.
[4] Artiles M. S., Rout C. S., Fisher T. S., "Graphene-based hybrid materials and devices for biosensing." *Adv. Drug Del. Rev.* 2011, vol. 63, pp. 1352–60.
[5] Bao H., Pan Y., Li L. "Recent advances in graphene-based nanomaterials for biomedical applications." *Nano Life*. 2012, vol. 2, pp. 1–15.
[6] ul Hasan K., Asif M. H., Nur O., Willander M. "Graphene-based hybrid materials and devices for biosensing." *J. Biosens. Bioelectron.* 2012, vol. 3, pp. 1–6.
[7] Pumera M. "Graphene in biosensing," *Materials Today*. 2011, vol. 14, pp. 308–15.
[8] Chua C. K., Pumera M. "Chemically modified graphenes as detectors in lab-on-chip device." *Electroanal.* 2011, vol. 25, pp. 945–50.
[9] Pumera M. "Graphene-based nanomaterials and their electrochemistry." *Chem. Soc. Rev.*2010, vol. 39, pp. 4146–57.
[10] Wilson G. S., Hu Y. "Enzyme-based biosensors for in vivo measurements." *Chem. Rev.* 2000, vol. 100, pp. 2693–704.
[11] Lu J., Drzal L. T., Worden R. M., Lee I. "Simple fabrication of a highly sensitive glucose biosensor using enzymes immobilized in exfoliated graphite nanoplatelets nafion membrane." *Chem. Mater.* 2007, vol. 19, pp. 6240–46.
[12] Wang Y., Shao Y., Matson D. W., Li J., Lin Y. "Nitrogen-doped graphene and its application in electrochemical biosensing." *ACS Nano* 2010, vol. 4, pp. 1790–98.
[13] Fu C., Yang W., Chen X., Evans D. G. "Direct electrochemistry of glucose oxidase on a graphite nanosheet–nafion composite film modified electrode." *Electrochem. Commun.* 2009, vol. 11, pp. 997–1000.
[14] Shan C., Yang H., Song J., Han D., Ivaska A., Niu L., "Direct electrochemistry of glucose oxidase and biosensing for glucose based on graphene." *Anal. Chem.* 2009, vol. 81, pp. 2378–82.
[15] Shan C., Yang H., Han D., Zhang Q., Ivaska A., Niu L. "Graphene/AuNPs/chitosan nanocomposites film for glucose biosensing." *Biosens. Bioelectron.* 2010, vol. 25, pp. 1070–74.
[16] Zhou M., Zhai Y., Dong S. "Electrochemical sensing and biosensing platform based on chemically reduced graphene oxide." *Anal. Chem.* 2009, vol. 81, pp. 5603–13.
[17] Lu Q., Dong X., Li L.-J., Hu X. "Direct electrochemistry-based hydrogen peroxide biosensor formed from single-layer graphene nanoplatelet–enzyme composite film." *Talanta*. 2010, vol. 82, pp. 1344–48.
[18] Xu H., Dai H., Chen G. "Direct electrochemistry and electrocatalysis of hemoglobin protein entrapped in graphene and chitosan composite film." *Talanta* 2010, vol. 81, pp. 334–38.
[19] Wang T., Zhu Y., Li G., *et al.* "Novel hydrogen peroxide biosensor based on the BPT/AuNPs/graphene/HRP composite." *Sci. China Chem.* 2011, vol. 54, pp. 1645–50.

[20] Zeng Q., Cheng J., Tang L., *et al.* "Self-assembled graphene-enzyme hierarchical nanostructures." *Adv. Funct. Mater.* 2010, vol. 20, pp. 3366–72.
[21] Dey R. S., Raj C. R., "Development of an amperometric cholesterol biosensor based on graphene–Pt nanoparticle hybrid material." *J. Phys. Chem. C.* 2010, vol. 114, pp. 21427–33.
[22] Nguyen H. B., Nguyen V. C., Nguyen V. T., *et al.* "Development of the layer-by-layer biosensor using graphene films: application for cholesterol determination." *Adv. Nat. Sci.: Nanosci. Nanotechnol.* 2013, vol. 4, 015013 (4pp) doi:10.1088/2043-6262/4/1/015013.
[23] Shan C., Yang H., Han D., Zhang Q., Ivaska A., Niu L. "Electrochemical determination of NADH and ethanol based on ionic liquid-functionalized graphene." *Biosens. Bioelectr.* 2010, vol. 25, pp. 1504–8.
[24] Guo K., Qian K., Zhang S., Kong J., Yu C., Liu B. "Bio-electrocatalysis of NADH and ethanol based on graphene sheets modified electrodes." *Talanta.* 2011, vol. 85, p. 1174–79.
[25] Israr M. Q., ul Hasan K., Sadaf J. R., *et al.* "Structural characterization and biocompatible applications of graphene nanosheets for miniaturization of potentiometric cholesterol biosensor." *J. Biosens. Bioelectron.* 2011, vol. 2:3. http://dx.doi.org/10.4172/2155-6210.1000109, 2011.
[26] Nikoleli G.-P., Israr M. Q., Tzamtzis N., Nikolelis D. P., Willander M., Psaroudakis N. "Structural characterization of graphene nanosheets for miniaturization of potentiometric urea lipid film based biosensors." *Electroanal.* 2012, vol. 24, pp. 1285–95.
[27] Nikoleli G.-P., Hussain Ibupoto Z., Nikolelis D. P., *et al.* "Potentiometric cholesterol biosensing application of graphene electrode with stabilized polymeric lipid membrane." *Centr. Eur. J. Chem.* 2011, vol. 11 (9), pp. 1554–61.
[28] Zhong Z., Wu W., Wang D., *et al.* "Nanogold-enwrapped graphene nanocomposites as trace labels for sensitivity enhancement of electrochemical immunosensors in clinical immunoassays: carcinoembryonic antigen as a model." *Biosens. Bioelectron.* 2010, vol. 25, pp. 2379–83.
[29] Du D., Wang L., Shao Y., Wang J., Engelhard M. H., Lin Y. "Functionalized graphene oxide as a nanocarrier in a multienzyme labeling amplification strategy for ultrasensitive electrochemical immunoassay of phosphorylated." *Anal. Chem.* 2011, vol. 83, pp. 746–52.
[30] Su B., Tang J., Yang H., Chen G., Huang J., Tang D. "A graphene platform for sensitive electrochemical immunoassay of carcinoembryoninc antigen based on gold-nanoflower biolabels." *Electroanalysis.* 2011, vol. 23, pp. 832–41.
[31] Tang J., Tang D., Li Q., Su B., Qiu B., Chen G. "Sensitive electrochemical immunoassay of carcinoembryonic antigen with signal dual-amplification using glucose oxidase and an artificial catalase." *Anal. Chim. Acta.* 2011, vol. 697, pp. 16–22.
[32] Wei Q., Xiang Z., He J., *et al.* "Dumbbell-like Au-Fe_3O_4 nanoparticles as label for the preparation of electrochemical immunosensors." *Biosens. Bioelectron.* 2010, vol. 26, pp. 627–31.

[33] Li H., Wei Q., He J., *et al.* "Electrochemical immunosensors for cancer biomarker with signal amplification based on ferrocene functionalized iron oxide nanoparticles." *Biosens. Bioelectron.* 2011, vol. 26, pp. 3590–95.
[34] Wie Q., Li T., Wang G., Li H., Qian Z., Yang M. "Fe_3O_4 nanoparticles-loaded PEG–PLA polymeric vesicles as labels for ultrasensitive immunosensors." *Biomaterials* 2010, vol. 31, pp. 7332–39.
[35] Cai Y., Li H., Du B., *et al.* "Ultrasensitive electrochemical immunoassay for BRCA1 using BMIM·BF_4-coated SBA-15 as labels and functionalized graphene as enhancer." *Biomaterials.* 2011, vol. 32, pp. 2117–23.
[36] Liu K., Zhang J.-J., Wang C., Zhu J.-J. "Graphene-assisted dual amplification strategy for the fabrication of sensitive amperometric immunosensor." *Biosens. Bioelectron.* 2011, vol. 26, pp. 3627–32.
[37] Wang G., Huang H., Zhang G., *et al.* "Gold nanoparticles/L-cysteine/graphene composite based immobilization strategy for an electrochemical immunosensor." *Anal. Meth.* 2010, vol. 2, pp. 1692–97.
[38] Su B., Tang J., Huang J., *et al.* "Graphene and nanogold-functionalized immunosensing interface with enhanced sensitivity for one-step electrochemical immunoassay of alpha-fetoprotein in human serum." *Electroanal.* 2010, vol. 22, pp. 2720–28.
[39] Zhuo Y., Chai Y.-Q., Yuan R., Mao L., Yuan Y.-L., Han J. "Glucose oxidase and ferrocene labels immobilized at Au/TiO_2 nanocomposites with high load amount and activity for sensitive immunoelectrochemical measurement of ProGRP biomarker." *Biosens. Bioelectron.* 2011, vol. 26, pp. 3838–44.
[40] Nikoleli G.-P., Nikolelis D. P., Tzamtzis N., Psaroudakis N. "A selective immunosensor for D-dimer based on antibody immobilized on a graphene electrode with incorporated lipid films." *Electroanalysis* 2014, vol. 26(7), pp. 1522–27.
[41] Paleček E., Fojta M. "Peer reviewed: detecting DNA hybridization and damage." *Anal. Chem.* 2001, vol. 73, pp. 74A–83A.
[42] Tosar J. P., Brañas G., Laíz J. "DNA hybridization sensors applied to real and complex biological samples." *Biosens. Biolectron.* 2010, vol. 26, pp. 1205–17.
[43] Lim C. X., Hoh H. Y., Ang P. K., Loh K. P. "Direct voltammetric detection of DNA and pH sensing on epitaxial graphene: an insight into the role of oxygenated defects." *Anal. Chem.* vol. 82, pp. 7387–93.
[44] Pumera M., Sasaki T., Iwai H. "Relationship between carbon nanotube structure and electrochemical behavior: heterogeneous electron transfer at electrochemically activated carbon nanotubes." *Chem. Asian J.,* 2008, vol. 3, pp. 2046–55.
[45] Ambrosi A., Pumera M. "Stacked graphene nanofibers for electrochemical oxidation of DNA bases." *Phys. Chem. Chem. Phys.,* 2010, vol. 12, pp. 8943–47.
[46] Jia Y., Yin X.-B., Zhang J., Zhou S., Song M., Xing K.-L. "Graphene oxide modified light addressable potentiometric sensor and its application for ssDNA monitoring." *Analyst*, vol. 137, pp. 5866–73.

Chapter 23

Sensing of nucleic acids and cancer cells using nanostructure-SPR integrated with microfluidic chip

Ji-Yen Cheng[1] *and Mansoureh Z. Mousavi*[1]

23.1 Introduction

The development of diagnostic methods that are sensitive, specific, rapid, robust and affordable is a priority for improving healthcare. According to World Health Organization (WHO), diagnostic devices for point-of-care (POC) testing are identified to be sensitive and specific to biological agents, user friendly, inexpensive and able to provide a rapid response to small sample volumes [1]. Several technologies are being used to detect biomarkers, including enzyme-linked immunosorbent assay (ELISA) for protein biomarkers and polymerase chain reaction (PCR) for nucleic acids. However, ELISA and PCR are both label-based and multistep methods that usually require significant sample preparation and experienced personnel to perform the test [2, 3]. Label-free techniques have attracted major interest for clinical analysis. There are different classes of label-free biosensors, but all are based upon the measurement of an inherent molecular property such as refractive index or mass [4].

Plasmonics is an enabling optical technology with applications in disease monitoring, diagnostics and imaging. Nanostructure transmission SPR, in particular, is an emerging technique with tremendous potential for clinical operation and development of POC testing. SPR sensors based on nanostructures enable chip-scale integration and allow high-throughput and label-free detections of biomarkers. Nanostructure SPR substrates can be fabricated with inexpensive and high-yield techniques and are therefore suitable candidates for low cost mass production and integration of disposable sensor cartridges. Integrating microfluidic chip with plasmonic sensors allows for the creation of a portable, stable and robust Lab-On-Chip system.

In this chapter we will discuss some of the most promising label-free technologies with significant impact on the field of biosensing and diagnostics, namely, conventional surface plasmon resonance (SPR), localized surface plasmon

[1]Research Center for Applied Sciences, Academia Sinica, Taiwan

resonance (LSPR) and nanostructure SPR arrays. Development of SPR biosensing technology is focused on improving sensitivity, miniaturizing the sensor system, tuning the operation range and high throughput detection [5]. We will discuss plasmonic-based biosensors and their integration with microfluidic chip. The application of SPR sensing platforms integrated with microfluidic chips for detection of nucleic acid and cells will be described in detail. Lastly, we will describe the current state of the art of plasmonic biosensors and give a perspective on the future of this technology for POC diagnostics.

23.2 Conventional SPR

SPR technology exploits propagating surface plasma waves (SPWs) excited on a metal plane. Surface plasmons are charge-density oscillations of electromagnetic excitations at the interface between two media with dielectric constants of opposite sign. Figure 23.1(a) illustrates how the electromagnetic wave decays evanescently into both media in the direction perpendicular to the interface. The field vectors reach their maxima at the boundary. These evanescent fields are asymmetrically distributed (larger decay in metal and small decay in the dielectric) [5]. The plasmon modes penetrate only few hundred nanometers into the dielectric medium, allowing subwavelength sensing. To excite surface plasmons on a metal-dielectric interface, the momentum and energy of incident photon and the plasmon modes must match. Attenuated total reflection (ATR) on a glass prism to excite SPR on a thin gold film is commonly used for sensing. ATR biosensors are sensitive to surface or environmental changes and are suitable for monitoring biological interactions. Monitoring the excitation resonance angle changes is used to detect and quantify the target molecule. However, there are limitations to using ATR as a biosensor platform. The ATR setup is bulky, expensive and requires a large amount of sample. Due to the optical configuration, ATR is rather difficult to be used for high-throughput and chip based detections [6, 7]. Despite these limitations, commercial systems based on ATR are already available. One of the first miniaturized and integrated SPR sensors was Spreeta by Texas Instruments. Spreeta SPR sensing chip contains an LED light source, a gold SPR surface, a reflecting mirror that directs the reflected light to a photodiode array and a temperature sensor. Application of Spreeta includes detection of analytes that range in size from small organics to analytes as large as whole cells [8]. Low sensitivity remains a major challenge of utilizing conventional SPR for clinical applications and as thus far restricted the deployment of such systems.

23.3 Localized surface plasmon resonance (LSPR)

LSPR technology is based on electromagnetic field enhancement at the position in close proximity to metallic nanoparticles. When light is incident on nanoparticles, collective electronic modes are excited so that the conduction band electrons oscillate and the nanoparticles scatter light in a specific wavelength range [9, 10].

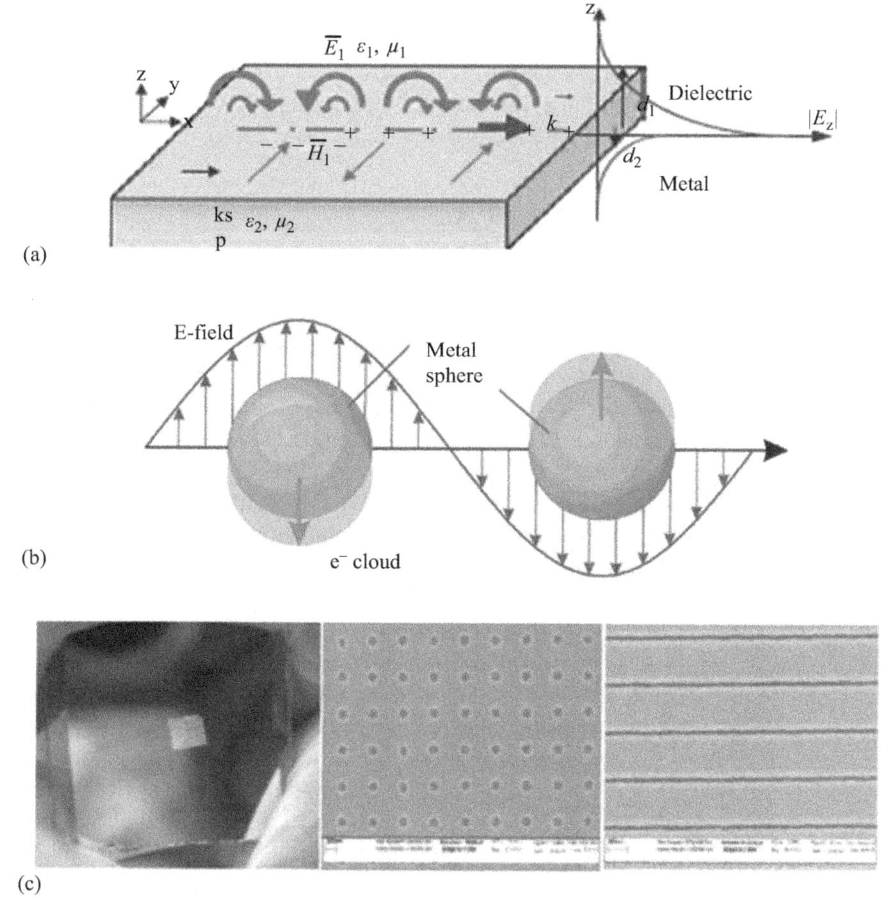

Figure 23.1 *(a) The schematic illustration of charge density oscillations at a metal–dielectric interface in x direction. The electromagnetic fields exponential decay from the interface into dielectric (d_1) and metal (d_2) shown on the right.* ***(b)*** *Schematic of plasmon oscillation illustrating the displacement of the conduction electron charge cloud.* ***(c)*** *(Left): The optical image of a 10 × 10 microarray on a glass slide. Each element in the array (dark square in the center of the chip) was consisted of a 600 nm-period gold nanoslit array. The area was 150 μm in square. (Middle): The SEM image of a 600 nm-period gold nanohole array. (Right): The SEM image of a 600 nm-period gold nanoslit array. Figure 23.1(a) and (c): Figures and captions adapted from Reference 5 with kind permission from Springer Science and Business Media. Figure 23.1(b) reprinted (adapted) with permission from Reference 9; Copyright (2003) American Chemical Society*

A scheme of plasmon oscillations is shown in Figure 23.1(b) [9]. In biosensing applications, the attachment of a target biomolecule to the nanoparticles results in a local refractive index change, which in turn produces a red or blue shift in the extinction peak wavelength [11, 12]. Coupled with compact spectrometers, LSPR technology is a suitable candidate for portable diagnostic applications.

23.4 Nanostructure array SPR

Gold nanostructures arrays with extraordinary optical transmission have been employed for biosensing applications [13–18]. Various nanostructure plasmonic arrays including nanoholes, nanodisk, nanoposts, nanotubes and nanopillars [19–28] have been reported as refractive-index-based sensors. Surface plasmon in nanostructure is excited directly by subwavelength metallic apertures. In periodic nanostructures, an extraordinary optical transmission (EOT) occurs when the surface plasmon wavelength meets the Bragg condition [18]. The resulting resonance modes are affected by the periodicity, size, and shape of nanostructure in the array [5, 29, 30]. Figure 23.1(c) shows SEM images of nanohole and nanoslit array fabricated by Lee *et al.* [5, 31]. Using the peak EOT wavelength as signal, high density sensing arrays have been reported [16, 17]. Array-based nanoplasmonic detection can be used for high-throughput biosensing applications and are also suitable for multiplexed detection. One type of nanostructure plasmonic array is nanohole arrays, which have been used as sensing platform for single and multiple detections. Nanohole array based sensors have been operated in two fluidic operation modalities; flow-over sensing mode and flow-through sensing mode [19]. In flow-over sensing mode the sample solution containing the analyte flows on top of the nanohole arrays. De Leebeeck *et al.* developed integrated nanohole arrays with a microfluidic chip sensing elements capable of chemical sensing and biomolecule adsorption monitoring for spatial/temporal measurements [16]. The design of the microfluidic chip integrated with nanohole array, SEM images of the nanohole array and schematic of the optical setup are shown in Figure 23.2(a) and (b). Multiple peaks in the transmission spectrum are observed using a broadband input. The periodicity of the nanohole determines the wavelength of SPRs. During the sensor operation, as shown in Figure 23.2(c) and (d), the spectrum is red-shifted in response to the increase of the refractive index of the solution.

Nanohole array based sensors operated in flow-through sensing mode combine the characteristics of nanohole arrays for both fluidic transport and plasmonic sensing. Ferreira *et al.* in 2009 explained the role of the in-hole gold surface in the plasmonic response [32]. The results suggested that the in-hole surface plays a dominant role in the peak shift employed in sensing. Eftekhari *et al.* reported a flow-through nanohole array based sensing platform which consisted of arrays of through nanoholes integrated into a microfluidic system [33]. This flow-through nanohole array sensor combines the benefits of nanofluidics and nanoplasmonics. Nanohole arrays served as fluidic element to parallelize the resistance and thus fluid handling and as optical elements to detect the adsorption of a monolayer and

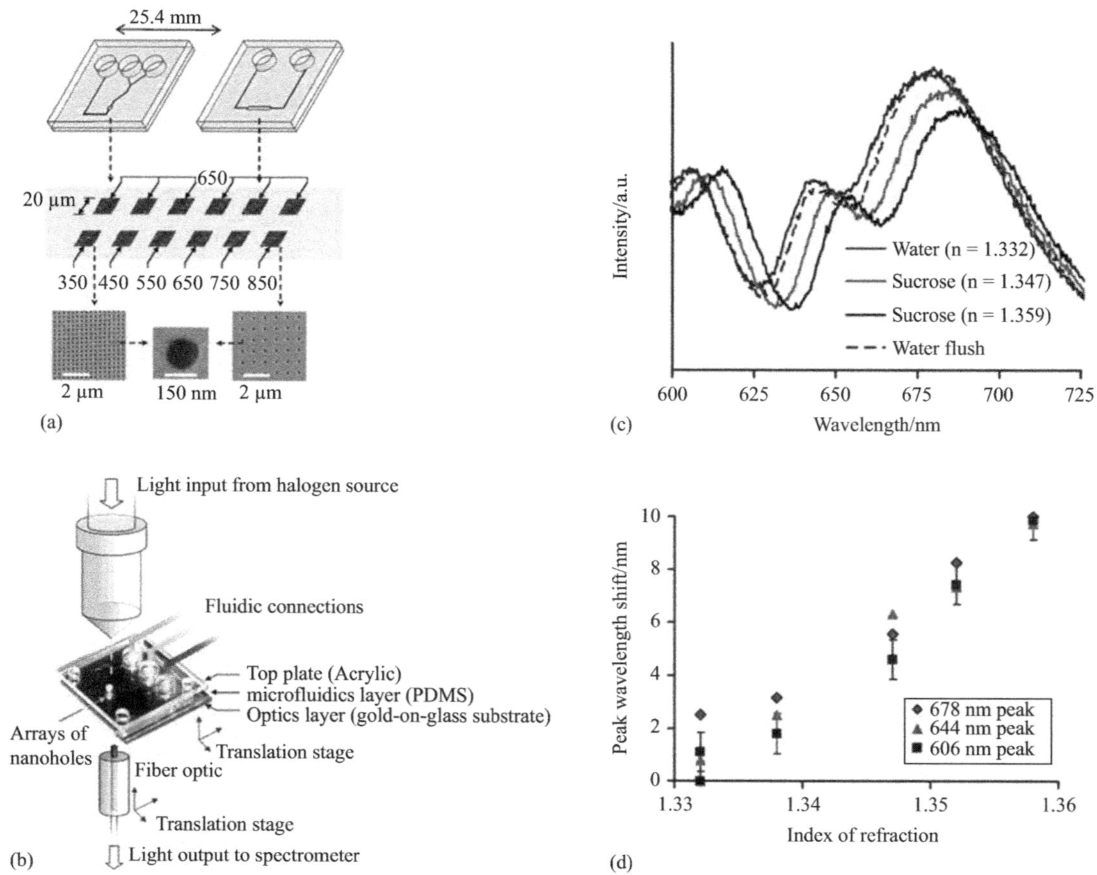

Figure 23.2 *(a) Schematic and images of the microfluidic chip with embedded nanohole arrays and SEM images of the nanoholes.* ***(b)*** *Optical setup and assembled microfluidic chip-integrated sensor.* ***(c)*** *Transmission spectra.* ***(d)*** *The red shift in peak wavelength as a function of refractive index. Reprinted (adapted) with permission from Reference 16; Copyright (2007) American Chemical Society*

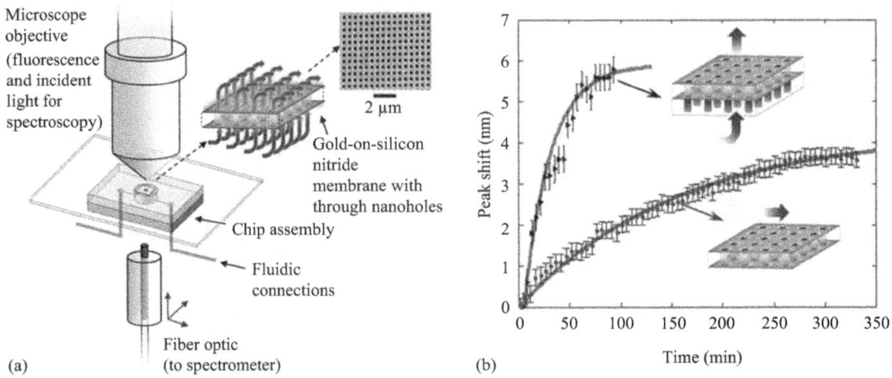

Figure 23.3 (a) Schematic of the optical and fluidic setup of flow-through nanohole array sensor (b) comparison of response obtained with flow-over and flow-through formats. Reprinted (adapted) with permission from Reference 33; Copyright (2009) American Chemical Society

multilayer assembly of biomolecules for sensing applications. Schematic of the experimental setup is demonstrated in Figure 23.3(a). The flow-through approach showed a 6-fold improvement in response time when compared to the established flow-over methodology. The comparison of responses of flow-through and flow over approaches are shown in Figure 23.3(b).

Techniques that are used for large-scale fabrication of arrays include top-down processes such as focused ion beam milling (FIB) and e-beam lithography [34]. These techniques require expensive fabrication methods that are not suitable for production of low-cost devices at high throughput. Developing low-cost fabrication techniques is one of the main issues that need to be addressed. Using nanoimprinting lithography, Lee *et al.* have developed a low-cost method to fabricate large-area uniform nanoslit arrays on a polymer substrate for sensitive detection. The development of nanoslit array platform has been described in Lee's publication [35]. Briefly, the gold nanoslits were fabricated on a polymer film using thermal-annealing-assisted template-stripping method. The template consists of nanogrooves on a silicon substrate that is fabricated using electron beam lithography and reactive ion etching method. The gold film is coated on the patterned silicon template. The template and polymer film are then pressed and heated to imprint the nano-structure pattern on the film. The schematic of fabrication process and SEM image of nanoslit chip are shown in Figure 23.4(a) and (b), respectively.

In nanostructure SPR, there exist cavity and SPR modes, which are resonances inside the nanoaperture and on the surface, respectively (Figure 23.4(c)). The Fano-resonance emerges from the coupling of the two modes [5, 36]. The constructive and destructive interferences of gap plasmon, i.e. cavity mode in the slits, and SPR mode result in the asymmetric Fano-resonance as shown in Figure 23.4(d). The SPR resonance mode and wavelength sensitivities of three kinds of nanostructures

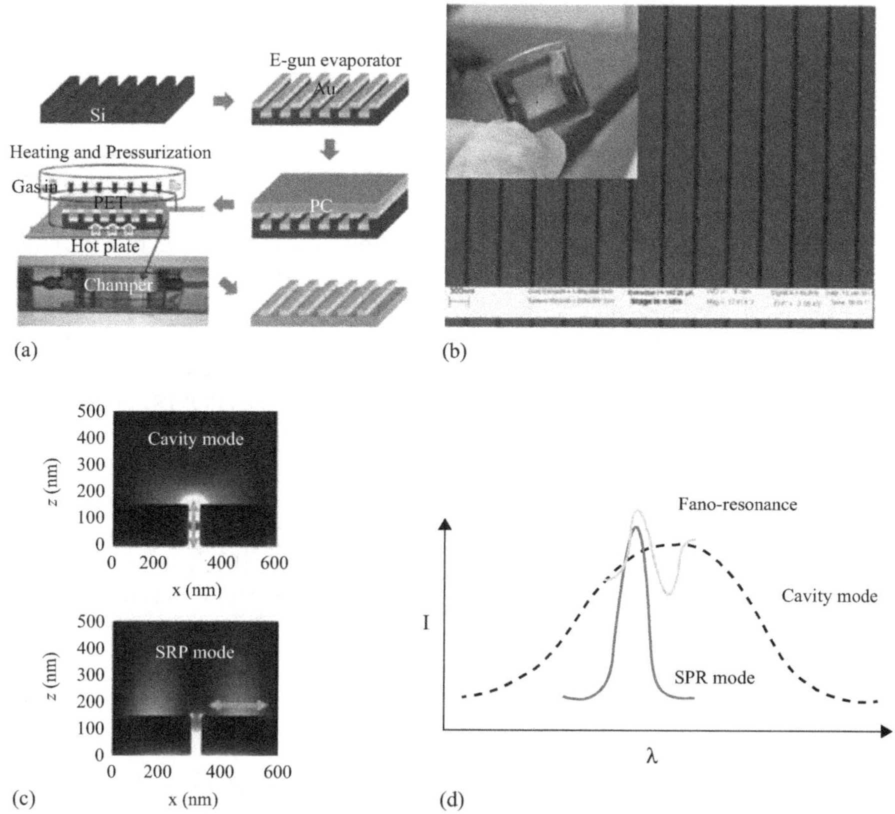

Figure 23.4 (a) Nanoimprinting lithography for fabrication of nanoslit array platform. (b) SEM and optical images of the nanoslits. (c) There are cavity mode and SPR mode which are inside the aperture and along the surface, respectively. (d) The schematic depiction of Fano-resonance is resulting from the coupling of cavity and SPR modes. Figure 23.4(a) and (b): Reprinted (adapted) with permission from Reference 35; Copyright (2012) American Chemical Society. Figure 23.4(c) and (d): Figure and caption adapted from Reference 5 with kind permission from Springer Science and Business Media

(nanoslits, nanoholes, and concentric circles) with various aperture sizes were studied and compared by Lee [30]. Increasing the period, decreasing dimension of the nano-apertures, optimizing the Fano resonance to reduce the resonance bandwidth and make a sharp slope, using the spectral integration analysis method to reduce the noise and enhance the S/N ratio and using thermally annealing nanoimprint method to fabricate smooth gold film are several ways mentioned by Lee to improve the detection resolution in gold nanostructures [5].

23.5 Integration of SPR sensors with microfluidic chip

Microfluidics provides a range of capabilities that are critically useful in biology, clinical analysis and sensing such as precise fluid manipulation, sample enrichment and multiplexing. Moreover, these tasks can be performed with a high degree of automation, enhanced efficiency, reduced requirements of sample and reagents and improved sensitivity in portable, compact and robust devices. Integrating microfluidics with plasmonic sensors allows for the creation of a portable, stable and robust Lab-On-Chip system for label-free detection [37–44]. Huang *et al.* demonstrated the integration of LSPR-based biosensing with microfluidic technologies, resulting in a portable biosensor device [45]. The schematic and image of LSPR-base microfluidic sensor developed by Huang is shown in Figure 23.5(a). Luo *et al.* fabricated a polydimethylsiloxane (PDMS) microfluidic device containing an array of gold spots to carry out immunoreactions with conventional SPR detection. SPR imaging was used to monitor the antibody–antigen recognition and binding events [46]. The schematic diagram of the microfluidic device is shown in Figure 23.5(b). The result showed that the combined microfluidic device and SPR imaging provide sensitive and efficient immunoassay and offers several advantages. The reaction time and sample consumption was reduced.

23.6 SPR sensors for multiplexing

Medical decision based on single biomarkers often results in a high possibility of false positives and false negatives. The combination of multiple biomarkers improves accuracy of disease diagnosis [47–49]. This demonstrates the importance of developing sensitive multiplexing assay of biomarkers to improve reliability of diagnosis. Array-based nanostructure plasmonic sensors can be used for high-throughput biosensing applications. The integration with microfluidic chips especially allows the development of high-throughput sensors. Bottazzi *et al.* have developed an imaging biosensing device (iNPx) which integrates the fluidics, the electronics, and the computing and data analysis unit resulting in a compact, standalone, and fully portable device. The iNPx system enables the real-time multiplexed detection of several analytes [50]. The nanoslits array fabricated by Lee's group is comparable with commercial DNA microarrays and can be used for the detection of a panel of biomarkers for better disease diagnosis [31]. A metallic nanohole-based SPR technology developed by Si Hoon Lee [51] combined the nanostructure SPR with a 50-channel microfluidic chip. This chip was used for high throughput full-spectral imaging and accurate quantification of receptor–ligand binding kinetics. Template stripping was used to fabricate large-area nanohole arrays having uniform optical properties to perform high-throughput SPR imaging spectroscopy of multiple parallel channels. The nanohole array substrate is attached to a PDMS microfluidic chip, which divided the nanohole array into 50 individual channels. Optical transmission or reflection spectra from all 50 channels were

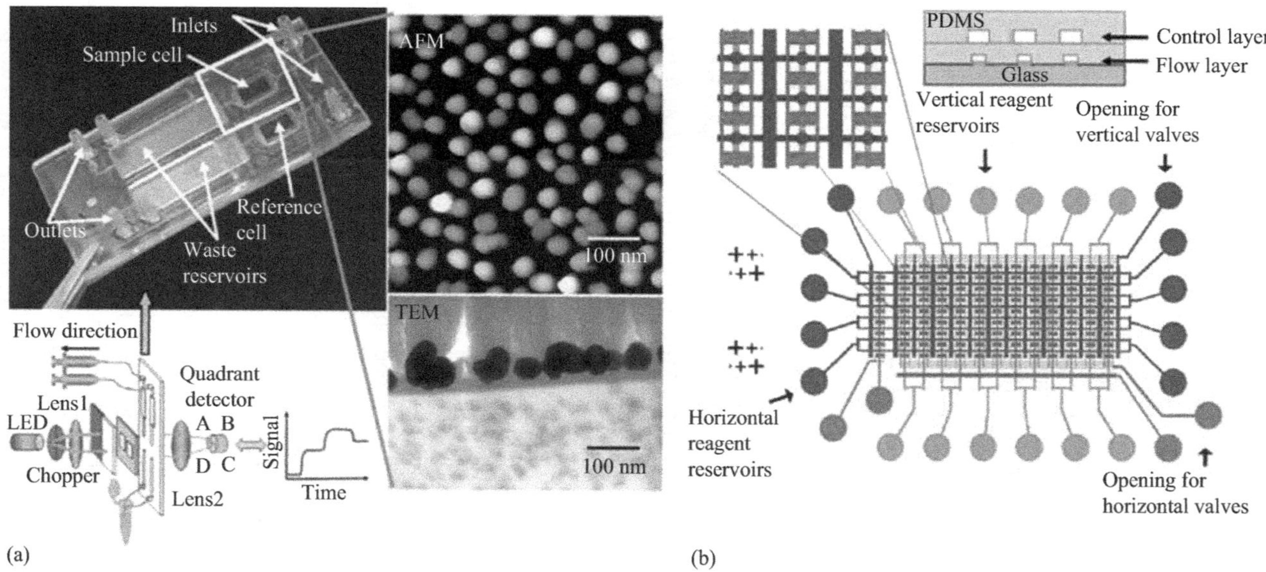

Figure 23.5 *(a) Schematic the transmission plasmon biosensing (TPB) readout platform and photograph of the microfluidic integrated LSPR biosensor. The inset shows the AFM and TEM images of the gold nanoparticle film with nanoparticle diameter = 43 nm. Scale bar = 100 nm, (b) microfluidic chip-integrated LSPR-imaging device. Figure 23.5(a): Figure and caption adapted from Reference 45 with kind permission from Springer Science and Business Media. Figure 23.5(b): Reproduced (adapted) from Reference 46 with permission of Royal Society of Chemistry*

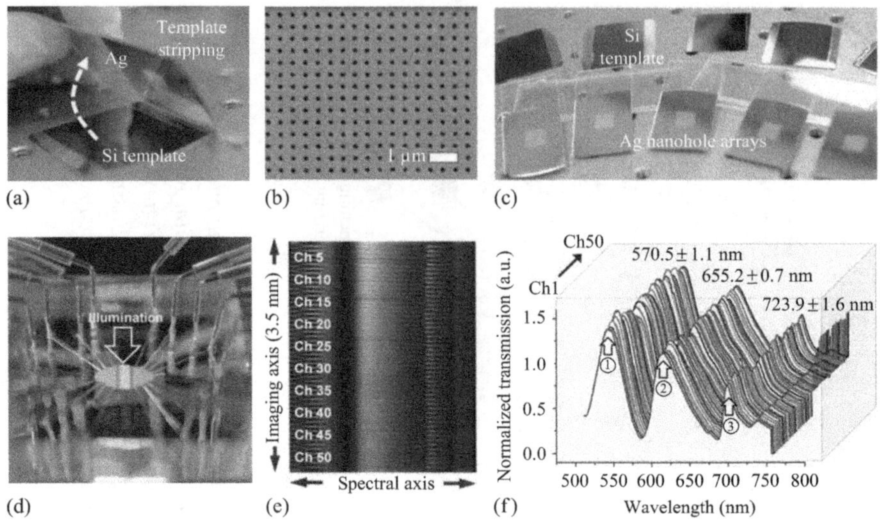

Figure 23.6 (a) Template stripping for fabrication of nanohole array. (b) SEM image of nanohole array. (c) Photograph of nanohole array templates. (d) Photograph of the microfluidic chip. (e) Full spectral from 50 parallel channels. (f) The transmission spectra from each channel. Reproduced (adapted) from Reference 51 with permission of Royal Society of Chemistry

monitored simultaneously (Figure 23.6). To demonstrate the application of multi-channel SPR spectral imaging, the binding kinetics of cholera toxin b (CTX-b) to ganglioside (GM1) receptors were measured [51]. For POC application, combination of nanostructure array SPR with microfluidic chips enables high-throughput sensing. Multiple arrays can be fabricated and by immobilizing different recognition molecule, each array can be used to probe specific target molecule and can be interrogated separately.

23.7 SPR-based biosensors

SPR biosensing has been used in a large range of applications, including detection of cells, nucleic acids, proteins, drugs, bacteria, viruses and monitoring of biomolecular interactions. One important potential clinical application of SPR is the diagnosis of early stage cancer. From the perspective of non-invasive diagnosis, detection of circulating biomarkers is an especially interesting application of SPR-based detection technology. The SPR sensing platforms could meet the main POC test requirements, including high sensitivity, high specificity, multiplexing, simplicity and low cost. Here, we focus on the application of SPR for detection of nucleic acids and cells.

23.7.1 SPR-based biosensors for detection of nucleic acids

The SPR-based sensors for nucleic acids can be classified into two categories of assay for the detection of chromosome anomalies (e.g., point mutations) and assay for the detection of genetic material as biomarkers (e.g. mRNAs, microRNAs).

Given that the SPR assay is based on a change in the refractive index near the sensor surface in response to a binding event, the sensitivity of detection can be improved by conjugating nanoparticles through mass and refractive index enhancement. Sandwich assays using proteins or enzymes that bind to the captured target or the target-probe complex to enhance the refractive index change have been used to improve the detection sensitivity [52–57].

23.7.1.1 Detection of DNA

SPR has been used for detection of point mutation and single nucleotide polymorphisms (SNPs) [57–59]. Jiang *et al.* reported a DNA-SPR-based sensing using portable instrumentation (Texas Instruments Spreeta) for detection of point mutation. The sensor was applied to PCR-amplified samples, DNA extracted from both normal and mutated, carrying the mutation at codon 248 of the TP53 cell lines. The biosensor distinguished between sequences differing by only one base in the SNP position using synthetic oligonucleotides or real samples [58]. Nanoparticle enhanced-SPR imaging for detection of single nucleotide polymorphisms in genomic DNA was developed by Li *et al.* [57]. The method utilize sequence-specific surface reactions of the enzyme *Taq* DNA ligase. The hybridization adsorption of complementary oligonucleotides attached to gold nanoparticles with the ligation products on the DNA microarray elements was detected using surface plasmon Resonance imaging (SPRI). The gold nanoparticles were shown to increase the sensitivity of the SPRI. The detection limit of the nanoparticle-enhanced SPRI single-base-pair identification was 1 pM, which is sufficient for the analysis of concentrated genomic DNA samples. The method was applied for the SNP genotyping of PCR products from human genomic DNA samples. Human genomic DNA samples were screened for a point mutation in the *BRCA*1 gene, which is linked with breast cancer. The scheme of the method is depicted in Figure 23.7(a). A sandwich-like assay for the detection of SNP in a 20 mer TP53 synthetic analogue with a four-channel SPR biosensor was developed by Sipova *et al.* The target DNA is recognized by the probe coupled with streptavidin oligonucleotide (SON) complexes ex situ, and when the mixture is introduced to the sensor, another part of the target DNA is recognized by the second probe immobilized on the sensor surface (Figure 23.7(b)). SON complexes are employed for enhancing the SPR sensor. Sensitivity down to 40 pM and a good specificity were achieved [59].

23.7.1.2 Detection of RNA

Several families of nucleic acid biomarkers (e.g. mRNA and miRNA) have been identified as diagnostic and prognostic biomarkers. Presence of nucleic acid biomarkers in human fluids (e.g. plasma, serum, urine) has been reported by various

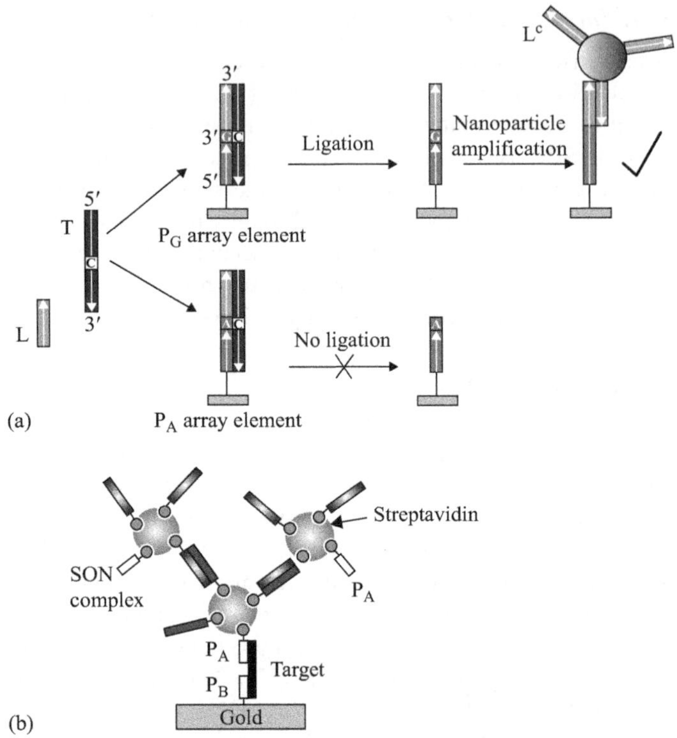

Figure 23.7 *(a) Schematic of the SNP genotyping method based on a combination of surface ligation chemistry and nanoparticle enhanced SPRI. The ligation only occurs if the duplex is perfectly complementary. (b) Assay based on streptavidin–oligonucleotide (SON) complexes: capture of SON–target complex by the DNA probes immobilized on the sensor surface. Figure 23.7(a): Reprinted (adapted) with permission from Reference 57; Copyright (2006) American Chemical Society. Figure 23.7(b): Figure and caption adapted from Reference 59 with kind permission from Springer Science and Business Media*

research groups [49]. Detection of nucleic acid biomarkers has many advantages over detecting protein biomarkers. Although immunoassays based on antibodies have been among the main diagnostic tools for clinical applications [60], they have several limitations. Antibodies are sensitive to temperature; many of commercially available antibodies are therefore unstable. The batch-related differences and varying affinity is another limitation of their usage as probes in biosensors [61]. In addition, proteins and antibodies are chemically and structurally complex, which makes them their interactions with the biosensor substrate unpredictable [62]. SPR-based sensors have been applied to detect nucleic acid biomarkers. Magnetic nanoparticle enhanced-nanostructure SPR for the detection of hnRNPB1 mRNA was reported by Mousavi *et al.* [63]. The approach for detection includes double

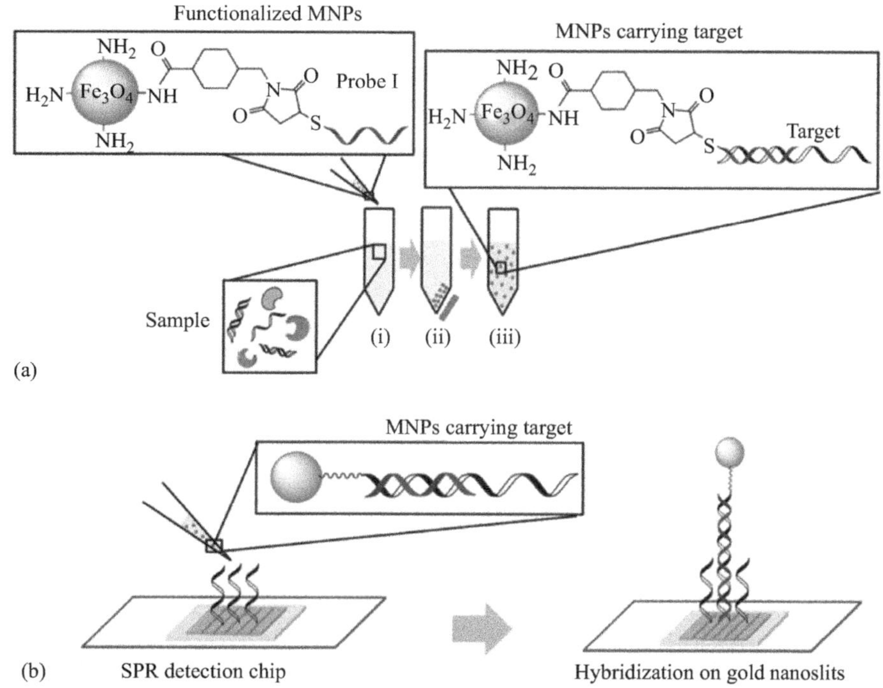

Figure 23.8 A schematic of the two-step method to detect the nucleic acid target. (a) First step includes capturing the target oligonucleotide on the magnetic nanoparticles (b) Second step: hybridizing the target molecule isolated on the MNPs with probe II on the gold nanoslits. Reproduced (adapted) from Reference 63; with permission of Royal Society of Chemistry

hybridization at two specific locations in two steps. First, the target mRNA is captured with MNPs, and second, MNPs carrying the target mRNA are introduced to the SPR chip for second hybridization on the gold nanoslits. MNPs were applied for two purposes; first to isolate the target molecule from the sample to prevent non-specific binding and second to enhance the SPR response. The schematic of method is shown in Figure 23.8. The method allows detection as low as 30 fM of the target mRNA without amplification and labeling.

Another family of nucleic acid biomarkers is micro-ribonucleic acids (miRNA), which have been used as diagnosis and prognosis biomarkers [64–66]. Weber *et al.* have shown the presence of miRNA in human fluids such as plasma, saliva, tears and urine and they have demonstrated the potential of theses extra-cellular miRNAs in human fluids as biomarker for detection of physiological conditions [67]. Given their high stability in body fluids, miRNAs are potential biomarkers for cancer diagnosis [68]. Sipova *et al.* developed a portable nucleic acid sensor based on a special diffraction grating called a surface plasmon coupler

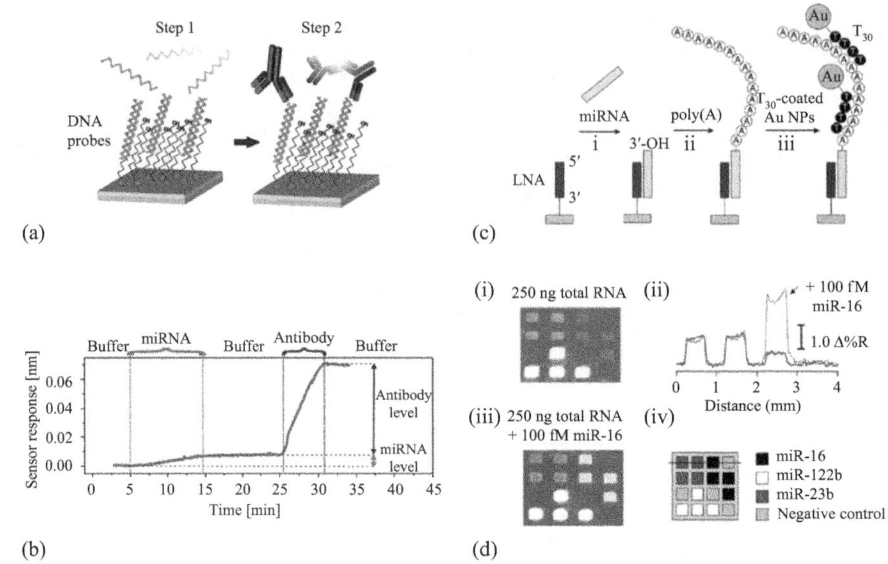

Figure 23.9 (a) Schematic illustrating the antibody-based assay for detection of miRNA. (b) temporal sensor response to the miRNA and antibody, (c) Schematic demonstrating the detection of microRNAs using a combination of surface polyadenylation chemistry and nanoparticle amplified SPRI detection (d) SPR difference image. Figure 23.9(a) and (b): reprinted (adapted) with permission from Reference 69; Copyright (2010) American Chemical Society. Figure 23.9(c) and (d): reprinted (adapted) with permission from Reference 72; Copyright (2006) American Chemical Society

and disperser (SPRCD) to detect miR-122 extracted from mouse liver tissue. The surface of the grating is functionalized with thiol-modified oligonucleotides to capture target miRNA from the sample. A specific antibody that recognizes DNA*RNA hybrids is introduced to bind to the DNA*RNA complex and enhances the response. Detection down to 2 pM was obtained. Schematic representation of the antibody-based assay for detection of miRNA is shown in Figure 23.9(a) and (b) [69]. A portable six channel SPR sensor was employed. The sensor system (SPRCD) was introduced in their previous work. The SPRCD sensor consists of a miniature cartridge integrating the diffraction grating and microfluidics which supports independent sensing channels [70]. Zhang *et al.* described a method using SPR to detect miR-122 in RNA extracted from human cancer cells. The senor system was a conventional SPR device Biacore X^{TM} analytical system. The target miRNA was captured by complementary DNA probe immobilized on the sensor surface and then an oligonucleotide probe linked to streptavidin was employed to bind with the target. The use of the streptavidin-oligonucleotide complex results in an ~5-fold increase in signal and therefore improving the detection sensitivity by a factor of ~24. With the introduction of streptavidin amplification, as low as 17 pM miRNA was detected [71]. Fang *et al.* introduced a method for the detection of miRNA, extracted from mouse liver tissue, based on thiol-modified LNA microarray immobilized on the gold chip surface (SPR imager, GWC Technologies). Schematic of the detection of microRNAs using a combination of surface polyadenylation chemistry and nanoparticle amplified SPRI detection is shown in Figure 23.9(c). SPRi transduction was enhanced with poly-(A) enzyme chemistry and T_{30}-coated Au nanoparticles [72]. The enzymatically amplified SPRI methodology was used to quantitatively measure miRNAs in total RNA samples down to femtomolar concentrations. The method was employed to simultaneously detect miR-16, miR-122b and miR-23b in a total RNA sample extracted from mouse liver tissue. Figure 23.9(d) shows SPR difference images obtained after the amplification of the adsorption of NPs onto a four-component array. The high sensitivity of the detection is due to the combination of surface enzyme chemistry and DNA-coated nanoparticles.

Despite the growing application of SPR for nucleic acid biomarkers, SPR-based sensor for detection of miRNAs in complex samples for clinical analysis are rather limited. Mousavi *et al.* demonstrated an SPR-based method that employs a capped gold nanoslit SPR sensing integrated in a microfluidic chip for the detection of a urinary miRNA biomarker [73]. The method utilizes magnetic nanoparticles (MNPs) for the isolation of target molecules and signal enhancement in conjunction with capped gold nanoslit transmission SPR. The capability of the method to detect urinary biomarker miRNA-16-5p in clinical sample was evaluated and the result was compared with quantitative PCR (qPCR). Without amplification and labeling, the method allows detection of miRNA biomarker in urine of patients with acute kidney injury (AKI). The approach includes double hybridization in two steps. As shown in Figure 23.10, in the first step, functionalized iron oxide MNPs functionalized with the complementary probe captures the target miRNA from the urine sample. In the second step the captured target molecule on the MNPs hybridize with the second complementary probe immobilized on the sensor surface. The gold nanoslit sensing chip was integrated with a novel microfluidic chip to provide an efficient way to capture the target molecules with minimal non-specific binding in a complex sample matrix such as urine. High specificity of the method was confirmed by applying the method to a sample containing high concentration of one-mismatch sequence. The SPR response of mismatched sequence was clearly distinguishable from the fully matched complementary target. The high specificity of the method is the result of pre-isolation of the target molecule, double hybridization and optimized flow of the sample to minimize the non-specific binding of non-target molecules. A novel fluidic chip, funnel chip, was designed and fabricated to integrate with the capped gold nanoslit film for the detection of rare miRNA biomarker in the urine sample. A nickel-coated ferritic iron needle attached to a cylindrical neodymium magnet was placed beneath the nanoslit to bring the MNPs carrying the target to the surface to bind with the probe immobilized on the gold nanoslits. This design provides an efficient way to capture target molecules with minimal non-specific binding.

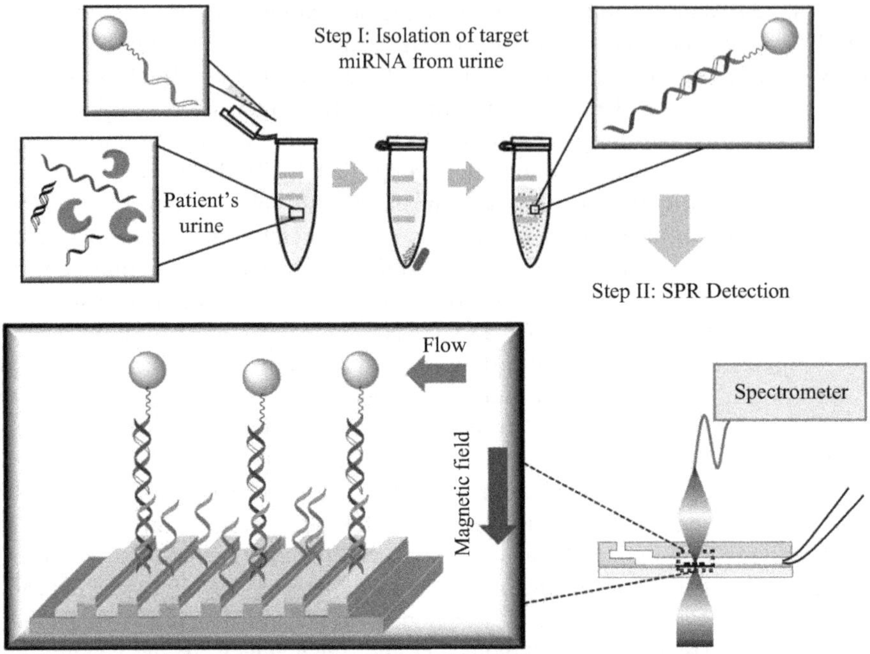

Figure 23.10 A schematic of the double hybridization method to detect the target miRNA in clinical urine sample. Reproduced (adapted) from Reference 73 with permission of Royal Society of Chemistry

As it was shown in Mousavi's work, designing a fluidic chip provides an efficient way to capture target molecules with minimal non-specific binding of non-target molecules due to shear forces produced by the fluid flow. Another approach to minimize the interference of complex clinical sample involves surface chemistry and surface functionalization techniques. The effect of the length and the terminating group of blocking thiols on the sensitivity and specificity of a DNA detection has been studied by Thipmanee *et al.* [74]. Polymeric blocking agents (e.g. Polyethylene glycol) also have been used to minimize the nonspecific interactions on the surface sensor. Lakshmipriya *et al.* showed that by using pentaethylenehexamine-terminated PEG (N6-PEG) on GNPs the sensitivity of detection was increased by 1000 times and completely prevents non-specific binding on the sensor surface [75]. Surface chemistry has a profound effect on the sensitivity of detection. Surface functionalization is a critical aspect of sensor development especially for detection of target biomolecules in complex clinical samples.

23.7.2 SPR-based biosensors for detection of cancer cells

Detection of rare cells is an important technology with a wide range of applications in clinical diagnosis and stem cell research [76–78]. To isolate the rare cells from biological samples, various methods have been developed. These techniques take

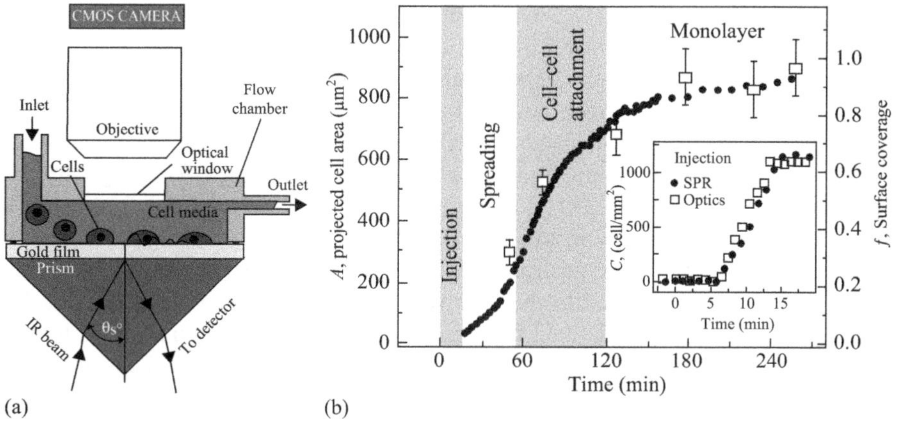

Figure 23.11 *(a) Infrared surface SPR-based technique for real time monitoring of cell–cell and cell–substrate interactions (b) Time dependence of the projected cell area estimated from the SPR shift. Reprinted from Reference 88*

advantage of different properties of cancer cells as compared to blood cells, such as expression of surface antigens, size and stiffness of cancer cells [79–87]. Among several techniques that are used for identification of captured cells, immunostaining of the isolated cancer cells and enumeration of labeled cells using a fluorescence microscope is one of the common methods [81, 82, 84]. Label-free conductivity measurement is another technique for detecting the captured cells [80, 87]. SPR as a label-free technology for detection of cells can be used to observe the kinetic of the cell binding in real time. Yashunsky *et al.* used an infrared surface SPR-based technique for real time monitoring of epithelial cell–cell and cell–substrate interactions (Figure 23.11). This study demonstrated the ability of FTIR-SPR to resolve different phases of cell–cell and cell–substrate adhesion [88]. Infrared SPR also has been used to monitor the submicron variations in cell layer morphology in real-time. The infrared SPR has relatively large sampling depth (several microns) and is sensitive to cell substrate region as well as more distant parts of the cell body. IR-SPR can provide information about the structure of adherent cells [89]. Hiragun *et al.* have demonstrated that cancer cell lines show various patterns of SPR signal (change in angle of resonance), which are different from pattern of SPR signal of normal cells. Therefore, by detecting SPR signal patterns and without any immunological labeling, the SPR biosensor may be used for diagnosis applications [90]. Yuhki *et al.* showed that PAM212 mouse keratinocytes showed a large SPR response when EGF-stimulated. Their results suggest that SPR response reflect intracellular events rather than changes in the size of the area to which cells adhere [91]. Tanaka *et al.* studied the relationship between the change of angle of SPR resonance and the antigen-induced signaling events in RBL-2H3 mast cells. The result of their study suggests that EGF induces the SPR signals via the phosphorylation of EGFR [92]. Different pattern of SPR signal induced by EGF may indicate a disorder in intracellular signal transductions of cancer cells [93]. An LSPR technique to detect oral epithelial cancer cells was reported by El-Sayed *et al.* The LSPR spectra from colloidal gold nanoparticles conjugated to monoclonal anti epidermal growth factor receptor (anti-EGFR) antibodies after incubation in cell cultures of nonmalignant cell line (HaCaT) and two malignant oral epithelial cell lines ((HOC 313 clone 8 and HSC 3) were measured. The specific and homogeneous binding of anti-EGFR antibody conjugated nanoparticles was found to give a sharper SPR absorption band with a red shifted maximum compared to that observed when added to the nonmalignant cells. These results suggest that SPR scattering imaging generated from antibody conjugated gold nanoparticles can be useful in molecular biosensor techniques for the diagnostic applications. SPR has been also used to study viability of cells [94]. Wu *et al.* have demonstrated label-free monitoring of cell viability by gold nanoslits-based Fano resonance biosensors (Figure 23.12). Gold nanoslits-based Fano resonance biosensors was used for label-free monitoring of adhesion cells viability [95].

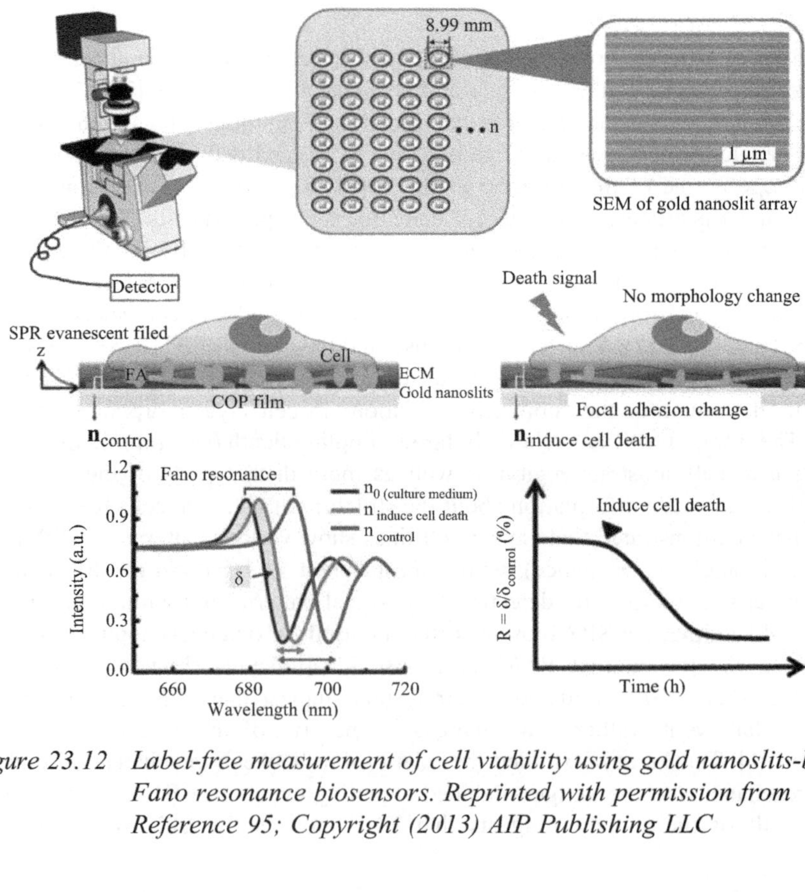

Figure 23.12 Label-free measurement of cell viability using gold nanoslits-based Fano resonance biosensors. Reprinted with permission from Reference 95; Copyright (2013) AIP Publishing LLC

Microfluidic devices for cell capturing provide efficient capturing of target cells with minimal non-specific binding owing to shear force produced by fluid flow. Mousavi *et al.* have developed a microfluidic chip integrated with gold nanoslit SPR platform for efficient immunomagnetic capturing and detection of rare cells in human blood [96]. The target cells first are captured by the first specific antibody on the magnetic nanoparticles, then introduced into a microfluidic chip integrated with a magnet. The gold nanoslit as sensing platform is embedded in the microfluidic chip. Cells captured on the magnetic nanoparticles bind with the second specific antibody immobilized on the surface of the gold nanoslit. The cell binding on the gold nanoslit was monitored by the wavelength shift of the SPR spectrum generated by the gold nanoslits. Short detection depth of SPR (400 nm) provides a sensitive method with minimum interference of non-targets in the biological samples. Their results highlight several advantages of double capturing method combined with SPR detection over some of the available technologies for rare cells detection. The scheme offers a simple way to capture and detect cancer cells in one chip. The double capturing results in a highly specific isolation of the target cells and minimizes the non-specific binding of non-target cells. The microfluidic chip with magnet was designed to minimize the non-specific binding of blood cells. The high velocity of the flow prevents the non-specific binding of non-target cells while the magnetic force from the integrated magnet brings down the MNPs captured target cells to the surface to bind with the second antibody on the gold nanoslits. At last, the use of SPR for detection allows for real time monitoring of the capturing process and for the discrimination between bound and unbound cells on the substrate. Combination of efficient rare cell isolation from blood with real-time SPR detection may be a valuable approach for high-throughput screening and early detection of cancer metastasis.

23.8 Conclusion

Development of technological platforms for POC is positioned at the intersection of multiple disciplines including chemistry, physics, electrical engineering, computer science, optics and biotechnology. Continued development of this technology requires close collaboration of researchers in a multitude of fields and the ability to bridge the terminology, knowledge and priorities gaps among disciplines. LOC devices with integrated plasmonic and microfluidic components for portable POC platforms are one prominent result of this cross-disciplinary collaboration. They are now at a mature stage for translating from research environment to the world of real, bed-side use in clinical environment. Integrated microfluidic-plasmonic technologies can be potentially used for various diseases and conditions, making them a broad-spectrum technology for the aid of medical professionals. Naturally, a number of final challenges have to be resolved and are in fact central to current research and development of POC-LOC plasmonics-based devices. Transition from prototype plasmonic technologies in laboratory settings to clinical application will require inexpensive and high-throughput fabrication strategies. In particular, if complete systems are to be integrated in portable devices, one should consider the requirements of interfacing the bio-sensor with appropriate optical systems, detectors and read-out electronics. System modularity will also need to be addressed in a complete system. Ideally, disposable and inexpensive microfluidic cartridges should be read by a portable instrument, thus facilitating operation in a clinical environment and limiting the PCO system running costs. Such challenges look almost trivial in comparison with what has already been achieved regarding plasmonic-based bio-sensors and will certainly present no obstacle for the deployment of this technology. We envision that robust and easy-to-operate plasmonic devices will support the bed-side technology and personalized medicine efforts in the near future.

References

[1] Mabey D, Peeling RW, Ustianowski A, Perkins MD: **Tropical infectious diseases: Diagnostics for the developing world**. *Nat Rev Micro* 2004, **2:**231–240.

[2] Hempen C, Karst U: **Labeling strategies for bioassays**. *Analytical and Bioanalytical Chemistry* 2006, **384:**572–583.

[3] Weiss JB: **DNA probes and PCR for diagnosis of parasitic infections**. *Clinical Microbiology Reviews* 1995, **8:**113–130.

[4] Qavi AJ, Washburn AL, Byeon JY, Bailey RC: **Label-free technologies for quantitative multiparameter biological analysis**. *Analytical and Bioanalytical Chemistry* 2009, **394:**121–135.

[5] Lee C-C, Lee K-L, Wu S-H, Wei P-K: **Plasmonic nanoslit arrays for sensitive biosensors**. In *The Current Trends of Optics and Photonics. Volume* **129:** Springer Netherlands; 2015: 447–468: *Topics in Applied Physics*.

[6] Schena M, Shalon D, Davis RW, Brown PO: **Quantitative monitoring of gene expression patterns with a complementary DNA microarray**. *Science* 1995, **270:**467–470.

[7] MacBeath G, Schreiber SL: **Printing proteins as microarrays for high-throughput function determination**. *Science* 2000, **289:**1760–1763.

[8] Soelberg SD, Chinowsky T, Geiss G, *et al.*: **A portable surface plasmon resonance sensor system for real-time monitoring of small to large analytes**. *Journal of Industrial Microbiology & Biotechnology* 2005, **32:**669–674.

[9] Kelly KL, Coronado E, Zhao LL, Schatz GC: **The optical properties of metal nanoparticles: The influence of size, shape, and dielectric environment**. *Journal of Physical Chemistry B* 2003, **107:**668–677.

[10] Eustis S, El-Sayed MA: **Why gold nanoparticles are more precious than pretty gold: Noble metal surface plasmon resonance and its enhancement of the radiative and nonradiative properties of nanocrystals of different shapes**. *Chemical Society Reviews* 2006, **35:**209–217.

[11] Schultz S, Smith DR, Mock JJ, Schultz DA: **Single-target molecule detection with nonbleaching multicolor optical immunolabels**. *Proceedings of the*

National Academy of Sciences of the United States of America 2000, **97:** 996–1001.

[12] Mock JJ, Smith DR, Schultz S: **Local refractive index dependence of plasmon resonance spectra from individual nanoparticles**. *Nano Letters* 2003, **3:**485–491.

[13] Brolo AG, Gordon R, Leathem B, Kavanagh KL: **Surface plasmon sensor based on the enhanced light transmission through arrays of nanoholes in gold films**. *Langmuir* 2004, **20:**4813–4815.

[14] Tetz KA, Pang L, Fainman Y: **High-resolution surface plasmon resonance sensor based on linewidth-optimized nanohole array transmittance**. *Optics Letters* 2006, **31:**1528–1530.

[15] Lesuffleur A, Im H, Lindquist NC, Oh SH: **Periodic nanohole arrays with shape-enhanced plasmon resonance as real-time biosensors**. *Applied Physics Letters* 2007, **90:**3.

[16] De Leebeeck A, Kumar LKS, de Lange V, Sinton D, Gordon R, Brolo AG: **On-chip surface-based detection with nanohole arrays**. *Analytical Chemistry* 2007, **79:**4094–4100.

[17] Pang L, Hwang GM, Slutsky B, Fainman Y: **Spectral sensitivity of two-dimensional nanohole array surface plasmon polariton resonance sensor**. *Applied Physics Letters* 2007, **91:**3.

[18] Ebbesen TW, Lezec HJ, Ghaemi HF, Thio T, Wolff PA: **Extraordinary optical transmission through sub-wavelength hole arrays**. *Nature* 1998, **391:**667–669.

[19] Escobedo C: **On-chip nanohole array based sensing: a review**. *Lab on a Chip* 2013, **13:**2445–2463.

[20] Maria J, Truong TT, Yao JM, *et al.*: **Optimization of 3D plasmonic crystal structures for refractive index sensing**. *Journal of Physical Chemistry C* 2009, **113:**10493–10499.

[21] Caldwell JD, Glembocki O, Bezares FJ, *et al.*: **Plasmonic nanopillar arrays for large-area, high-enhancement surface-enhanced Raman scattering sensors**. *ACS Nano* 2011, **5:**4046–4055.

[22] Aksu S, Yanik AA, Adato R, Artar A, Huang M, Altug H: **High-throughput nanofabrication of infrared plasmonic nanoantenna arrays for vibrational nanospectroscopy**. *Nano Letters* 2010, **10:**2511–2518.

[23] Lee SW, Lee KS, Ahn J, Lee JJ, Kim MG, Shin YB: **Highly sensitive biosensing using arrays of plasmonic Au nanodisks realized by nanoimprint lithography**. *ACS Nano* 2011, **5:**897–904.

[24] Lindquist NC, Lesuffleur A, Im H, Oh SH: **Sub-micron resolution surface plasmon resonance imaging enabled by nanohole arrays with surrounding Bragg mirrors for enhanced sensitivity and isolation**. *Lab on a Chip* 2009, **9:**382–387.

[25] Yanik AA, Huang M, Kamohara O, *et al.*: **An optofluidic nanoplasmonic biosensor for direct detection of live viruses from biological media**. *Nano Letters* 2010, **10:**4962–4969.

[26] Lee SW, Lee KS, Ahn J, Lee JJ, Kim MG, Shin YB: **Highly sensitive biosensing using arrays of plasmonic Au nanodisks realized by nanoimprint lithography**. *ACS Nano* 2011, **5**:897–904.

[27] Truong TT, Maria J, Yao J, *et al.*: **Nanopost plasmonic crystals**. *Nanotechnology* 2009, **20**:8.

[28] McPhillips J, Murphy A, Jonsson MP, *et al.*: **High-performance biosensing using arrays of plasmonic nanotubes**. *ACS Nano* 2010, **4**:2210–2216.

[29] Gordon R, Sinton D, Kavanagh KL, Brolo AG: **A new generation of sensors based on extraordinary optical transmission**. *Accounts of Chemical Research* 2008, **41**:1049–1057.

[30] Lee KL, Wang WS, Wei PK: **Comparisons of surface plasmon sensitivities in periodic gold nanostructures**. *Plasmonics* 2008, **3**:119–125.

[31] Lee KL, Wu SH, Wei PK: **Intensity sensitivity of gold nanostructures and its application for high-throughput biosensing**. *Optics Express* 2009, **17**:23104–23113.

[32] Ferreira J, Santos MJL, Rahman MM, Brolo AG, Gordon R, Sinton D, *et al.*: **Attomolar protein detection using in-hole surface plasmon resonance**. *Journal of the American Chemical Society* 2009, **131**:436–437.

[33] Eftekhari F, Escobedo C, Ferreira J, *et al.*: **Nanoholes as nanochannels: Flow-through plasmonic sensing**. *Analytical Chemistry* 2009, **81**: 4308–4311.

[34] Lindquist NC, Nagpal P, McPeak KM, Norris DJ, Oh SH: **Engineering metallic nanostructures for plasmonics and nanophotonics**. *Reports on Progress in Physics* 2012, **75**:61.

[35] Lee KL, Chen PW, Wu SH, Huang JB, Yang SY, Wei PK: **Enhancing surface plasmon detection using template-stripped gold nanoslit arrays on plastic films**. *ACS Nano* 2012, **6**:2931–2939.

[36] Miroshnichenko AE, Flach S, Kivshar YS: **Fano resonances in nanoscale structures**. *Reviews of Modern Physics* 2010, **82**:2257–2298.

[37] Chin CD, Linder V, Sia SK: **Lab-on-a-chip devices for global health: Past studies and future opportunities**. *Lab on a Chip* 2007, **7**:41–57.

[38] Myers FB, Lee LP: **Innovations in optical microfluidic technologies for point-of-care diagnostics**. *Lab on a Chip* 2008, **8**:2015–2031.

[39] Dittrich PS, Manz A: **Lab-on-a-chip: microfluidics in drug discovery**. *Nature Reviews Drug Discovery* 2006, **5**:210–218.

[40] Wang SQ, Inci F, Chaunzwa TL, *et al.*: **Portable microfluidic chip for detection of Escherichia coli in produce and blood**. *International Journal of Nanomedicine* 2012, **7**:2591–2600.

[41] Ozcan A, Demirci U: **Ultra wide-field lens-free monitoring of cells on-chip**. *Lab on a Chip* 2008, **8**:98–106.

[42] Wan Y, Tan JF, Asghar W, Kim YT, Liu YL, Iqbal SM: **Velocity effect on aptamer-based circulating tumor cell isolation in microfluidic devices**. *Journal of Physical Chemistry B* 2011, **115**:13891–13896.

[43] Tokel O, Inci F, Demirci U: **Advances in Plasmonic Technologies for Point of Care Applications**. *Chemical Reviews* 2014, **114**:5728–5752.

[44] Nahavandi S, Baratchi S, Soffe R, Tang SY, Mitchell A, Khoshmanesh K: **Microfluidic platforms for biomarker analysis**. *Lab on a Chip* 2014, **14:**1496–1514.

[45] Huang C, Bonroy K, Reekmans G, *et al.*: **Localized surface plasmon resonance biosensor integrated with microfluidic chip**. *Biomedical Microdevices* 2009, **11:**893–901.

[46] Luo Y, Yu F, Zare RN: **Microfluidic device for immunoassays based on surface plasmon resonance imaging**. *Lab on a Chip* 2008, **8:**694–700.

[47] Kozak KR, Su F, Whitelegge JP, Faull K, Reddy S, Farias-Eisner R: **Characterization of serum biomarkers for detection of early stage ovarian cancer**. *PROTEOMICS* 2005, **5:**4589–4596.

[48] Oikonomopoulou K, Li L, Zheng Y, *et al.*: **Prediction of ovarian cancer prognosis and response to chemotherapy by a serum-based multiparametric biomarker panel**. *British Journal of Cancer* 2008, **99:** 1103–1113.

[49] Chen X, Ba Y, Ma L, *et al.*: **Characterization of microRNAs in serum: a novel class of biomarkers for diagnosis of cancer and other diseases**. *Cell Research* 2008, **18:**997–1006.

[50] Bottazzi B, Fornasari L, Frangolho A, *et al.*: **Multiplexed label-free optical biosensor for medical diagnostics**. *Journal of Biomedical Optics* 2014, **19:**017006–017006.

[51] Lee SH, Lindquist NC, Wittenberg NJ, Jordan LR, Oh SH: **Real-time full-spectral imaging and affinity measurements from 50 microfluidic channels using nanohole surface plasmon resonance**. *Lab on a Chip* 2012, **12:**3882–3890.

[52] Tamada K, Nakamura F, Ito M, Li X, Baba A: **SPR-based DNA detection with metal nanoparticles.** *Plasmonics* 2007, **2:**185–191.

[53] He L, Musick MD, Nicewarner SR, *et al.*: **Colloidal Au-enhanced surface plasmon resonance for ultrasensitive detection of DNA hybridization**. *Journal of the American Chemical Society* 2000, **122:**9071–9077.

[54] Long MS, Keating CD: **Nanoparticle conjugation increases protein partitioning in aqueous two-phase systems**. *Analytical Chemistry* 2006, **78:**379–386.

[55] Kim S, Lee J, Lee SJ, Lee HJ: **Ultra-sensitive detection of IgE using biofunctionalized nanoparticle-enhanced SPR**. *Talanta* 2010, **81:**1755–1759.

[56] Goodrich TT, Lee HJ, Corn RM: **Direct detection of genomic DNA by enzymatically amplified SPR imaging measurements of RNA microarrays**. *Journal of the American Chemical Society* 2004, **126:**4086–4087.

[57] Li YA, Wark AW, Lee HJ, Corn RM: **Single-nucleotide polymorphism genotyping by nanoparticle-enhanced surface plasmon resonance imaging measurements of surface ligation reactions**. *Analytical Chemistry* 2006, **78:**3158–3164.

[58] Jiang TS, Minunni M, Wilson P, Zhang J, Turner APF, Mascini M: **Detection of TP53 mutation using a portable surface plasmon resonance DNA-based biosensor**. *Biosensors & Bioelectronics* 2005, **20:**1939–1945.

[59] Sipova H, Springer T, Homola J: **Streptavidin-enhanced assay for sensitive and specific detection of single nucleotide polymorphism in TP53**. *Analytical and Bioanalytical Chemistry* 2011, **399:**2343–2350.

[60] Nelson PN, Reynolds GM, Waldron EE, Ward E, Giannopoulos K, Murray PG: **Monoclonal antibodies**. *Journal of Clinical Pathology-Molecular Pathology* 2000, **53:**111–117.

[61] Ohara R, Knappik A, Shimada K, Frisch C, Ylera F, Koga H: **Antibodies for proteomic research: Comparison of traditional immunization with recombinant antibody technology**. *Proteomics* 2006, **6:**2638–2646.

[62] Briand E, Salmain M, Compere C, Pradier CM: **Immobilization of Protein A on SAMS for the elaboration of immunosensors**. *Colloids and Surfaces B-Biointerfaces* 2006, **53:**215–224.

[63] Mousavi MZ, Chen HY, Wu SH, *et al.*: **Magnetic nanoparticle-enhanced SPR on gold nanoslits for ultra-sensitive, label-free detection of nucleic acid biomarkers**. *Analyst* 2013, **138:**2740–2748.

[64] Lu J, Getz G, Miska EA, *et al.*: **MicroRNA expression profiles classify human cancers**. *Nature* 2005, **435:**834–838.

[65] Mlcochova H, Hezova R, Stanik M, Slaby O: **Urine microRNAs as potential noninvasive biomarkers in urologic cancers**. *Urologic Oncology: Seminars and Original Investigations* 2014, **32:**41.e41–41.e49.

[66] Li JB, Tan SB, Kooger R, Zhang CY, Zhang Y: **MicroRNAs as novel biological targets for detection and regulation**. *Chemical Society Reviews* 2014, **43:**506–517.

[67] Weber JA, Baxter DH, Zhang SL, *et al.*: **The MicroRNA spectrum in 12 body fluids**. *Clinical Chemistry* 2010, **56:**1733–1741.

[68] Kosaka N, Iguchi H, Ochiya T: **Circulating microRNA in body fluid: a new potential biomarker for cancer diagnosis and prognosis**. *Cancer Science* 2010, **101:**2087–2092.

[69] Sipova H, Zhang SL, Dudley AM, Galas D, Wang K, Homola J: **Surface plasmon resonance biosensor for rapid label-free detection of microribonucleic acid at subfemtomole level**. *Analytical Chemistry* 2010, **82:**10110–10115.

[70] Piliarik M, Vala M, Tichý I, Homola JĆ: **Compact and low-cost biosensor based on novel approach to spectroscopy of surface plasmons**. *Biosensors and Bioelectronics* 2009, **24:**3430–3435.

[71] Zhang DC, Yan YR, Cheng W, *et al.*: **Streptavidin-enhanced surface plasmon resonance biosensor for highly sensitive and specific detection of microRNA**. *Microchimica Acta* 2013, **180:**397–403.

[72] Fang SP, Lee HJ, Wark AW, Corn RM: **Attomole microarray detection of MicroRNAs by nanoparticle-amplified SPR imaging measurements of surface polyadenylation reactions**. *Journal of the American Chemical Society* 2006, **128:**14044–14046.

[73] Mousavi MZ, Chen HY, Lee KL, *et al.*: **Urinary micro-RNA biomarker detection using capped gold nanoslit SPR in a microfluidic chip**. *Analyst* 2015, **140:**4097–4104.

[74] Thipmanee O, Samanman S, Sankoh S, *et al.*: **Label-free capacitive DNA sensor using immobilized pyrrolidinyl PNA probe: Effect of the length and terminating head group of the blocking thiols**. *Biosensors and Bioelectronics* 2012, **38:**430–435.

[75] Lakshmipriya T, Fujimaki M, Gopinath SCB, Awazu K, Horiguchi Y, Nagasaki Y: **A high-performance waveguide-mode biosensor for detection of factor IX using PEG-based blocking agents to suppress non-specific binding and improve sensitivity**. *Analyst* 2013, **138:**2863–2870.

[76] Chaffer CL, Weinberg RA: **A perspective on cancer cell metastasis**. *Science* 2011, **331:**1559–1564.

[77] Bidard FC, Fehm T, Ignatiadis M, *et al.*: **Clinical application of circulating tumor cells in breast cancer: overview of the current interventional trials**. *Cancer and Metastasis Reviews* 2013, **32:**179–188.

[78] Maheswaran S, Haber DA: **Circulating tumor cells: a window into cancer biology and metastasis**. *Current Opinion in Genetics & Development* 2010, **20:**96–99.

[79] Talasaz AH, Powell AA, Huber DE, *et al.*: **Isolating highly enriched populations of circulating epithelial cells and other rare cells from blood using a magnetic sweeper device**. *Proceedings of the National Academy of Sciences of the United States of America* 2009, **106:**3970–3975.

[80] Adams AA, Okagbare PI, Feng J, *et al.*: **Highly efficient circulating tumor cell isolation from whole blood and label-free enumeration using polymer-based microfluidics with an integrated conductivity sensor**. *Journal of the American Chemical Society* 2008, **130:**8633–8641.

[81] Stott SL, Hsu CH, Tsukrov DI, *et al,*: **Isolation of circulating tumor cells using a microvortex-generating herringbone-chip**. *Proceedings of the National Academy of Sciences of the United States of America* 2010, **107:**18392–18397.

[82] Nagrath S, Sequist LV, Maheswaran S, *et al.*: **Isolation of rare circulating tumour cells in cancer patients by microchip technology**. *Nature* 2007, **450:**1235–U1210.

[83] Zheng S, Lin H, Liu JQ, *et al.*: **Membrane microfilter device for selective capture, electrolysis and genomic analysis of human circulating tumor cells**. *Journal of Chromatography A* 2007, **1162:**154–161.

[84] Hou HW, Warkiani ME, Khoo BL, *et al.*: **Isolation and retrieval of circulating tumor cells using centrifugal forces**. *Scientific Reports* 2013, **3:**8.

[85] Hou HW, Li QS, Lee GYH, Kumar AP, Ong CN, Lim CT: **Deformability study of breast cancer cells using microfluidics**. *Biomedical Microdevices* 2009, **11:**557–564.

[86] Tan SJ, Yobas L, Lee GYH, Ong CN, Lim CT: **Microdevice for the isolation and enumeration of cancer cells from blood**. *Biomedical Microdevices* 2009, **11:**883–892.

[87] Dharmasiri U, Balamurugan S, Adams AA, Okagbare PI, Obubuafo A, Soper SA: **Highly efficient capture and enumeration of low abundance prostate cancer cells using prostate-specific membrane antigen**

aptamers immobilized to a polymeric microfluidic device. *Electrophoresis* 2009, **30:**3289–3300.

[88] Yashunsky V, Lirtsman V, Golosovsky M, Davidov D, Aroeti B: **Real-time monitoring of epithelial cell-cell and cell-substrate interactions by infrared surface plasmon spectroscopy**. *Biophysical Journal* 2010, **99:**4028–4036.

[89] Yashunsky V, Lirtsman V, Zilbershtein A, *et al.*: **Surface plasmon-based infrared spectroscopy for cell biosensing**. *Journal of Biomedical Optics* 2012, **17:**8.

[90] Hiragun T, Yanase Y, Kose K, *et al.*: **Surface plasmon resonance-biosensor detects the diversity of responses against epidermal growth factor in various carcinoma cell lines**. *Biosensors and Bioelectronics* 2012, **32:**202–207.

[91] Yanase Y, Suzuki H, Tsutsui T, Hiragun T, Kameyoshi Y, Hide M: **The SPR signal in living cells reflects changes other than the area of adhesion and the formation of cell constructions**. *Biosensors & Bioelectronics* 2007, **22:**1081–1086.

[92] Tanaka M, Hiragun T, Tsutsui T, Yanase Y, Suzuki H, Hide M: **Surface plasmon resonance biosensor detects the downstream events of active PKCĪ^{2} in antigen-stimulated mast cells**. *Biosensors and Bioelectronics* 2008, **23:**1652–1658.

[93] Yanase Y, Hiragun T, Ishii K, *et al.*: **Surface plasmon resonance for cell-based clinical diagnosis**. *Sensors* 2014, **14:**4948.

[94] El-Sayed IH, Huang X, El-Sayed MA: **Surface plasmon resonance scattering and absorption of anti-EGFR antibody conjugated gold nanoparticles in cancer diagnostics: Applications in oral cancer**. *Nano Letters* 2005, **5:**829–834.

[95] Wu SH, Hsieh SY, Lee KL, Weng RH, Chiou A, Wei PK: **Cell viability monitoring using Fano resonance in gold nanoslit array**. *Applied Physics Letters* 2013, **103:**4.

[96] Mousavi M, Chen H-Y, Hou H-S, *et al.*: **Label-free detection of rare cell in human blood using gold nano slit surface plasmon resonance**. *Biosensors* 2015, **5:**98.

Chapter 24

Surface plasmon resonance based miniaturized biosensors for medical applications

Dmitriy V. Sotnikov[1], *Anatoly V. Zherdev*[1] *and Boris B. Dzantiev*[1]

24.1 Introduction

Optical biosensors based on the phenomenon of surface plasmon resonance (SPR) have been successfully applied to solve various analytical tasks for more than 30 years [1–6]. SPR is the resonant oscillation of conduction electrons at the interface between two media one of which has negative real part of dielectric permeability. Quanta of such oscillations of electronic gas are named surface plasmons [7]. Conditions for SPR excitation are extremely sensitive to composition of the environment near the media interface and this makes it possible to detect intermolecular complexes by means of SPR.

Nowadays, among other optical biosensors, systems based on SPR registration have leading position [8–10]. This is caused, first of all, by high sensitivity of the method and the method adaptability for detection of wide range of objects, from small molecules to whole cells. Use of SPR in analytical systems allows full fulfilling of the biosensor approach advantages and makes it possible to register ligand–receptor interactions in real time, without use of labels and with the minimal sample preparation [11].

Creation of theoretical base for such devices development began at the beginning of the twentieth century when in 1902 Wood described diffracted light spectra anomalies caused by surface plasmon wave [12]. And as late as in 1968 Otto [13], Kretschmann and Raether [14] showed excitation of surface plasmons by light using a method of attenuated total reflection.

Various SPR-biosensor types are generally classified by applied surface plasmons excitation methods. Main existing types of plasmons excitation methods are those which use prisms with high refraction index (Otto–Kretschmann method), wave guides and diffraction gratings. Rarer are other methods, for example, with use of photonic crystals. Combination of several excitation schemes in one device

[1]A.N. Bach Institute of Biochemistry, Research Center of Biotechnology of the Russian Academy of Sciences. Leninsky prospect 33, Moscow 119071, Russia

is also possible [15]. Methods based on localized surface plasmon resonance (LSPR) phenomenon and methods using SPR/LSPR influence over such optical processes as adsorption, fluorescence or Raman scattering [16] should be particularly mentioned.

Current trends in area of SPR-biosensor development are increase of detectors sensitivity [17], increase of analysis productivity [8], development of portable low-cost devices and their adaptation for application in point of care [15].

In this chapter, short description of concept being a basis of the method, SPR-systems classification, methods for sensor surface functionalization are given; structure of present-day SPR-sensors market is described. Special attention is paid to methods of SPR-sensors miniaturization and to assessment of these methods efficiency for medical applications, including prospects of SPR-sensors use for on-site diagnostics.

24.2 Principle of SPR-sensors work

As it was already noted, SPR-methods are based on interaction of electromagnetic wave, reached interface of two media, with electronic gas located in thin film of conducting material laid between these media. In most cases, metal is used as a conducting material because real part of dielectric permeability is negative for metals and this is a necessary condition for surface electromagnetic waves generation in wavelength range from ultraviolet to infrared [18]. SPR generation is possible only at a certain ratio of contacting media permeability values. In visible and near infrared parts of spectra, gold, silver, aluminum and copper possess suitable characteristics [19]. In addition to ability to generate distinctive SPR, gold is chemically inert therefore sensor surfaces made of gold are characterized by high stability and low level of nonspecific interactions [20]. These factors were the cause of the common solution that the substance used as a cover of sensitive surfaces of SPR-sensors is gold. Transparent materials with high refraction index are used as the dielectric medium, for example, silica [21].

For SPR excitation, it is necessary that the exciting ray fell on media interface from the media with large refraction index with such direction which provides full internal reflection [7].

If conducting material is placed on media interface, electromagnetic field can cause oscillations of free electrons in it. The electromagnetic wave energy is partially absorbed and dissipated, and partially transferred to generated reflected ray and surface electromagnetic wave in conducting film. If energy transmission to one of these ways is increased, then energy transferred to another, obviously, is decreased.

Result of electromagnetic emission interaction with conductor is determined by a ratio of the emission frequency and own frequency of electronic gas density oscillation – plasma frequency (PF). For light with a frequency above PF, conductor is transparent since electrons are not able to shield a wave. Light with a frequency below PF is reflected because of electrons shielding effect [22, 23].

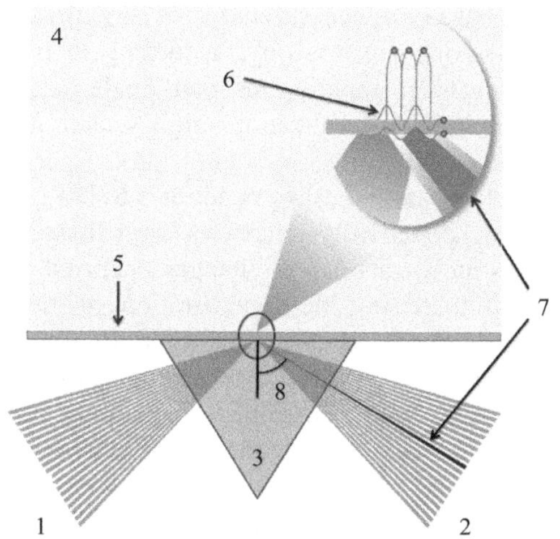

Figure 24.1 *Principle of surface plasmon resonance exciting. 1 – exciting light; 2 – reflected light; 3 – dielectric prism made of material with high refraction index; 4 – analyzed media; 5 – metal film; 6 – surface plasmon; 7 – decreasing of reflected light intensity; 8 – surface plasmon resonance angle*

For majority of metals PF lays in ultra-violet area of spectra and this is a reason of their characteristic gloss in visible range. For SPR excitation, light with frequency below PF is used.

Despite effective light shielding at frequency below PF, if conductor layer thickness is rather small (less than a wavelength of exciting light), part of light energy passes through the layer and excites a surface plasmon. Value of photon impulse projection to media interface depends on its frequency and angle of incidence, and impulse of surface plasmon depends on the conductor properties and indices of refraction of the adjoining media. If the surface plasmon impulse is equal to photon impulse projection to media interface, part of photons is absorbed by electronic oscillation surface waves (surface plasmon resonance) and this leads to reduction of reflected light intensity (Figure 24.1) [16].

SPR is extremely sensitive to the smallest changes of refraction index in interface area. This allows real time detecting of various complexes presence in the media interface by change of wave parameters at which resonance takes place. Those parameters can be:

- resonant wavelength of exciting light for fixed angle of incidence,
- resonant angle of ray falling for fixed frequency,
- amplitude of light wave,
- phase of light.

Accordingly, all registering devices are divided in four types of based on measured parameter: angle of reflection, frequency, intensity and phase shift of light.

SPR-analysis methods based on measurement of the first two parameters are also named surface plasmons spectroscopy, according to frequency and angular spectra [24]. Nowadays, sensors applying resonant angle measurement method are mostly used due to simplicity of realization, high sensitivity and wide working range [25, 26].

Electromagnetic field of surface wave penetrates to both media, and amplitude of plasmon wave field exponentially decreases with distance from the surface. Therefore the method is most sensitive to changes occurred directly on the media surface. As wavelength increases, field penetration depth decreases. The last parameter is a distance from the surface at which field amplitude decreases by ***e*** times (***e*** – the basis of natural logarithm). For example, for system gold-dielectric (with refraction index 1.32) field penetration depth increases from 100 nm for wavelength of 600 nm to 600 nm for wavelength of 1000 nm [25].

Two types of plane polarized light wave exist: s-wave and p-wave. s-Polarized wave (s – senkrecht) has a vector of electric field E perpendicular to plane of incidence. s-Polarized wave also is called σ-polarized, sagittal wave, E-type wave, a TE wave (Transverse Electric). p-Polarization (p – parallel) means the wave which has electric field vector parallel to plane of incidence. p-Polarized wave is also called π-polarized, H-type wave, TM wave (Transverse Magnetic). Generally, electric component of electromagnetic wave interacts with electrons of substance atoms. Thus the surface plasmon is a cross wave with electric field intensity vector perpendicular to the media interface. Therefore, p-polarized wave interacts with surface plasmon more strongly. For this reason p-polarized light is mostly used for SPR-sensors [27]. However, recently SPR registration techniques based on phase modulation of reflected light, applying both p- and s-light wave components, are used often [26]. In such techniques, difference in s- and p-component interaction with plasmons are applied for analytical measurements.

To make binding with sensor surface specific, the surface is modified with sorbents and binding molecules, such as antibodies, aptamers, etc. [25].

24.3 Types of SPR-sensors

As it was noted earlier, to achieve conditions for SPR excitation, it is necessary that plasmon wave vector and projection of exciting light wave vector to surface were equal. But, as impulse of oscillating electrons wave is always more than that of photons with zero weight, an additional impulse should be given to light wave for wave vectors equality [23]. For this purpose, special devices are used which are named coupling devices. Generally those devices are prisms, waveguides and diffraction gratings [15, 25].

24.3.1 SPR-sensors with prismatic coupling devices (couplers)

In pioneer devices for SPR excitation, proposed by Otto [13] and Kretschmann [14], special prisms made of dielectric with high refraction index were used for coupling. Otto and Kretschmann schemes are different in geometry and relative

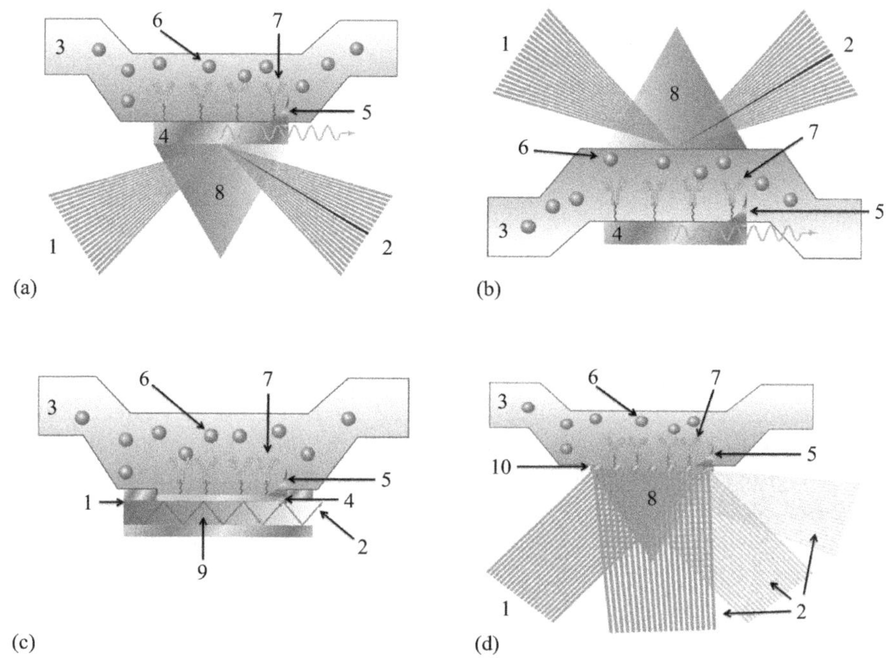

Figure 24.2 Schemes of SPR-sensors with various types of coupling devices: (a) with dielectric prism in Kretschmann's configuration; (b) with dielectric prism in Otto's configuration; (c) with waveguide; (d) with diffraction grating. 1 – exciting light; 2 – reflected light; 3 – analyzed media; 4 – metal film; 5 – plasmon field intensity; 6 – analyte; 7 – receptor; 8 – dielectric prism with high refraction index; 9 – waveguide; 10 – diffraction grating

positioning of conducting and dielectric layers. In Kretschmann's geometry, a metal film is placed between a prism and dielectric media (Figure 24.2a), and in Otto's geometry the dielectric media is placed between a prism and metal layer (Figure 24.2b). Nowadays, in SPR-sensors, prismatic scheme of Kretschmann's geometry is mainly used. In this scheme, thin metal film is applied on the base of the prism made of dielectric. The light wave passes through the prism and gets the basis, and this causes emergence of attenuating wave. This wave penetrates though the film and excites a surface plasmon. Opposite side of the film either directly contacts to the analyzed media, or is exposed to additional modifications to enable specific interaction and/or improvement of analytical parameters of sensor device [28]. The conducting surface is lit with monochromatic light with various angles of incidence being in the range of total internal reflection. After reflection from the metal film, light gets to the detector. If wave vectors are equal for one of angles of incidence (resonant angle) and one of frequencies (resonant wavelength), photons' energy is absorbed by the plasmon, leading to decrease of the reflected light intensity. Change of media composition near the sensor surface leads to change of conditions for SPR excitation and shift of resonant angle, resonant frequency, reflected waves phase and light intensity registered by the detector.

24.3.2 SPR-sensors with waveguide coupling devices

Dielectric material with high refraction index can be used for manufacturing of waveguide-directing channel in which the wave propagates. The metal film is applied on the surface of such channel. Electromagnetic field is concentrated in the central part of waveguide, but small part of the attenuating wave penetrates into the layer with low refraction index (analyzed media) through a metal film and excites a surface plasmon on its external border (Figure 24.2c). Fiber-optical channels with metal covering in sensing area are most often used for this purpose. Light propagation in such channels is possible due to full internal reflection effect [29]. In SPR-biosensors with waveguide coupling devices the following parameters can be used as registered signal: SPR resonant frequency shift as a result of interaction of the sensor surface with analyte (frequency modulation), phase shift (phase modulation) or change of transmitted light intensity at a certain wavelength (intensity modulation) [30].

24.3.3 SPR-sensors with diffraction gratings

Plasmons excitation is also possible when light falls from dielectric media to metal diffraction grating with a period less than the light wavelength. Plasmon excitation takes place under the light diffracted on the grating provided wave vectors of light and surface plasmon are matched. Matching of wave vectors depends not only on parameters of exciting light (frequency and angle of incidence) and a refraction index of the analyzed media, but also on the grating period and a diffraction maximum order. SPR-sensors with diffraction gratings can work both in the transmission mode and in the reflection mode [31–33]. Scheme of SPR-sensor with diffraction grating for reflection mode is given in Figure 24.2d, as an example. SPR measurements with such sensors can be performed on the basis of registration of frequency, phase, amplitude or angular characteristics.

24.3.4 Localized SPR (LSPR)

Electric field, interacting with electronic gas in metal particles with size less than a wavelength of exciting light, causes collective oscillations of electrons relative to positively charged nuclei. Unlike surface plasmons in the conducting films, electrons oscillation does not propagate in nanoparticles. Such oscillations are similar to those of harmonious oscillator. Excitation of such oscillations is called an LSPR.

At excitation of electronic oscillation at resonant frequency, strong increase of light scattering by nanoparticles is observed. The calculation of LSPR conditions by use of Mie's theory shows that localized surface plasmon can be excited by electromagnetic wave directly, without use of additional coupling devices. Similar to SPR, this phenomenon is extremely sensitive to changes of refractive index of media near the metal surface. It makes it possible to monitor processes occurred on nanoparticles' surface by shift of the extinction peak in spectrum of the light passing through nanoparticles solution [34].

24.4 Analytical parameters of SPR-sensors

Main characteristics used for SPR-sensors assessment and comparison are sensitivity, resolution, limit of detection and dynamic range [25].

Sensor sensitivity is a ratio of sensor signal change to the change of a measured value. Quantitatively, sensitivity is equal to the slope of the calibration curve [35]. As in various types of sensors different signal parameters are measured (angle, wavelength, intensity, phase shift), sensitivity can be expressed in different units of measurement. In SPR-sensors, change of refraction index is a measured parameter which is expressed in RIU (refractive index unit). Depending on a sensor type, RIU, nm/RIU, per cent/RIU, rad/RIU [17] can be the sensitivity measurement units, respectively.

SPR-sensor resolution is the minimum measurable change of refraction index. This value is equal to a ratio of standard noise deviation to sensitivity of the SPR-sensor. As the standard deviation is measured in the same units as the sensor signal, resolution, unlike sensitivity, for all types of SPR-sensors is measured in one unit – RIU. For this reason different SPR-sensors are usually compared by resolution, but not by sensitivity [26, 35]. Since at the same noise level, increase of sensor sensitivity results in a reduction of its resolution, sensors with the smaller resolution are usually more sensitive.

Another important parameter – the lower detection limit of analyte (which is often called just a detection limit) – directly depends on resolution of the sensor. In most cases, this parameter is defined as analyte concentration which causes change of the sensor signal equal to three (more rare – to two) standard deviations of a background signal. A detection limit in SPR-analysis is directly proportional to the sensor resolution, but it also depends on analyte properties, first of all on its molecular weight, thickness of sensitive layer, and also on constant of interaction with receptor [35]. Sometimes, one more parameter, upper detection limit, is defined. It is the highest analyte concentration, different from top plateau of concentration dependence. The lower detection limit is more important sensor characteristic as the upper detection limit can be easily overcome by sample dilution.

One more important characteristic is the dynamic range of a sensor – a range of measured parameter values between the lower and the upper detection limits [36, 37]. Dynamic range can be defined as values dispersion, difference between the upper and the lower detection limits, ratio of these two limits or logarithm of this ratio. Definition, which sometimes is incorrectly used as a synonym of dynamic range – working range (measuring range) – a range of values of the parameter which can be measured with specified accuracy [37]. Working range is usually less than dynamic range.

24.5 Sensor surface functionalization

As it was noted earlier, SPR-analysis is preceded by functionalization of sensor surface necessary for specific binding of a target substance. Methods of immobilization of specific binding molecules (ligands) on the surface of optical chips are similar to those of other carriers' modification (e.g., chromatographic sorbents, nano- and microparticles). Selection of an appropriate immobilization method depends on the chemical nature of the ligands. Antibodies and, more rarely, other proteins, peptides or nucleic acids (e.g., in the form of aptamer) as well as molecular imprinted polymers are used as ligands [38–41]. If antibodies are used as an analyte (in serodiagnostics), sensor surface is modified by antigen or its derivative. In inhibiting analysis scheme (see Section 24.6.) ligand itself serves as an analyte (native or modified). In serodiagnostics and inhibiting analysis, composition of any chemical nature can potentially be a ligand.

There are different functionalization methods depending on the type of the formed bonds.

24.5.1 Covalent binding

Taking into account that the vast majority of SPR-chips are made of gold that has high reactivity to sulfur, a surface of gold chips can be directly modified by sulfur-containing compounds. N-alkylthiols and disulfides which form self-assembled monolayer on a gold surface are most often used for this purpose [42]. Such modification can be the first stage of chip functionalization allowing attachment to its surface of various chemical groups for further modification.

For covalent coupling of ligands containing amine groups, chips covered with carboxylated dextran layer are usually used. They can be activated with mix of N-hydroxysuccinimide and ethyl-(dimethylaminopropyl) carbodiimide (carbodiimide reaction). As a result, highly reactive ether groups which further interact with amine groups of ligands with formation of amide bond are formed. In case of protein ligands, lysine amino groups or N-terminal amino groups can be reactive. In some cases, modifications of this reaction are used with immobilization of ligands by thiol and aldehyde groups [28,38].

For covalent immobilization of nucleic acids and their derivatives, 11-mercaptoundecylamine, dithiobis (N-succinimidyl propionate) or other reagents can be used [43–45].

Methods of covalent binding of saccharide fragments are of great interest. Using such methods, it is possible not only to immobilize saccharide molecules but also to perform site-directed immobilization of antibodies as the majority of antibodies are glycated protein with a pair of oligosaccharide chains on CH2 domain of Fc fragment. Since the oligosaccharide chain is located far from antigen-binding Fab fragments, this approach reduces probability of the decrease in antibodies binding ability after immobilization. Oligosaccharide chains can be oxidized to aldehydes chemically or enzymatically and then covalently coupled to amine, hydrazine, semicarbazide and other groups [46]. For covalent binding of saccharides, 3-aminophenylboronic acid is also used. First, amino group of 3-aminophenylboronic acid binds covalently on the carboxylated chip surface by means of carbodiimide reaction described above. Then free – $B(OH)_2$ groups interact with saccharide fragments, forming cyclic ether through cis-1,2 or 1,3-diol groups [47].

Covalent immobilization is almost irreversible therefore covalently modified chips are very stable, but, as a rule, they are suitable only for analysis of one analyte.

24.5.2 Non-covalent binding

Ligands immobilized by non-covalent methods can be removed from the surface using rather simple methods, for example, by changing pH of solution. This provides possibility of multiple regeneration of the surface, but also results in reducing the stability of the surface composition and strong dependence on environment factors.

A significant part of non-covalent immobilization methods is based on various affine interactions. In this case, one of two interacting reagents is bound covalently on a chip surface, and the second reagent non-covalently interacts with the bound one. Among such pairs antibodies – secondary antibodies; avidin (or streptavidin, NeutrAvidin, traptavidin, etc.) – biotinylated ligands; IgG – IgG-binding proteins (e.g., protein A *Staphylococcus aureus*, protein G *Streptococcus* spp.); complementary DNA fragments are the most widely used [48–52].

Method of immobilization of protein ligands containing so-called Histag (sequence of 6 histidines) is quite widespread [53]. These proteins are immobilized on the chip with surface modified by an ion-exchange NTA compound (nitrilotriacetate), due to formation of three chelate complexes consisting of two histidine residues, one bivalent metal ion and one NTA molecule. The resulting complex can be destroyed by addition of the competing ligand (e.g., imidazole) or a chelate reagent (e.g., ethylenediaminetetraacetic acid, EDTA).

A separate group includes immobilization methods based on hydrophobic interactions. Immobilization of lipidic mono- and bilayers, lipid micelles and liposomes is carried out on the chip with hydrophobic acyl spacers by means of such methods [28].

24.6 SPR-analysis formats

There are four main formats of analysis performed in SPR-sensors. They differ in the structure of the complexes formed on the sensor surface and in the order of components binding (Figure 24.3) [8].

Change of a refraction index near the sensor surface increases with the increase of mass of molecules bound with the surface. Therefore a direct analysis (Figure 24.3a) is, in most cases, carried out if the analytes have rather large mass (as a rule, more than 5 kDa, exact threshold value depends on technical characteristics of the sensor) [10]. Binding of such objects with a functionalized surface of the sensor leads to a considerable change of refraction index in the interface area. Therefore binding can be directly registered by a detector with a high sensitivity.

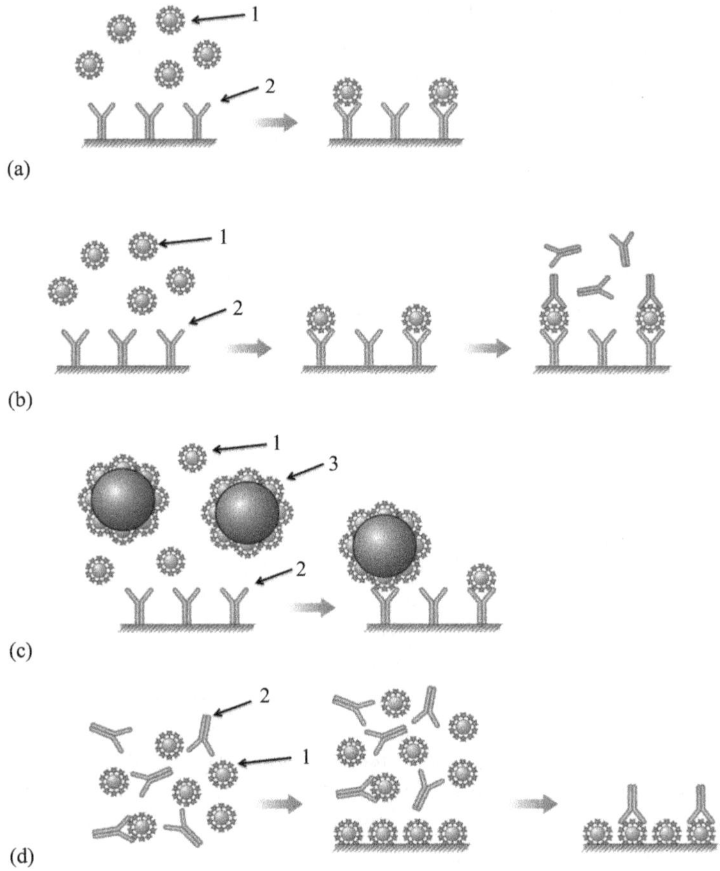

Figure 24.3 SPR-analysis formats: (a) direct; (b) 'sandwich'; (c) competitive; (d) inhibiting. Growth in analyte concentration results in an increase of the registered signal for (a) and (b) formats, and in a decrease for (c) and (d) formats. 1 – analyte; 2 – receptor (antibodies); 3 – antigen conjugate with a high-molecular carrier

If an analyte has several potential binding sites with receptor molecules, it still has free valences after formation of the complex on the chip surface. Usually this is applicable to large molecules and their complexes. Free valences can interact with a receptor added to solution, and this leads to additional growth of a signal caused by increase in a receptor mass bound with the surface. As a result, an analyte complex is located between two (or more) receptor molecules (Figure 24.3b). This so-called 'sandwich'-format is applied to achieve a higher sensitivity of detection.

Binding of low-molecular compounds causes weak change of refraction index. Therefore it is difficult to detect small molecules by SPR method directly. In such cases, in addition to analyte in the sample, a modified analyte is also added into the system [25]. Two formats of analysis are possible with such reagents. In the first case an analyte is conjugated with a larger carrier, and a receptor is immobilized on the sensor surface. Conjugated and free analyte are mixed up and compete for binding with the immobilized receptor (Figure 24.3c). In the second case, a receptor in a fixed concentration is added to the solution, and the analyte or its conjugate is immobilized on the surface. Free analyte in the solution is bound with the receptor, preventing interaction of the receptor with the modified surface (Figure 24.3d). Inhibiting analysis is a kind of the competitive analysis, but it is often regards as a separate format.

24.7 Mass-produced SPR-sensors

The first commercially available SPR-biosensor was presented by Swedish company Pharmacia Biosensor AB in 1990. In 1996, the company changed its name to Biacore AB Corporation and now it is the absolute leader in SPR-biosensor market [54]. Since the first SPR-biosensor presentation, the company has developed more than 10 modifications and improved the equipment parameters – analysis sensitivity and accuracy, and also productivity due to use of multiplex technologies and automation.

Despite overwhelming domination of Biacore in SPR-biosensor market, recently an increasing number of the companies present their production in this area. Main present-day models of SPR-sensors available in the modern market are listed in Table 24.1. Other SPR-platforms, which are at different development and commercialization stages, are mentioned in scientific literature [7, 55].

New projects reflect the main tendency in the area of the development of SPR-equipment – intention to create multichannel devices. Within this frame, special attention should be paid to SPR imaging (SPRi) – technology of simultaneous detection of multiple interactions on the surface of the sensor chip formed as a matrix of sensitive elements with various affinity [56]. This technology allows for simultaneous registration by CCD camera of interactions with large – up to several hundred – number of binding zones which differ from each other by immobilized reagents.

Today, mass-produced SPR-sensors are successfully applied for medical diagnostics of hormonal status of organism, to detect markers of cardiovascular diseases, immune disorders, genetic diseases, and inflammatory processes, onco-markers, virus and bacterial pathogens, etc. [10].

24.8 SPR-sensors for non-laboratory diagnostics

24.8.1 Commercial portable SPR-sensors

The key factor defining possibility of the sensor to be applied for local diagnostics are the sensor dimensions. The majority of analytical platforms available in the market are expensive stationary devices which can be used only in laboratories. However in ninetieth, Texas Instruments company (USA) developed and

Table 24.1 Present-day models of commercial SRP-sensors

Company	Country	Present-day models	Reference	Note
Accurion	Germany	Nanofilm_ep3se	www.accurion.com	Company is a result of merge of Halcyonics GmbH and Nanofilm Technology GmbH. Produces multi-functional ellipsometer with option of SPR imaging
Analytical μ-Systems	Germany	BIOSUPLAR 6	www.biosuplar.de	Branch of Mivitec
Biacore AB Corporation	Sweden/ USA	Biacore 4000, Biacore S200, Biacore T200, Biacore X100, Biacore C, Biacore 3000, Biacore Q	www.biacore.com	In 2006, the company was purchased by General Electric Healthcare (USA)
BioNavis	Finland	SPR Navi 200; SPR Navi 210A; SPR Navi 220A	www.bionavis.com	
BiOptix	USA	BiOptix 404pi	www.bioptixinc.com	
Bio-Rad Laboratories	USA	ProteOn XPR36	www.bio-rad.com	
Biosensing Instrument	USA	BI-4500 SERIES; BI-4000 SERIES; BI-3000 SERIES; BI-2000 SERIES	biosensingusa.com	
China Medical Technologies	China	SPR-960	ccsunostik.en.china.cn	
GWC Technologies	USA	The SPRimagerII; SPR100	www.gwctechnologies.com	
HORIBA Scientific	Japan	XelPleX; OpenPlex SuPRa-MS	www.horiba.com	In 2009, company Horiba purchased company GenOptics (France) – producer of SPR and SPRi systems
IBIS Technologies	Netherlands	IBIS-MX96	www.ibis-spr.nl	

Kinetic Evaluation Instruments	Netherlands	Esprit ESPR; TWINGLE; SPRINGLE	bcf.assic.sinica.edu.tw	A spin-out from Metrohm Autolab. Up to 2009 it was called Eco Chemie
Korea Materials & Analysis Corp. (K-MAC)	Korea	SPRmicro; SPRi; SPR LAB;	www.kmac.com.tw	
Nano SPR	USA	NanoSPR1; NanoSPR6 321; NanoSPR8 481	nanospr.com	
Nicoya Lifesciences	Canada	OpenSPR	www.nicoyalife.com	
Nippon Telegraph and Telephone Corporation – Advanced Technology (NTT-AT)	Japan	SPR SS-1001	www.ntt-at.com	
Optrel	Germany	The Multiskop	www.optrel.de	Produces multi-functional optical platforms with option '*surface plasmons*'
Plexera	USA	PlexArray	www.plexera.com	
Reichert Technologies	USA	Reichert4SPR; SR7500DC	www.reichertspr.com	Part of AMETEK, predecessor – Leica Microsystems
Seattle Sensor Systems	USA	SPIRIT	www.seattlesensors.com	SPR-sensors apply chips Spreeta2000 (Texas Instruments)
Sensia	Spain	Indicator; Indicator-G	www.sensia.es	Part of MONDRAGON Corporation Cooperative Group
SensiQ Technologies	USA	SensiQ Pioneer FE; SensiQ Pioneer AE; SensiQ	www.sensiqtech.com	Earlier – branch of ICx Nomadics/FLIR Systems
Sierra Sensors	Germany	SPR-2	www.sierrasensors.com	
Texas Instruments	USA	Spreeta/Spreeta 2000	www.ti.com	Manufacturer – ICx Nomadics/FLIR Systems
XanTec bioanalytics	Germany	SR7500DC SR7000DC	www.xantec.com	

commercialized a tiny SPR-sensor Spreeta™ [57], with dimensions of $3 \times 1.5 \times 4$ cm and price about US$50 (manufacturer – ICx Nomadics/FLIR Systems) [7]. Later, the company presented even smaller device – Spreeta2000™ with dimensions of $1.5 \times 0.7 \times 3$ cm. Despite the sizes, this sensor is a full SPR-platform consisting of light source, polarizer, prism, sensor surface and angular detector [58]. The sensor refraction index resolution is 5×10^{-6} RIU. One of the limiting factors in SPR-sensors miniaturization is resonance sensitivity to temperature changes. Spreeta does not stabilize temperature in the cell, but uses a signal correction protocol taking into account temperature deviation. SPRmicro analyzer produced by Korean company K-MAC (Korea Materials & Analysis Corp.) has a similar design though a little bigger dimensions: $4.5 \times 14 \times 13$ cm. This design seems very promising for portable systems of point of care diagnostics.

Spreeta SPR-sensor is successfully applied for various analytical purposes, including medical diagnostics. Jiang *et al.* used Spreeta sensor for detection of mutation of gene-suppressor of TP53 tumors. For this purpose, on the gold surface of the sensor chip, thiolated derivatives of complementary nucleotides (26 pairs) were immobilized. Analysis of DNA taken from mutated and unmutated cells demonstrated that the presence of only one substitute in a nucleotide sequence resulted in a 34% decrease in the sensor signal. This analysis allowed revealing TP53 mutations with high specificity within 2 min. The binding ability of the sensor chip remained unchanged even after 50 cycles of regeneration [59].

Serodiagnostics – a detection of anti-pathogen specific antibodies in blood – is considered to be the one of the most universal approaches in the diagnostics of infectious diseases. Chung *et al.* used such approach for diagnostics of human hepatitis B by means of Spreeta [60]. The results obtained by testing of patients' sera well correlated with the ones obtained by a traditional ELISA as a reference method.

Later, SPIRIT™ system (Seattle Sensor Systems, USA) which allows carrying out simultaneous analysis on 8 Spreeta2000 chips was developed. Each chip has 3 channels and it is possible to carry out an analysis in 24 channels simultaneously [61]. This device is rather compact for point of care use (weight – 3 kg, dimensions – $28 \times 22 \times 13$ cm). Its efficiency for the analysis of several analytes from small molecules (2,4-Dinitrophenol-l-lysine (MW 349)) to viruses (Norwalk virus) and whole bacteria (*Francisella tularensis* LVS) was demonstrated. The SPIRIT™ system also has own temperature control system (to 0.01 °C) which enhances measurements accuracy.

Large number of studies shows considerable progress in the development of portable devices suitable for application out of the laboratory. Among SPR-sensors available in the market, the following sensors sufficiently small for application in non-laboratory conditions should be mentioned: NanoSPR1 – $19 \times 11.5 \times 11.5$ cm, NanoSPR6 321 – $21.5 \times 13 \times 10$ cm; NanoSPR8 481 – $21.5 \times 13 \times 10$ cm (NanoSPR Devices, USA); BIOSUPLAR 6 – $20 \times 9 \times 8$ cm (Analytical μ-Systems, Germany); SPRmicro – $4.5 \times 14 \times 13$ cm (K-MAC, Korea); Handy-SPR PS-0109 – $17 \times 10 \times 5$ cm (NTT Advanced Technology Corporation, Japan); OpenSPR – $16 \times 21 \times 12$ cm (Nicoya Lifesciences, Canada). These devices use

SPR effect for conducting films as a rule. Only the last of them applies LSPR principle on gold nanoparticles.

24.8.2 Recent works in portable SPR-sensors development

Besides commercial portable SPR-sensors, some prototypes promising for local application are under development. For example, the development of a hand-held SPR-sensor with dimensions of 15 × 8 cm and weight of 600 g is described in the study of Feltis *et al.* [62]. Application of this sensor was shown on the example of highly toxic protein detection – ricin. Sensitivity of measurement considerably conceded to sensitivity of stationary commercial SPR-sensor: the prototype detection limit is 200 ng/ml vs. 10 ng/ml for Biacore-1000. However, portability and integrated power supply do this platform very perspective for use in beyond the laboratory.

Development of portable SPR-sensors attracts an increasing attention of researchers, expanding proposals of new products in the field. The group of researchers from Montreal University (Canada) has recently developed a portable SPR-sensor P4SPR for screening of medicines [63]. Dimensions of this device are 17.5 × 15.5 × 5.5 cm, and weight is less than 1.3 kg. This efficiency of this device was demonstrated in the analysis of methotrexate as potentially toxic anticarcinogenic medicine. The sensor measured the amount of medicine in the patients' blood for less than in 1 min. The accuracy was higher than that of stationary equipment and allowed calculating the optimum dose of the medicine thus reducing of potential risks for the patient.

Considerable success has been achieved in the field of integration of microfluid chips and SPRi technologies. This made it possible to create compact and, at the same time, high-performance SPR-systems. Ouellet *et al.* developed a compact microfluid matrix for SPR-analysis having 264 chambers with size of 700 pL and sensitive elements [64]. The microfluid matrix is made of glass workpieces with size of 2.5 × 7.5 × 0.11 cm using soft lithography technology. Possibility of simultaneous interactions registration in separate cameras has been shown for the interaction of human α-thrombin and IX human factor with specific antibodies.

Size reduction of a sensitive element often leads to an increase of analyte detection limit. Therefore, SPRi-systems often concede on sensitivity to non-multiplex SPR-systems. For sensitivity increase, additional stages of signal amplification are often used. It is known that the signal of SPR-sensors directly depends on the mass of the object bound with the sensor surface and a field of the surface wave penetrates into media on distance up to several hundred nanometers. Therefore, an obvious way to enhance SPR-analysis sensitivity is use of various nanoparticle as labels. Gold nanoparticles are mostly used due to their high stability, well developed functionalization techniques, and a possibility to produce particles with a controlled size and shape [65–68]. One more advantage of metal nanoparticles is the double mechanism of SPR enhancement: due to increase of the mass on the sensor surface and due to interaction of surface plasmons fields exited on the sensor metal film with own electrons of metal nanoparticle (combination of SPR-LSPR) [68].

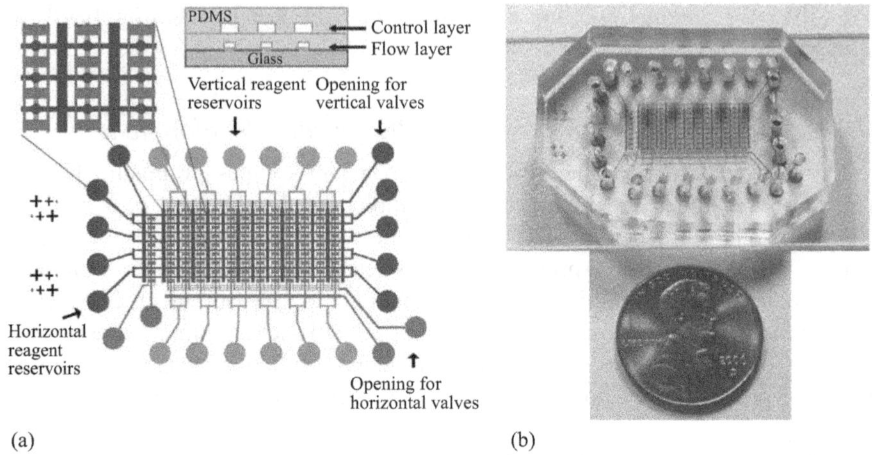

Figure 24.4 Microfluidic SPRi platform. (a) Schematic representation of the microfluidic system of the chip. (b) Picture of the microfluidic system shown on the top displays the vertical positioning of the control and flow layers with channels filled by dyes for visualization. The figure from Reference 69 is published with the kind permission of the Royal Society of Chemistry

Luo *et al.* proposed SPRi-system with signal enlargement by means of conjugates of gold nanoparticles with secondary antibodies for simultaneous detection of interactions on 96 sensor elements (Figure 24.4) [69]. Signal amplification stage allowed for a decrease of detection limit from 0.21 nM to 38 pM for model analyte – biotinylated bovine serum albumin. However, the duration of the analysis increases from 10 min to 1 h. The presented system is of great interest for potential application in non-laboratory diagnostics as it combines compactness, productivity and high sensitivity of the analysis.

In recent years, a new type of the optical sensors having great prospects for non-laboratory application – sensors on the basis of smart phones [70] – has been developed. Overall application and affordable price make these mobile devices an ideal platform for the development of devices for personalized and local diagnostics. One of such devices proposed by Preechaburana et al. is a tiny SPR-sensor with angular modulation [71]. This device is fixed to the smart phone screen so that light reflected from a sensor surface goes to the smart phone camera which becomes the sensor detector (Figure 24.5). A light source is the glow of the screen on which red rectangle is displayed. The coupling device is a replaceable optical element made of polymethylsiloxane (PDMS) and epoxy rubber. Light from the screen is focused on the gold sensor chip by a plano-cylindrical optical element made of PDMS, and, after reflection from sensor, goes to the camera through lenses system. The angle of light ray incidence to the surface depends on location of the pixel which emits this ray. Due to SPR excitation, dark spot is observed on the camera image; and this spot shift is a sensor signal. For reagents supply to the

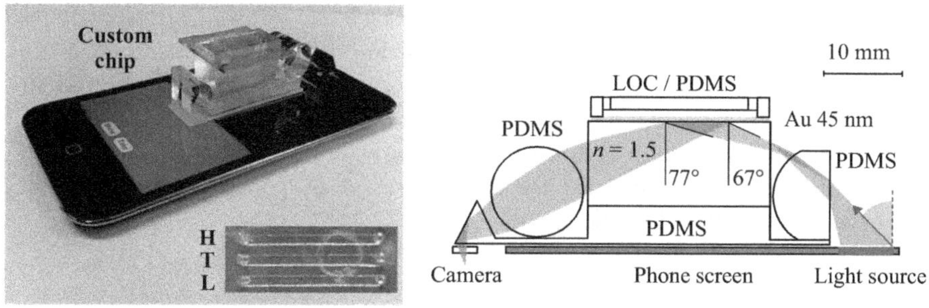

(a) (b)

Figure 24.5 (a) Appearance of SPR-sensor based on cell phone; (b) Raytrace of the experimental arrangement showing the light path from screen to camera (PDMS – polydimethylsiloxane, LOC – lab-on-a-chip). The figure from Reference 71 is published with the kind permission of the Wiley-VCH publisher

sensor surface, special microchannel system is provided in the device. By means of this device, detection of β_2 microglobulin – marker of cancer, inflammatory diseases and diseases of kidneys – has been shown. The sensor resolution is 2.14×10^{-6} RIU and it can compete with resolutions of other portable SPR-sensors.

Smart phones can be used as a basis of portable SPR-sensors with other types of the coupling devices and registration methods. For example, Gallegos *et al.* created an SPR-sensor with wavelength modulation, with plasmons excitation system on the basis of photon crystal – periodic structure with variable refraction index. The device is a smart phone accessory and it can be easily placed in one hand. Application of the developed sensor was shown for detection of immunoglobulin G with concentrations up to 4.25 nM [72].

24.9 Conclusion

Since the first appearance in the market, SPR-sensors have been used extensively in various analytical areas, including medical diagnostics. Possibility of analysis without use of labels, in complex multicomponent matrices, including biological fluids, made this method extremely attractive for identification of pathogens and detection of markers of various diseases. Besides, SPR-sensors allow carrying out of highly efficient analysis with high sensitivity, accuracy and reproducibility. The minimum sample preparation, possibility of automation and replaceable chips with immobilized specific reagents reduces the analysis procedure to a set of simple, not labor-consuming manipulations, which do not require high professional training.

The majority of SPR-analyses is carried out in a laboratory and requires an expensive stationary equipment. However, one of the main tendencies in the development of modern SPR-analytics is an intention to develop miniature and cheap SPR-sensors for non-laboratory application. The last achievements in areas of nanoplasmonics, microfluidics and microelectronics allowed creation of inexpensive and compact devices suitable for application in points of care.

Simplicity of modern portable SPR-devices design and possibility of their integration into widespread mobile devices, make plasmon technologies potentially affordable for a wide range of consumers. Significant progress in the field made in recent years gives opportunities for application of SPR-analysis for local diagnostics and personalized medicine.

Acknowledgments

Authors are grateful to A.E. Urusov (A.N. Bach Institute of Biochemistry, Research Center of Biotechnology of the Russian Academy of Sciences) for preparation of Figures 24.1–24.3 for this manuscript.

This work was financially supported by the Russian Science Foundation (project No 14-14-01131).

References

[1] Pockrand I., Swalen J.D., Gordon J.G., Philpott M.R. 'Surface plasmon spectroscopy of organic monolayer assemblies'. *Surface Science*. 1978;74 (1):237–44.

[2] Gordon J.G., Ernst S. 'Surface plasmons as a probe of the electrochemical interface'. *Surface Science*. 1980;101:499–506.

[3] Nylander C., Liedberg B., Lind T. 'Gas detection by means of surface plasmons resonance'. *Sensors and Actuators*. 1982–1983;3:79–88.

[4] Hart R.M., Bergman J.G., Wokaun A. 'Surface-enhanced Raman scattering from silver particles on polymer-replica substrates'. *Optics Letters*. 1982;7 (3):105–7.

[5] Liedberg B., Nylander C., Lundstrom I. 'Surface plasmons resonance for gas detection and biosensing'. *Sensors and Actuators*. 1983;4:299–304.

[6] Cullen D.C., Brown R.G., Lowe C.R. 'Detection of immuno-complex formation via surface plasmon resonance on gold-coated diffraction gratings'. *Biosensors*. 1987–1988;3(4):211–25.

[7] Schasfoort R.B.M., Tudos A.J. (eds.). *Handbook of Surface Plasmon Resonance*. Cambridge: The Royal Society of Chemistry; 2008, p. 403.

[8] Situ C., Buijs J., Mooney M.H., Elliott C.T. 'Advances in surface plasmon resonance biosensor technology towards high-throughput, food-safety analysis'. *Trends in Analytical Chemistry*. 2010;29(11):1305–15.

[9] Rich R.L., Myszka D.G. 'Grading the commercial optical biosensor literature—class of 2008: 'The Mighty Binders'. *Journal of Molecular Recognition*. 2010;23(1):1–64.

[10] Mariani S., Minunni M. 'Surface plasmon resonance applications in clinical analysis'. *Analytical and Bioanalytical Chemistry*. 2014;406(9):2303–23.

[11] Choi I., Choi Y. 'Plasmonic nanosensors: review and prospect'. *IEEE Journal of Selected Topics in Quantum Electronics*. 2012;18(3):1110–21.
[12] Wood R.W. 'On a remarkable case of uneven distribution of light in a diffraction grating spectrum'. *Philosophical Magazine Series 6*. 1902;4 (21):396–402.
[13] Otto A. 'Excitation of nonradiative surface plasma waves in silver by the method of frustrated total reflection'. *Zeitschrift für Physik*. 1968;216 (4):398–410.
[14] Kretschmann E., Raether H. 'Radiative decay of non-radiative surface plasmons excited by light'. *Zeitschrift für Naturforschung*. 1968;23A:2135–36.
[15] Tokel O., Inci F., Demirci U. 'Advances in plasmonic technologies for point of care applications'. *Chemical Reviews*. 2014;114(11):5728−52.
[16] Li M., Cushing S.K., Wu N. 'Plasmon-enhanced optical sensors: a review'. *Analyst*. 2015;140(2):386–406.
[17] Shalabney A., Abdulhalim I. 'Sensitivity-enhancement methods for surface plasmon sensors'. *Lasers and Photonics Reviews*. 2011;5(4):571–606.
[18] Daghestani H.N., Day B.W. 'Theory and applications of surface plasmon resonance, resonant mirror, resonant waveguide grating, and dual polarization interferometry biosensors'. *Sensors*. 2010;10(11):9630–46.
[19] Palik E. (ed.). *Handbook of Optical Constants of Solids*. New York: Academic Press; 1998; vol. 3, p. 999.
[20] *Biacore Sensor Surface Handbook*. BR-1005-71 edn. Uppsala: GE Healthcare Bio-Sciences AB; 2005.
[21] Yuk J., Hong D.-G., Jung J.-W., *et al.* 'Sensitivity enhancement of spectral surface plasmon resonance biosensors for the analysis of protein arrays'. *European Biophysics Journal*. 2006;35(6):469–76.
[22] Oates T.W.H., Wormeester H., Arwin H. 'Characterization of plasmonic effects in thin films and metamaterials using spectroscopic ellipsometry'. *Progress in Surface Science*. 2011;86(11–12):328–76.
[23] Lakowicz J.R. 'Plasmonics in biology and plasmon-controlled fluorescence'. *Plasmonics*. 2006;1(1):5–33.
[24] De Mol N.J., Fischer M.J.E. (eds.). *Surface Plasmon Resonance. Methods and Protocols*. New York: Springer Science; 2010, p. 286.
[25] Homola J. 'Surface plasmon resonance sensors for detection of chemical and biological species'. *Chemical Reviews*. 2008;108(2):462–93.
[26] Huang Y.H., Ho H.P., Wu S.Y., Kong S.K. 'Detecting phase shifts in surface plasmon resonance: a review [online]'. *Advances in Optical Technologies*. 2012;2012:12. Article ID 471957. Available from http://dx.doi.org/10.1155/2012/471957.
[27] Brongersma M.L., Kik P.G. (eds.). *Surface Plasmon Nanophotonics*. Springer series in optical sciences. vol. 131. Berlin: Springer Science; 2007, p. 268.
[28] Nagata K., Handa H. (eds). *Real-Time Analysis of Biomolecular Interactions: Applications of BIACORE*. Tokio: Springer Science; 2000, p. 256.

[29] Jorgenson R.C., Yee S.S. 'A fiber-optic chemical sensor based on surface plasmon resonance'. *Sensors and Actuators B: Chemical*. 1993;12(3):213–20.

[30] Homola J., Yee S.S., Gauglitz G. 'Surface plasmon resonance sensors: review'. *Sensors and Actuators B: Chemical*. 1999;54(1–2):3–15.

[31] Cullen D.C., Brown R.G., Lowe C.R. 'Detection of immunocomplex formation via surface plasmon resonance on gold coated diffraction gratings'. *Biosensors*. 1987;3(4):211–25.

[32] Cullen D.C., Lowe C.R. 'A direct surface plasmon-polariton immunosensor: preliminary investigation of the non-specific adsorption of serum components to the sensor interface', *Sensors and Actuators B: Chemical*. 1990;1 (1–6):576–79.

[33] Jory M.J., Vukusic P.S., Sambles J.R. 'Development of a prototype gas sensor using surface plasmon resonance on gratings'. *Sensors and Actuators B: Chemical*. 1994;17(3):203–9.

[34] Mayer K.M., Hafner J.H. 'Localized surface plasmon resonance sensors'. *Chemical Reviews*. 2011;111(6):3828–57.

[35] Homola J. (ed.). *Surface Plasmon Resonance Based Sensors*. Springer series on chemical sensors and biosensors. *Series 4*. Berlin: Springer Science; 2006, p. 252.

[36] McNaught A.D., Wilkinson A. (eds). *IUPAC. Compendium of Chemical Terminology (the "Gold Book")*. 2nd edn. Oxford: Blackwell Scientific Publications; 1997, p. 1622.

[37] Inczedy J., Lengyel T., Ure A.M. (eds.). *IUPAC. Compendium of Analytical Nomenclature (the "Orange Book")* [online]. 3rd edn. Oxford: Blackwell Science Publications; 1998, p. 964. Available from http://iupac.org/publications/analytical_compendium/

[38] Hermanson G.T. *Bioconjugate Techniques*. 2nd edn. San Diego: Academic Press; 2008, p. 1202.

[39] D'Agata R., Spoto G. 'Artificial DNA and surface plasmon resonance'. *Artificial DNA: PNA & XNA*. 2012;3(2):45–52.

[40] Luzi E., Minunni M., Tombelli S., Mascini M. 'New trends in affinity sensing: aptamers for ligand binding'. *Trends in Analytical Chemistry*. 2003;22 (11):810–18.

[41] Haupt K., Mosbach K. 'Molecularly imprinted polymers and their use in biomimetic sensors'. *Chemical Reviews*. 2000;100(7):2495–504.

[42] Knoll W., Liley M., Piscevic D., Spinke J., Tarlov M.J. 'Supramolecular architectures for the functionalization of solid surfaces'. *Advances in Biophysics*. 1997;34:231–51.

[43] Brockman J.M., Frutos A.G., Corn R.M. 'A multistep chemical modification procedure to create DNA arrays on gold surfaces for the study of protein-DNA interactions with surface plasmon resonance imaging'. *Journal of the American Chemical Society*. 1999;121(35):8044–51.

[44] D'Agata R., Corradini R., Grasso G., Marchelli R., Spoto G. 'Ultrasensitive detection of DNA by PNA and nanoparticle-enhanced surface plasmon

resonance imaging'. *Chembiochem: A European Journal of Chemical Biology*. 2008;9(13):2067–70.
[45] Fang S., Lee H.J., Wark A.W., Corn R.M. 'Attomole microarray detection of microRNAs by nanoparticle-amplified SPR imaging measurements of surface polyadenylation reactions'. *Journal of the American Chemical Society*. 2006;128(43):14044–6.
[46] Makaraviciute A., Ramanaviciene A. 'Site-directed antibody immobilization techniques for immunosensors'. *Biosensors and Bioelectronics*. 2013;50:460–71.
[47] Egawa Y., Miki R., Seki T. 'Colorimetric sugar sensing using boronic acid-substituted azobenzenes'. *Materials*. 2014;7(2):1201–20.
[48] Chivers C.E., Crozat E., Chu C., Moy V.T. Sherratt D.J., Howarth M., 'A streptavidin variant with slower biotin dissociation and increased mechanostability'. *Nature Methods*. 2010;7(5):391–3.
[49] Šípová H., Homola J. 'Surface plasmon resonance sensing of nucleic acids: a review'. *Analytica Chimica Acta*. 2013;773:9–23.
[50] Luppa P.B., Sokoll L.J., Chan D.W. 'Immunosensors—principles and applications to clinical chemistry'. *Clinica Chimica Acta*. 2001;314(1):1–26.
[51] Mullett W.M., Lai E.P., Yeung J.M. 'Surface plasmon resonance-based immunoassays'. *Methods*. 2000;22(1):77–91.
[52] D'Agata R., Spoto G. 'Surface plasmon resonance imaging for nucleic acid detection'. *Analytical and Bioanalytical Chemistry*. 2013;405(2–3):573–84.
[53] Zhen G., Falconnet D., Kuennemann E., *et al.* 'Nitrilotriacetic acid functionalized graft copolymers: a polymeric interface for selective and reversible binding of histidine-tagged proteins'. *Advanced Functional Materials*. 2006;16(2):243–51.
[54] Rich R.L., Myszka D.G. 'Survey of the year 2007 commercial optical biosensor literature'. *Journal of Molecular Recognition*. 2008;21(6):355–400.
[55] Baird C.L., Myszka D.G., 'Current and emerging commercial optical biosensors'. *Journal of Molecular Recognition*. 2001;14(5):261–8.
[56] Kodoyianni V. 'SPR principles'. *Biotechniques*. 2011;50(1):32–40.
[57] Melendez J.L., Carr R.A., Keller R.C. *Integrally Formed Surface Plasmon Resonance Sensor*. *U.S. Patent* No 5912456. 1997.
[58] Soelberg S.D., Chinowsky T., Geiss G., *et al.* 'A portable surface plasmon resonance sensor system for real-time monitoring of small to large analytes'. *Journal of Industrial Microbiology and Biotechnology*. 2005;32 (11–12):669–74.
[59] Jiang T., Minunni M., Wilson P., Zhang J., Turner A.P., Mascini M. 'Detection of TP53 mutation using a portable surface plasmon resonance DNA-based biosensor'. *Biosensors and Bioelectronics*. 2005;20 (10):1939–45.
[60] Chung J., Kim S., Bernhardt R., Pyun J. 'Application of SPR biosensor for medical diagnostics of human hepatitis B virus (hHBV)'. *Sensors and Actuators B: Chemical*. 2005;111:416–22.

[61] Chinowsky T.M., Soelberg S.D., Baker P., *et al.* 'Portable 24-analyte surface plasmon resonance instruments for rapid, versatile biodetection'. *Biosensors and Bioelectronics*. 2007;22(9):2268–75.
[62] Feltis B., Sexton B., Glenn F., Best M., Wilkins M., Davis T. 'A hand-held surface plasmon resonance biosensor for the detection of ricin and other biological agents'. *Biosensors and Bioelectronics*. 2008;23(7):1131–6.
[63] Zhao S.S., Bukar N., Toulouse J.L., *et al.* 'Miniature multi-channel SPR instrument for methotrexate monitoring in clinical samples'. *Biosensors and Bioelectronics*. 2015;64:664–70.
[64] Ouellet E., Lausted C., Lin T., Yang C.W.T., Hood L., Lagally E.T. 'Parallel microfluidic surface plasmon resonance imaging arrays'. *Lab on a Chip*. 2010;10(5):581–8.
[65] Unser S., Bruzas I., He J., Sagle L. 'Localized surface plasmon resonance biosensing: current challenges and approaches'. *Sensors*. 2015;15(7): 15684–716.
[66] Kwon M.J., Lee J., Wark A.W., Lee H.J. 'Nanoparticle-enhanced surface plasmon resonance detection of proteins at attomolar concentrations: comparing different nanoparticle shapes and sizes'. *Analytical Chemistry*. 2012;84(3):1702–7.
[67] Urusov A.E., Kostenko S.N., Sveshnikov P.G., Zherdev A.V., Dzantiev B.B. Ochratoxin A immunoassay with surface plasmon resonance registration: lowering limit of detection by the use of colloidal gold immunoconjugates. *Sensors and Actuators B: Chemical*. 2011;156(1):343–9.
[68] Zeng S., Baillargeat D., Hod H.-P., Yong K.-T. 'Nanomaterials enhanced surface plasmon resonance for biological and chemical sensing applications'. *Chemical Society Reviews*. 2014;43(10):3426–52.
[69] Luo Y., Yu F., Zare R.N. 'Microfluidic device for immunoassays based on surface plasmon resonance imaging'. *Lab on a Chip*. 2008;8(5):694–700.
[70] Zhang D., Liu Q. 'Biosensors and bioelectronics on smartphone for portable biochemical detection'. *Biosensors and Bioelectronics*. 2016;75: 273–84.
[71] Preechaburana P., Gonzalez M.C., Suska A., Filippini D. 'Surface plasmon resonance chemical sensing on cell phones'. *Angewandte Chemie*. 2012;124 (46):11753–6.
[72] Gallegos D., Long K.D., Yu H., *et al.* 'Label-free biodetection using a smartphone'. *Lab on a Chip*. 2013;13(11):2124–32.

Chapter 25

Methods for monitoring oxidative stress using conventional and advanced nanodiagnostics methods

Pawan Kumar Maurya[1,2], Prabhanshu Kumar[2], Pradeep Kumar[3] and Elisa Brietzke[1]

25.1 Introduction

Oxidative stress (OS) is the imbalance between oxidant producing system and antioxidant defense mechanism resulting in an excessive production of reactive oxygen species (ROS) [1]. Under normal physiological conditions aerobic cells use oxygen as terminal electron acceptor in electron transport chain (ETC) in mitochondria. Mitochondria are the greatest source of ROS [2]. OS is widely recognized as a central feature of many biological processes and diseases, due to their impact on cell injury and death, being involved in aging, neurodegenerative disease, such as Alzheimer's and Parkinson's, neuropsychiatric diseases such as schizophrenia, bipolar, major depressive disorder, cancer [3]. Oxidative adducts derived from carbohydrates, proteins, lipids and DNA, are widely used to measure OS level in biological samples. This includes malonaldehyde (MDA), which is an indicator of lipid peroxidation [4], reduced glutathione (GSH) as an antioxidant and 8-hydroxy-2'-deoxyguanosine (8OHdG) as an indicator of DNA oxidation. Nowadays, the methods used to quantify biomarkers involve complex, expensive and non-portable techniques, which impair a more effective utilization of OS biomarkers as a predictive tool for disease installation.

25.1.1 Oxidants

Oxidants encompass ROS and reactive nitrogen species (RNS), sulfur-centered radicals and various others. ROS/RNS may be radical's or non-radical's (Table 25.1). Generally, the ROS/RNS mediating OS in biological system are

[1]Interdisciplinary Laboratory of Clinical Neuroscience (LiNC), Department of Psychiatry, Federal University of São Paulo, São Paulo, Brazil
[2]Amity Institute of Biotechnology, Amity University Uttar Pradesh, Noida 201303, India
[3]Avram and Stella Goldstein-Goren Department of Biotechnology Engineering, Ben Gurion University, Beer Sheva 84105, Israel

Table 25.1 Reactive oxygen/nitrogen species (ROS/RNS)

Radicals	Non-radicals
Superoxide (O_2^{*-})	Hydrogen peroxide (H_2O_2)
Hydroxyl ($^*OH$)	Singlet oxygen ($^1\Delta O_2$)
Hydroperoxyl (HOO^*)	Hypochlorite (^-OCl)
Alkoxyl {L(R)O^*}	Hydroperoxide {L(R)OOH}
Peroxyl {L(R)OO^*}	Peroxynitrite ($ONOO^-$)
Nitric oxide (NO^*)	

thought to be radicals. These reactive molecules contain one or more unpaired electrons, which react with biomolecules (lipids, proteins, sugars and nucleic acids). There are certain other reactive molecules which are derived from oxygen and lack unpaired electrons are referred as non-radical molecules, such as hydrogen peroxide (H_2O_2), singlet oxygen ($^1\Delta O_2$), having anti-parallel spin of two electrons, is highly reactive molecule [5]. They are as follow:

The ROS/RNS can be generated in both endogenous and exogenous ways.

25.1.1.1 Endogenous

i. Formation of ROS by incomplete reduction of oxygen in ETC of mitochondria.
ii. The host defense system, which includes the 'oxidative burst' mediated by nicotinamide adenine dinucleotide phosphate hydrogen (NADPH) oxidase, generating superoxide radicals, and myeloperoxidase, leading to the formation of hypochlorous acids.
iii. Nitric oxide is synthesized by group of enzymes referred as nitric oxide synthase, which catalyses the conversion of an amino acid, L-arginine into nitric oxide radical (NO^*) and L-citrulline. In the presence of oxygen and superoxide, NO^* is converted to more reactive species, such as nitrogen dioxide and peroxynitrite.

25.1.1.2 Exogenous

Ultraviolet radiation, smoking, various drugs

25.1.2 Antioxidants

According to definition, antioxidants are molecules which, when present in small concentration compared to the biomolecules they are supposed to protect, can prevent or reduce the extent of oxidative destruction of biomolecules [6] (Table 25.2).

The assay of OS parameters has brought significant insight into pathophysiology of many diseases in humans by signifying the involvement of ROS/RNS and/or the decrease of antioxidant status of organism [7]. Free radicals/ROS/RNS represents a significant mechanism of tissue damage, which often operated synergistically with proteases and leukocytes phagocytes.

Table 25.2 List of antioxidants and their mechanism of action

S. No.	Antioxidants (enzymatic & non-enzymatic)	Mechanism of action
1	Super oxide dismutase (SOD)	Catalyses conversion of superoxide radical into hydrogen peroxide (H_2O_2)
2	Catalase (CAT)	Convert H_2O_2 in to H_2O
3	Glutathione peroxidase (GPx)	Convert H_2O_2 in to H_2O by utilizing reduced glutathione (GSH)
4	Glutathione reductase (GR)	Reduction of oxidized glutathione (GSSG) to reduced form (GSH)
5	Glutathione (GSH)	Radical scavenger and substrate for GPx
6	Ascorbic acid (AA)	Radical scavenger
7	Uric acid	Radical scavenger
8	Bilirubin	Radical scavenger
9	Albumin	Binds heme, Cu^{2+}, scavenger of HOCl
10	α & γ- Tocopherol	Peroxyl radical scavenger

Monitoring OS in humans can be done indirectly by assaying product of oxidative damage or by investigating the antioxidant potential of an organism, tissue or body fluids to withstand further oxidation. Recent advances in nanotechnology lead to development on new diagnostic methods for monitoring OS status of organism using nanodiagnostic methods [8, 9]. In this chapter, we will therefore deal with both conventional and nanodiagnostic methods for measuring OS. We will restrict our self to the more recent development in this field.

25.2 Conventional methods for monitoring oxidative stress

25.2.1 Determination of total antioxidant activity

Antioxidant status of the body is an indicator of OS, and in many cases reduced antioxidant capacity of the body is a consequence of increased OS.

25.2.1.1 Ferric reducing ability of plasma (FRAP) assay

The basic principle behind this method is the reduction of ferric ion a complex with 2,4,6- tri[2-pyridyl]-s-triazine to a colored ferrous complex. Hence this assay measures the ability of sample to reduce ferric ion complex. This method can be easily automated, highly reproducible, and linear. It is not so much influenced by protein albumin, which is an important antioxidant in plasma.

The ferric reducing ability of plasma (FRAP) values were determined following the method of Benzie and Strain [10]. Working FRAP reagent was prepared by mixing acetate buffer (300 mM, pH 3.6], 2,4,6- tri[2-pyridyl]-s-triazine (10 mM in 40 mM HCl) solution and $FeCl_3.6H_2O$ (20 mmol/l) solution in 10:1:1 ratio, respectively. Three milliliter of FRAP reagent was mixed with 100 μl of plasma; the content was mixed vigorously for making uniform solution. The absorbance was read at 593 nm at the interval of 30 s for 4 min. Aqueous solution of known

Fe^{2+} concentration in the range of 100–1000 μmol/l was used for calibration. Using the regression equation the FRAP values (μmol Fe (II) per liter) of the plasma is calculated.

25.2.1.2 Total peroxyl radical-trapping potential (TRAP) assay

This assay measures the time required to use up the antioxidant in the sample challenged with a constant flux of peroxyl radical generated by ABAP, AAPH or AMVN. This method was originally proposed by Wayner *et al.* [11].

25.2.2 Method for monitoring lipid peroxidation

Lipid peroxidations are generally free radical chain reaction which induces the oxidation of polyunsaturated fatty acids (PUFA) [12]. PUFAs (linoleic, linolenic and arachidonic acid) are the fatty acids having double bond in there structure and are ready target for free radicals. Cell membranes are made of protein lipid bilayer structure and lipids constitute major portion of PUFA. Lipid peroxidation is initiated by abstraction of hydrogen atom from reactive methylene group of PUFA. The initiation is usually performed by a radical (R^*). Molecular oxygen rapidly adds to the carbon-centered radical (R^*) forming lipid peroxyl radical (LOO^*), which in turn can abstract a hydrogen from another PUFA and form comparatively stable lipid hydroperoxide (LOOH). The reaction scheme is shown in (25.1).

$$\begin{aligned} &LH + R^* \longrightarrow L^* + RH \\ &L^* + O2 \longrightarrow LOO^* \\ &LH + LOO^* \longrightarrow L^* + \end{aligned} \tag{25.1}$$

MDA is one of the lipid peroxidation products. MDA was measured according to the method of Esterbauer and Cheeseman [13]. Packed erythrocytes/plasma/serum were suspended in 3 ml Krebs'–Ringer phosphate buffer (KRP), pH 7.4. The lysate (1 ml) was added to 1 ml of 10% trichloroacetic acid (TCA) and mixture was centrifuged for 5 min at 1000 g. The supernatant (1 ml) was added to 1 ml of 0.67% thiobarbituric acid (TBA) in 0.05 mol/l NaOH and boiled for 20 min at temperature greater than 900 °C, cooled and the absorbance read at 532 nm (OD1) and 600 nm (OD2). The net optical density (OD) was calculated after subtracting absorbance at OD2 from that at OD1. The concentration of MDA in erythrocytes was determined from a standard plot.

25.2.3 Measurement of redox status – reduced glutathione (GSH)/oxidized glutathione (GSSG) ratio

Reduced glutathione (GSH; γ-Glu-Cys-Gly) is a tripeptide, made up of glutamic acid, cysteine and glycine amino acids. It is a major intracellular non-protein sulfhydryl compound and is accepted as the most important intracellular hydrophilic antioxidant. It is present intracellularly in millimolar concentration, in human plasma in micromolar concentration [14]. Reduced glutathione has many biological functions, including maintenance of membrane protein –SH groups in the reduced form, the oxidation of which can otherwise cause altered cellular structure and function. GSH is oxidized to its disulfide (GSSG); hence, this ratio may be used in the identification of OS in cells/tissues. GSH/GSSG ratio has been linked to OS in various diseases including Alzheimer's disease, cancer and aging [15].

Total GSH was determined using a kinetic assay involving continuous reduction of 5, 5'-dithiobis, 2-nitrobenzoic acid (DTNB) by GSH in the presence of NADPH, forming 2-nitro-5-thiobenzoic acid, which was read at 412 nm. GSSG was determined in hemolysate following the method of Tietze [16]. GSH and GSSG levels are reported in μM/g Hb. Standard curve was determined with freshly prepared standard solution of 33 mM GSSG.

25.3 Measurement of oxidative status using various oxidative stress biomarkers

25.3.1 Determination of acetylcholinesterase activity

Acetylcholinesterase plays a crucial role in memory, learning and movement [17]. Broadly acetylcholinesterase can be divided into two major classes based on their solubilization properties into a hydrophilic or asymmetric (collagen tailed) and hydrophobic or globular form of the enzyme. Asymmetric form of the enzyme contains a collagen like tail and is soluble only in buffers of high ionic strength. The tail is responsible for the attachment of the active sites of the enzymes to the basement membrane and also to form aggregate of the enzymes, these cleaved globular forms of enzymes are soluble in buffers of low ionic strength. Hydrophobic or globular form of the enzyme acetylcholinesterase is the one, which is soluble only in buffers supplemented with detergent, and these do not contain collagen like tails. It is found that acetylcholinesterase is dependent on amphiphilic surrounding for its full catalytic activity. Enzyme acetylcholinesterase is considered as a proteinase-activated protein kinase and its activity is maintained by the surrounding medium of proteins containing hydrophobic segments. At higher concentration, more than 2.5 mg/ml the acetylcholinesterase do not need amphiphile for their maximum catalytic activity, they themselves aggregate with proteins to form acetylcholinesterase-protein-micelles which gives them the hydrophobic interaction for the full catalytic activity. It is considered as an important biomarker of OS.

Acetylcholinesterase activity was estimated as described previously [18]. The final assay mixture (5 ml) contained 0.1 M Tris-HCl, 0.5 mM EDTA (pH 8.0), 0.025 mM DTNB in 0.1% sodium citrate and 0.05 ml of 1:20 red cell hemolysate. After pre-incubation for 10 min at 37 °C the reaction was initiated by adding 0.25 ml of 10 mM acetylthiocholine iodide. The increase in the OD of the system was measured against that of the blank at 412 nm for 10–15 min.

The OD of the blank prepared by substituting the volume of hemolysate used by 1:10 diluted β−mercaptoethanol-EDTA stabilizing solution was also read for 5–10 min at 412 nm and the blank rate was subtracted from the rate measured in the presence of hemolysate. The reaction process is shown in (25.2).

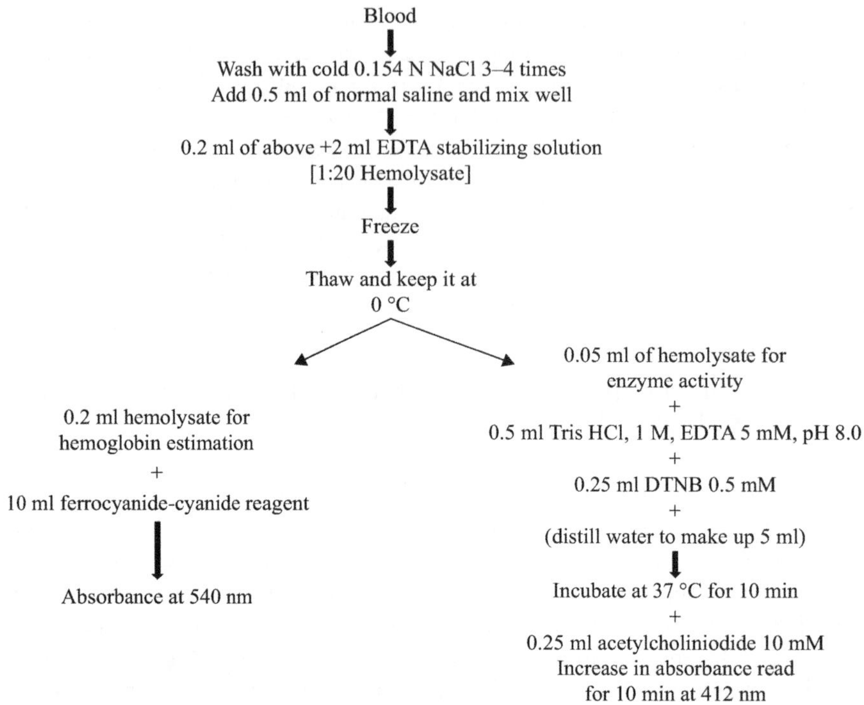

Figure 25.1 Flow chart for estimation of acetylcholinesterase activity

$$\begin{aligned}
&\text{Acetylthiocholinesterase}\\
&\text{Acetylthiocholineiodide} \longrightarrow \text{thiocholineiodide} + \text{acetate ion}\\
&\text{Thiocholineiodide} + \text{DTNB} \longrightarrow \text{5-thio-2-nitrobenzoic acid}\\
&\qquad\qquad\qquad\qquad\qquad + \text{oxidized thiocholineiodide}
\end{aligned} \tag{25.2}$$

5-thio-2-nitrobenzoate ion imparts yellow color to the assay medium having maximum absorption at 412 nm. A molar extinction coefficient of 1.36×10^{-4} l/mol/cm was used for the thionitrobenzoate ion at 412 nm. Activity of acetylcholinesterase is expressed as I.U., i.e., micro-mole of acetylthiocholineiodide hydrolyzed per gram of hemoglobin at 37 °C per hour. A detailed flow diagram for the estimation of acetylcholinesterase activity is shown in Figure 25.1.

25.3.2 Determination of membrane sulfhydryl (–SH) group

The importance of the –SH group in overall cellular redox balance has been emphasized. Membrane oxidative damage has a considerable effect on membrane mechanical properties. Membrane –SH group oxidative damage may be an important molecular mechanism inducing changes in the membrane microelasticity or whole cell deformability under conditions of physiological and pathological OS [4].

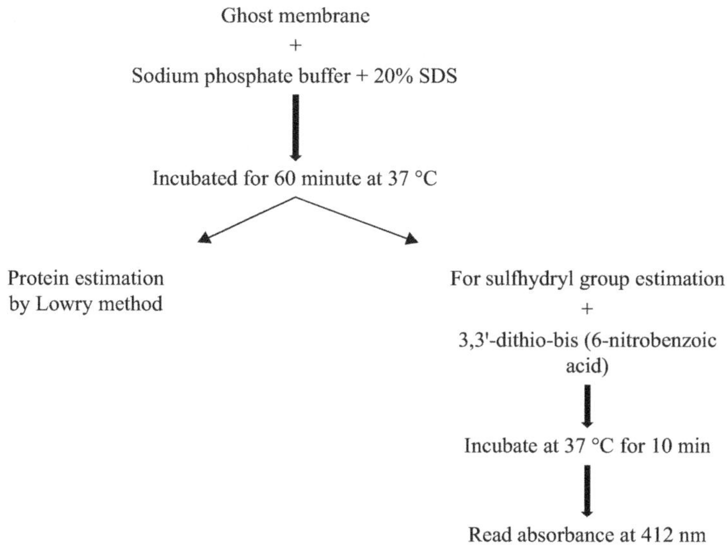

Figure 25.2 Flow chart for the estimation of membrane sulfhydryl (–SH) group

Membrane –SH was determined following the method as described by Kitajima *et al.* [19]. Ghost membrane (0.2 ml) was mixed with 2.8 ml of 0.1 M sodium phosphate buffer containing 0.1m MEDTA pH (8.0). To this was added 0.3 ml of 20 % SDS mixed and the above mixture was incubated at 37 °C for 60 min. After incubation the solution was divided into two parts of 3 ml and 0.3 ml. To 3 ml, of the solution 0.1 ml of DTNB (0.1M) was added and again incubated for 15 min at 37 °C and its observation was read at 412 nm against reference blank which did not contain ghost membrane. 0.3 ml of solution was used for estimation of protein content following the method of Lowry *et al.* [20], using bovine serum albumin as the standard whose absorbance was read at 620 nm. Sulfhydryl group in membrane reduces 5'5-dithiobis 2-nitrobenzoic acid (DTNB) forming a yellow colored anionic product, whose OD is measured at 412 nm. A molar extinction coefficient of 13600 was used when –SH group reacts with DTNB. The concentration of –SH group is expressed in terms of nanomoles per milligram of protein (nM/mg of protein). The process for the estimation of membrane sulfhydryl (–SH) group is shown in Figure 25.2.

25.3.3 Determination of protein carbonyl content

Proteins are targets of various post-translational deleterious modifications, which are altering their biological functions. ROS and RNS, originating from oxidative metabolism as well as other toxic compounds such as dicarbonyl and reactive aldehydes, are mainly responsible for these damages [21]. Increased protein carbonyl content is a hallmark of cellular and organismal aging [22]. Protein damage leading to the formation of carbonyl groups derives from direct oxidation of several amino acid side chains but can also derive through protein adducts formation with lipid peroxidation products and dicarbonyl glycating compounds.

Carbonyl group content was determined following the method as described by Levine *et al.* [23], using the 2'4 di-nitro phenyl hydrazine (DNPH) assay with slight modification. Approximately 1 mg of protein was precipitated with 20% TCA (1:1 vol/vol) in Eppendorf tube and vortexed for 30 s. After centrifugation the clear supernatant was discarded and pellet was re-suspended with 0.5 ml of 10 mM DNPH in 2 M HCl and allowed to stand at room temperature for 60 min. Vortexing at every 5 min intervals, to facilitate the reaction of DNPH with pellet proteins. The protein was precipitated again with 20% TCA and then the precipitated protein (pellet) was washed three times with 1.0 ml of 1:1(vol/vol) ethanol: ethyl acetate mixture. Finally the pellets were dissolved in 0.7 ml of 6 M guanidine hydrochloride at 37 °C. After centrifugation for 5 min at 6000 g to precipitate the insoluble material, the clear supernatant was read against a complimentary blank at their maximum absorbance of 365 nm. Parallel blank was also run with the same procedure using 2 M HCl alone instead of 2,4 DNPH reagent. Carbonyl group content is expressed in nanomoles per milligram of protein using a molar absorbance coefficient of 22000 mol/l/cm. The process for the estimation of protein carbonyl content is shown in Figure 25.3.

Ghost membrane
+
Sodium phosphate buffer + 20% SDS

↓

Incubated for 60 min at 37 °C

↓

20% TCA
Vortexed and centrifuged
Supernatant discarded

↓

Pellets suspended in 10 mM DNPH (0.5 ml)

↓

Incubate at room temperature for 60 min
(Vortexed at 5 minute intervals)

↓

Precipitated with 1 ml 20% TCA
Pellets wash three times with Ethanol:Ethyl acetate mixture (1:1)

↓

Pellets dissolved in 1ml 6 M Guanidine hydrochloride
Centrifuge at 5000 rpm for 5 min

↓

Read absorbance at 365 nm

Figure 25.3 Flow chart for the estimation of protein carbonyl content

25.3.4 Determination of red blood cell osmotic fragility

Erythrocyte membrane stability can be affected by various factors. It may be the osmolarity of suspending medium, hemoglobin content, hematocrit value and turn over. OS results, in change in composition of membrane i.e. breakdown of lipids, proteins and other component of membrane which decreases the membrane stability.

Osmotic fragility (OF) experiments were performed by preparing hypotonic phosphate buffer solutions (PBS) equivalent to 0.10% to 0.85% NaCl by diluting stock phosphate buffer saline. Phosphate buffer saline was prepared and experiment performed according to the method of Dacie and Lewis [24], except that the extent of hemolysis was measured colorimetrically at 540 nm instead of a yellow green filter. Stock Phosphate buffer saline was made by dissolving 25 g NaCl, 6.825 g Na_2HPO4 and 1.215 g $NaH_2PO_4{\cdot}2H_2O$ in 500 ml distilled water to make a solution osmolarity equivalent to 10% NaCl which was diluted by distilled water to make hypotonic solution of varying concentration. Heparinized blood was added to hypotonic solutions of varying concentrations of NaCl (PBS) in the proportion of 1 to 100. Generally 0.5 ml of the blood was added to 5.0 ml of the phosphate buffer saline and thoroughly mixed. After keeping it at room temperature for 30 min the hypotonic solutions were centrifuged for 5 min at 3500 rpm in a clinical centrifuge. The OD of the supernatant was determined at 540 nm by using supernatant of 0.85% NaCl (PBS) hypotonic solution in which undetectable lysis took place as blank. The supernatant of 0.1% NaCl (PBS) hypotonic solution in which maximum lysis took place was arbitrarily delimited to have shown 100% lysis. Extent of hemolysis was calculated by dividing the absorbance of varying hypotonic solution by absorbance of solution showing maximum hemolysis (0.1 % NaCl (PBS)) (25.3).

$$\text{Extent of hemolysis} = \frac{\text{OD of supernatant of NaCl (PBS)}\,\% \times 100}{\text{OD of supernatant with maximum lysis}(0.1\%\,\text{NaCl})} \tag{25.3}$$

The erythrocyte hemolysis curve was prepared by plotting percent of NaCl solution on *X*-axis and percent hemolysis on *Y*-axis the osmolytic curve represents the cumulative frequency of the individual erythrocyte fragility present in the blood under study and on the osmolarity curve the percent of NaCl (PBS) in which 50% hemolysis of the cells take place represents the fragility of the maximum numbers of the cell and is expressed as mean erythrocyte fragility.

25.4 Advanced nanodiagnostic methods for monitoring oxidative stress

The OS is associated with the diminished capacity of antioxidant system to counteract an overproduction of free radicals in the form of ROS/RNS. Since OS damages biomolecules and leads to genetic disorders, diabetes, cancer, Alzheimer's and Parkinson's disease, there is urging need for OS monitoring using advanced nanodiagnostic methods, so that its prevention can be possible. Several biomarkers of OS have been identified, including glutathione (GSH), membrane –SH group, 3-nitrotyrosine (NT), homocysteine (Hcys), and cysteine (Cys) [25]. While these biomarkers can be accurately determined using advanced instrumental assay, a wide screening would require the development of small, inexpensive, rapid and simple in operation platforms for biomarker analysis.

Electrochemical methods have also been used to their simplicity, rapidity, high sensitivity, and low cost. These include the reduction of GSSG on a hanging mercury drop electrode, carbon nanotube modified electrode and a nanoscale copper hydroxide composite carbon ionic liquid electrode. The advantage of electrochemical method is that they can be miniaturized for in vivo measurement. Micro-biosensors for in vivo measurement offer several advantages such as rapid response time of a few second, small feature sizes, capable of running a small sample volume. In recent years, considerable progress has been made in the application of enzyme-based micro-biosensors to neurophysiology measurements such as dopamine, ATP and adenosine. Though these micro-biosensors provide a unique way to explore the microenvironments, there are limitations to be considered when designing them.

25.4.1 Gold nanoparticle based assay for biomarker of oxidative stress

The biomolecule-induced gold nanoparticles assembly process can be monitored using surface plasmon (SP) absorbance and SP band shift. The oscillation frequency of the local SP is very sensitive to the change in dielectric environment of nanoparticles and distance between nanoparticle [9]. The collective oscillation of local SPs is excited when the distance between d between gold nanoparticles (AuNP) is: $d < 5r$, where r is the AuNP radius. Theoretical studies of plasmonic oscillations and SP absorbance spectra have enabled the understanding of mechanisms leading to the absorbance maximum shifts associated with the assembly process.

25.4.2 Detection of glutathione using biosensor

Glutathione is an important thiol tripeptide consisting of three amino acids, viz., glutamic acid, cysteine and glycine. It exists in two forms, reduced form (GSH) and other is in oxidized form (GSSG). In healthy living cells more than 90% of glutathione exist in reduced state, however, pathological conditions causing OS result in the conversion of GSH to GSSG. The high concentration of GSSG is associated with asthma and even during normal aging [15]. The analysis of these biomarkers of OS becomes key factor for preventive treatment [26]. Since the main redox potential maintaining system in eukaryotic cell homeostasis is the ratio of GSH/GSSG redox couple, therefore, the analysis of the GSH and GSSG concentration in the body is important because it provides a sensitive index of whole body OS, as well as being helpful in the diagnosis of certain clinical disorder. A range of methods have been used to detect GSH and GSSG which include the microplate reader assay, fluorometry, calorimetry and high performance liquid chromatography (HPLC). However these methods require an additional, time consuming derived step.

The pioneering works in developing immunosensors for GSH have been done by Cliffel and coworkers [27]. They have immobilized the anti-GSH antibody (Ab) on a protein. A layer adsorbed nonspecifically on a gold electrode. The response to GSH conjugate was monitored by recording the oscillation frequency of the quartz piezoresonator substrate. Immunosensor design is based on the bio-recognition principle with an anti-GSH monoclonal Ab immobilized covalently with AHT basal SAM through an EDC-activated reaction. The anti-GSH Ab molecule were immobilized on a thiol SAM via amide bond between carboxylic groups of the fragment crystallizable region (Fc) stem of an Ab and amine groups of the thiol. To control nonspecific binding, the electrodes were incubated with 0.001% BSA solution.

In vivo detection of GSSG using biosensor was reported by Noh *et al.* [26]. The microbiosensor was examined to detect in vivo GSSG. It has been reported that GSSG is reduced to GSH in the presence of β-nicotinamide adenine dinucleotide phosphate (NADPH) and glutathione reductase (GR). Thus, NADPH and GR can be used as material to fabricate a biosensor for GSSG detection. Conducting polymers are widely used in the fabrication of biosensors because biomolecules can be covalently immobilized onto the conjugated polymer layers as they contain functional groups such as carboxylic (–COOH) or amine ($-NH_2$). The polymers, though biocompatible, are limited in use as base substrate for biosensors due to their low conductivity. Hence gold nanoparticles (AuNPs) can be used for modifying the polymer layers to enhance the sensitivity of the biosensor. The biosensor probe was fabricated by immobilizing GR and NADPH through covalent bonding on a carboxylic acid group-functionalized conducting polymers layer on the AuNPs deposited glassy carbon electrode (GCE). The immobilization of GR and NADPH on the conducting polymer layer was confirmed using X-ray photon spectroscopy (XPS), a quartz crystal microbalance (QCM), cyclic voltammetry (CV) and linear sweep voltammetry (LSV). The fabricated biosensor was applied to detect GSSG with LSV and chronoamperometry. Experimental parameters were optimized and the detection limit of GSSG was determined. The developed biosensor was successfully examined for spiked GSSG concentration in plasma samples. An in vivo microbiosensors was also fabricated by similar fabrication steps using a Pt microelectrode and successfully applied for GSSG detection in Sprague-Dawley rats treated with diquat and t-butyl hydroperoxide (t-BHP) to monitor OS, which was reflected by high concentration of GSSG.

25.4.3 Detection of 3-nitro-L-tyrosine (3NT) using solid phase extraction (SPE) sorbent material

The 3-nitro-L-tyrosine (3NT) is an OS biomarker associated with neurodegenerative disorders (Figure 25.4). Nitration of aromatic ring of free and protein-bound tyrosine residue is a major product of the peroxinitrite attack, a powerful oxidant produced by inflammatory cells, compromising the integrity and the functionality of proteins causing DNA damage and cell dysfunction. As a result, 3NT is a stable end product proposed as biomarker of oxidative damage mediated by peroxinitrite. Increased levels of free 3NT have been detected in neurodegenerative

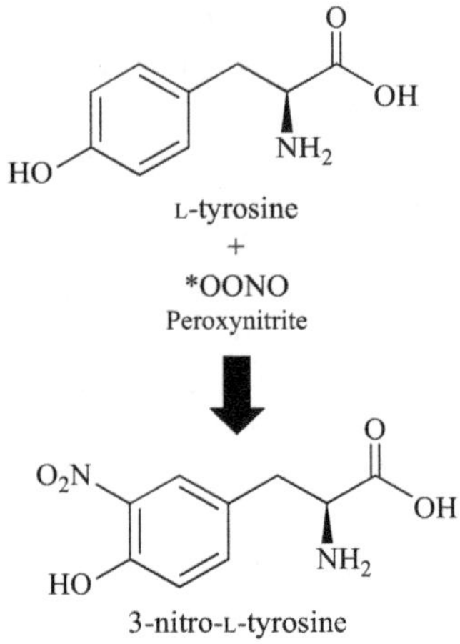

Figure 25.4 Nitration of tyrosine by peroxynitrite

tissue and also in biological fluids of patients with neurological disorders such as Parkinson's disease. Recent studies suggest a direct neurotoxic role of this modified amino acid that can cause a selective loss of dopamine neurons, but the molecular mechanism of this toxic effect in unknown.

Several highly sensitive methodologies have been employed to identify and quantify 3NT both in biological fluids and tissue including gas chromatography-mass spectrometry, gas chromatography-tandem mass spectrometry and high performance liquid chromatography coupled to mass, tandem mass or electrochemical detectors.

Immunological techniques have been widely used to detect 3NT mainly in tissue and biological fluids but their use can only be semiqualitative due to the cross-reactivity with other compounds present in the complex matrices such as biological fluids and the natural antibodies exhibit poor stability and require long production time and high cost. Researchers are focusing on the production of artificial antibodies able to selectively bind a target analyte with the same sensitivity of the natural antibodies but with simple steps and low cost production. Molecular imprinting technology (MIT) is today a viable synthetic approach to design robust molecular recognition elements able to recognize target biomolecules at molecular level, mimicking natural recognition entities, such as antibodies and biological receptors. Mergola *et al.* for the first time reported that the synthesis of a selective molecularly imprinted polymer (MIP) used as solid phase extraction (SPE) sorbent for the selective clean up and pre-concentration of 3NT from biological samples [28]. The polymer was prepared by bulk polymerization using methacrylic acid (MAA) as functional monomer and acetonitrile (MeCN) as porogen with traces of acetic acid (HoAc) and trifluroacetic acid (TFA). In order to evaluate its binding properties, the MIP was analyzed by batch rebinding experiments and subsequently used as SPE sorbent for the selective extraction of 3NT from human urine

25.4.4 Microsensor arrays

Analysis of glutathione OS biomarker can be done with accurate advanced instrumental techniques; there is a need for the development of inexpensive, field-deployable analytical platforms for disease screening and protection against environmental exposure [29]. The application of microsensor for monitoring of OS has been discussed [30].

Each of the microsensors consisted of interdigitated electrode and one reference electrode. The entire chip surface was isolated with the exception of small exposed area for contact with electrolyte. The sensor was arranged in a group of sis sensor on chip. One of the electrodes of each interdigitated pair was connected to the common and the other had an independent connection. This arrangement enabled measurements of voltametric characteristics, as well as monitoring of lateral conductance independently in each sensory film with reduced number of interconnections.

25.4.5 Detection of 8-hydroxy-2'-deoxyguanosine (8OHdG) using immunosensor

Immunosensors combine an Ab as biological recognition element with a transducer signaling device that follows the binding of free antigen (Ag) present in the solution under analysis and the Ab anchored to a solid support. The transducer convert electrical, optical, mass or heat changes of the solution into a measurable signal. A critical step in immunosensor design is the immobilization of the Ab on the solid support. Many approaches for immobilizing antibodies on a solid support lead to random orientation of these proteins all over the modified surface, creating supports of low density binding sites and decreased binding affinity. Ferreira and Sales propose a different and simpler immunosensor design, by activating the carboxylic groups at Fc region and coupling these directly to an amine functionalized surface [31]. This carboxylic activation process has been employed for decades for protein covalent binding and is expected to be compatible with protein structure, therefore preventing significant loss of activity of Ab. This concept is applied to an electrochemical impedance spectroscopy (EIS) transduction, a direct and label-free method for probing protein binding events such as those from Ab–Ag interactions. It offers fast, accurate, sensitive and selective and quantitative responses, coupled with portability, low cost and minimal power requirements. EIS is also independent from sample turbidity or optical pathway, widening the range of sample to which it may be applied.

25.5 Conclusion and the future

In hospitals and clinical laboratories, practically no measurements of OS parameters are the part of routine analysis for the diagnosis of diseases. Gaps exist between the findings from experimental data and clinical research and application of free radical activity measurement in various disease conditions. We have demonstrated conventional and advanced nanodiagnostic methods for monitoring biomarkers of the OS. The interaction of small molecules such as glutathione, malonaldehyde, membrane –SH groups with nanoparticles are important in view of novel biomedical applications of nanoparticles for diagnosis and therapeutic purpose, as well as for the development of biosensors with metal nanoparticle enhanced responsiveness. Novel sensing platform have been explored for the detection of OS biomarkers.

Acknowledgment

PKM acknowledges support by fellowship (Science without Borders – Level A) from coordination of Improvement of Higher Education Personnel (CAPES), National Counsel of Technological and Scientific Development (CNPq), Brazil.

List of abbreviations

ROS	reactive oxygen species
RNS	reactive nitrogen species
OS	oxidative stress
H_2O_2	hydrogen peroxide
$^1O_2$	singlet oxygen
Q_2^*	superoxide radical
$^*OH$	hydroxyl radical
NO	nitric oxide
FRAP	ferric reducing ability of plasma
8OHdG	8-hydroxy-2’-deoxyguanosine
MDA	malonaldehyde
AuNP	gold nanoparticle
SP	surface plasmon
XPS	X-ray photon spectroscopy
QCM	quartz crystal microbalance
CV	cyclic voltammetry
LSV	linear sweep voltammetry

References

[1] Harman D. Origin and evolution of the free radical theory of aging: a brief personal history, 1954–2009. *Biogerontology*. 2009;10(6):773–81.

[2] Miles SL, McFarland M, Niles RM. Molecular and physiological actions of quercetin: need for clinical trials to assess its benefits in human disease. *Nutr Rev*. 2014;72(11):720–34.

[3] Maurya PK, Noto C, Rizzo LB, et al. The role of oxidative and nitrosative stress in accelerated aging and major depressive disorder. *ProgNeuropsychopharmacolBiol Psychiatry*. 2016;65:134–44.

[4] Rizvi SI, Maurya PK. Markers of oxidative stress in erythrocytes during aging in humans. *Ann N Y Acad Sci*. 2007;1100:373–82.

[5] Phaniendra A, Jestadi DB, Periyasamy L. Free radicals: properties, sources, targets, and their implication in various diseases. *Indian J Clin Biochem*. 2015;30(1):11–26.

[6] Halliwell B. How to characterize a biological antioxidant. *Free Radic Res Commun*. 1990;9(1):1–32.

[7] Bhat AH, Dar KB, Anees S, *et al*. Oxidative stress, mitochondrial dysfunction and neurodegenerative diseases; a mechanistic insight. *Biomed Pharmacother*. 2015;74:101–10.

[8] Elgrabli D, Dachraoui W, Menard-Moyon C, *et al*. Carbon nanotube degradation in macrophages: live nanoscale monitoring and understanding of biological pathway. *ACS Nano*. 2015;9(10):10113–24.

[9] Yasmin Z, Khachatryan E, Lee YH, Maswadi S, Glickman R, Nash KL. In vitro monitoring of oxidative processes with self-aggregating gold nanoparticles using all-optical photoacoustic spectroscopy. *Biosens Bioelectron*. 2015;64:676–82.

[10] Benzie IF, Strain JJ. The ferric reducing ability of plasma (FRAP) as a measure of "antioxidant power": the FRAP assay. *Anal Biochem*. 1996;239 (1):70–6.

[11] Wayner DD, Burton GW, Ingold KU, Locke S. Quantitative measurement of the total, peroxyl radical-trapping antioxidant capability of human blood plasma by controlled peroxidation. The important contribution made by plasma proteins. *FEBS Lett*. 1985;187(1):33–7.

[12] Ansari FA, Ali SN, Mahmood R. Sodium nitrite-induced oxidative stress causes membrane damage, protein oxidation, lipid peroxidation and alters major metabolic pathways in human erythrocytes. *Toxicol In Vitro*. 2015;29 (7):1878–86.

[13] Esterbauer H, Cheeseman KH. Determination of aldehydic lipid peroxidation products: malonaldehyde and 4-hydroxynonenal. *Methods Enzymol*. 1990;186:407–21.

[14] Szabo S, Nagy L, Plebani M. Glutathione, protein sulfhydryls and cysteine proteases in gastric mucosal injury and protection. *Clin Chim Acta*. 1992;206 (1–2):95–105.

[15] Kumar P, Maurya PK. L-cysteine efflux in erythrocytes as a function of human age: correlation with reduced glutathione and total anti-oxidant potential. *Rejuvenation Res*. 2013;16(3):179–84.

[16] Tietze F. Enzymic method for quantitative determination of nanogram amounts of total and oxidized glutathione: applications to mammalian blood and other tissues. *Anal Biochem*. 1969;27(3):502–22.

[17] Swapna I, SathyaSaikumar KV, Murthy Ch R, Gupta AD, Senthilkumaran B. Alterations in kinetic and thermotropic properties of cerebral membrane-bound acetylcholineesterase during thioacetamide-induced hepatic encephalopathy: correlation with membrane lipid changes. *Brain Res*. 2007;1153:188–95.

[18] Antokhin AM, Gainullina ET, Ryzhikov SB, Taranchenko VF, Yavaeva DK. Rapid method for measurement of acetylcholinesterase activity. *Bull Exp Biol Med*. 2009;147(1):109–10.

[19] Kitajima H, Yamaguchi T, Kimoto E. Hemolysis of human erythrocytes under hydrostatic pressure is suppressed by cross-linking of membrane proteins. *J Biochem*. 1990;108(6):1057–62.

[20] Lowry OH, Rosebrough NJ, Farr AL, Randall RJ. Protein measurement with the Folin phenol reagent. *J Biol Chem*. 1951;193(1):265–75.

[21] Fedorova M, Bollineni RC, Hoffmann R. Protein carbonylation as a major hallmark of oxidative damage: update of analytical strategies. *Mass Spectrom Rev*. 2014;33(2):79–97.

[22] Baraibar MA, Ladouce R, Friguet B. Proteomic quantification and identification of carbonylated proteins upon oxidative stress and during cellular aging. *J Proteomics*. 2013;92:63–70.

[23] Levine RL, Garland D, Oliver CN, et al. Determination of carbonyl content in oxidatively modified proteins. *Methods Enzymol*. 1990;186:464–78.

[24] Delano MD. Simple physical constraints in hemolysis. *J Theor Biol*. 1995;175(4):517–24.

[25] Stobiecka M, Hepel M. Effect of buried potential barrier in label-less electrochemical immunodetection of glutathione and glutathione-capped gold nanoparticles. *Biosens Bioelectron*. 2011;26(8):3524–30.

[26] Noh HB, Chandra P, Moon JO, Shim YB. In vivo detection of glutathione disulfide and oxidative stress monitoring using a biosensor. *Biomaterials*. 2012;33(9):2600–7.

[27] Gerdon AE, Wright DW, Cliffel DE. Quartz crystal microbalance detection of glutathione-protected nanoclusters using antibody recognition. *Anal Chem*. 2005;77(1):304–10.

[28] Mergola L, Scorrano S, Del Sole R, Lazzoi MR, Vasapollo G. Developments in the synthesis of a water compatible molecularly imprinted polymer as artificial receptor for detection of 3-nitro-L-tyrosine in neurological diseases. *Biosens Bioelectron*. 2013;40(1):336–41.

[29] Yang L, Guiseppi-Wilson A, Guiseppi-Elie A. Design considerations in the use of interdigitated microsensor electrode arrays (IMEs) for impedimetric characterization of biomimetic hydrogels. *Biomed Microdevices*. 2011;13 (2):279–89.

[30] Kanai AJ, Strauss HC, Truskey GA, Crews AL, Grunfeld S, Malinski T. Shear stress induces ATP-independent transient nitric oxide release from vascular endothelial cells, measured directly with a porphyrinic microsensor. *Circ Res*. 1995;77(2):284–93.

[31] Ferreira NS, Sales MG. Disposable immunosensor using a simple method for oriented antibody immobilization for label-free real-time detection of an oxidative stress biomarker implicated in cancer diseases. *Biosens Bioelectron*. 2014;53:193–9.

Chapter 26

Metallic nanobiosensors for biological analysis and medical diagnostics

Yen Nee Tan[1], Xin Ting Zheng[1] and Yong Yu[1]

26.1 Introduction

Metallic nanoparticles (NPs), such as gold and silver nanoparticles (AuNPs and AgNPs) in the size range of 1–100 nm, have attracted immense interest for biological analysis due to their comparable size with biomolecules of interest and unique optical, chemical, electrical and catalytic properties. To be more specific, there are two size regimes (2–100 nm and <2 nm) which are of particular interest for metallic NPs (Scheme 26.1a). Particles of 2–100 nm show bright colors due to localized surface plasmon resonance (LSPR), which refers to the resonant oscillation of free electrons across metallic NPs excited at a particular frequency of light [1, 2]. On the other hand, particles of size falling below 2 nm, which is comparable to the Fermi wavelength of electrons (~0.5 nm for Au and Ag), do not show LSPR due to their strong quantum confinement effects [3]. The number of metal atoms in each particle is so few (<150) that their electronic levels become discrete and highly size-dependent, leading to unique optical properties such as molecular-like absorptions [4, 5] and strong luminescence [6, 7] (Scheme 26.1b), which are distinctly different from large metal NPs or single atoms. In this book chapter, we will exclusively use metal NPs hereafter for particles of 2–100 nm and metal nanoclusters (NCs) for the particles with size <2 nm [8–11] for the convenience of description.

Metal NPs absorb and scatter intensely at its LSPR wavelength [12]. The LSPR spectrum and solution color of metal NPs largely depends on their size, shape and composition (Scheme 26.1c and d) [12]. For example, spherical AuNPs with average size of 10 nm absorb maximally at 520 nm in water, whereas their Ag analogues of the same diameter absorb mainly at 390 nm [1]. In addition, the LSPR of metal NPs is also highly sensitive to the change of their environment such as solvent, surface ligand, temperature and interparticle distance, which properties can be utilized for sensing application [2]. In particular, colloidal metal NPs drastically change color upon aggregation (i.e., change of interparticle distance). When these

[1]Institute of Materials Research and Engineering, the Agency for Science, Technology and Research (A*STAR), 2 Fusionopolis Way, #08-03, Innovis 138634, Singapore

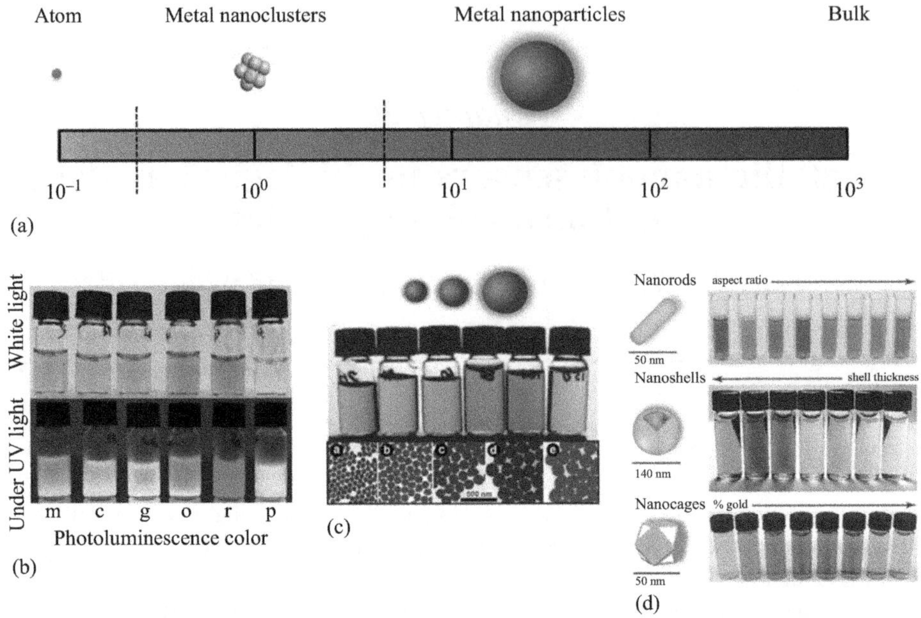

Scheme 26.1 (a) Hierarchy of materials from atoms to bulk. (b) Photos of different gold nanoclusters synthesized in our lab under white light (top) and UV excitation (bottom). The yellowish brown color of AuNCs are increasingly intense from left to right, except for the one on the extreme right, which is almost colorless. Photoluminescence colors of the AuNCs are magenta(m), cyan(c), green(g), orange(o), red(r), and pink(p) from left to right. (c) Representative transmission electron microscope (TEM) images of Au spheres (bottom) with their respective color solution (top). The colors of the Au sphere solutions are orange, tangerine, coral, pink, violet and gray from left to right. Average diameters are 66, 100, 139, 157 and 181 nm from left to right. Reprinted with permission from [13] Copyright (2012) Springer. (d) Light absorption and consequently color of gold nanorods, silica–gold core–shell NPs, and gold nanocages varies with aspect ratio, shell thickness or per cent gold. For the top row, colors of the gold nanorods are blue, cyan, grayish blue, grey, brown, copper, orange, red from left to right as the aspect ratio increases. For the middle row, colors of gold nanoshells are orange, purple, blue, cyan, green, light green, colorless from left to right as the shell thickness increases. For the bottom row, colors of the gold nanocages are yellow, orange, brown, purple, blue, dark blue, light blue, gray from left to right as the % gold increases. The actual colors can be viewed in the respective references. Reprinted with permission from Reference 14 Copyright (2010) Royal Society of Chemistry

metal NPs are coupled with organic ligands, the change of dielectric constant also leads to the shift of LSPR peak. Such color change of metal NPs is straightforward and highly visible, which make them as powerful sensing probes that can convert the 'invisible' biomolecular interactions, e.g., antigen-antibody recognition, complementary DNA base pairings and/or sequence-specific DNA-protein binding into a detectable optical signal.

Besides LSPR, metal NPs have been observed to enhance or quench nearby fluorophores depending on the distance between the fluorophore and the metal NPs. Metal-enhanced fluorescence (MEF) comprises of two cooperative mechanisms, a near-field effect and an induced plasmon effect. Ten times enhancement in fluorescence has been reported from fluorophores that are placed at least 11 nm away from the surface of metal NPs, which has been mainly observed with AgNPs [15]. On the other hand, AuNPs have been found to effectively quench the fluorescence of fluorophores appended to their surfaces when the emission spectrum of fluorophore overlaps with the LSPR band. The process of quenching can be nanosurface energy transfer (NSET) which covers a distance of 15 nm or photoinduced electron transfer (PET) [2].

In contrast to metal NPs, the strong and tunable luminescence is one of the most intriguing properties of the ultrasmall metal NCs. Compared to common fluorophores such as organic dyes and quantum dots, luminescent metal NCs are featured by their ultrasmall size (<2 nm, in contrast to quantum dots), good biocompatibility, negligible toxicity (in contrast to quantum dots), good photo (in contrast to organic dyes) and colloidal stability, which render them as ideal optical probes for use in a variety of biomedical applications, such as sensing [16–19] and imaging [20–24]. Particularly, luminescent metal NCs have been used for detection of a wide range of biologically occurring species, including adenosine triphosphate (ATP) [25, 26], cocaine [27], cysteine [16], dopamine [28, 29], proteins [30, 31], enzymes [32, 33], DNA [34], siRNA [35], etc.

Starting from next section, we will introduce how the unique optical properties of metal NPs and metal NCs are utilized to construct sensing probes to signal the presence of biological species of interest. First of all, the design of colorimetric and refractive index nanobiosensors based on the absorption properties of metal NPs will be presented in Section 26.2.1. After that, the light scattering properties of plasmonic particles and its applications for biological sensing will be discussed in Section 26.2.2. In Section 26.2.3, we will describe how metal NPs alters the optical properties of neighboring fluorophores for fluorescent nanobiosensor construction. In Section 26.2.4, the concept of metal NC based nanobiosensor will be introduced with a few typical examples to demonstrate how the interaction with biological species of interest alters the intrinsic luminescence of metal NCs. We will also give examples on the latest development of metallic nanobiosensors into paper-based point-of-care (POC) diagnostic devices in Section 26.3. Last but not the least, the commercialization potentials and the future challenges of metallic nanobiosensors will be concluded in Section 26.4.

26.2 Sensing principles

A wide array of detection mechanisms is available for metallic NP-based nanobiosensor due to their unique optical properties as illustrated in the Introduction. The underlying sensing principles can be categorized based on the light absorption/scattering properties of the metal NPs or the interaction between the metal NPs and the fluorophore/Raman active reporter appended to the surface. We will also highlight a new class of metallic fluorophore, i.e., metal NCs that possess interesting luminescence properties for their applications in biological sensing.

26.2.1 Sensing based on absorption of metal NPs

The LSPR of metal NPs is sensitive to their size, shape, interparticle distance as well as the dielectric constant of the environment. The changes in LSPR caused by target analyte binding can be detected by light absorption techniques which include colorimetric- and refractive index-based metallic nanobiosensors. The colorimetric assay is designed based on the interparticle-distance changes induced by a specific target binding in homogenous solution. In contrast, the refractive index-based nanobiosensing is due to the adsorption of biomolecules onto the metal surface and is typically performed in heterogeneous format.

26.2.1.1 Interparticle-distance dependent color change

Colorimetric detection, a method based on interparticle-distance dependent color change is the most popular method due to its simplicity and easy readout. As metal NPs approach each other closer than their diameter, a red-shift of the LSPR peak and a drastic color change can be observed due to inter-particle coupling [36]. The key in colorimetric assay design is to carefully control NP aggregation and dispersion as guided by the interparticle attractive and repulsive forces [37].

'Interparticle crosslinking' and 'non-crosslinking aggregation' are the two common approaches of utilizing the interparticle-distance dependent color change properties of metal NPs to design colorimetric assays for a wide range of analytes including ions, DNA, proteins and small molecules [2, 37]. The milestone work reported by Mirkin *et al.* shows the first attempt of applying the 'interparticle crosslinking' mechanism for the colorimetric detection of target DNA. In the assay design, two sets of AuNPs, each grafted with a complementary strand of single-stranded (ss) DNA to a part of the target DNA were prepared. In the presence of target DNA, hybridization induces ssDNA-conjugated AuNP to crosslink and aggregate, which results in a rapid color change from red to blue with femtomoles detection sensitivity [38]. More recently, Mizuo *et al.* designed a non-crosslinking colorimetric method for detecting target DNA based on the differential salt stability between ssDNA-AuNPs and double-stranded (ds) DNA-AuNPs. While the ssDNA-AuNPs could withstand high salt concentration up to 2.5 M NaCl, the complementary target DNA hybridized dsDNA-AuNPs aggregated quickly even at a low salt concentration of 0.5 M. The probe is highly sequence sensitive and is able to detect single base mismatch at the terminus opposite to the anchored site [39]. Aggregation process in this method is faster than the crosslinking system due to the

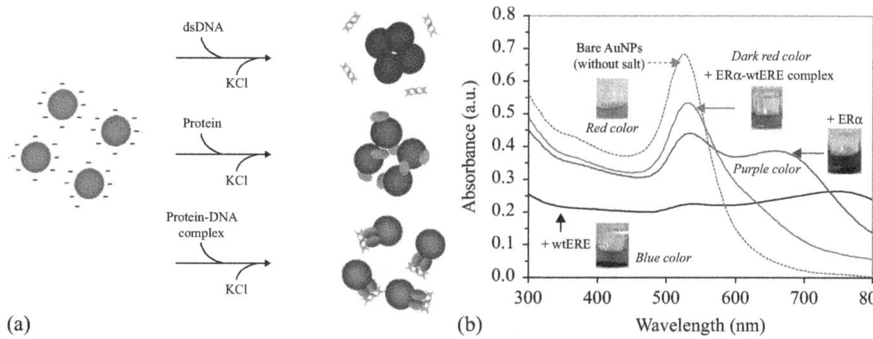

Figure 26.1 *(a) Schematic illustration of AuNPs' stability against salt-induced aggregation in the presence of double-stranded (ds) DNA, protein and protein-dsDNA complex, respectively. (b) UV-visible adsorption spectra and grayscale color photographs of AuNPs exposed to wtERE (50 nM, blue color), ERα (100 nM, purple color), and ERα-wtERE complex (preincubation of 100 nM ERα and 50 nM wtERE, dark red color), taken at 10 min upon salt addition (final KCl concentration is 20 mM). Result for a stable citrate-anion capped AuNP solution without addition of salt is shown as a reference (red color). Reprinted with permission from Reference 40 Copyright (2010) American Chemical Society*

quick reduction of repulsive forces upon duplex formation, however, it will require more target DNAs for effective signal transduction.

While in most of the colorimetric bioassay designs, metal NPs are first modified with probe biomolecules such as DNAs, antibodies or aptamers, Tan *et al.* reported another non-crosslinking colorimetric assay utilizing unmodified AuNPs to study the interaction between various DNA-binding proteins and their DNA response elements. A first example is the study of interaction between human estrogen receptors (ERα and ERβ) and their estrogen response elements (EREs). As shown in Figure 26.1, the pre-formed protein-DNA complexes could stabilize the citrate anion-capped AuNPs against salt-induced aggregation better than the protein or the DNA alone due to synergistic electrosteric protection [40]. This bioassay design has been later extended to study the interaction between ssDNA binding (SSB) protein and different ssDNA variations [41]. This straightforward and versatile colorimetric assay not only detected the formation of SSB complexes with ssDNAs of different lengths and nucleotide compositions but also allowed rapid evaluation of their corresponding binding properties. Furthermore, the same strategy has also been used to study other transcription factor-DNA pairs such as forkhead box protein A1 (FoxA1)-DNA binding [42]. More interestingly, the addition of a spin filtration step allowed the study of ligand inhibition of protein–DNA interactions which can be further generalized to study protein-ligand binding [43]. Fourteen small ligands were tested against two transcription factors, FoxA1 and AP-2γ (activating enhancer binding protein 2 gamma) to identify binder and non-binders, proving the assay robustness.

While colorimetric assays is advantageous to allow fast, low-cost and label-free detection in homogeneous solution that only requires simple instrument such as spectrometer or even naked eyes, it has its own drawbacks. For instance, metal NPs tend to aggregate under various external stimulations such as changes in ionic strength, temperature and pH, thus careful control of the environmental condition and a novel assay design involving target analytes-enabled stabilization of metal NPs is crucial. To conquer this problem, Tan *et al.* have recently developed an 'analyte' stabilized metal NPs-based fast colorimetric assay for measuring sequence-specific protein-DNA interactions using a specially designed dsDNA-metal NP conjugates to prevent false positive results from particle aggregation [44]. In the assay, a model DNA sequence containing the wildtype estrogen receptor response element (ERE) was segmented into two half site dsDNA (v1 and v2) and was conjugated with AuNPs to form complementary dsERE-AuNPs conjugates. They have demonstrated that ERE-sequence specific ERα proteins could serve as the unique stabilizers to retard the aggregation of complementary v1-AuNPs and v2-AuNPs mixture by synergistic effect of base-pairing and charge screening by salt ions (Figure 26.2).

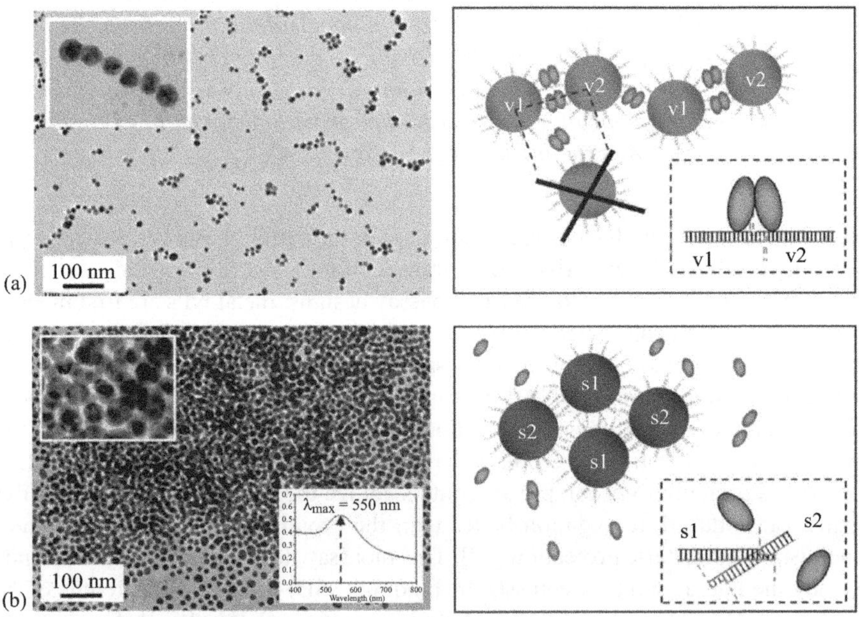

Figure 26.2 TEM images (left) and corresponding particle aggregation mechanism (right) for the complementary mixture of (a) wildtype ERE containing v1-AuNPs and v2-AuNPs (1:1 ratio) and (b) scrambled DNA containing s1-AuNPs and s2-AuNPs (1:1 ratio), in the protein binding buffer containing 0.1 M PBS, 25 mM KCl, 0.1 mM EDTA, 0.2 mM DTT and 1% of glycerol, in the presence of ER (100 nM, final concentration). All the TEM images were sampled after 20 min of reaction with ER in salt buffer. Reprinted with permission from Reference 44 Copyright (2010) American Chemical Society

A further study on the segmented DNA design principles has been reported to provide a general guideline for versatile metal NPs-based bioassay development [45].

Low sensitivity is another common disadvantage of colorimetric nanobiosensors. One feasible way to achieve signal amplification and sensitivity improvement is to combine colorimetric detection with thermal cycling as proposed by Kato and Oishi [46]. They developed an ultrasensitive colorimetric DNA/RNA assay using a combination of enzyme-free click chemical ligation chain reaction (CCLCR) on AuNPs and a magnetic separation with streptavidin-modified magnetic beads. This ultrasensitive assay is able to detect down to 50 zM of target DNA, to discriminate singe base mismatches and to specifically detect target DNA or RNA from cell lysate.

26.2.1.2 Refractive index change

The LSPR of metal NPs is sensitive to changes in the dielectric constant, i.e., refractive index, of the surrounding medium or adsorbents on the surfaces. When molecules bind to metal NPs, the refractive index around metal NPs will change, causing the LSPR wavelength to shift. Local refractive index changes induced by biomolecular interactions can be monitored via the LSPR peak shift, offering a simple, selective and label-free way of molecular detection [47]. The plasmonic sensitivity is defined as the plasmon wavelength shift per refractive index unit change (nm/RIU). Moreover, the distance-dependent nature of this plasmonic sensitivity allows only interactions in close proximity to the NP surface to result in an LSPR shift.

The refractive index sensitivity is dependent on both the shape and size of the metal NPs. For example, Au nanospheres exhibit the smallest refractive index sensitivity of 44 nm/RIU and Au nanobranches have the larger sensitivity of 703 nm/RIU [48]. A hollow Au nanotube is found to be exceptionally sensitive to refractive index with a sensitivity of 1568 nm/RIU [49]. Recently, Au core – palladium shell NPs are found to be more sensitive to refractive index than AuNPs and AgNPs of similar size, thus they are considered as a promising candidate for refractive index sensing [50]. With the latest development in colloidal chemistry, it is now feasible to engineer the nanostructure of the metal NPs to achieve the optimal refractive index sensitivity, thus significantly improving the sensor performance.

The refractive index change based sensing is simple, label-free, fast, and specific. It requires no separation/purification steps and only common laboratory equipment is needed for detection. Different from the colorimetric assay, refractive index-based LSPR biosensor mainly utilizes a heterogeneous assay format, which can be easily incorporated onto chips to allow miniaturization and multiplexing detection. For example, Frederix *et al.* constructed a transmission plasmon biosensor by immobilizing AuNPs or AgNPs on a transparent substrate, and successfully detected human serum albumin (HSA) [51]. Zhang *et al.* fabricated a plasmonic gold nanostructure array to monitor refractive index changes with a sensitivity of 255 nm/RIU. The biotin-functionalized LSPR chip could detect as low as 10 nM of streptavidin in PBS buffer [52]. The feasibility of a homogeneous assay have been demonstrated using antibody-coated AuNP probes [53]. However, the sensitivity, detection limits and multiplex capability of this method need further improvement before the realization of practical application in POC diagnostics [54].

26.2.2 Sensing based on light scattering of metal NPs

Metal NPs have large light scattering cross-section. For instance, the light scattering cross-section of an 80 nm AuNP is about a million-fold larger than that of typical fluorophores or quantum dots. The strong scattered light intensity from metal NPs helps to avoid the background interference from the biological sample matrix [12], thus allowing easy detection in whole blood, serum, cells and tissues. Furthermore, the scattered light from metal NPs is not susceptible to quenching or photobleaching under repeated/continuous exposure to light. Here, we will discuss two types of metal NPs-enabled light scattering based detection techniques which show a higher sensitivity than the light-absorption based NPs assays.

26.2.2.1 Scattered light intensity or wavelength change

Direct measurement of the scattered light intensity or wavelength change of metal NPs upon biomolecular binding is probably the most well-known light scattering based detection method. Upon analyte binding with the metal NP probes, the scattered light intensity or wavelength change observed using an optical microscope or spectrophotometer can be correlated to analyte concentration.

Storhoff *et al.* have demonstrated the detection of unamplified genomic DNAs based on scattering of ssDNA conjugated-AuNP probes [55]. As illustrated in Figure 26.3, the target DNA binding introduces clustering of ssDNA-Au NP probes and the scattered light from the AuNP probes is imaged or captured by a CMOS detector. While individual AuNPs scatter a green light, the AuNP clusters scatter yellow to orange light, due to a plasmon band red-shift. This method enables detection of zeptomole quantities of nucleic acid targets without signal amplification, offering four orders of magnitude improvement in sensitivity than the typical absorption-based techniques. It is also possible to directly monitor the light scattering intensity change. According to Rayleigh scattering theory, the scattered light intensity is proportional to the sixth power of the NP radius. Target-induced NP cluster formation could increase the scattered light intensity drastically. Zhang *et al.* have successfully applied this sensing principle to detect adenosine from urine using aptamer modified AuNPs with a detection limit of 1.8 nM [56]. The nanobiosensing based on scattered light intensity or wavelength change are simple, rapid and sensitive.

26.2.2.2 NP-enabled dynamic light scattering (DLS)

DLS measures particle size by monitoring the scattered light intensity fluctuation of particles undergoing Brownian motion in solution. Utilizing metal NPs as sensing probes, DLS can measure both aggregation-induced *particle* size change and/or individual particle size change. Specific binding of analyte to biofunctionalized metal NP probes will result in cross-linking and aggregation of NPs, thus leading to average particle size increase. For large biomacromolecules, DLS can be applied to trace individual particle size change.

In 2008, Huo *et al.* first reported a homogenous one-step AuNP-enabled DLS immunoassay for prostate-specific antigen (PSA) detection [57]. This technique couples the use of AuNP probes as a light-scattering enhancer and DLS as a signal read-out system. The assay is based on the antibody–antigen interaction induced

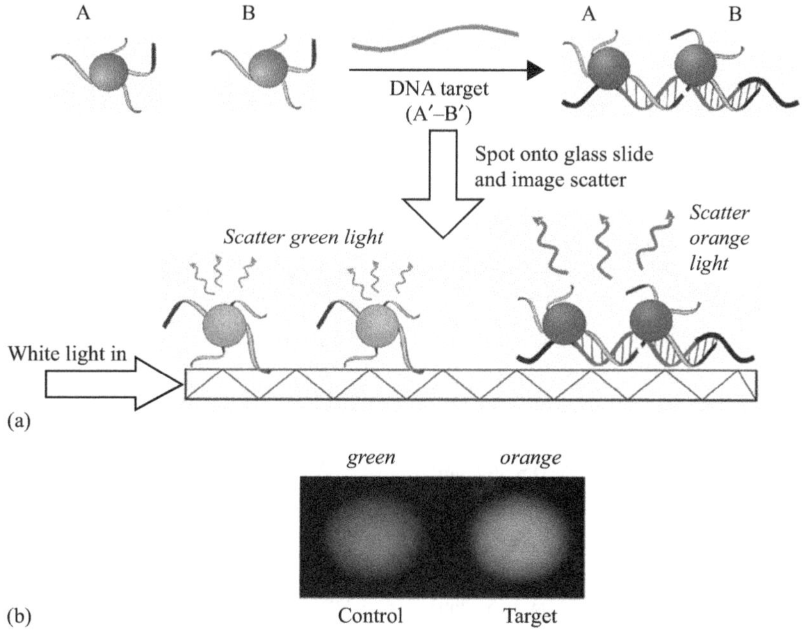

Figure 26.3 (a) Step 1: ssDNA-AuNP probes (A and B) are hybridized to a DNA target in solution. Step 2: The samples are spotted onto a glass slide which is illuminated with white light in the plane of the slide. The evanescent induced scatter from the AuNPs is visually observed or imaged by a CMOS detector. Individual 40- to 50-nm diameter gold probes scatter green light, whereas complexed probes scatter yellow to orange light. (b) When spotted onto an illuminated glass slide, the color of evanescent light induced scatter from the control sample is green; in contrast, the color is orange for the target sample. Reprinted with permission from Reference 55 Copyright (2004) Nature Publishing Group

AuNPs aggregation, and the subsequent increase in average particle size can be measured by DLS and then correlated to the analyte concentration. The same group then extended this NP-enabled DLS detection concept for target DNA measurement using two sets of DNA-functionalized AuNP probes. As shown in Figure 26.4a, hybridization with the complementary target DNAs will induce AuNPs aggregation, which can then be detected as average diameter increase by DLS. The detection limit is estimated to be ~1 pM, which is 4 orders of magnitude lower than the absorption based methods. Moreover, this highly selective assay is capable of discriminating single base pair mismatch [58]. The binding between protein A and human IgG was later monitored in real time using the protein A-conjugated AuNPs coupled with DLS technique [59].

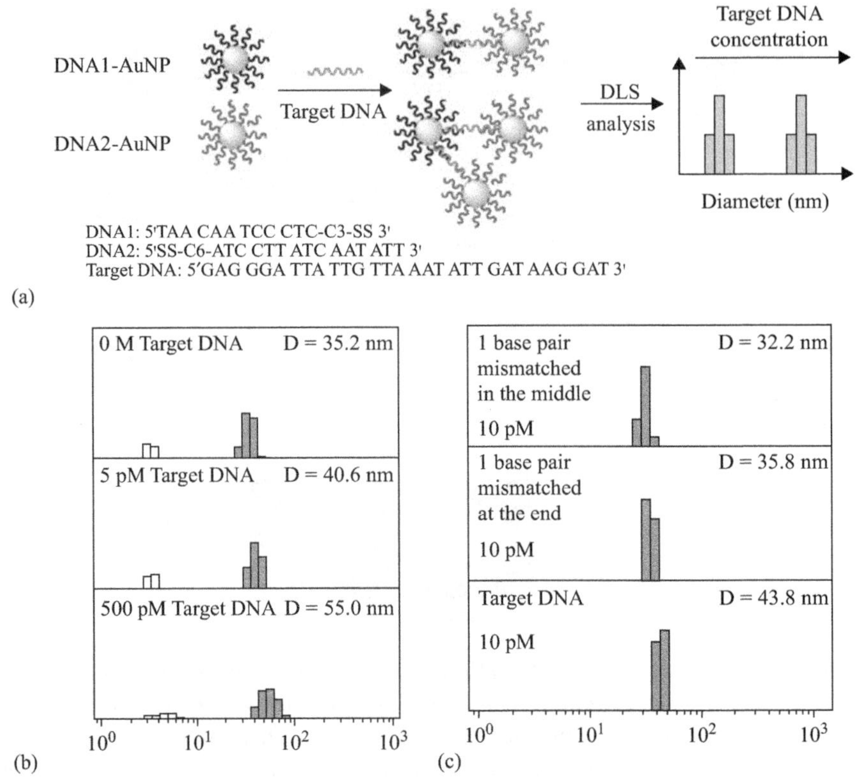

Figure 26.4 (a) Schematic illustration of a homogeneous detection of DNA using AuNP probes and DLS; the size and size distribution (in diameter, nm) of DNA-AuNP assay solutions in the presence of (b) perfectly matched target DNAs; and (c) single base pair mismatched DNAs at a concentration of 10 pM. Reprinted with permission from Reference 58 Copyright (2008) American Chemical Society

More recently, an AuNP nanoassembly-based system has been developed for sensitive and selective detection of let7 miRNA with single base discrimination sensitivity. Two sets of ssDNA conjugated AuNPs were synthesized in a carefully controlled manner to exhibit only 2–5 strands of ssDNAs per particle as compared to previously reported ssDNA-AuNPs that are usually fully saturated with ssDNAs on the NP surface. The addition of target let7 miRNA causes the formation of defined nanoassemblies such as AuNP dimers, trimers or higher order mers, which can be detected in DLS with a distinct size [60].

In summary, NP-enabled DLS detection offers better sensitivity as compared to the light absorption based method. They are usually single step homogeneous assay with good reproducibility, allows real-time kinetic studies and are amenable to high-throughput analysis when performed using multi-well plates.

26.2.3 Sensing based on interaction between metal NPs and fluorophore/reporter

As discussed in the Introduction, metal NPs have been observed to either enhance or quench the luminescence of nearby fluorophores depending on the distance between the metal NPs and the fluorophore. Metal-induced fluorescence quenching or enhancement can thus be exploited to detect various biological species of interest. Other than the spectral properties of fluorophore, the inelastic scattering of photons from the vibrational states of fluorophore (i.e., Raman reporter) can also be influenced by plasmonic nanostructures. In this section, three different types of nanobiosensor designs based on different interactions between the metal NPs and fluorophore/reporter, viz., metal-induced fluorescence quenching, metal-enhanced fluorescence and surface-enhanced Raman scattering will be discussed.

26.2.3.1 Metal-induced fluorescence quenching

Metal NPs can be used to construct Förster resonance energy transfer (FRET)-based nanobiosensor. FRET is the non-radiative energy transfer from an excited fluorophore (donor) to another fluorophore (acceptor) by means of intermolecular dipole–dipole coupling. There are two prerequisites to make FRET happen: the donor and acceptor must be sufficiently close (< 10 nm) and the absorption band of the acceptor overlaps with the emission band of the donor. Metal NPs are excellent acceptor to construct FRET-based nanobiosensors thanks to their large extinction coefficient as well as their broad and tunable absorption in the visible range. A wide variety of luminescent species have been used as donor for FRET-based biosensors, including organic dyes [61], quantum dots [62], upconversion NPs [63] and metal NCs [64, 65].

As shown in Figure 26.5, there are two types of metal NP constructed FRET-based nanobiosensors. In the first type (a), analyte molecules showing strong affinity to both the fluorophore and metal NPs bring the donor molecule to the proximity of metal NPs. The energy transfer from the donor to metal NPs thus occurs and the fluorescence of the donor molecule is turned off. For example, Li *et al.* used biotin-modified upconversion NPs as donors and biotin-modified AuNPs as acceptors to construct a sensor system for avidin detection [63]. The specific

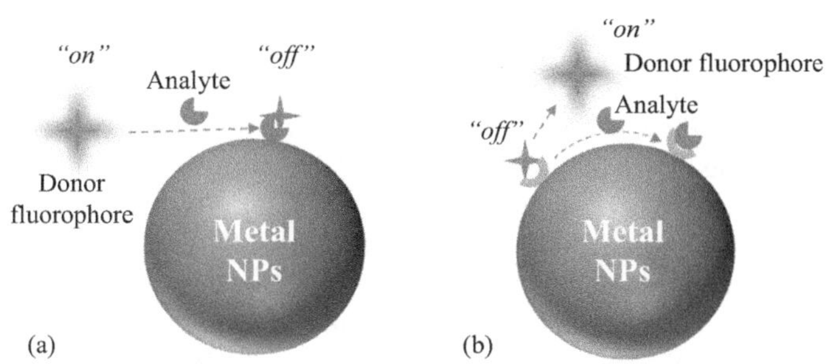

Figure 26.5 FRET-based metal nanobiosensor designs via fluorescence (a) turn-off and (b) turn-on sensing mechanisms

interaction between biotin and avidin brought the upconversion NPs and AuNPs closely together, leading to the quenching of upconversion luminescence. More recently, Yang *et al.* designed a novel FRET sensor for the detection of specific *Staphylococcus aureus* gene sequence [66]. Graphene quantum dots (GQDs) modified with capture probe oligonucleotide and AuNPs conjugated with reporter probe oligonucleotide were used as donor and acceptor, respectively. The target oligos co-hybridized with the capture and receptor oligonucleotides brought the GQDs and AuNPs to close proximity and a luminescence quenching efficiency of up to 87% was observed, reaching the limit of detection of 1 nM for *S. aureus* gene.

In the second type (b), the donor molecule is effectively quenched by metal NPs in the proximity in the absence of target molecules. The quenched fluorescence can be turned on upon the addition of target molecules which bind stronger to metal NPs. The donor fluorophore is thus released to restore its fluorescence. The analyte concentration can be quantified by monitoring the recovered fluorescence proportionally. For example, Yan *et al.* designed a heparin sensor using metal NCs as energy donor [67]. The nanobiosensor was constructed by linking trypsin-stabilized AuNCs with cysteamine-modified AuNPs via electrostatic interactions to trigger FRET effect. In the presence of target molecules, i.e., heparin, trypsin-stabilized AuNCs were replaced since heparin had more negative charges than trypsin and it would bind preferentially to cysteamine-modified AuNPs. The luminescence of trypsin-stabilized AuNCs was finally recovered. This method gave a linear response range of 0.1–4.0 $\mu g \cdot mL^{-1}$ and a detection limit of 0.05 $\mu g \cdot mL^{-1}$ for heparin.

26.2.3.2 Metal-enhanced fluorescence

Metal-enhanced fluorescence (MEF) occurs when a fluorophore is placed in the near field of metal NPs, the interaction between the fluorophore dipole and the metal NP LSPR increases the brightness of the fluorophore, decreases its lifetime and enhances its photostability [68]. MEF is highly desirable in life science as it overcomes the intrinsic weakness of organic dyes such as weak brightness and poor photostability. MEF is distance-dependent and the enhanced fluorescence decreases exponentially from the surface of SPR supporting materials, resembling the exponential electric field near-field decay above the NP surface [69].

There are mainly two types of MEF structures reported in literature, including NP deposits on substrate and periodic metal nanostructure [70, 71]. NP deposits are usually synthesized by wet chemistry with a low cost for production. However, the MEF performance is less than impressive due to difficulty in precisely controlling the size of metal NPs and distance between the metal NPs and the fluorophore. Early studies using Ag nanoislands produced by simply reducing silver nitrate achieved a net increase of 2–3 fold enhancement [72]. Electrochemical deposition of AgNP film achieved 17-fold enhancement with 300-fold enhancement at hot spots [73]. Gold and silver nanorods synthesized by seed-mediated growth have shown 40~50-fold enhancement [74]. Gold nanorods have also been demonstrated in constructing a dual mode sensor detecting both MEF and SERS signals (see Section 26.2.3.3 on SERS principles). The fluorescence and SERS signals were enhanced by 2.2 and 1.7×10^5 times, respectively.

Periodic structure is usually fabricated by electron beam lithography [75, 76], nanoimprint lithography [77, 78] and colloidal lithography [79]. Periodic structure is more expensive to fabricate but shows a much better MEF performance due to its well defined structure. Using gold bowties with 10 nm spacing fabricated by electron beam lithography, Kinkhabwala *et al.* observed 1340-fold enhancement for a single fluorophore molecule [76]. The main problem of using electron beam lithography to fabricate MEF structure is the difficulty in making plasmonic nanostructure patterns in large scale. Nanoimprint lithography is a good way to make MEF structures in large scale. Chou *et al.* combined nanoimprint, guided self-assembly and self-alignment to successfully fabricate highly ordered plasmonic nanodots on a 4-inch wafer, which has been demonstrated to enhance the average fluorescence of immunoassay of protein A and Immunoglobulin G by 7400 times [77]. A 4×10^6-fold enhancement was even observed for a single fluorophore molecule at the hot spot. Colloidal lithography usually obtains a lower fluorescence enhancement but is promising in low cost fabrication.

26.2.3.3 Surface-enhanced Raman scattering

Surface-enhanced Raman scattering (SERS) is an ultrasensitive spectroscopic technique to detect biomolecules in the proximity of plasmonic nanostructures. Raman scattering describes the inelastic scattering of incident photons and contains useful information of molecules' vibrational states. The intensity of Raman scattering is inherently weak. When the elastic scattering of photons occurs in the vicinity of plasmonic nanostructure, however, the intensity of Raman scattering can be greatly enhanced (up to 10^{14}-fold). This phenomenon is termed as surface enhanced Raman scattering (SERS) and forms the basis of constructing an ultrasensitive spectroscopic technique for the detection of biological species. Compared to fluorescence-based biosensors, SERS is a rapid, non-destructive technique that can provide compound specific information, achieve multicomponent analysis and possess superior detection limit and sensitivity.

A SERS tag is usually constructed by combining metal NPs (substrates) with specific organic Raman active molecules (reporters) whereby the design of metal substrates is more extensively studied. The enhancement of Raman scattering signal is highly dependent on the size, shape, orientation and aggregation states of metal NP substrates. Individual particles of Au and Ag nanospheres [80, 81], Au nanoshell coated on silica [82], Au nanorods [83], multibranched AuNPs such as nanostars [84] and nanoflowers [85], and bimetallic Au-Ag NPs [86] are widely used as SERS substrates. The clustering of NPs generates intense electromagnetic field at the junction of adjacent NPs (which are generally called 'hot spots') is favored in the preparation of SERS substrates. Salt- or dye-induced aggregation or immobilization on support materials (such as silica, polystyrene, and polymer beads) are common ways to make NP clusters suitable for SERS substrates.

SERS has been used for detection of a wide range of species in biological systems, such as chloride ions [87], small molecules such as glucose [88] and ATP [89], proteins such as IgG [90, 91] and avidin [92], and DNA [93]/RNA targets [94]. Future direction of SERS sensor will focus on increasing the reproducibility of SERS signal, expanding the multiplex labeling ability, reducing the size of SERS tag for subcellular imaging, and development of multifunctional nanoplatforms with fluorescent, magnetic and therapeutic properties.

26.2.4 Sensing based on intrinsic luminescent properties of metal NCs

Metal NCs adopt a core-shell structure where metal core of <2 nm are surrounded by an outer shell of organic ligand. The ligand shell separates the metal NCs core from the surroundings and readily meets incoming biological species. Specific interactions between the analyte and organic ligand shell are thus necessary for the development of nanobiosensor. Such interactions usually modify the compactness of the ligand shell and return exposure of the volatile metal core to atmosphere, which results in luminescence quenching. Some analytes may penetrate through the ligand shell and directly break down the metal core, showing similar effect of luminescence quenching. The signal of luminescence turn-off can thus be used for the detection of biological species. Luminescent metal NCs are a special type of fluorophore. The principle of metal-induced fluorescence quenching may also apply to metal NCs and a competitive assay can thus be used to construct luminescence turn-on biosensors. This section will summarize the progress of utilizing metal NCs as probes for developing nanobiosensor based on the luminescence turn-off or turn-on. The chemistry underlined the interaction between the analyte and the metal NCs will be discussed. Finally, a unique design of utilizing the formation kinetics of AuNCs to probe the interaction between protein and protein-binding drugs will be introduced.

26.2.4.1 NC luminescence turn-off

Luminescence turn-off is a common configuration adopted in the development of fluorescent metal NCs as sensing probes for biological detection. In this configuration, the biological species of interest interacts specifically with either the organic ligand shell or the metal core of the NCs. In the former case, the interaction between the analyte and the ligand shell leads to insufficient protection of the NC core, and thus exposes the volatile NC core to air. In the latter case, the analyte interacts directly with the NC core and breaks it down. Both cases lead to luminescence quenching and the bioanalytes can thus be detected by correlating the fluorescence intensity to the concentration of analyte.

Figure 26.6 shows a typical design of utilizing the interaction of analyte with the ligand shell of metal NCs for the detection of post translational modification (PTM) enzymes, such as histone deacetylase 1 and protein kinase A [33]. Peptide-templated luminescent AuNCs were used as the optical probe. The peptide formed a compact ligand shell and prevented the direct contact of AuNC core from atmosphere oxygen. When the analyte enzymes came to contact with the peptide-based ligand shell, chemical modifications (i.e., enzymatic deacetylation) altered the configuration of peptide and thus decreased the compactness of the ligand shell, leading to direct contact of AuNC core with atmosphere oxygen and thus

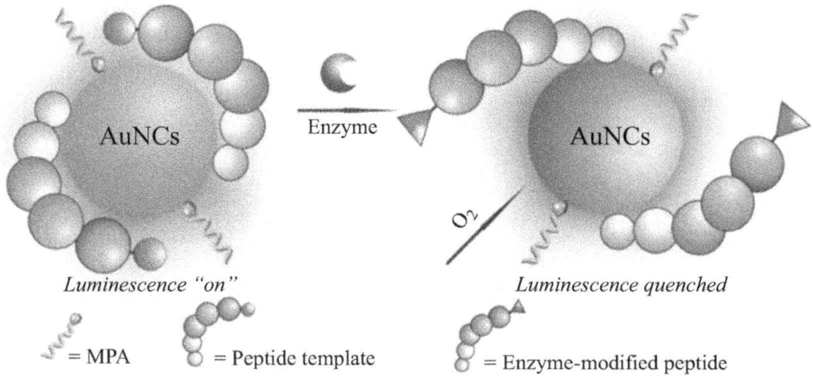

Figure 26.6 Schematic of peptide-templated AuNCs as probe for protein post-translational modifications enzyme sensing. Reprinted with permission from Reference 33 Copyright (2013) American Chemical Society

luminescence quenching via energy transfer. Due to the high reaction activity of an enzymatic reaction, detection limit down to subpicomolar was achieved. A similar approach has been employed to detect protease [78] by using protein-templated AuNCs as protease can degrade the protein shell to allow atmosphere oxygen to contact with the AuNC core, thus quenching the luminescence. In another research, human serum albumin (HSA)-stabilized AuNCs were used as sensing element for the detection of free bilirubin in blood based on the high affinity of bilirubin to bind onto HSA to induce structure change of HSA and the resultant insufficient protection of AuNC core against atmosphere oxygen [95]. Modification of luminescent AuNC by mixing with urease has also been demonstrated for the detection of urea [96].

The direct interaction of analyte with the core of luminescent metal NCs can also be used to design effective biosensors. Yuan *et al.* recently developed a luminescence quenching method for selective detection of cysteine among other biothiols and non-thiol-containing amino acids [16]. This method integrated the specific steric hindrance of the ligand shell and the unique thiol-Ag interaction. As shown in Figure 26.7, luminescent AgNCs protected by glutathione (GSH-AgNCs) was used as the optical probe. GSH prevented large biothiols (GSH) and proteins from penetrating through the ligand shell due to the bulkiness of GSH, while small biothiols such as cysteine and amino acids were able to pass through the GSH layer. Due to strong thiol-Ag interactions, AgNCs were broken down in the case of cysteine and fluorescence quenching could be observed. Therefore, the concentration of cysteine in the system were specifically determined by the luminescence intensity of AgNCs. Notably a linear response range of 0–500 nM for cysteine was achieved in this method and the limit of detection was 3 nM (S/N = 3).

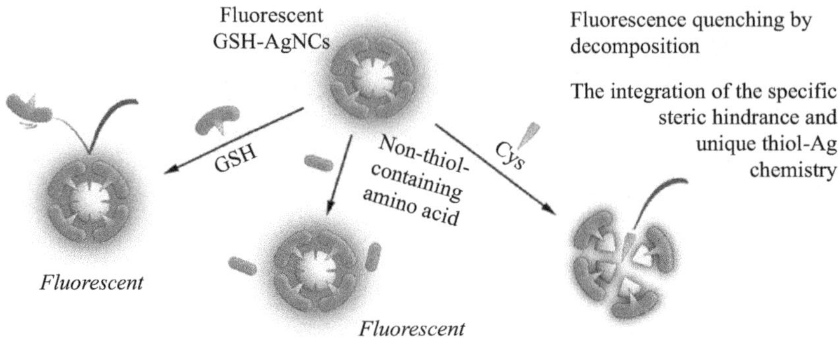

Figure 26.7 Schematic of selective detection of cysteine based on thiol-induced decomposition of AgNC core. Reprinted with permission from Reference 16 Copyright (2012) American Chemical Society

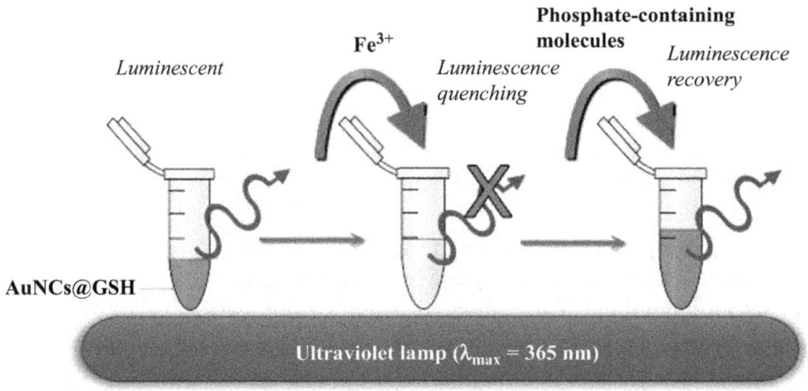

Figure 26.8 Schematic showing luminescence turn-on detection of phosphate-containing molecules using GSH-AuNCs complexed with Fe^{3+} as probe. Reprinted with permission from Reference 97 Copyright (2012) American Chemical Society

26.2.4.2 NC luminescence turn-on

Luminescence turn-on is another configuration adopted in developing metal NCs-based nanobiosensors. In this type of sensor design, a certain type of quencher is first introduced to attach to luminescent metal NCs and induces fluorescence quenching via electron or energy transfer. When bioanalytes with a stronger affinity is present, luminescent metal NCs will be replaced and released to restore the luminescence. The more analyte molecules presented in the system, the more metal NCs can be replaced and the stronger luminescence can be recovered. The concentration of analyte can thus be correlated to the fluorescence intensity of the reaction mixture.

The nanobiosensor can be constructed using metal ions as luminescence quencher. Figure 26.8 shows the detection of phosphate-containing molecules by using GSH-protected AuNCs complexed with Fe^{3+} as the sensing probe [97]. Fe^{3+} is a well-known quencher for many fluorophores. In this study, Fe^{3+} was first introduced to complex with GSH-AuNCs by coordinating Fe^{3+} with the COOH groups on the surface of AuNCs via electrostatic interactions. The initial red emission of AuNCs was quenched by Fe^{3+} in the proximity via electron transfer. When phosphate-containing metabolites such as adenosine-5'-triphosphate (ATP) and pyrophosphate were present in the sensor system, AuNCs were released to recover the luminescence as the complex formed by phosphate and Fe^{3+} had a larger formation constant. This study demonstrated that the designed sensor was effective for the detection of ATP and pyrophosphate, which optical signal is readily observable by naked eye. The linear response range for both ATP and pyrophosphate was 50 μM to sub-millimolar and the limit of detection for ATP and pyrophosphate reached ~43 and ~28 μM, respectively. Other than Fe^{3+}, a separate study also demonstrated the fluorescence turn-on detection of ATP and pyrophosphate by using Cu^{2+} as quencher to complex with the egg white ovalbumin templated AuNCs [98].

26.2.4.3 Formation process of luminescent metal NCs

Aforementioned are examples of luminescent nanobiosensors utilizing as-synthesized metal NCs as sensing elements. In this section, we introduce a novel design of utilizing the formation process of luminescent AuNCs to probe the binding interactions of small molecules to protein and its application in drug screening [99]. Albumin proteins such as bovine serum albumin (BSA) [7] and HSA [100] have been widely used as biotemplates to direct the synthesis of fluorescent AuNCs. The typical synthesis involves the encapsulation of Au ions inside the protein, and the subsequent reduction of Au ions to form AuNCs. Specific functional groups of the protein, such as tyrosine residuals, are speculated to serve as reducing agent at alkaline condition. The amount of tyrosine residuals, which is closely related to protein unfolding degree, is thus correlated to the formation rate of luminescent AuNCs. The unfolding process of the albumin protein, on the other hand, can be controlled by either temperature or denaturing agents. Higher temperature or inclusion of denaturing agents could accelerate protein unfolding, thus increasing the formation rate of AuNCs and leading to amplified fluorescence signal. Small molecular drugs that bind to albumin proteins, however, could stabilize the protein from unfolding by altering the midpoint denaturation temperature and enthalpy of unfolding of the protein, thus retarding the formation of AuNCs and leading to lower fluorescence intensity.

The study of protein-drug binding was carried out by incubating the protein (HSA as a model) with different small molecular drugs, followed by the synthesis of AuNCs using the drug-loaded protein as template at a higher temperature (60 °C) (Figure 26.9). The binding strengths of different drugs were differentiated by their relative fluorescence intensities. The lower fluorescence intensity, the stronger the drug bound to the protein. Four small drugs (i.e., sulfanilamide, phenytoin, warfarin and ibuprofen) were selected as model drugs and their relative binding strengths were differentiated using this principle. The binding constants (K_D) of warfarin and ibuprofen on HSA were also calculated by varying the loading amount of respective drug, which were similar to the values reported in the literature and validated the feasibility of applying this unique method in clinical diagnostics.

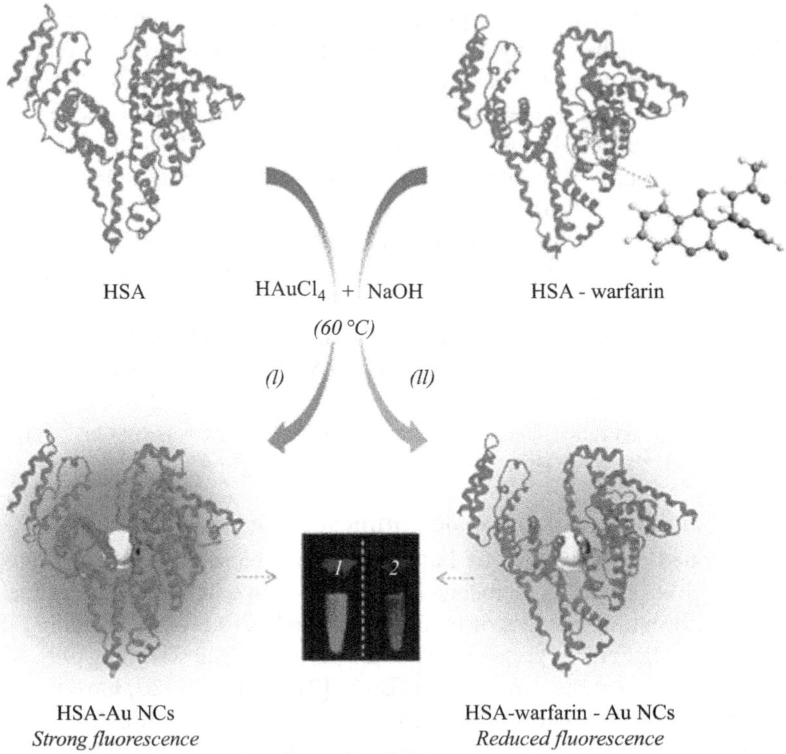

Figure 26.9 Schematic demonstrating the study of protein-drug binding by synthesizing AuNCs using drug-loaded protein as template. Reprinted from Reference 99 with permission from The Royal Society of Chemistry

26.2.5 Summary/outlook

A myriad of assay formats are available for nanobiosensing applications. The key to select a particular one is based on the requirement of target detection. When sensitivity is of primary concern, the fluorescence and DLS methods usually offer lower detection limits than the colorimetric and refractive index sensing. SERS can even detect at single molecule level. In terms of simplicity and reliance on equipment, the colorimetric method outperforms DLS and SERS since it can be viewed by even the naked eyes. It might be noteworthy to highlight that metal NCs which represent a new class of fluorophore has the potential to outperform the conventional organic dyes in fluorescence-based nanobiosensors development.

26.3 Development of paper-based POC diagnostic devices

The major hurdle in monitoring and controlling disease is the design and delivery of simple, low-cost and robust diagnostic tests. At present, biomarker tests are usually conducted at centralized laboratories with sophisticated equipment and require long waiting time as well as high cost. The development of smaller, faster and cheaper POC devices that is able to make medical test results available at the patient's bedside or in doctor's office is therefore important for rapid and routine diagnosis of diseases. It is envisioned that POC devices will greatly improve patient care in both underdeveloped regions as well as developing countries by providing affordable healthcare solutions. While POC devices are expected to have a revolutionary impact on global health, intense research has been underway to design and develop POC devices with all the desirable features as pointed out below.

First and foremost, a POC device should be a miniaturized, portable, self-containing system that allows biomarker detection in a complex sample. It should be affordable, sensitive, specific, user-friendly, rapid, robust, equipment-free or require only simple instrumentation. Reduced sample volume and minimized user intervention are also desirable for a POC diagnostic device. Among the different diagnostic platforms, paper-based nanobiosensors, which possess most of the desired features, are considered one of the answers to these demands. In particular, the metallic nanobiosensors as described in this book chapter are highly amenable to develop into paper-based POC devices. In this section, three types of paper-based nanobiosensors including the dipstick assay, the lateral flow assay (LFA) and the paper-based microfluidics (μPADs) as well as their advantages and disadvantages for POC applications will be briefly discussed.

26.3.1 Dipstick assays

Dipstick assay represents one of the most established formats for POC diagnostics. Dipstick assays are very simple, requiring only introduction of sample onto a paper pre-stored with reagents and subsequent comparison with the colorimetric chart. A well-known example is the pH strip. The first dipstick test for glucose quantification in urine was proposed in 1950s and commercialized in 1960s. After the urine sample is introduced onto the dipstick, the reagent in the dipstick reacts and changes color. The color is then compared against a colorimetric chart to semi-quantify the glucose level. Today, commercial urinalysis dipsticks have been widely adapted to a number of analytes.

Although dipstick tests are simple, lightweight, low-cost and equipment-free, the detection is usually not quantitative and it is almost impossible to design sophisticated assays. Here we show an example of metal NP-based dipstick assay. As shown in Figure 26.10, a one-step AuNPs-based competitive immunoassay was developed to detect a pesticide-dichlorodiphenyltrichloroethane (DDT) on a nitrocellulose (N.C.) dipstick [101]. The Au NP-conjugated anti-DDT antibodies were first mixed with free DDTs to form immunocomplexes. When the DDA-BSA conjugates immobilized strips were dipped into the immunocomplex solution, the free AuNP-conjugated anti-DDT antibodies will bind competitively with DDA-BSA. The color intensity obtained is inversely proportional to the DDT concentrations.

26.3.2 Lateral flow assays

Similar to dipstick assays, LFAs have all the reagents pre-stored in the strip. In addition, LFAs integrate the sample flow to allow versatile assay designs like sandwich and competitive formats. An LFA typically consists of a sample pad, a conjugation pad, a reaction membrane/detection pad, and an absorbent pad. The most well-known

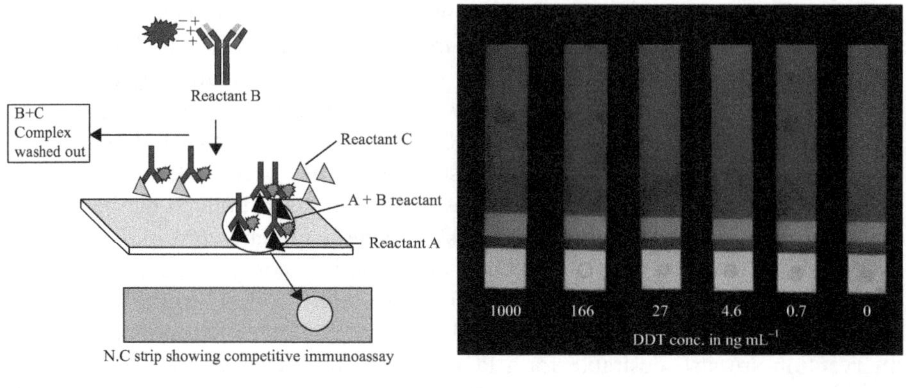

(a) (b)

Figure 26.10 (a) Schematic diagram of AuNP based competitive immunoassay for DDT detection. Reactant A-immobilized 1,1,1-trichloro-2,2-bis (chlorophenyl) acetic acid) (DDA)- BSA conjugate; Reactant B-AuNP conjugated IgY; Reactant C-free DDT. (b) DDT detection with dipsticks. Reprinted with permission from Reference 101 Copyright (2009) Elsevier

LFA is the commercially available pregnancy test strip. In this sensor strip, AuNPs and micro-latex beads are used, both functionalized with specific antibodies to β-hCG, a hormone released by pregnant women. Upon mixing these particles with urine samples containing β-hCG, pink aggregates appear at the test line [12].

Although LFAs offer many advantages such as low-cost, lightweight, portability, minimal sample preparation, and allow different assay designs, its main drawback is the difficulty in performing multiplex and quantitative analysis with high sensitivity and selectivity [102]. To improve the detection sensitivity, He *et al.* recently described an ultrasensitive nucleic acid LFA based on the introduction of AuNP-horseradish peroxidase (HRP) dual labels, with which the detection limit for DNA is markedly lowered by 1000 times. The deposition of insoluble enzymatic product greatly intensifies the color of the captured AuNPs at the test zone as shown in Figure 26.11, leading to significant signal amplification. This LFA strip is capable of detecting as low as 0.01 pM target DNA without instrumentation, thus offering a rapid, sensitive and low-cost DNA detection tool for POC diagnosis of genetic diseases or infectious agents [103]. Multiplexing has also been demonstrated in recent reports. A multiplexed lateral flow POC platform using multicolored AgNPs has been designed to simultaneously detect three pathogens including Yellow Fever, Ebola and Dengue in a single strip, achieving a detection limit of 150 ng mL^{-1} for each infectious disease [104].

26.3.3 Microfluidic paper analytical devices

Recently, functionalized papers have been applied to construct microfluidic devices called μPADs, by patterning paper into hydrophilic channels separated by

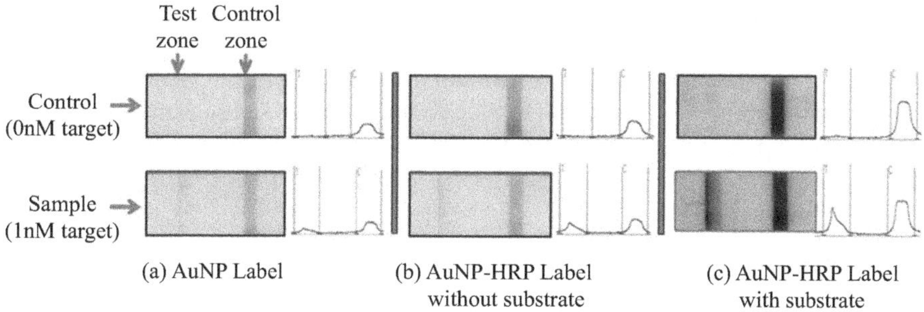

Figure 26.11 *Typical images and recorded responses of LFAs. (a) AuNP label based LFA, assay time: 24 min; (b) AuNP-HRP dual label-based LFA without applying enzymatic substrate, assay time: 24 min; (c) AuNP-HRP dual label-based LFA with enzymatic substrate. Enzymatic reaction time: 6 min, the total assay time: 30 min. Reprinted with permission from Reference 46 Copyright (2011) Elsevier*

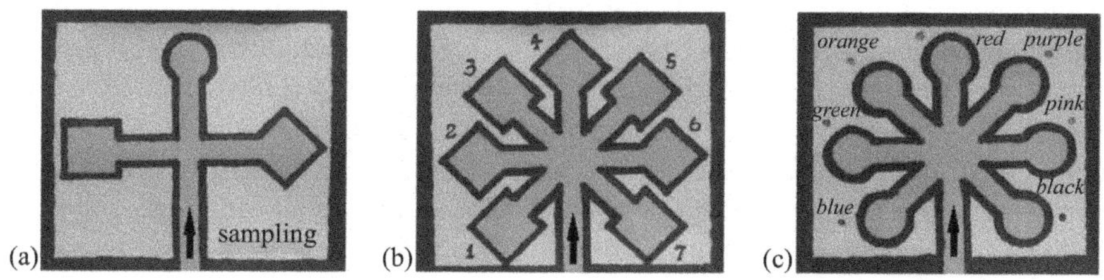

Figure 26.12 *(a) Shape-, (b) number- and (c) color-coded μPADs capable of performing multianalyte bioassays. The original color codes are represented by the different colored small dots next to each well. The actual color is labeled in this grayscale image for clear representation. Reprinted with permission from Reference 106 Copyright (2012) American Chemical Society*

hydrophobic barriers. As shown in Figure 26.12, the sample can be introduced and detected simultaneously at different test zones to achieve multianalytes detection [105]. The μPADs depicted in Figure 26.12c was used for colorimetric detection of PSA based on gold-enhanced immunogold sandwich assays [106]. An ideal paper-based microfluidic device would require only sample addition and readout interpretation by the user, thus minimizing user manipulation and effort. Paper-based microfluidic devices are capable of simultaneously performing multiple functions thus offering a distinct advantage over the traditional dipstick and LFAs. In general, μPADs allow multiplex and quantitative analysis with low sample requirement.

26.3.4 Summary/outlook

Dipstick and LFAs are the dominant formats in rapid POC diagnostics over the past few decades, due to their compactness, portability, low-cost and easy interpretation without sophisticated instrumentation. However, these two types of POC usually have low sensitivity and generally lack of quantitative measurement and multiplex detection, thus their potential in consumer markets is limited. Although still in its early development stage, μPADs that enables fluid handling and quantitative analysis holds the promise of being the future leading technology in the field of POC diagnostics.

26.4 Future perspectives

26.4.1 Commercialization potentials

The global in vitro diagnostics (IVD) market was valued at almost $50 billion in 2012 with a high compound annual growth rate (CAGR) of 7.8% [107]. POC testing constitutes the largest share of the IVD global market and is currently the fastest growing area. Therefore, not only is POC urgently needed for providing healthcare solutions, there is also a huge market demand for such devices.

Although metallic nanobiosensors have been proven promising for POC development based on abundant proof-of-principle studies in laboratory settings, commercialization has generally been slow with glucose monitoring and pregnancy tests as the two exemplary large-scale consumer products [108]. Effective technology transfers are still necessary for commercial and clinical translation to achieve widespread use and exert an impact. Intensive effort is currently ongoing to transform the prototypes built in laboratories into a highly reproducible diagnostic platform that can be mass manufactured in factories.

26.4.2 Future challenges

Although metallic nanobiosensors have been shown to be excellent tools for biological analysis and medical diagnostics, there are still major hurdles to overcome. The main challenges include the reproducible synthesis of high-quality metallic NPs and the optimization of nanobiosensor performance in physiological solution. The application of metallic nanobiosensors in complex biological fluids such as urine, serum and blood need to be carefully verified for real-world applications. In addition, the trend of metallic nanobiosensor design is to further improve robustness, sensitivity and multiplex capability. In terms of detection sensitivity, the intrinsic nanobiosensor sensitivity as well as the detector signal-to-noise ratio needs to be improved. Multiplexing capability is proven feasible but need to be upgraded in the regards of handling and reproducibility. Their lightweight, portable and easy-to-use nature makes them ideal for POC applications. However, most of metallic nanobiosensors are developed at the laboratory level and they need to be transformed into practical platforms with better reproducibility, reusability and stability. In addition, higher sensitivity and lower detection limits need to be achieved by integrating these nanobiosensors with a portable reader for facile quantification. The intrinsic advantages of metallic NPs have attracted an intense interest in nanobiosensing applications, which will continue to revolutionize the field of medical diagnostics in the years to come.

References

[1] Jain PK, Huang X, El-Sayed IH, El-Sayed MA. 'Noble metals on the nanoscale: optical and photothermal properties and some applications in imaging, sensing, biology, and medicine'. *Acc. Chem. Res.* 2008;41(12):1578–86.

[2] Saha K, Agasti SS, Kim C, Li X, Rotello VM. 'Gold nanoparticles in chemical and biological sensing'. *Chem. Rev.* 2012;112(5):2739–79.

[3] Zheng J, Nicovich PR, Dickson RM. 'Highly fluorescent noble-metal quantum dots'. *Annu. Rev. Phys. Chem.* 2007;58(1):409–31.

[4] Negishi Y, Nobusada K, Tsukuda T. 'Glutathione-protected gold clusters revisited: bridging the gap between gold (I)–thiolate complexes and thiolate-protected gold nanocrystals'. *J. Am. Chem. Soc.* 2005;127(14):5261–70.

[5] Yu Y, Chen X, Yao Q, Yu Y, Yan N, Xie J. 'Scalable and precise synthesis of thiolated Au_{10-12}, Au_{15}, Au_{18}, and Au_{25} nanoclusters via pH controlled CO reduction'. *Chem. Mater.* 2013;25(6):946–52.

[6] Yu Y, Luo Z, Chevrier DM, *et al.* 'Identification of a highly luminescent $Au_{22}(SG)_{18}$ nanocluster'. *J. Am. Chem. Soc.* 2014;136(4):1246–49.

[7] Xie J, Zheng Y, Ying JY. 'Protein-directed synthesis of highly fluorescent gold nanoclusters'. *J. Am. Chem. Soc.* 2009;131(3):888–89.

[8] Jin R. 'Quantum sized, thiolate-protected gold nanoclusters'. *Nanoscale.* 2010;2(3):343–62.

[9] Shang L, Dong SJ, Nienhaus GU. 'Ultra-small fluorescent metal nanoclusters: synthesis and biological applications'. *Nano Today.* 2011;6(4):401–18.

[10] Diez I, Ras RHA. 'Fluorescent silver nanoclusters'. *Nanoscale.* 2011;3 (5):1963–70.

[11] Luo Z, Zheng K, Xie J. 'Engineering Ultrasmall water-soluble gold and silver nanoclusters for biomedical applications'. *Chem. Commun.* 2014;50 (40):5143–55.

[12] Jans H, Huo Q. 'Gold nanoparticle-enabled biological and chemical detection and analysis'. *Chem. Soc. Rev.* 2012;41(7):2849–66.

[13] Chanana M, Mateo C, Salgueirino V, Correa-Duarte M. Synthesis of Gold Nanoparticles. In: Bhushan B, editor. *Encyclopedia of Nanotechnology*, Springer Netherlands; 2012. p. 2621–30.

[14] Skrabalak SE, Au L, Li X, Xia Y. 'Facile synthesis of Ag nanocubes and Au nanocages'. *Nat. Protocols.* 2007;2(9):2182–90.

[15] Beqa L, Singh AK, Khan SA, Senapati D, Arumugam SR, Ray PC. 'Gold nanoparticle-based simple colorimetric and ultrasensitive dynamic light scattering assay for the selective detection of Pb(II) from paints, plastics, and water samples'. *ACS Appl. Mater. Interfaces.* 2011;3(3):668–73.

[16] Yuan X, Tay Y, Dou X, Luo Z, Leong DT, Xie J. 'Glutathione-protected silver nanoclusters as cysteine-selective fluorometric and colorimetric probe'. *Anal. Chem.* 2012;85(3):1913–19.

[17] Xie J, Zheng Y, Ying JY. 'Highly selective and ultrasensitive detection of Hg^{2+} based on fluorescence quenching of Au nanoclusters by Hg^{2+}–Au^{+} interactions'. *Chem. Commun.* 2010;46(6):961–63.

[18] Shang L, Dong S. 'Silver nanocluster-based fluorescent sensors for sensitive detection of Cu(II)'. *J. Mater. Chem.* 2008;18(39):4636–40.

[19] Chang H-Y, Chang H-T, Hung Y-L, Hsiung T-M, Lin Y-W, Huang C-C. 'Ligand effect on the luminescence of gold nanodots and its application for detection of total mercury ions in biological samples'. *RSC Adv.* 2013;3 (14):4588–97.

[20] Petty JT, Story SP, Juarez S, *et al.* 'Optical sensing by transforming chromophoric silver clusters in DNA nanoreactors'. *Anal. Chem.* 2011;84 (1):356–64.

[21] Yu J, Patel SA, Dickson RM. 'In vitro and intracellular production of peptide-encapsulated fluorescent silver nanoclusters'. *Angew. Chem., Int. Ed.* 2007;46(12):2028–30.

[22] Wang Y, Cui Y, Zhao Y, *et al.* 'Bifunctional peptides that precisely biomineralize Au clusters and specifically stain cell nuclei'. *Chem. Commun.* 2012;48(6):871–73.

[23] Tao Y, Li Z, Ju E, Ren J, Qu X. 'Polycations-functionalized water-soluble gold nanoclusters: a potential platform for simultaneous enhanced gene delivery and cell imaging'. *Nanoscale.* 2013;5(13):6154–60.

[24] Shang L, Dorlich RM, Brandholt S, *et al.* 'Facile preparation of water-soluble fluorescent gold nanoclusters for cellular imaging applications'. *Nanoscale.* 2011;3(5):2009–14.

[25] Liu D, Wang Z, Jiang X. 'Gold nanoparticles for the colorimetric and fluorescent detection of ions and small organic molecules'. *Nanoscale.* 2011;3(4):1421–33.

[26] Zhang M, Guo S-M, Li Y-R, Zuo P, Ye B-C. 'A label-free fluorescent molecular beacon based on DNA-templated silver nanoclusters for detection of adenosine and adenosine deaminase'. *Chem. Commun.* 2012;48(44): 5488–90.

[27] Zhou Z, Du Y, Dong S. 'DNA–Ag nanoclusters as fluorescence probe for turn-on aptamer sensor of small molecules'. *Biosens. Bioelectron.* 2011;28 (1):33–37.

[28] Ban R, Abdel-Halim ES, Zhang J, Zhu J-J. 'β-Cyclodextrin functionalised gold nanoclusters as luminescence probes for the ultrasensitive detection of dopamine'. *Analyst.* 2015;140(4):1046–53.

[29] Kwak K, Kumar SS, Lee D. 'Selective determination of dopamine using quantum-sized gold nanoparticles protected with charge selective ligands'. *Nanoscale.* 2012;4(14):4240–46.

[30] Li J, Zhong X, Zhang H, Le XC, Zhu J-J. 'Binding-induced fluorescence turn-on assay using aptamer-functionalized silver nanocluster DNA probes'. *Anal. Chem.* 2012;84(12):5170–74.

[31] Huang Y, Li H, Zhang Y, Li W, Sun L, Li G. 'Ultrasensitive and feasibly achieved protein detection based on the integration of three signal amplification reactions via sharing a DNA sequence'. *Chem. Commun.* 2015;51 (55):11004–07.

[32] Teng Y, Jia X, Li J, Wang E. 'Ratiometric fluorescence detection of tyrosinase activity and dopamine using thiolate-protected gold nanoclusters'. *Anal. Chem.* 2015;87(9):4897–902.

[33] Wen Q, Gu Y, Tang L-J, Yu R-Q, Jiang J-H. 'Peptide-templated gold nanocluster beacon as a sensitive, label-free sensor for protein post-translational modification enzymes'. *Anal. Chem.* 2013;85(24):11681–85.

[34] Ma J-L, Yin B-C, Le H-N, Ye B-C. 'Label-free detection of sequence-specific DNA based on fluorescent silver nanoclusters-assisted surface plasmon-enhanced energy transfer'. *ACS Appl. Mater. Interfaces*. 2015;7 (23):12856–63.

[35] Shah P, Thulstrup PW, Cho SK, *et al.* 'In-solution multiplex mirna detection using dna-templated silver nanocluster probes'. *Analyst*. 2014;139 (9):2158–66.

[36] Ghosh SK, Pal T. 'Interparticle coupling effect on the surface plasmon resonance of gold nanoparticles: ? from theory to applications'. *Chem. Rev.* 2007;107(11):4797–862.

[37] Zhao W, Brook MA, Li Y. 'Design of gold nanoparticle-based colorimetric biosensing assays'. *ChemBioChem*. 2008;9(15):2363–71.

[38] Mirkin CA, Letsinger RL, Mucic RC, Storhoff JJ. 'A DNA-based method for rationally assembling nanoparticles into macroscopic materials'. *Nature*. 1996;382(6592):607–09.

[39] Sato K, Hosokawa K, Maeda M. 'Rapid aggregation of gold nanoparticles induced by non-cross-linking DNA hybridization'. *J. Am. Chem. Soc.* 2003;125(27):8102–03.

[40] Tan YN, Su X, Liu ET, Thomsen JS. 'Gold-nanoparticle-based assay for instantaneous detection of nuclear hormone receptor−response elements interactions'. *Anal. Chem.* 2010;82(7):2759–65.

[41] Tan YN, Lee KH, Su X. 'Study of single-stranded DNA binding protein–nucleic acids interactions using unmodified gold nanoparticles and its application for detection of single nucleotide polymorphisms'. *Anal. Chem.* 2011;83(11):4251–57.

[42] Aung KMM, New SY, Hong S, *et al.* 'Studying forkhead box protein A1–DNA interaction and ligand inhibition using gold nanoparticles, electrophoretic mobility shift assay, and fluorescence anisotropy'. *Anal. Biochem.* 2014;448(0):95–104.

[43] New SY, Aung KMM, Lim GL, *et al.* 'Fast screening of ligand-protein interactions based on ligand-induced protein stabilization of gold nanoparticles'. *Anal. Chem.* 2014;86(5):2361–70.

[44] Tan YN, Su X, Zhu Y, Lee JY. 'Sensing of transcription factor through controlled-assembly of metal nanoparticles modified with segmented DNA elements'. *ACS Nano*. 2010;4(9):5101–10.

[45] Tan YN, Lee KH, Su X. 'A study of DNA design dependency of segmented DNA-induced gold nanoparticle aggregation towards versatile bioassay development'. *RSC Adv.* 2013;3(44):21604–12.

[46] Kato D, Oishi M. 'Ultrasensitive detection of DNA and RNA based on enzyme-free click chemical ligation chain reaction on dispersed gold nanoparticles.' *ACS Nano*. 2014;8(10):9988–97.

[47] Sepúlveda B, Angelomé PC, Lechuga LM, Liz-Marzán LM. 'LSPR-based nanobiosensors'. *Nano Today*. 2009;4(3):244–51.

[48] Chen H, Kou X, Yang Z, Ni W, Wang J. 'Shape- and size-dependent refractive index sensitivity of gold nanoparticles'. *Langmuir*. 2008;24 (10):5233–37.

[49] Bridges CR, DiCarmine PM, Seferos DS. 'Gold nanotubes as sensitive, solution-suspendable refractive index reporters'. *Chem. Mater.* 2012;24 (6):963–65.

[50] Sugawa K, Tahara H, Yamashita A, *et al.* 'Refractive index susceptibility of the plasmonic palladium nanoparticle: potential as the third plasmonic sensing material'. *ACS Nano*. 2015;9(2):1895–904.

[51] Frederix F, Friedt J-M, Choi K-H, *et al.* 'Biosensing based on light absorption of nanoscaled gold and silver particles'. *Anal. Chem.* 2003;75 (24):6894–900.

[52] Zhang N, Su X, Free P, *et al.* 'Plasmonic metal nanostructure array by glancing angle deposition for biosensing application'. *Sensor. Actuat. B Chem.* 2013;183:310–18.

[53] Englebienne P, Van Hoonacker A, Verhas M, Khlebtsov NG. 'Advances in high-throughput screening: biomolecular interaction monitoring in real-time with colloidal metal nanoparticles'. *Comb. Chem. High Throughput Screen.* 2003;6(8):777–87.

[54] Zhou X, Wong T, Song H, *et al.* 'Development of localized surface plasmon resonance-based point-of-care system'. *Plasmonics*. 2014;9(4):835–44.

[55] Storhoff JJ, Lucas AD, Garimella V, Bao YP, Muller UR. 'Homogeneous detection of unamplified genomic DNA sequences based on colorimetric scatter of gold nanoparticle probes'. *Nat Biotech*. 2004;22(7):883–87.

[56] Zhang J-Q, Wang Y-S, He Y, *et al.* 'Determination of urinary adenosine using resonance light scattering of gold nanoparticles modified structure-switching aptamer'. *Anal. Biochem.* 2010;397(2):212–17.

[57] Liu X, Dai Q, Austin L, *et al.* 'A one-step homogeneous immunoassay for cancer biomarker detection using gold nanoparticle probes coupled with dynamic light scattering'. *J. Am. Chem. Soc.* 2008;130(9):2780–82.

[58] Dai Q, Liu X, Coutts J, Austin L, Huo Q. 'A one-step highly sensitive method for DNA detection using dynamic light scattering'. *J. Am. Chem. Soc.* 2008;130(26):8138–39.

[59] Jans H, Liu X, Austin L, Maes G, Huo Q. 'Dynamic light scattering as a powerful tool for gold nanoparticle bioconjugation and biomolecular binding studies'. *Anal. Chem.* 2009;81(22):9425–32.

[60] Seow N, Tan YN, Yung L-YL. 'Gold nanoparticle–dynamic light scattering tandem for the rapid and quantitative detection of the let7 microRNA family'. *Part. Part. Syst. Charact.* 2014;31(12):1260–68.

[61] Zhang Y, Wei G, Yu J, Birch DJS, Chen Y. 'Surface plasmon enhanced energy transfer between gold nanorods and fluorophores: application to endocytosis study and RNA detection'. *Faraday Discuss.* 2015;178(0):383–94.

[62] Mandal G, Bardhan M, Ganguly T. 'Occurrence of förster resonance energy transfer between quantum dots and gold nanoparticles in the presence of a biomolecule'. *J. Phys. Chem. C.* 2011;115(43):20840–48.

[63] Wang L, Yan R, Huo Z, *et al.* 'Fluorescence resonant energy transfer biosensor based on upconversion-luminescent nanoparticles'. *Angew. Chem., Int. Ed.* 2005;44(37):6054–57.

[64] Qin L, He X, Chen L, Zhang Y. 'Turn-on fluorescent sensing of glutathione S-transferase at near-infrared region based on FRET between gold nanoclusters and gold nanorods'. *ACS Appl. Mater. Interfaces.* 2015;7 (10):5965–71.

[65] Morishita K, MacLean JL, Liu B, Jiang H, Liu J. 'Correlation of photobleaching, oxidation and metal induced fluorescence quenching of DNA-templated silver nanoclusters'. *Nanoscale.* 2013;5(7):2840–49.

[66] Shi J, Chan C, Pang Y, *et al.* 'A fluorescence resonance energy transfer (FRET) biosensor based on graphene quantum dots (GQDs) and gold nanoparticles (AuNPs) for the detection of meca gene sequence of Staphylococcus aureus'. *Biosens. Bioelectron.* 2015;67:595–600.

[67] Liu J-M, Chen J-T, Yan X-P. 'Near infrared fluorescent trypsin stabilized gold nanoclusters as surface plasmon enhanced energy transfer biosensor and in vivo cancer imaging bioprobe'. *Anal. Chem.* 2013;85(6):3238–45.

[68] Geddes CD. 'Metal-enhanced fluorescence'. *Phys. Chem. Chem. Phys.* 2013;15(45):19537–37.

[69] Dragan A, Bishop E, Casas-Finet J, *et al.* 'Distance dependence of metal-enhanced fluorescence'. *Plasmonics.* 2012;7(4):739–44.

[70] Darvill D, Centeno A, Xie F. 'Plasmonic fluorescence enhancement by metal nanostructures: shaping the future of bionanotechnology'. *Phys. Chem. Chem. Phys.* 2013;15(38):15709–26.

[71] Deng W, Xie F, Baltar HTMCM, Goldys EM. 'Metal-enhanced fluorescence in the life sciences: here, now and beyond'. *Phys. Chem. Chem. Phys.* 2013;15(38):15695–708.

[72] Chen I, Ting AY. 'Site-specific labeling of proteins with small molecules in live cells'. *Curr. Opin. Biotechnol.* 2005;16(1):35–40.

[73] Zhang J, Matveeva E, Gryczynski I, Leonenko Z, Lakowicz JR. 'Metal-enhanced fluoroimmunoassay on a silver film by vapor deposition'. *J. Phys. Chem. B.* 2005;109(16):7969–75.

[74] Aslan K, Leonenko Z, Lakowicz JR, Geddes CD. 'Fast and slow deposition of silver nanorods on planar surfaces: ? application to metal-enhanced fluorescence'. *J. Phys. Chem. B.* 2005;109(8):3157–62.

[75] Acuna GP, Möller FM, Holzmeister P, Beater S, Lalkens B, Tinnefeld P. 'Fluorescence enhancement at docking sites of dna-directed self-assembled nanoantennas'. *Science.* 2012;338(6106):506–10.

[76] Kinkhabwala A, Yu Z, Fan S, Avlasevich Y, Mullen K, Moerner WE. 'Large single-molecule fluorescence enhancements produced by a bowtie nanoantenna'. *Nat. Photon*. 2009;3(11):654–57.

[77] Li W-D, Ding F, Hu J, Chou SY. 'Three-dimensional cavity nanoantenna coupled plasmonic nanodots for ultrahigh and uniform surface-enhanced Raman scattering over large area'. *Opt. Express*. 2011;19(5):3925–36.

[78] Wang Y, Wang Y, Zhou F, Kim P, Xia Y. 'Protein-protected Au clusters as a new class of nanoscale biosensor for label-free fluorescence detection of proteases'. *Small*. 2012;8(24):3769–73.

[79] Xie F, Centeno A, Ryan MR, Riley DJ, Alford NM. 'Au nanostructures by colloidal lithography: from quenching to extensive fluorescence enhancement'. *J. Mate. Chem. B*. 2013;1(4):536–43.

[80] Lee PC, Meisel D. 'Adsorption and surface-enhanced Raman of dyes on silver and gold sols'. *J. Phys. Chem.* 1982;86(17):3391–95.

[81] Leopold N, Lendl B. 'A new method for fast preparation of highly surface-enhanced Raman scattering (sers) active silver colloids at room temperature by reduction of silver nitrate with hydroxylamine hydrochloride'. *J. Phys. Chem. B*. 2003;107(24):5723–27.

[82] Wang H, Kundu J, Halas NJ. 'Plasmonic nanoshell arrays combine surface-enhanced vibrational spectroscopies on a single substrate'. *Angew. Chem., Int. Ed.* 2007;46(47):9040–44.

[83] Huang X, El-Sayed IH, Qian W, El-Sayed MA. 'Cancer cell imaging and photothermal therapy in the near-infrared region by using gold nanorods'. *J. Am. Chem. Soc.* 2006;128(6):2115–20.

[84] Pazos-Pérez N, Barbosa S, Rodríguez-Lorenzo L, *et al*. 'Growth of sharp tips on gold nanowires leads to increased surface-enhanced Raman scattering activity'. *J. Phys. Chem. Lett.* 2010;1(1):24–27.

[85] Xie J, Zhang Q, Lee JY, Wang DIC. 'The synthesis of SERS-active gold nanoflower tags for in vivo applications'. *ACS Nano*. 2008;2(12):2473–80.

[86] Philip D, Gopchandran KG, Unni C, Nissamudeen KM. 'Synthesis, characterization and SERS activity of Au–Ag nanorods'. *Spectrochim. Acta Mol. Biomol. Spectrosc.* 2008;70(4):780–84.

[87] Tsoutsi D, Montenegro JM, Dommershausen F, *et al*. 'Quantitative surface-enhanced Raman scattering ultradetection of atomic inorganic ions: the case of chloride'. *ACS Nano*. 2011;5(9):7539–46.

[88] Vangala K, Yanney M, Hsiao C-T, *et al*. 'Sensitive carbohydrate detection using surface enhanced Raman tagging'. *Anal. Chem.* 2010;82(24): 10164–71.

[89] Li M, Zhang J, Suri S, Sooter LJ, Ma D, Wu N. 'Detection of adenosine triphosphate with an aptamer biosensor based on surface-enhanced Raman scattering'. *Anal. Chem.* 2012;84(6):2837–42.

[90] Wang C, Chen Y, Wang T, Ma Z, Su Z. 'Monodispersed gold nanorod-embedded silica particles as novel Raman labels for biosensing'. *Adv. Funct. Mater.* 2008;18(2):355–61.

[91] Chen S, Yuan Y, Yao J, Han S, Gu R. 'Magnetic separation and immunoassay of multi-antigen based on surface enhanced Raman spectroscopy'. *Chem. Commun.* 2011;47(14):4225–27.
[92] Han XX, Chen L, Guo J, Zhao B, Ozaki Y. 'Coomassie brilliant dyes as surface-enhanced Raman scattering probes for protein−ligand recognitions'. *Anal. Chem.* 2010;82(10):4102–06.
[93] Zhang H, Harpster MH, Park HJ, Johnson PA, Wilson WC. 'Surface-enhanced Raman scattering detection of DNA derived from the west nile virus genome using magnetic capture of Raman-Active gold nanoparticles'. *Anal. Chem.* 2011;83(1):254–60.
[94] Cao YC, Jin R, Mirkin CA. 'Nanoparticles with Raman spectroscopic fingerprints for dna and RNA detection'. *Science.* 2002;297(5586): 1536–40.
[95] Santhosh M, Chinnadayyala SR, Kakoti A, Goswami P. 'Selective and sensitive detection of free bilirubin in blood serum using human serum albumin stabilized gold nanoclusters as fluorometric and colorimetric probe'. *Biosens. Bioelectron.* 2014;59(0):370–76.
[96] Nair LV, Philips DS, Jayasree RS, Ajayaghosh A. 'A near-infrared fluorescent nanosensor (AuC@Urease) for the selective detection of blood urea'. *Small.* 2013;9(16):2673–77.
[97] Li P-H, Lin J-Y, Chen C-T, *et al.* 'Using gold nanoclusters as selective luminescent probes for phosphate-containing metabolites'. *Anal. Chem.* 2012;84(13):5484–88.
[98] Selvaprakash K, Chen Y-C. 'Using protein-encapsulated gold nanoclusters as photoluminescent sensing probes for biomolecules'. *Biosens. Bioelectron.* 2014;61(0):88–94.
[99] Yu Y, New SY, Xie J, Su X, Tan YN. 'Protein-based fluorescent metal nanoclusters for small molecular drug screening'. *Chem. Commun.* 2014;50 (89):13805–08.
[100] Yan L, Cai Y, Zheng B, *et al.* 'Microwave-assisted synthesis of BSA-stabilized and HSA-protected gold nanoclusters with red emission'. *J. Mater. Chem.* 2012;22(3):1000–05.
[101] Lisa M, Chouhan RS, Vinayaka AC, Manonmani HK, Thakur MS. 'Gold nanoparticles based dipstick immunoassay for the rapid detection of dichlorodiphenyltrichloroethane: an organochlorine pesticide'. *Biosens. Bioelectron.* 2009;25(1):224–27.
[102] Yetisen AK, Akram MS, Lowe CR. 'Paper-based microfluidic point-of-care diagnostic devices'. *Lab. Chip.* 2013;13(12):2210–51.
[103] He Y, Zhang S, Zhang X, *et al.* 'Ultrasensitive Nucleic acid biosensor based on enzyme–gold nanoparticle dual label and lateral flow strip biosensor'. *Biosens. Bioelectron.* 2011;26(5):2018–24.
[104] Yen C-W, de Puig H, Tam JO, *et al.* 'Multicolored silver nanoparticles for multiplexed disease diagnostics: distinguishing dengue, yellow fever, and ebola viruses'. *Lab. Chip.* 2015;15(7):1638–41.

[105] Kumar A, Hens A, Arun RK, *et al.* 'A paper based microfluidic device for easy detection of uric acid using positively charged gold nanoparticles'. *Analyst*. 2015;140(6):1817–21.
[106] Nie J, Zhang Y, Lin L, *et al.* 'Low-cost fabrication of paper-based microfluidic devices by one-step plotting'. *Anal. Chem.* 2012;84(15):6331–35.
[107] In vitro Diagnostics (IVD) Market (Applications, End-users & Types) Trends & Global Forecasts (Major & Emerging Markets – G7, Japan & BRIC): *Markets and Markets*; 2011.
[108] Howes PD, Chandrawati R, Stevens MM. 'Colloidal nanoparticles as advanced biological sensors'. *Science*. 2014;346(6205).

Chapter 27

Carbon nanomaterial based biosensors for onsite biomedical diagnosis

Jian Zhang[1] and Zhen Yuan[1]

27.1 Introduction

Biosensor is considered as an analytical device that combines a sensitive biomedical component in direct spatial contact with a transduction element [1–3]. To date, advances in biosensor are experiencing a transition from in vitro sensing to in vivo targeting and imaging the lesion of live animals and human.

In particular, due to recent advances in nanomaterials and associated fabrication technologies, nanomaterial-based biosensors shed light on the biological events detection [4–6]. Interestingly, among all these nanomaterials, carbon nanomaterials (CNMs) are considered to be ideal candidates to interact with biological systems because of their excellent physical and chemical properties including high carrier mobility, high surface-to-volume ratio, and robustness [7, 8]. CNMs have shown superior potential for the development and improvement of biosensors, for example, a multitude of CNMs-based biosensors have been explored and applied in ultrasensitive biosensing.

Advances in CNMs-based biosensors are growing so quickly that we are not able to introduce all the perspectives in this field. In this chapter, we only pay particular attention to the recent technique developments in single-walled carbon nanotubes (SWNTs) and graphene-based biosensors and focus on the introduction of their in vitro and in vivo applications.

27.2 Basic instruction about carbon nanomaterials (CNMs)

CNMs including fullerenes, carbon nanotubes, graphene and so on [9] are defined as carbon materials that have structural features with at least one dimension of 100 nm or less. As shown in Figure 27.1, both SWNTs and graphene consist of sp_2 hybridized carbon atoms that can be conceptually visualized as graphene sheet derivatives [10, 11].

[1]Faculty of Health Sciences, University of Macau, Av. Padre Tomás Pereira, Taipa, Macau

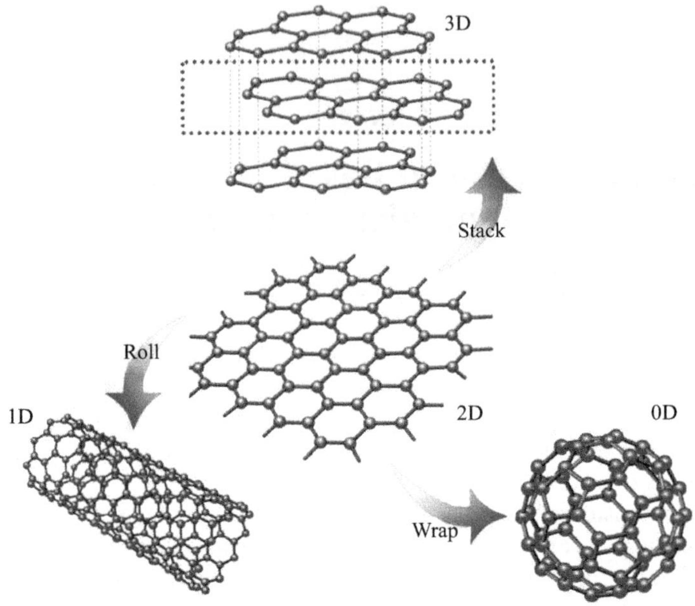

Figure 27.1 Graphene: the basic building block for other carbon allotropes, graphite (3D), fullerene (0D), and SWNT (1D). Reprinted with permission from Reference 1; Copyright (2015), American Chemical Society

Due to the significance and extensive application of SWNTs, new synthesis processes as displayed in Figure 27.2 are being developed for different purposes [12]. Briefly, synthesis of SWNTs can be conducted based on different approaches including laser ablation, arc discharge, and chemical vapour deposition (CVD) [13]. If solid form is used for carbon source, sublimation of graphite needs high temperature manners that the temperature will be up to 3200 °C. However, for liquid or gaseous carbon sources, the generic term of 'medium temperature methods' or 'low temperature methods' is generally utilized. The different categories of synthesis methods for SWNTs are due to the fact that all ingredients may be provided in various ways. So far, all these synthesis methods involve three major components: (1) catalyst nanoparticles, (2) carbon sources, (3) the energy input [14].

In addition, the synthesis process based on mechanical cleavage or chemical synthesis methods is usually adopted for graphene. Although free-standing graphene was in the beginning made by mechanical cleavage of graphite [15], mechanical exfoliation in throughput is low and the generated graphene size is also small. In contrast, chemical synthesis method is the best option for low cost mass production of graphene. The typical process includes exfoliating graphite through oxidation to yield graphite oxide (GO), and then sonicating this material to generate GO. GO can be subsequently reduced by chemical method (hydrazine method), thermal reduction, photothermal reduction, or electrochemical reduction so that RGO (reduced graphene oxide) is produced [16]. Importantly, it is noted that large-size graphene is

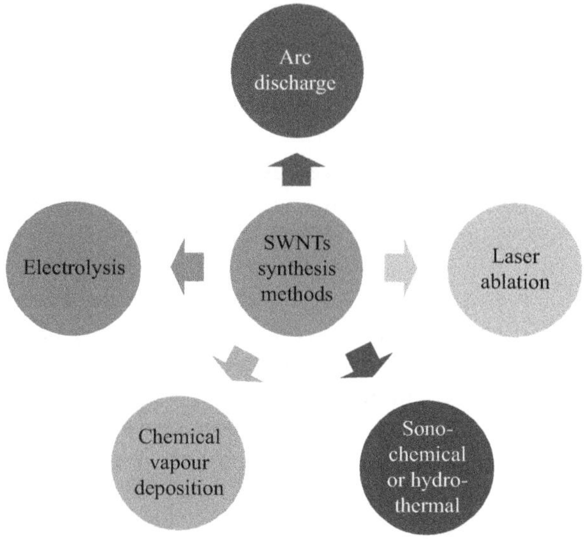

Figure 27.2 Methods currently being employed for SWNTs synthesis

often used for device fabrication, in which CVD growth can control the size and shape of the graphene film. Another advantage of chemical synthesis method is that it allows the in situ doping of heteroatoms into the carbon lattice and consequently the electronic property of the graphene film can be tuned. However, this method may suffer from the disadvantages of existence of defects, impurities and post-CVD transfer of the graphene film [17].

Importantly, to make the reinforcements most effective in advanced composites, a good chemical bond to CNMs must be present to improve and enhance their mechanical properties. In addition, covalent functionalization is robust and versatile, which has been used to functionalize carbon nanotubes and graphene for biosensing and drug delivery [18–20]. However, the oxygen-containing groups existing upon the graphene basal plane may disrupt the π-conjugation, which would affect the conductivity of graphene. As a result, recent investigations on the development of noncovalent functionalization methods have provided another impetus towards extending the scope of their application spectrum. Various molecules can be used to noncovalently functionalize SWNTs and graphene via hydrophobic binding or π–π stacking interactions [13, 21]. Interestingly, noncovalent functionalization has the advantage of without generating defects on the SWNT or graphene surface, which thus preserves their intrinsic electronic properties.

27.3 CNMs-based biosensor and its applications

27.3.1 In vitro application of CNMs biosensor

One of the most important functions of the biosensor for in vitro applications is continuous monitoring for bimolecular interactions with excellent sensitivity and attractive selectivity. Because CNMs owns the excellent mobility, it is an ideal option to use CNMS for ultra-small sensors such as glucose, DNAs and so on.

27.3.1.1 Single-walled carbon nanotube based biosensor for in vitro detection

Due to the extremely small sizes as well as unique electronic properties, SWNTs have utilized as field-effect-transistor (FET)-based biosensors. For example, semiconducting SWNTs have been employed to be configured into FET devices for the construction of novel biosensor as shown in Figure 27.3 [22, 23].

The detection and management of diabetes disease need continuous glucose monitoring. SWNTs was first introduced into the biosensing of glucose based on FET in 2003 [24]. Glucose oxidase (GOD) was attached in a controlled way to the nanotube sidewall, which could be performed via one linking molecule as shown in Figure 27.4a. Real-time recordings were conducted in which the conductance of a GOx-coated semiconducting SWNT in milli-Q water varied as a function of time. If milli-Q water (MQW) was put into the liquid (dash arrow in Figure 27.4b), the change in conductance was not that obvious. When 0.1 M glucose in MQW was put into the liquid (hard arrow in Figure 27.4b), increased conductance of the tube up to 10% would be found. However, issues related to GOD have to be resolved for later extensive applications, which include high cost and insufficient long-term stability. For example, SWNTs-based biosensors are easily influenced by pH value, temperature, toxic chemicals and humidity because of the nature of enzymes [25]. In addition, metal/metal oxide based catalysts including Cu [26], CuO [27], MnO_2 [28] and Ni [29] are often utilized to modify the electrodes for non-enzymatic determination.

So far the work in biological processes such as DNA hybridization would result in the electrostatic interaction as well as charge transfer, which enables electronic detection using biosensor devices. In 2006, SWNTs FETs were first assembled for the investigation of the interaction among the single-stranded DNA oligonucleotide, SWNTs and the following processes of DNA hybridization which would appear upon the device's surfaces [30]. The findings suggested that SWNT

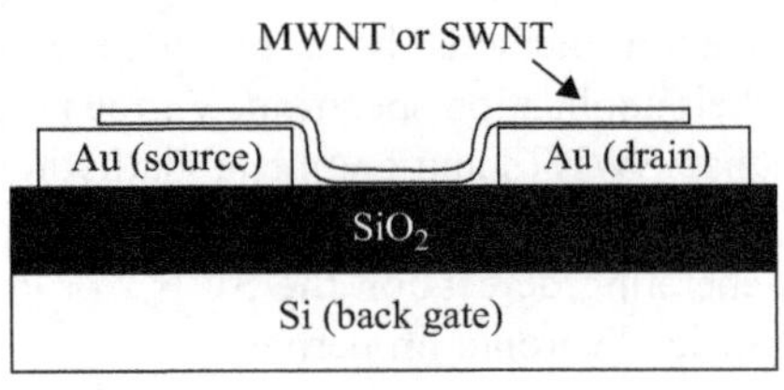

Figure 27.3 Schematic cross-section of the FET devices. A single carbon nanotube of either multi-wall (MW) or single-wall (SW) type bridges the gap between two gold electrodes. The silicon substrate is used as back gate. Reprinted with permission from Reference 23; Copyright [2015], AIP Publishing LLC

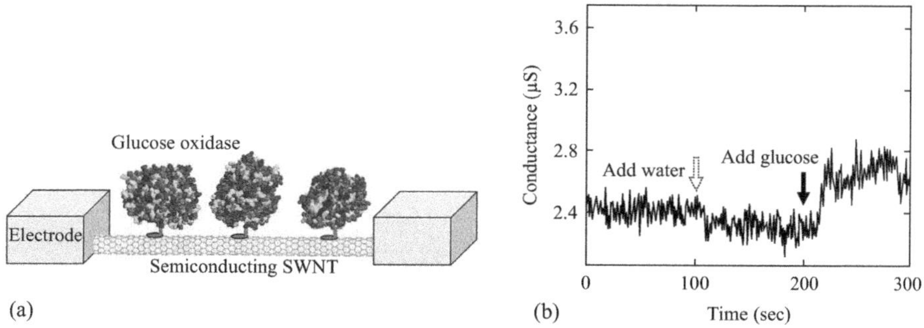

Figure 27.4 *(a) Schematic picture of two electrodes connecting a semiconducting SWCNT with GOD enzymes immobilized on its surface. (b) Real-time electronic response of the SWNT sensor to glucose, the substrate of GOx. Reprinted with permission from Reference 24; Copyright (2015), American Chemical Society*

FETs were able to be selectively changed with the DNA oligonucleotide and would keep the specificity of hybridization. In particular, a novel method for building functionalized SWNT FET arrays to identify DNA hybridization was implemented for the goal of the specific adsorption of DNA to SWNTs as shown in Figure 27.5a [31]. After hybridization, statistically significant changes were observed in key transistor parameters (Figure 27.5b and c). To further improve the sensitivity, 'nanoparticle enhancement' approach was performed, in which the target DNAs were hybridized with probe DNAs on the device, and reporter DNAs labelled with Au nanoparticles flanked a segment of the target DNA sequence [32].

Besides the biosensor mentioned above, an aptamer-modified SWNTs FET biosensor for the detection of thrombin was also presented [33], which had a linear sensitivity in the thrombin physiological ranged from 70 pM to 70 nM. Recently SWNTs-based FET biosensors have been conducted to be responsive to pH and sodium [34–36].

27.3.1.2 Graphene-based biosensor for in vitro detection

Graphene is able to offer excellent electron transfer properties, which plays an essential role in the performance of sensors [37]. The early graphene FET-based biosensors composed of graphene transistors were produced from chemically modified graphenes (CMGs). CMGs included GOs and graphene amines (GAs) [38]. The functional groups on GOs or GAs were also explored to fabricate three CMG-based biosensors: (i) a single-bacterium biodevice, (ii) a label-free DNA sensor and (iii) a bacterial DNA/protein, and a polyelectrolyte chemical transistor. It is interesting to find that the bacteria biodevice had excellent sensitivity. For example, one bacterium attachment could improve the conductivity up to 40% (Figure 27.6a). This is because of p-type properties from CMGs. As such, the attachment of a negatively charged species, such as bacteria, is equivalent to a negative potential gating, which will further enhances the whole density and the

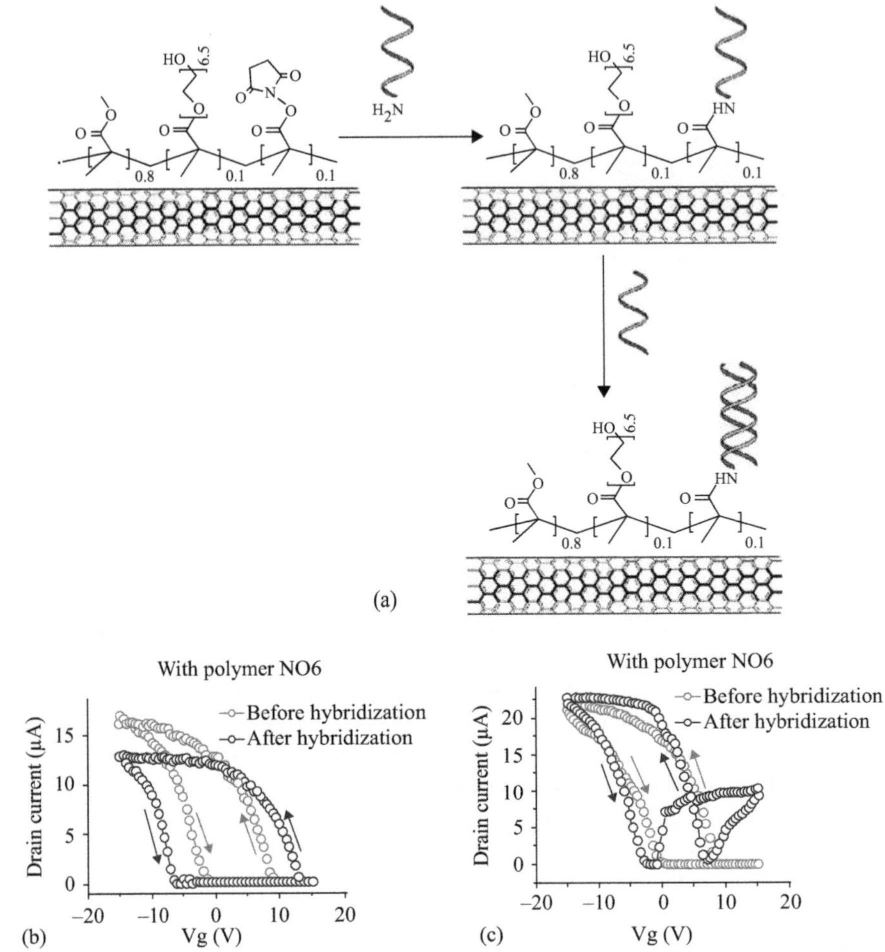

Figure 27.5 (a) Schematic representation of the bonding of the polymer to SWNT (top right and left) and DNA hybridization (lower right). (b) I_d–V_g curve of a device functionalized with NO6 polymer, before and after DNA hybridization. (c) I_d–V_g curve of a device without the NO6 polymer before and after DNA hybridization. Reprinted with permission from Reference 31, Copyright (2015), American Chemical Society

conductivity of CMG. Likewise, single-stranded DNA tethered on graphene reversibly increases the device conductance during cycles of dehybridization and rehybridization with its complementary DNA strand (Figure 27.6b). In the end, the results revealed that adsorption of polyelectrolyte molecules on the modified graphenes could cause polarity-dependent changes in electrical conductivity.

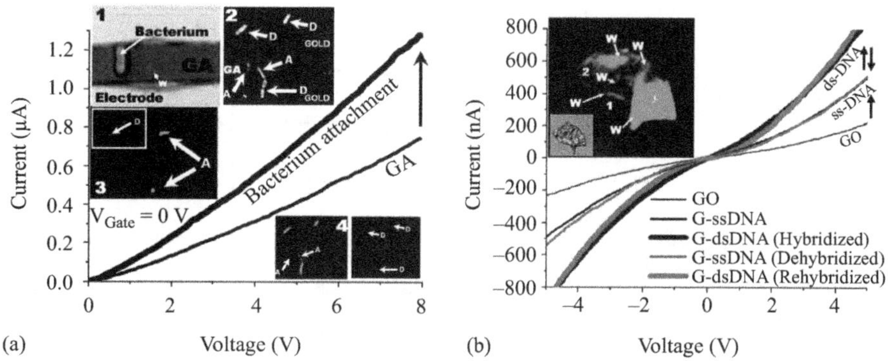

Figure 27.6 *(a) The conductivity of the p-type GA device increases upon attachment of a single bacterial cell on the surface of GA (inset 1). LIVE/DEAD confocal microscopy test on the bacteria deposited on GA confirmed that most of the bacteria were alive after the electrostatic deposition (inset 3). A = alive and D = dead. The LIVE/DEAD test conducted immediately after the electrical measurements on the GA–gold–bacteria device (inset 2 and inset 4) showed that the bacterial cells on GA atop silica remain alive, while the bacteria deposited on the GA atop gold electrodes die after electrical measurements (inset 4 (right)). (b) DNA transistor: ss-DNA tethering on GO increases the conductivity of the device. Successive hybridization and dehybridization of DNA on the G-DNA device results in completely reversible increase and restoration of conductivity. Inset shows a G-DNA (ds) sheet with wrinkles and folds clearly visible. Reprinted with permission from Reference 38, Copyright (2015), American Chemical Society*

The implementation of graphene in aqueous electrolytes for the application in biosensors has been extensively explored [35, 39–47]. The utilization of solution-gated epitaxial graphene as pH sensors has been presented and discussed [39] and the electrolyte-gated graphene field-effect transistors were also developed for the detections of pH values and the absorption of protein [35]. Recent work demonstrated that the biocompatibility of reduced GOs with proteins. After protein functionalization, biosensors were generated for the detection of various metals with high sensitivity [42].

Moreover, graphene-based biosensor is capable of detecting action potentials generated from electrically active neurons for its application in neuroscience. For example, the arrays of CVD-grown graphene FETs have been used for the extracellular recordings of action potentials from electrogenic cells (Figure 27.7a and b) [45]. The action potentials of cardiomyocyte-like HL-1 cells could be effectively measured and tracked across the transistor array as plotted in Figure 27.7c. The graphene FETs combined with the large transconductive sensitivity of these devices clearly

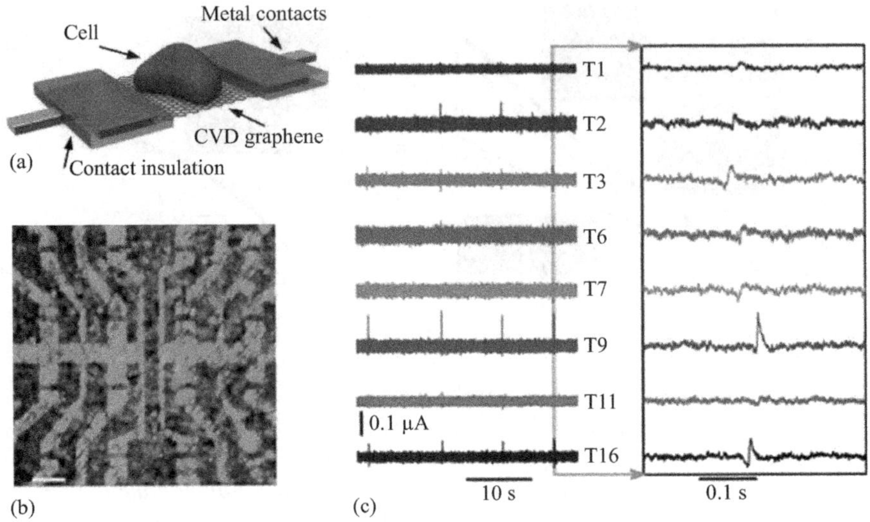

Figure 27.7 *(a) Schematic view of a G-SGFET with a cell on the gate area. The graphene is shown between the drain and source metal contacts, which are protected by a chemically resistant layer. (b) Combination of an optical microscopy image of a transistor array and a fluorescence image of the calcein-stained cell layer on the same array. The scale bar is 100 μm. (c) Simultaneous current recordings of eight transistors in one FET array over tens of seconds and hundreds of milliseconds. Reprinted with permission from Reference 45, Copyright (2015), John Wiley and Sons*

exhibited the advantages of graphene FETs according to the high signal-to-noise ratio. The findings also revealed the high-performance graphene FETs integrated with graphene electronics may bring a true breakthrough in bioelectronics.

27.3.2 In vivo application of CNMs-based biosensor

27.3.2.1 CNMs-based biosensor for tumour detection

Cancer including lung cancer, rectal and prostate cancer, colon cancer and breast cancer remains a leading cause of morbidity and mortality. The use of imaging technique to detect cancers at an early stage provides better opportunities for patients to obtain more effective treatment with fewer side effects. In consideration of the absence of acute toxicity, relatively long circulation time, and rapid renal clearance, CNMs have been developed into attractive tumour diagnostic and therapeutic nanodevices. To date, CNMs-based tumour detection technologies have been explored for various in vivo imaging approaches from positron emission tomography (PET) to optical molecular imaging.

Radiolabelling is a much more sensitive method, which is able to accurately track the labelled substances in vivo in a quantitative manner. The biodistribution of radio-labelled SWNTs in mice has been quantified by using in vivo PET [48]. It is found that SWNTs that are functionalized with phospholipids bearing poly-ethylene-glycol (PEG) are surprisingly stable in live animal body (Figure 27.8a). In addition, the effect of PEG chain length on the biodistribution and circulation of the SWNTs were also studied (Figure 27.8b). The findings suggested that effectively PEGylated SWNTs exhibit relatively long blood circulation times and low uptake by the reticuloendothelial system (RES). In particular, efficient targeting of integrin positive tumour in mice is achieved with SWNTs coated with PEG chains linked to an arginine–glycine–aspartic acid (RGD) peptide (Figure 27.8c).

In 2011, Yang *et al.* reported a method that labelled NGO–PEG with ^{125}I by anchoring iodine atoms on the defects and edges of GO [49–51]. ^{64}Cu-labelled NGO–PEG were also developed for in vivo PET imaging, in which active tumour targeting by conjugating NGO–PEG with an antibody TRC105 was utilized to target vasculatures in 4T1 tumour. Moreover, CNMs have been used as novel contrast agents for in vivo optical molecular imaging of animals. For example, SWNT as contrast agents have been employed for two-dimensional fluorescence and bioluminescence imaging or three-dimensional tomography using different animal models. The first ever imaging of nanotubes inside a living animal was performed in 2007 [52], in which, Drosophila larvae were fed by food containing SWNTs and imaged by NIR fluorescence microscopy. The biodistribution of SWNTs in live larvae was monitored by the nanotube fluorescence signals. Recently, RGD conjugated PEGylated SWNTs was also implemented as Raman probes for in vivo tumour imaging in live mice [53, 54]. After intravenous injection of targeted SWNTs to living mice bearing a tumour xenograft, strong SWNT Raman signals were observed in the tumour, while little signals was identified in the tumour after injection of non-targeted SWNTs.

SWNTs as contrast agent can also be utilized in photoacoustic molecular imaging. Photoacoustic imaging, in which sounds are generated as a result of local heating by the absorption of laser light, has higher spatial resolution than traditional fluorescence imaging methods [55]. RGD-conjugated SWNTs as the contrast agent have been employed for photoacoustic molecular imaging of cancer in a mouse tumour model (Figure 27.9) [56].

27.3.2.2 CNMs-based biosensor for cancer therapy

Toxicity studies reveal that highly water soluble and serum stable CNMs are bio-compatible and nontoxic. They can be used for both molecular imaging and cancer therapy. Targeted drug delivery with CNMs requires conjugation of both targeting molecules and drug molecules to the same CNMs. In 2008, Liu *et al.*, showed in vivo SWNT drug delivery for tumour suppression in mice. They conjugate paclitaxel (PTX), a widely used cancer chemotherapy drug, to branched poly-ethylene glycol chains on SWNTs via a cleavable ester bond to obtain a water-soluble SWNT-PTX conjugate [57]. SWNT-PTX is able to afford higher efficacy in suppressing tumour growth than clinical Taxol in a murine 4T1 breast cancer

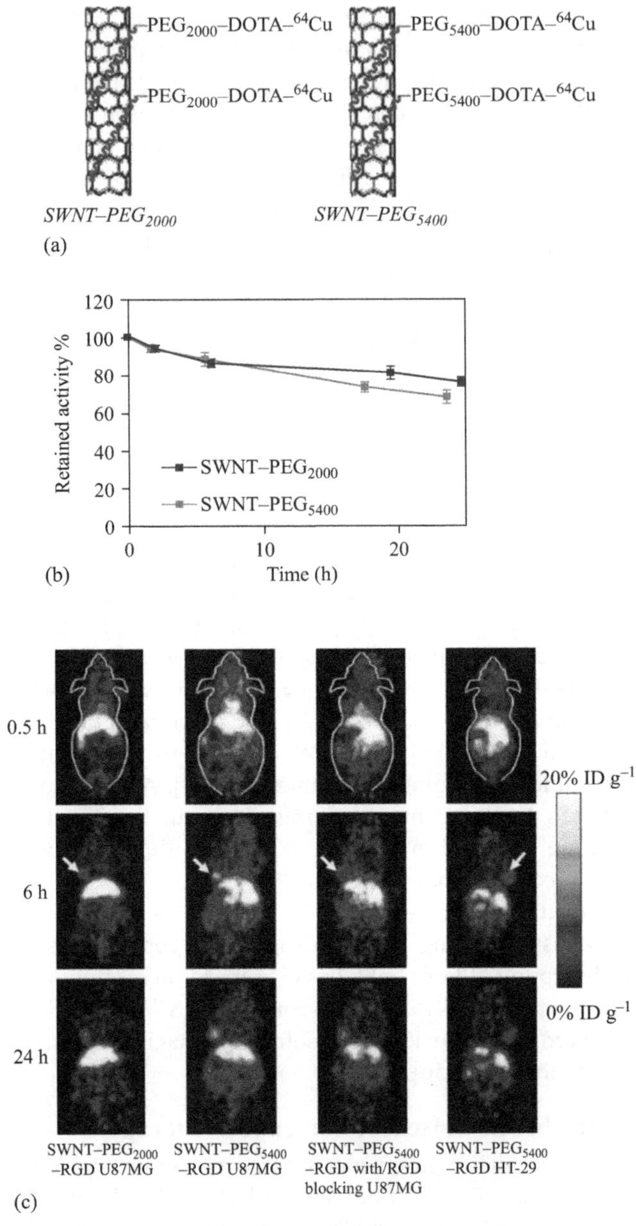

Figure 27.8 *(a) Schematic drawings of non-covalently functionalized SWNT–PEG_{2000}, SWNT–PEG_{5400} with DOTA–^{64}Cu. (b), Total ^{64}Cu activity left in the mice at different time points of the two different SWNT conjugates. (c) Targeting of integrin avb3-positive U87MG tumour in mice by RGD-functionalized SWNTs. The arrows point to the tumour. Reprinted with permission from Reference 48, Copyright (2015), Nature Publishing Group*

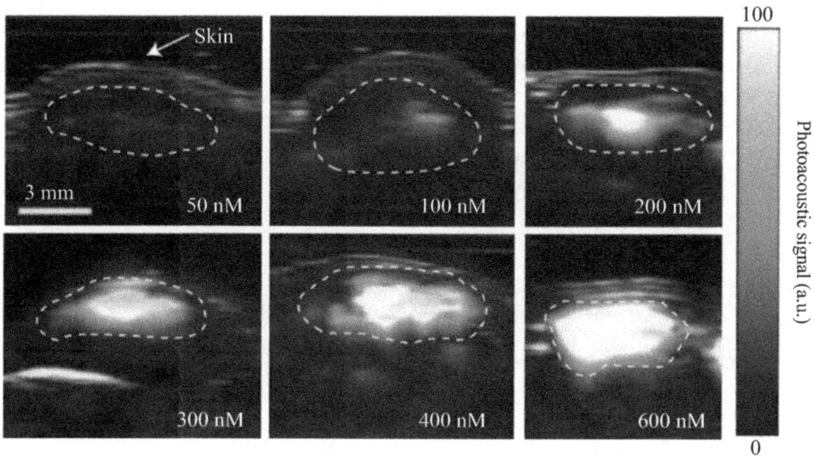

Figure 27.9 Photoacoustic detection of SWNTs in living mice. Mice were injected subcutaneously with single-walled carbon nanotubes at concentrations of 50–600 nM. Dotted line labeled areas show the photoacoustic image of single-walled nanotubes under the skin tissues of mouse with different concentration that were overlaid on corresponding ultrasound image. The surface of skin is visible in the ultrasound image that was labeled with white arrow. Reprinted with permission from Reference 56, Copyright (2015), Nature Publishing Group

model, due to the prolonged blood circulation and 10-fold higher tumour PTX uptake by SWNT delivery likely through enhanced permeability and retention. Drug molecules carried into the RES are released from SWNTs and excreted via biliary pathway without causing obvious toxic effects to normal organs.

Interestingly, NGO after PEGylation showed excellent physiological stability, which can be utilized for the loading of water-insoluble aromatic drug SN38 via π–π stacking [58]. Further, the synthesized NGO–PEG–SN38 agent was able to exhibit an enhanced cancer cell killing ability than the water soluble pro-drug CPT1118 (Figure 27.10). This excellent drug loading ability of GO has also been confirmed by several other groups in their respective studies [59, 60].

27.4 Conclusions

CNMs biosensors could offer enormous advantages over the present gold standards, which paves the way to realize direct and real-time detection of biomolecules in a multiplexed and label-free manner with the superior sensitivity and selectivity. Chemically functionalized CNMs have exhibited and will continue to show their potential in tumour-targeted accumulation with little toxicity, excretion and biocompatibility for preclinical study.

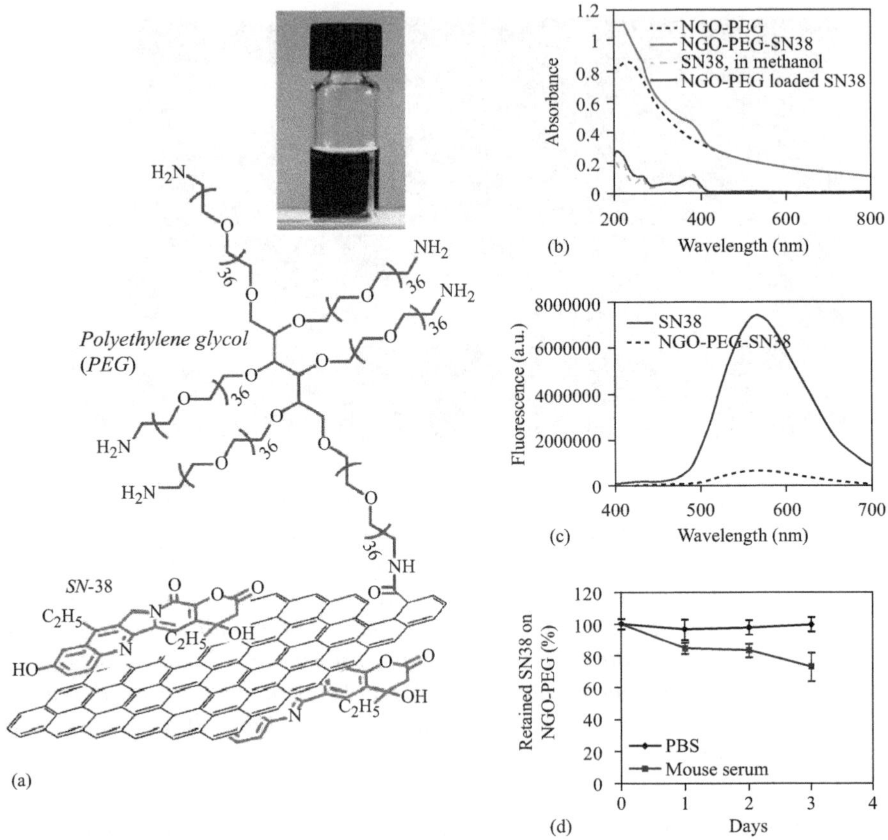

Figure 27.10 *SN38 loading on NGO–PEG: (a) schematic draw of SN38 loaded NGO–PEG; (inset) a photo of NGO–PEG–SN38 water solution. (b) UV–vis absorption spectra of NGO–PEG, NGO–PEG–SN38, SN38 in methanol, and difference spectrum of NGO–PEG and NGO–PEG–SN38. The SN38 absorbance at 380 nm was used to determine the loading. (c) Fluorescence spectra of SN38 and NGO–PEG–SN38 at [SN38] = 1 μM. Significant fluorescence quenching was observed for SN38 adsorbed on NGO. (d) Retained SN38 on NGO–PEG over time incubated in PBS and serum respectively. SN38 loaded on NGO–PEG was stable in PBS and released slowly in serum. Error bars were based on triplet samples. Reprinted with permission from Reference 58, Copyright (2015), American Chemical Society.*

References

[1] Aryal BP. *Protein-nanoparticle Conjugates: Developing Biosensors for Small Molecule Detection*. ProQuest; 2008.

[2] Clark LC, Lyons C. 'Electrode systems for continuous monitoring in cardiovascular surgery'. *Annals of the New York Academy of Sciences* 1962;102 (1):29–45.

[3] Eggins BR, Hickey C, Toft SA, Zhou DM. 'Determination of flavanols in beers with tissue biosensors'. *Analytica Chimica Acta* 1997;347(3):281–88.

[4] Wang J. 'Nanomaterial-based electrochemical biosensors'. *Analyst* 2005;130(4):421–26.

[5] Pandey P, Datta M, Malhotra B. 'Prospects of nanomaterials in biosensors'. *Analytical Letters* 2008;41(2):159–209.

[6] Chopra N, Gavalas VG, Bachas LG, Hinds BJ, Bachas LG. 'Functional one–dimensional nanomaterials: applications in nanoscale biosensors'. *Analytical Letters* 2007;40(11):2067–96.

[7] Gogotsi Y, Presser V. *Carbon Nanomaterials*. CRC Press; 2013.

[8] Dai L. *Carbon Nanotechnology: Recent Developments in Chemistry, Physics, Materials Science and Device Applications*. Elsevier; 2006.

[9] Cao G. *Nanostructures & Nanomaterials: Synthesis, Properties and Applications*. World Scientific; 2004.

[10] Odom TW, Huang J-L, Kim P, Lieber CM. 'Atomic structure and electronic properties of single-walled carbon nanotubes'. *Nature* 1998;391(6662):62–64.

[11] Wan X, Huang Y, Chen Y. 'Focusing on energy and optoelectronic applications: a journey for graphene and graphene oxide at large scale'. *Accounts of Chemical Research* 2012;45(4):598–607.

[12] Prasek J, Drbohlavova J, Chomoucka J, *et al.* 'Methods for carbon nanotubes synthesis—review'. *Journal of Materials Chemistry* 2011;21(40):15872–84.

[13] Dai H. 'Carbon nanotubes: synthesis, integration, and properties'. *Accounts of Chemical Research* 2002;35(12):1035–44.

[14] Journet C, Picher M, Jourdain V. 'Carbon nanotube synthesis: from large-scale production to atom-by-atom growth'. *Nanotechnology* 2012;23 (14):142001.

[15] Novoselov KS, Geim AK, Morozov S, *et al.* 'Electric field effect in atomically thin carbon films'. *Science* 2004;306(5696):666–69.

[16] Kotchey GP, Allen BL, Vedala H, *et al.* 'The enzymatic oxidation of graphene oxide'. *ACS Nano* 2011;5(3):2098–108.

[17] Liu Y, Dong X, Chen P. 'Biological and chemical sensors based on graphene materials'. *Chemical Society Reviews* 2012;41(6):2283–307.

[18] Peng X, Wong SS. 'Functional covalent chemistry of carbon nanotube surfaces'. *Advanced Materials* 2009;21(6):625–42.

[19] Chen Y, Star A, Vidal S. 'Sweet carbon nanostructures: carbohydrate conjugates with carbon nanotubes and graphene and their applications'. *Chemical Society Reviews* 2013;42(11):4532–42.

[20] Hong SY, Tobias G, Ballesteros B, *et al.* 'Atomic-scale detection of organic molecules coupled to single-walled carbon nanotubes'. *Journal of the American Chemical Society* 2007;129(36):10966–67.

[21] Loh KP, Bao Q, Ang PK, Yang J. 'The chemistry of graphene'. *Journal of Materials Chemistry* 2010;20(12):2277–89.

[22] Tans SJ, Devoret MH, Dai H, *et al.* 'Individual single-wall carbon nanotubes as quantum wires'. *Nature* 1997;386(6624), 474–477.

[23] Martel Ra, Schmidt T, Shea H, Hertel T, Avouris P. 'Single-and multi-wall carbon nanotube field-effect transistors'. *Applied Physics Letters* 1998;73 (17):2447–49.

[24] Besteman K, Lee J-O, Wiertz FG, Heering HA, Dekker C. 'Enzyme-coated carbon nanotubes as single-molecule biosensors'. *Nano Letters* 2003;3 (6):727–30.

[25] Wilson R, Turner A. 'Glucose oxidase: an ideal enzyme'. *Biosensors and Bioelectronics* 1992;7(3):165–85.

[26] Kang X, Mai Z, Zou X, Cai P, Mo J. 'A sensitive nonenzymatic glucose sensor in alkaline media with a copper nanocluster/multiwall carbon nanotube-modified glassy carbon electrode'. *Analytical Biochemistry* 2007;363 (1):143–50.

[27] Jiang L-C, Zhang W-D. 'A highly sensitive nonenzymatic glucose sensor based on CuO nanoparticles-modified carbon nanotube electrode'. *Biosensors and Bioelectronics* 2010;25(6):1402–07.

[28] Chen J, Zhang W-D, Ye J-S. 'Nonenzymatic electrochemical glucose sensor based on MnO 2/MWNTs nanocomposite'. *Electrochemistry Communications* 2008;10(9):1268–71.

[29] Lu L-M, Zhang L, Qu F-L, *et al.* 'A nano-Ni based ultrasensitive nonenzymatic electrochemical sensor for glucose: enhancing sensitivity through a nanowire array strategy'. *Biosensors and Bioelectronics* 2009;25(1):218–23.

[30] Star A, Tu E, Niemann J, Gabriel J-CP, Joiner CS, Valcke C. 'Label-free detection of DNA hybridization using carbon nanotube network field-effect transistors'. *Proceedings of the National Academy of Sciences of the United States of America* 2006;103(4):921–26.

[31] Martínez MT, Tseng Y-C, Ormategui N, Loinaz I, Eritja R, Bokor J. 'Label-free DNA biosensors based on functionalized carbon nanotube field effect transistors'. *Nano Letters* 2009;9(2):530–36.

[32] Dong X, Lau CM, Lohani A, *et al.* 'Electrical detection of femtomolar DNA via gold-nanoparticle enhancement in carbon-nanotube-network field-effect transistors'. *Advanced Materials* 2008;20(12):2389–93.

[33] SuáKim K, KwangáHahn S. 'Real-time, step-wise, electrical detection of protein molecules using dielectrophoretically aligned SWNT-film FET aptasensors'. *Lab on a Chip* 2010;10(16):2052–56.

[34] Lee D, Chander Y, Goyal SM, Cui T. 'Carbon nanotube electric immunoassay for the detection of swine influenza virus H1N1'. *Biosensors and Bioelectronics* 2011;26(8):3482–87.

[35] Ohno Y, Maehashi K, Yamashiro Y, Matsumoto K. 'Electrolyte-gated graphene field-effect transistors for detecting pH and protein adsorption'. *Nano Letters* 2009;9(9):3318–22.
[36] Sofue Y, Ohno Y, Maehashi K, Inoue K, Matsumoto K. 'Highly sensitive electrical detection of sodium ions based on graphene field-effect transistors'. *Japanese Journal of Applied Physics* 2011;50(6).
[37] Zeng G, Xing Y, Gao J, Wang Z, Zhang X. 'Unconventional layer-by-layer assembly of graphene multilayer films for enzyme-based glucose and maltose biosensing'. *Langmuir* 2010;26(18):15022–26.
[38] Mohanty N., Berry V. 'Graphene-based single-bacterium resolution biodevice and DNA transistor: interfacing graphene derivatives with nanoscale and microscale biocomponents'. *Nano Letters* 2008;8(12):4469–76.
[39] Ang PK, Chen W, Wee ATS, Kian PL. 'Solution-gated epitaxial graphene as pH sensor'. *Journal of the American Chemical Society* 2008;130(44): 14392–93.
[40] Ohno Y, Maehashi K, Matsumoto K. 'Label-free biosensors based on aptamer-modified graphene field-effect transistors'. *Journal of the American Chemical Society* 2010;132(51):18012–13.
[41] He Q, Sudibya HG, Yin Z, *et al.* 'Centimeter-long and large-scale micropatterns of reduced graphene oxide films: fabrication and sensing applications'. *ACS Nano* 2010;4(6):3201–08.
[42] Sudibya HG, He Q, Zhang H, Chen P. 'Electrical detection of metal ions using field-effect transistors based on micropatterned reduced graphene oxide films'. *ACS Nano* 2011;5(3):1990–94.
[43] Dankerl M, Hauf MV, Lippert A, *et al.* 'Graphene solution-gated field-effect transistor array for sensing applications'. *Advanced Functional Materials* 2010;20(18):3117–24.
[44] Cohen-Karni T, Qing Q, Li Q, Fang Y, Lieber CM. 'Graphene and nanowire transistors for cellular interfaces and electrical recording'. *Nano Letters* 2010;10(3):1098–102.
[45] Hess LH, Jansen M, Maybeck V, *et al.* 'Graphene transistor arrays for recording action potentials from electrogenic cells'. *Advanced Materials* 2011;23(43):5045–49.
[46] Cao X, He Q, Shi W, *et al.* 'Graphene oxide as a carbon source for controlled growth of carbon nanowires'. *Small* 2011;7(9):1199–202.
[47] Yin Z, He Q, Huang X, *et al.* 'Real-time DNA detection using Pt nanoparticle-decorated reduced graphene oxide field-effect transistors'. *Nanoscale* 2012;4(1):293–97.
[48] Liu Z, Cai W, He L, *et al.* 'In vivo biodistribution and highly efficient tumour targeting of carbon nanotubes in mice'. *Nature Nanotechnology* 2007;2(1):47–52.
[49] Yang K, Wan J, Zhang S, Zhang Y, Lee S-T, Liu Z. 'In vivo pharmacokinetics, long-term biodistribution, and toxicology of PEGylated graphene in mice'. *ACS Nano* 2010;5(1):516–22.

[50] Yang K, Wan J, Zhang S, Tian B, Zhang Y, Liu Z. 'The influence of surface chemistry and size of nanoscale graphene oxide on photothermal therapy of cancer using ultra-low laser power'. *Biomaterials* 2012;33(7):2206–14.

[51] Yang K, Hu L, Ma X, *et al.* 'Multimodal imaging guided photothermal therapy using functionalized graphene nanosheets anchored with magnetic nanoparticles'. *Advanced Materials* 2012;24(14):1868–72.

[52] Leeuw TK, Reith RM, Simonette RA, *et al.* 'Single-walled carbon nanotubes in the intact organism: near-IR imaging and biocompatibility studies in Drosophila'. *Nano Letters* 2007;7(9):2650–54.

[53] Keren S, Zavaleta C, Cheng Z, de La Zerda A, Gheysens O, Gambhir S. 'Noninvasive molecular imaging of small living subjects using Raman spectroscopy'. *Proceedings of the National Academy of Sciences* 2008;105 (15):5844–49.

[54] Zavaleta C, De La Zerda A, Liu Z, *et al.* 'Noninvasive Raman spectroscopy in living mice for evaluation of tumour targeting with carbon nanotubes'. *Nano Letters* 2008;8(9):2800–05.

[55] Xu M, Wang LV. 'Photoacoustic imaging in biomedicine'. *Review of Scientific Instruments* 2006;77(4):041101.

[56] De La Zerda A, Zavaleta C, Keren S, *et al.* 'Photoacoustic molecular imaging in living mice utilizing targeted carbon nanotubes'. *Nature Nanotechnology*2008;3:557–62.

[57] Liu Z, Chen K, Davis C, *et al.* 'Drug delivery with carbon nanotubes for in vivo cancer treatment'. *Cancer Research* 2008;68(16):6652–60.

[58] Liu Z, Robinson JT, Sun X, Dai H. 'PEGylated nanographene oxide for delivery of water-insoluble cancer drugs'. *Journal of the American Chemical Society* 2008;130(33):10876–77.

[59] Sahoo NG, Bao H, Pan Y, *et al.* 'Functionalized carbon nanomaterials as nanocarriers for loading and delivery of a poorly water-soluble anticancer drug: a comparative study'. *Chemical Communications* 2011;47(18):5235–37.

[60] Sun X, Liu Z, Welsher K, *et al.* 'Nano-graphene oxide for cellular imaging and drug delivery'. *Nano Research* 2008;1(3):203–12.

Chapter 28

Nanoparticle-based sensing of oligonucleotides and proteins

Virendra Majarikar[1], Ashish Ranjan[2] and Amit Jaiswal[2]

28.1 Introduction

Nanotechnology has opened new horizons for highly sensitive, selective, rapid and cost-effective analysis of biomolecules which plays inevitably important role in sensing, diagnostics and treatment. Unique properties of nano-scale materials and advancement of technology have certainly enhanced the sensitivity and the limit of detection. Depending on their composition, nanoparticles (NPs) have different physico-chemical properties such as high electron density and strong optical absorption (e.g., gold nanoparticles, Au NPs), magnetic moment (e.g., iron oxide nanoparticles, IONPs) and photoluminescence (e.g., semiconductor quantum dots, QDs) [1]. Recent ongoing research involves synthesis of novel nanomaterials (NMs), study of material properties, its characterization, miniaturization of outmoded existing devices, establishment of new methodological routes and fundamental perceptions into the understanding of materials and their interaction with biological systems are key components in the development of an ideal sensing strategy for a biomolecule. The bioaffinity and biocatalytic properties of NMs are generally exploited to engineer biosensors in order to make selective interactions with the analyte of interest and the detection mechanism is based on the electronic and optical properties or the signal transduction ability of the NPs [2a].

Biosensors are having extensive applications in the areas of life science, electronics, drug delivery and nanomedicine, plasmonics and nanocatalysis. Several label-free methods have been used to identify (in some cases also quantify) biomolecules [3]. Research is focused on bioconjugated NPs for molecular imaging, molecular screening and targeted therapy. The easy functionalization of NMs with biomolecules imparts them the ability to sense an analyte molecule specifically. Even though there are thousands of different biomolecules in a biological cell, majority of it can be classified into proteins, nucleic acids, lipids and carbohydrates.

[1]Department of Biomedical Engineering, Indian Institute of Technology Hyderabad, Telangana, India
[2]School of Basic Sciences, Indian Institute of Technology Mandi, Mandi 175001, Himachal Pradesh, India

These classes of biomolecules are crucial to a wide range of biochemical processes in the human body. These biomolecules are either building blocks or the carrier of genetic information or play a role in signal transduction process. They also play a significant role in maintaining homeostasis, various physiological functions, and are responsible for catalyzing each biochemical reactions to sustain life.

This chapter deals with the application of NMs mainly Au NPs for the sensing of oligonucleotides and proteins. The chapter is not an exhaustive review of all the NM-based sensors for biomolecules reported till date. However, this provides information on the few of the different types of NM-based nanosensors developed for sensing of nucleic acids and proteins.

28.2 Sensing of oligonucleotides

NM-based sensing systems have been developed for monitoring the levels of various nucleotides in environmental and biological samples. Various point of care devices have been developed for sensing the nucleotide analyte in the sample. Functionalization of NMs with oligonucleotides is the analytical tool for biological sensing.

Oligonucleotides are normally characterized by the sequence of nucleotide residues that make up the entire molecule or short fragments of nucleic acids with defined confirmation and sequence. They regulate gene expression and have a wide range of applications in genetic testing, research and forensics. A significant challenge in biosensing of the nucleotide is the simple, sensitive and specific detection of oligonucleotide sequences. The detection of these short DNA or RNA molecules can be used to diagnose and monitor disease, identify infectious agents and genetic predispositions to disease. There are many established techniques for oligonucleotide detection; none of them are without some limitations. The techniques developed to address this challenge, such as Southern and Northern Blotting, are insensitive, labor-intensive, expensive and can only test for a single oligonucleotide at a time.

The first report on sensing of oligonucleotide can be traced back to Shimidzu *et al.*'s [4] work in 1992, in which a novel method for sensing of oligonucleotide, by fluorescence quenching via photo-induced electron transfer between the P(V) porphyrin- and pyrene-labeled oligonucleotide was reported. In this method, two types of oligonucleotide derivatives were synthesized and hybridization capabilities of them with complementary oligonucleotides were evaluated subsequently. Later in 1994, Kumar *et al.* [5] monitored the hybridization of oligonucleotide using light-addressable potentiometric and evanescent wave fluorescence sensor. One biotinylated and the other FITC-labeled oligonucleotide hybridized together by Watson–Crick pairing were captured on streptavidin-coated surfaces via biotin–streptavidin binding. The fluoresceinated probe was detected potentiometrically by light-addressable potentiometric sensing (LAPS) which utilizes urease-conjugated anti-fluorescein antibodies and by evanescent wave spectroscopy (EWS) based on total internal reflection. The method provided 50 ng limit of detection using EWS and 20 pg fluoresceinated oligonucleotide could be detected using the LAPS,

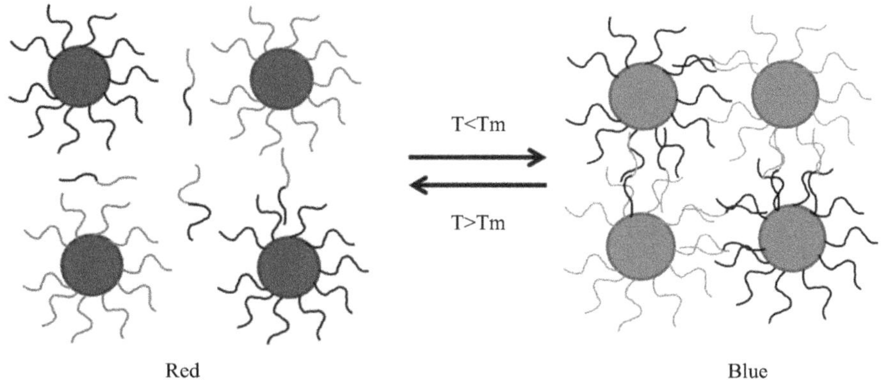

Figure 28.1 Schematic showing the aggregation of Au NPs in the presence of the target oligonucleotide and at a temperature less than that of the melting temperature of the probe-target oligonucleotide. Redrawn with permission from Reference 2b. Copyright © 2005, published by the American Chemical Society

whereas a dose-dependent reduction of signal was observed in the presence of a non-fluoresceinated oligonucleotide of identical sequence as that of the fluoresceinated target.

In 1996, Mirkin *et al.* [6] demonstrated an oligonucleotide sensor by exploiting DNA-meditated Au NP assembly (Figure 28.1). In this work, Au NPs were functionalized with thiolated DNA strand of two different sequences. The sequence on one of the NP was designed in order to match with half of the sequence of the target oligonucleotide, while the sequence on the other NP matches with other half sequence of the target. The addition of the target analyte led to oligonucleotide-directed Au NP aggregation due to the Watson–Crick pairing. This hybridization of the target oligonucleotide led to the assembly of Au NPs, forming its aggregates and leading to the red shift in the LSPR spectra and enabling visual colorimetric identification of the presence of analyte. This oligonucleotide induced aggregation of Au NPs change the color of the solution from red to blue and thus can easily be identified by naked eye. Further the process can be reversed by thermal denaturation. Interestingly, the aggregation of oligonucleotide-Au NPs depends on the specificity of DNA interactions to direct the interactions between particles of different size and composition.

Similarly, Gang *et al.* [7] have reported a time-resolved optical sensing of oligonucleotide hybridization using Au NPs. The shift in the LSPR peak enabled the distinction between the target and the non-target analyte in a time-dependent manner.

A very recent approach to oligonucleotide sensing was reported by Pascual *et al.* [8] in 2015. Mesoporous silica nanoparticles (mSi NPs) capped with oligonucleotides were synthesized which acted as DNA-responsive dye delivery system and were used for genomic DNA detection (Figure 28.2). Uncapping and delivery were then selectively achieved only in the presence of a target analyte. The dye

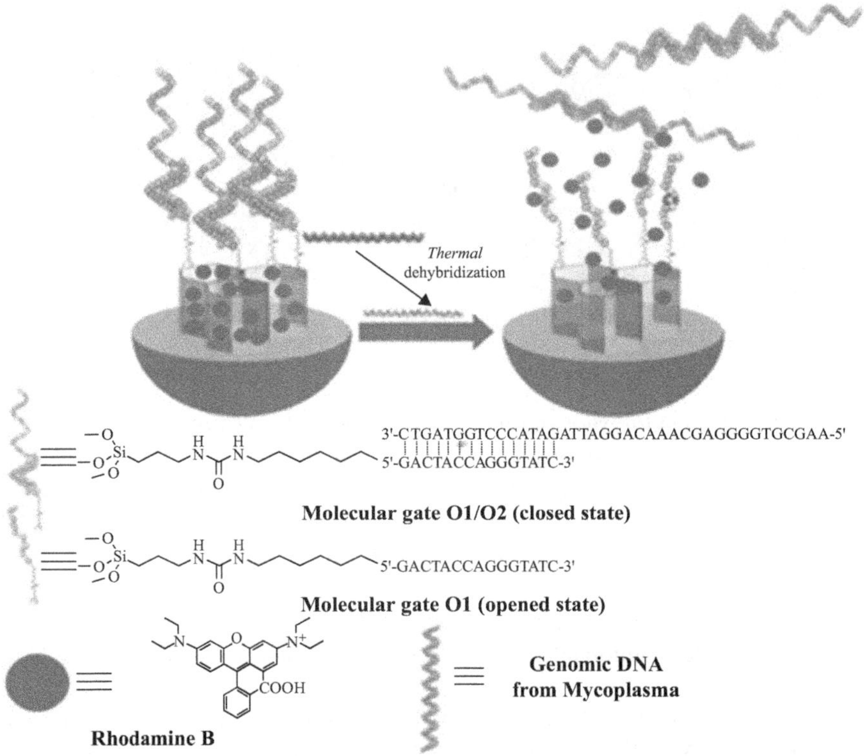

Figure 28.2 Schematic representation of the gated material S1-O1/O2 capped with a dsDNA. Release of the fluorescent dye rhodamine B occurs only in the presence of a single strand of Mycoplasma genomic DNA. Reproduced with permission from Reference 8. Copyright © 2015, published by the Royal Society of Chemistry

rhodamine B was loaded into the mSi NPs and then the external surface was functionalized with (3-isocyanato-propyl) triethoxysilane. Two single stranded DNA sequences (O1 & O2) with an O2 overhang were first hybridized and then covalently attached to the surface of the mSi NPs which created a lock for the pores. Presence of a single strand of Mycoplasma genomic DNA displaces the O2 strand from the solid because of sequence complementarity with the O2 overhang. This leads to opening of the pore and release of dye which can be monitored spectrophotometrically.

28.3 Sensing of protein

The sensing/detection of protein can govern the metabolic state of the organism. The detection of a particular peptide or protein is used in various diagnostic applications. Conventionally, ELISA and Western Blot are used for the identification of the protein of interest (POI). With the advent of nanotechnology, several nanosensors were fabricated to sense the POI.

Thanh *et al.* [9] have reported the sensing of proteins in serum sample using Au NPs aggregation-based immunoassay for anti-protein A in 2002. Au NP-based immunoassay provides extraordinary properties with respect to immunoassay such as more stable suspensions, are less susceptible to non-specific aggregation and less scattering of visible light, resulting in reduced background signal in turbidometric assays and lower detection limit. Au NPs coated with protein A were used to determine the level of anti-protein A. The system worked both in aqueous and serum solutions. This immunoassay involved the aggregation of Au NPs bearing protein antigens with anti-protein A. The rate of aggregation for this immunoassay was monitored by measuring the absorption of the gold colloid suspension at 620 nm using absorption spectroscopy. The limit of detection of this immunoassay was about 1 μg/mL of anti-protein A in serum sample. The sensitivity of this assay was comparable to the conventional ELISA technique, however the reported method was much simpler to perform as it involved only one step in contrast to ELISA.

On similar principle of analyte-induced aggregation of NP, Medcalf *et al.* [10] developed an aggregation-based immune-turbidimetric assay for urine albumin. In their assay, poly-(vinyl naphthalene) NPs were coated with chloromethylstyrene polymer, which was subsequently used to immobilize anti-human serum albumin. This aggregation-based immunoassay for urine albumin was detected using absorption spectrometry by measuring the change in light scattering intensity at 340 nm.

Tsai *et al.* [11] have reported protein–protein interaction detection using Au NP-based competitive colorimetric assay. It incorporates an assembly of protein A (albumin) and protein B (thrombin) functionalized Au NPs to determine their binding affinity. The presence of protein A crosslinks another coated Au NPs with concomitant red shift in the LSPR spectrum. Due to prevailing weak non-covalent interaction between Au NPs and protein A functionalize to it, another protein in analyte sample is able to dislocate Au NPs resulting strong protein–protein interaction and its subsequent detection via colorimetric assay. Figure 28.3 shows the schematic of colorimetric competitive binding assay to study the interaction between two proteins. Au NPs are functionalized with a ligand which can be identified by a protein molecule denoted by X. Thus in the presence of this protein X the Au NPs form aggregates due to ligand–protein interaction leading to a change in color of the Au NP solution from red to blue. However, the addition of another protein, denoted by Y, capable of interacting with protein X, could influence the binding between X and Au NPs. It is therefore possible to undo the agglomeration of Au NPs and cause the segregation of Au NPs. This results in the shift in the color of the Au NPs solution back to the ruby red color.

One of the striking methods for detection and identification of proteins involve "Chemical Nose" (Figure 28.4) approach using NP–fluorescent polymer by You *et al.* [12] in early 2007. Researchers demonstrated that differential selective interactions between molecules can be used to generate patterns based on fluorescence signal, which can then be used to identify analytes or changes in complex mixtures. In this work six structurally related cationic Au NPs were synthesized and they were

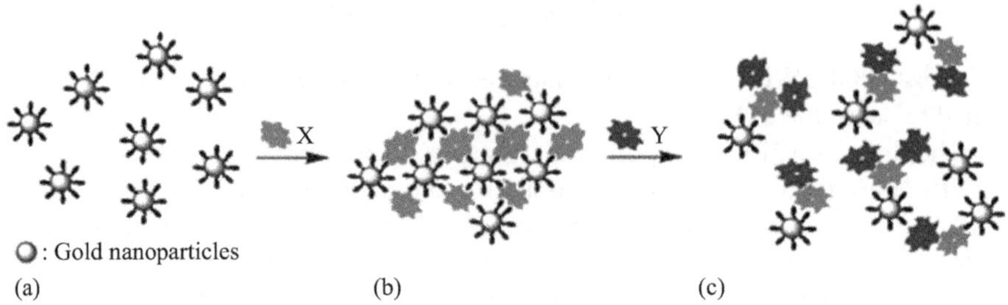

Figure 28.3 *Schematic illustration of the colorimetric detection of protein-protein interaction based on the aggregation of Au NPs. (a) Protein X binds to the ligands present on the surface of Au NPs and promotes agglomeration of the particles via multivalent ligand -protein interactions (b). Addition of another protein Y, influence the binding between X and Au NPs reversing the agglomeration of Au NPs. As a result, the color of the solution can change from blue to the deep red color (c). Please refer to the cited article for colour image. Reproduced with permission from Reference 11. Copyright © 2007, published by the Royal Society of Chemistry*

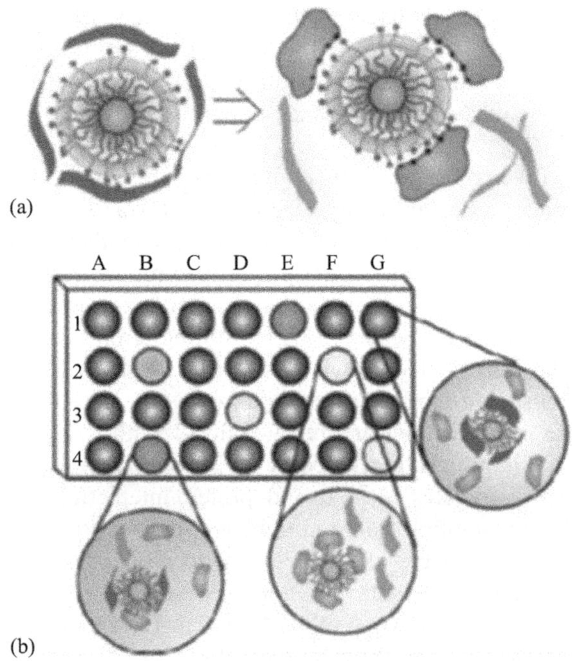

Figure 28.4 *Schematic representation of (a) "Chemical Nose" sensor array: displacement of the quenched fluorescent protein by the analyte protein from the Au NP surface and the restoration of fluorescence and (b) pattern generation through differential release of fluorescent polymers from gold nanoparticles. Please refer to the cited article for colour image. Reproduced with permission from Reference 12. Copyright © 2007, published by Macmillan Publishers Ltd: [Nature nanotechnology]*

made to interact with fluorescent polymer. The fluorescence of the polymer was quenched due to their presence in close vicinity to the Au NPs. The addition of analyte proteins disrupts the NP–polymer interaction, enabling the regain of fluorescence from the polymer and thus creating a distinct fluorescence response pattern. Owing to the fact that protein–NP interactions are differential, it leads to a fingerprint fluorescence response pattern for individual proteins which was characterized using linear discriminate analysis resulting in successful unknown sample identification with an overall accuracy of 94.2%.

An analogous method was developed by De *et al.* [13] in 2009 based on the above-mentioned principle. Here, investigators have reported an array of sensor for proteins sensing at bio-relevant concentrations in buffer and human serum using conjugates of NPs-green fluorescent protein. Final fluorescence response pattern for individual proteins at different concentrations or mixtures was characterized using linear discriminant analysis with accuracy of 100% and 97% in buffer and human serum respectively.

Wei *et al.* [14] have described aptamer-based colorimetric sensing of protein using unmodified Au NP probes in 2007 (Figure 28.5). Aptamers are single-stranded oligonucleotide-based binding molecules produced using an in vitro selection process. These DNA or RNA aptamers have specific structures which can bind to a wide variety of targets with high affinity and specificity. Differential selective interaction has been reported between aptamers and small organic molecule, e.g., proteins in biological sample. The aggregation of Au NPs probes in presence of analyte molecule results in visible color change from red to blue at nanomolar concentrations due to plasmonic coupling, providing a practical platform for protein sensing.

In early 2008 Wang *et al.* [15] developed protein biosensors using DNA-modified Au NPs. The aptameric DNA was hybridized to a probe sequence tagged

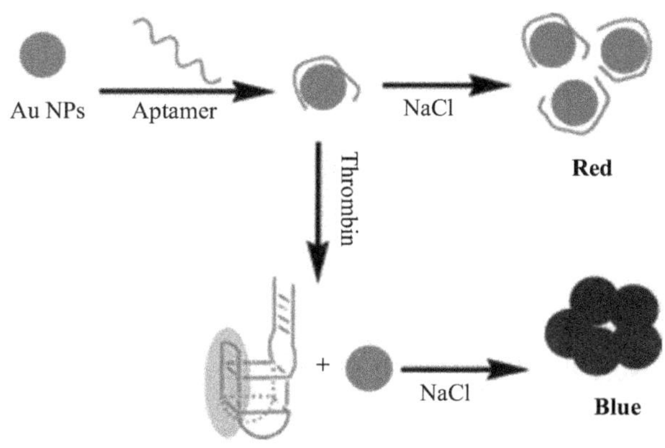

Figure 28.5 Schematic illustration of aptamer-based colorimetric sensing of protein using gold nanoparticle probes. Please refer to the cited article for colour image. Reproduced with permission from Reference 14. Copyright © 2007, published by the Royal Society of Chemistry

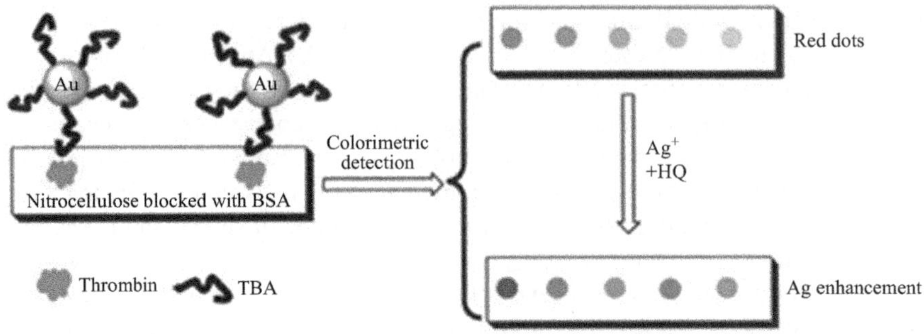

Figure 28.6 Illustration of dot-blot assay colorimetric detection of protein by aptamer–Au NPs conjugates. Please refer to the cited article for colour image. Reproduced with permission from Reference 16. Copyright © 2008, published by the Royal Society of Chemistry

with a fluorescent dye. The presence of an analyte protein enables the change in the structure of the aptameric DNA allowing the release of the probe strand which can be detected spectrophotometrically. Later in 2008, Wang *et al.* [16] have reported colorimetric detection of protein by aptamer–Au NPs conjugates based on a dot-blot assay (Figure 28.6). Au NPs demonstrate a unique optical properties enabling colorimetric detection of proteins in real time without the need of any sophisticated instrument using a dot-blot assay which represents a simplified biomolecule detection method. This assay involves preparation of mixture containing the protein molecule (thrombin), to be detected and is applied directly on a membrane (nitrocellulose) as a dot. This assay makes use of binding affinity or interaction property between aptamer functionalized with Au NPs and thrombin. Au NPs were functionalized with thrombin sensitive aptamer that can bind to the analyte thrombin protein which was immobilized on a membrane. This binding results in accumulation of Au NPs at the sites where the analyte protein is present and enables visual identification due to the formation of red color. Colorimetric detection is spotted through circular templates directly onto the membrane substrate which improves thrombin detection sensitivity via silver enhancement solution.

28.4 Conclusion

This chapter presented a few of the different sensing methodologies developed for sensitive and selective sensing of proteins and nucleic acids using NPs. Au NPs because of their brilliant color due to the LSPR and the sensitivity of this LSPR spectra to size and agglomeration enables the detection and identification of analyte molecules. This chapter is not a comprehensive review on the sensors developed using NMs but it presents few of the interesting sensing methodology for the detection of nucleic acids and proteins using NMs.

References

[1] Verderio P., Avvakumova S., Alessio G., *et al.* Delivering Colloidal Nanoparticles to Mammalian Cells: A Nano–Bio Interface Perspective. *Advanced Healthcare Materials*. 2014; **3**: 957–976.

[2a] Ansari A.A., Alhoshan M., Alsalhi S.M., Aldwayyan S.A. Prospects of Nanotechnology in Clinical Immunodiagnostics. *Sensors*. 2010; **10**: 6535–6581.

[2b] Rosi N.L., Mirkin C.A. Nanostructures in Biodiagnostics. *Chemical Reviews*. 2005; **105**(4): 1547–1562.

[3] Lane A.L., Qian X., Nie S. SERS Nanoparticles in Medicine: From Label-Free Detection to Spectroscopic Tagging. *Chemical Reviews*. 2015; **115**: 10489–10529.

[4] Shimidzu T., Segawa H., Kitamura M., Nimura A. Syntheses of Oligonucleotide Derivatives with P(V) Porphyrin and Their Properties. *Nucleic Acids Symposium Series*. 1992; **27**: 97–108.

[5] Kumar P., Willson C.R., Valdes J.J., Chambers C.J. Monitoring of Oligonucleotide Hybridization Using Light-Addressable Potentiometric and Evanescent Wave Fluorescence Sensing. *Materials Science and Engineering*: C. 1994; **1**(3): 187–192.

[6] Mirkin A.C., Letsinger L.R., Mucic C.R., Storhoff J.J. A DNA-Based Method for Rationally Assembling Nanoparticles into Macroscopic Materials. *Nature*. 1996; **382**: 607–609.

[7] Liu G.L., Rodriguez V.B., Lee L.P. Time-Resolved Optical Sensing of Oligonucleotide Hybridization via Au Colloidal Nanoparticles. *Journal of Nanoscience and Nanotechnology*. 2005; **5**(11): 1933–1937.

[8] Pascual L., Baroja I., Aznar E., *et al.* Oligonucleotide-Capped Mesoporous Silica Nanoparticles as DNA-Responsive Dye Delivery Systems for Genomic DNA Detection. *Chemical Communications*. 2015; **51**: 1414–1416.

[9] Thi N., Thanh K., Rosenzweig Z. Development of an Aggregation-Based Immunoassay for Anti-Protein A Using Gold Nanoparticles. *Analytical Chemistry*. 2002; **74**: 1624–1628.

[10] Medcalf E.A., Newman D.J., Gorman E.G., Price C.P. Rapid, robust method for measuring low concentrations of albumin in urine. *Clinical Chemistry*. 1990; **36**(3): 446–449.

[11] Tsai S.C., Yu B.T., Chen T.C. Gold Nanoparticle-Based Competitive Colorimetric Assay for Detection of Protein–Protein Interactions. *Chemical Communication*. 2005; **34**: 4273–4275.

[12] You C.C., Miranda O.R., Gider B., *et al.* Detection and Identification of Proteins Using Nanoparticle-Fluorescent Polymer "Chemical Nose" Sensors. *Nature Nanotechnology*. 2007; **2**: 318–323.

[13] De M., Rana S., Akpinar H. Sensing of proteins in human serum using conjugates of nanoparticles and green fluorescent protein. *Nature Chemistry*. 2009; **1**: 461–465.

[14] Wei H., Li B., Li J., Wang E., Dong S. Simple and Sensitive Aptamer-Based Colorimetric Sensing Of Protein Using Unmodified Gold Nanoparticle Probes. *Chemical Communications*. 2007; **36**: 3735–3737.

[15] Wang W., Chen C., Qian M., Zhao S.X. Aptamer Biosensor for Protein Detection Using Gold Nanoparticles. *Analytical Biochemistry*. 2008; **373**: 213–219.

[16] Wang Y., Li D., Ren W., Liu Z., Dong S., Wang E. Ultrasensitive Colorimetric Detection of Protein by Aptamer–Au Nanoparticles Conjugates Based on a Dot-Blot Assay. *Chemical Communications*. 2008; **22**: 2520–2522.

Index

absorbance 348–9
  detection 426–7
absorption of metal NPs, sensing based on 540
  interparticle-distance dependent color change 540–3
  refractive index change 543
AC electrokinetics-based capacitive biosensor 317
  devices and methods 324
    interdigitated microelectrode sensors 324
    measurement procedure 326
    sample preparation and electrode functionalization 324–6
  experiments 326
    capacitance changes due to protein binding and detachment 327–8
    capacitive sensing for rapid analysis of surface quality control 326
    effect of AC frequency 329–32
    effect of electrode designs 332–4
    selectivity in complex fluids 334–6
    sensitive and quantitative detection 328–9
  mechanisms 319
    ACEK enhancement of affinity sensing 321–4
    capacitive detection of biomolecular binding on electrode surface 319–20
    direct detection of interfacial capacitance 320–1
AC electro-osmosis (ACEO) 319, 322
AC electrothermal (ACET) effect 319, 322–3, 334
acetylcholinesterase (AChE)
  activity, determination of 525–6
  -based electrochemical sensors 43
acid-labile surfactant (ALS) 60
acrylamide 51
acrylamide polymer-based HydroMIP 450
acute kidney injury (AKI) 487
acute-phase proteins 353
adaptive immune response, process of 211–12
adenosine-5'-triphosphate (ATP) 552
adrenaline 111
adsorption approach 346
affinity-based biosensors 295
affinity-based immobilization 453
affinity chromatographic purification 214
affinity sensing, ACEK enhancement of 321–4
affordability 423
Affymetrix gene chip 355
a*IIb*b3 integrins 173–4
alcohol dehydrogenase (ADH) 464
aldehyde-intermediate 451
alginate-encapsulated FMNS (Alg-FMNS) 370
alkaline phosphatase 41, 295
alternating current electrokinetics (ACEK) 318–19, 332–3
  affinity sensing, ACEK enhancement of 321–4

Alzheimer's disease biomarkers, detection of 12
3-aminophenylboronic acid 506–7
(3-aminopropyl) triethoxysilane (APTES) 324, 326
aminopterin 215
amperometric biosensors 129, 299–300, 464
amperometric detection 26, 28, 427
amperometry 37, 112
analog-front end (AFE) circuitry 382, 387
analog-to-digital converter (ADC) block 382
analyte-specific biosensors 115–22
antenna characterization for NCVS sensor 405–6
antibodies 184
  classification of 209
  in immunoassays 257–8
antibody generation for use in biosensors 209–11
antibody-mediated immunity 211–12
antibody optimisation for biosensor applications 221
  immobilisation strategies 224–5
  specificity, sensitivity and affinity 221–2
  stability for biosensor applications 223–4
antigen-antibody interaction 453
antigen-specific affinity purification 215
anti-gliadin antibody as biomarker 50
antioxidant activity, determination of 523
  ferric reducing ability of plasma (FRAP) assay 523–4
  total peroxyl radical-trapping potential (TRAP) assay 524
antioxidants 522–3
apolipoprotein E gene 6
Aptamer–gD interactions 102
aptamers 45, 74, 184, 257, 371, 450, 589
  for detection of cancer cells 75–9
  for *in vitro* cancer cells 76–9
aptasensors 45, 77–8
  electrochemical 45
arc-tangent demodulation 402
  for NCVS sensors 401–2
array-based nanoplasmonic detection 476
arrhythmias 384
artificial electron acceptors 22, 113
artificial redox mediators 113–14
AS1411 aptamer 284–5
as-prepared N-doped graphene 462
attenuated total reflection (ATR) 95, 474, 499
auto-fluorescent protein (AFP) 189
Autolab SPR 96
Avalanche Photodiode (APD) 347
Avian Influenza Virus (AIV) 145, 148–9
Avidin-Alkaline Phosphatase (ALP) conjugate 41–2
avidity 258
Azospirillum brasilense 327

backscattering interferometer 199
bacterial cells, *in vitro* detection of 79
  electrochemical and optical nanobiosensors for 79–80
  lab-on-a-chip and chip-plate based nanobiosensors for 83
  microfluidics for bacterial cells detection 81
  paper-based nanobiosensors for 82
  perspectives of nanobiosensors in 83–4
baryodynia 277, 279
basal-plane pyrolytic graphite (BPG) electrode 53
base stacking (BS) technique 57
BD™ Directigen™ EZ Flu A+B kit 265
Beer-Lamberts law 348
benzene 51
Beta-Glo assay system 433
β-nicotinamide adenine dinucleotide phosphate (NADPH) 531

biacore 95
  biomolecular interactions on biacore chips 101
  biomolecular recognition in 102
  kinetic analyses 99, 103
  principle in 97–8
  recommendations for controlled experiments 105
  refunctioning and regeneration of chip surfaces 103–5
  sensing surfaces 99–101
    non-fouling on 101–2
Biacore 4000 219–20
BIAcore T100 102–3
Biacore X^{TM} analytical system 486
BIAlite 97
bioaffinity 262, 346, 469, 583
biocatalyst 43, 345
biochemiluminescent detection-based SP-IVD 242
biocompatibility 7, 9, 47, 110, 122–6, 352, 463, 573
biocompatible hydrophilic outer membranes 24
biofouling 26–7, 109, 121, 122–6, 128
bioluminescence resonance energy transfer (BRET) 189
biomarker protein, quantitative detection of 328–9
biomarkers detection 76–9
biomolecular binding, capacitive detection of
  on electrode surface 319–20
biomolecular interactions, biacore chip-surfaces for 101
biomolecular recognition in biacore system 102
biomolecule immobilization 262–3
biomolecules 7–8, 42, 97, 112, 247
  coverage on the tracker 264
  immobilization of 142, 262, 448–53
  proper vs poor orientation of 143
bio-optrodes: *see* fibre optical biosensors (FOBS)
bioreceptors 79, 345–6
biorecognition techniques 184
biosensor design 387, 465, 547, 558
biosensor fabrication 63, 65, 129
biosensors, defined 1, 342
biosignal instrumentation amplifier (INA) 389–90
  design consideration 390–1
  fully differential folded-cascode based chopper stabilized INA 391–8
  state-of-the-art performance comparison 398
biotin-strept (avidin) system 149, 453
bivalent antibody 224
black boxes 166, 347
block copolymer micelle nanolithography 169
blood, analysis of drugs in 432
  illicit drugs analysis 437
  therapeutical drugs analysis 432–7
blood glucose monitoring 49, 352
B-lymphocyte-derived plasma cells 209
BMP-7 (bone morphogenetic protein-7) 281
Bode plot 329
Boltzmann constant 299
bovine serum albumin (BSA) 60, 112, 514, 527, 553
Bragg condition 476
breast cancer 354, 483
breast cancer susceptibility gene (BRCA1) 466, 483
BUN analyser 112
1-butyl-3-methylimidazolium dodecanesulfonate (BAS) 60

calcium alginate 452
calicivirus 182
calorimetric transducers 74
Campylobacter jejuni, detection of 52
cancer biomarker 6–7, 13–14, 354–5
  biosensors for 52
  detection 267
cancer cells
  in vitro detection of 75
    aptamers for 75–9

SPR-based biosensors for detection of 488–91
cancer disease, biosensors in 355
cancer therapy, CNMs-based biosensor for 575–7
capacitance 301
changes due to protein binding and detachment 327–8
dipolar capacitance of molecular layers 304–6
double-layer capacitance 302–4
electrochemical capacitance 306–9
electrostatic/geometrical capacitance 302
interfacial 319–21, 326, 336
capacitive biosensors 309–13
capacitive-coupling based non-contact wearable ECG sensors 381–2
capacitive detection of biomolecular binding on electrode surface 319–20
capacitive sensing for rapid analysis of surface quality control 326
capillarity restricted modification (CARM) method 430
capillary array electrophoresis (CAE) system 66
capillary electrophoresis (CE) technique 55
capillary flow rate 258
carbamate insecticides 43
carbodiimide-intermediate 451
carbohydrate antigen (CA)
CA 125 295
CA 15-13 295
CA-19-19 295
carbon nanomaterials (CNMs) 567–9
in electrochemical biosensors 47–8
carbon nanomaterials (CNMs)-based biosensor and its applications 569
in vitro application of CNMs biosensor 569
graphene-based biosensor for in vitro detection 571–4
single-walled carbon nanotube based biosensor for in vitro detection 570
in vivo application of CNMs-based biosensor 592
CNMs-based biosensor for cancer therapy 575–7
CNMs-based biosensor for tumour detection 574–5
carbon nano strings 260
carbon nanostructures 148–9, 150
carbon nanotubes (CNT) 47, 114, 155, 200–2
CNT deposited onto Si/SiO_2 substrate 156
CNT–DNA core-shell 155
CNT-FET 148
CNT loaded with silver nanoparticles 152
carbon particles 260
carbonyl-di-imidazole (CDI) 451–2
carboxyl-terminated QDs605 153
carcinoembryonic antigen (CEA) 9, 295
cardiac troponin 353
cardiac troponin I (cTnI) 353–4
cardiomyocyte-like HL-1 cells 573
cardiovascular disease, biosensors in 353–4
cardiovascular disease biomarkers 353
CdSe hollow nanostructures onto GCE 153
celiac disease sensor 50
cell adhesion kinetics, dependence of on surface density of integrin ligands 170–4
cell adhesion on tailored surfaces 169–70
cell adhesion research, label-free optical biosensors in 165–8
cell-based biorecognition 184
cell-based biosensors 75
cellobiose dehydrogenase 114
cell penetrating peptides (CPPs) 286–7
Cell-SELEX 76

cellulose nanocrystals (CNC)-based hydrogels 450
chemically modified graphenes (CMGs) 571
chemically reduced graphene oxide (CRGO) 460, 462, 467
chemical vapor deposition (CVD) growth 460
chemiluminescence detection 427
CH-Fe_3O_4 nanocomposite onto ITO electrode 153
chicken IgY purification 215
chip-plate based nanobiosensors 83
chip surfaces
  refunctioning and regeneration of 103–5
chitosan (CS) nanoparticles 285
chitosan/AuNP nanocomposite 6
chitosan nanoparticle surface 372
cholesterol biosensors 49, 464
cholesterol esterase 295, 463
cholesterol oxidase (ChOx) 43, 49, 295, 463
choline oxidase (ChOX) 45, 452
circularly permuted (CP) AFP-based biosensors 189
circulating tumor cells (CTCs) detection, nanobiosensors for 363
  nanostructured interfaces designed for 364
    from artificial to biomimetic 366–8
    from micro to nano 364–6
    from traditional to smart 368–70
  purification and isolation strategy based on nanostructured interfaces 371–3
click chemical ligation chain reaction (CCLCR) 542
clinical diagnosis
  conventional techniques for 141
  nanomaterials for 141
    carbon nanostructures 148–9, 150
    magnetic nanoparticles (MGNPs) 146–8
    metal nanoparticles (MNPs) 144–5
    nanostructured conducting polymers (NCPs) 149, 151
    nanostructured metal oxide (NMO) 151–7
    quantum dots (QDs) 145–6
  nanoparticles based biosensors for 152–7
cloud computing 247
CM3 chip 99
CM4 chip 99
CM5 chip 99
codeine 428, 431–2
collective diffusion coefficient 447
colloidal lithography 549
colorimetric, fluorescent and luminescent detection 232–3, 243–4
colorimetric detection-using SP-IVD 232–3
commercial-of-the-shelf (COTS) antennas 406
commercial portable SPR-sensors 509–13
common-mode rejection ratio (CMRR) 390
competitive immunoassay 255–6, 437
complementary sequence (CS) 371
complex fluids, selectivity in 334–6
concanavalin A (Con A) 29
conducting polymers 6–7, 45–7
  nanostructured 149–51
conductometric biosensors 39, 112
conductometric microbiosensors 111
conductometry 39, 427
confinement length 173
contact-based ECG sensors 381
continuous glucose monitoring (CGM) systems 120, 122
continuous glucose monitoring systems (CGMS) 22–4
continuous tapered fibre 344
continuous wave (CW) incident wave 400
conventional SPR 474

Cottrel's equation 23
covalent binding 506–7
covalent bonding 347
covalent immobilization 450–2, 507
covalent-orientated antibody immobilisation strategy 225
C-reactive protein (CRP) 6, 353
CTC-chip 363
CuHCF nanoparticles onto Au electrode 152
Cu hexacyanoferrate 145
culture 141
Cy3-extravidin and Cy3-IgG 60
cyanine dye 3 (Cy3) 194
cyclic olefin copolymer (COC) 424
cyclic voltammetry (CV) 531
cytochrome c (Cyt c) 119
cytometry 239–40, 245

D-dimer antibody 466–7
Debye–Huckel Theory 319
Debye length 307, 319
defibrillation 384–6, 415
delipidation-and-precipitation 215
demountable direct injection high efficiency nebulizer (D-DIHEN) 63
Dexcom and Medtronic biosensors 22
diabetes applications, biosensors for 352
- biosensors for glucose measuring 352–3
- glucose as diabetes biomarker 352

DiCAST 218–19
dielectrophoresis (DEP) 81–2, 319, 322–3, 332
differential pulse voltammetry (DPV) 52, 467
diffraction gratings, SPR-sensors with 504
diffusion immunoassay (DIA) 433, 435
digital microfluidics (DMF) 428, 432, 437
2,3-dihydroxypropyl methacrylate 124
2'4 di-nitro phenyl hydrazine (DNPH) 528
dipolar capacitance of molecular layers 304–6
dipstick assays 555
diquat 531
direct-conversion receiver and range correlation in NCVS sensors 403–5
direct electron transfer (DET) 25, 42, 48, 114, 461–2
disease biomarkers, detection of 1
disposable microfluidic device 426
disulfides 506
5,5'-dithiobis, 2-nitrobenzoic acid (DTNB) 525, 527
DL-TBOA 116
DNA
- -based biosensors 184
- DNA biosensor 144
- DNA hybridization assay 12
- DNA sensors 6, 467–8
- separation and extraction of 57–8
- SPR-based biosensors for detection of 483

dopamine 25, 116–17
Doppler-based non-contact vital signs (NCVS) sensor 381, 398
- antenna characterization for 405–6
- direct-conversion receiver and range correlation in 403–5
- Doppler radar principle 400–1
- experimental results and analysis 411–15
- fourth-generation NCVS sensor hardware 404
- NCVS system evaluated with several antennas 406–11
- quadrature receiver and arc-tangent demodulation for NCVS sensors 401–2

Doppler effect 400
Doppler shift 400
double hybridization method 487–8
double-layer capacitance 302–4
double-stranded DNA (dsDNA) 467
- dsDNA-AuNPs 540
- ds-DNA fragments 57

dried blood spots (DBS) 436
droplet-based microfluidics 58
dry film photoresist 425
dummy IDMEs 326, 334
dynamic light scattering (DLS) 545–6
dynamic mass redistribution (DMR) 167–8
dynamic solid phase extraction (dSPE) 58

easy-to-use portable devices 73
e-beam lithography 478
edge-plane pyrolytic graphite (EPPG) 468
electric double layer (EDL) 304, 319
electrocardiogram (ECG)/elektro-kardiogram (EKG) 379
electrocardiogram (ECG) signal 380
electrochemical biosensors 1–2, 120, 185, 295, 299, 451, 459
  aptasensors 45
  for cancer 52
  for environmental monitoring 50
    genotoxicants 51
    heavy metals 51
    pesticides 50
    toxic gases 51
  enzymatic biosensor 42
    direct detection of analytes 42–3
    indirect detection of analytes via inhibition of enzyme activity 43
  in food industry 51–2
  functions of AuNPs in 4
    immobilization of biological recognition element 7
    improvement of electron transfer efficiency 5–7
    nanocarrier for signal amplification 8–10
    nanocatalyst for signal amplification 10–14
    signal generation 8
  graphene nanomaterials used in fabrication of 460–1
  of healthcare 49
    celiac disease sensor 50
    cholesterol 49–50
    glucose 49
    oxidative stress 50
  immunosensors 43
    direct 44
    indirect 43–4
  materials used in construction of 45
    carbon nanomaterial 47–8
    conducting polymers 45–7
    nanoparticles 48–9
  miniaturized graphene 461–8
  nucleic acid sensors 39
    detection of genotoxicants/pesticide 40
    detection of hybridisation 40–2
  for pathogens 52–3
  principle of 37
    conductometry 39
    potentiometry 38
    surface charge using field-effect transistors 38–9
    voltammetry 37
  smartphone (SP)-based 242
  whole cells based sensors 44
    based on cellular activity of the cell 45
    based on cellular barrier behaviour 45
electrochemical capacitance 306–9
Electrochemical Capacitance Spectroscopy (ECS) 310
electrochemical capacitive biosensors for point-of-care diagnostics
  amperometric principles 299–300
  capacitance and capacitive phenomena, types of 301
    dipolar capacitance of molecular layers 304–6
    double-layer capacitance 302–4
    electrochemical capacitance 306–9
    electrostatic/geometrical capacitance 302
  capacitive biosensors 309–13
  electrochemistry and biosensors 293–8

impedimetric principles 300–1
potentiometric principles 299
summarization and perspectives 313–14
electrochemical detection 236–9, 244–5, 427–8
enzymes as an aid to 41–2
electrochemical detector (ECD) 431
electrochemical immunosensor 1–2, 6, 43–4, 295, 453
electrochemical impedance 300
electrochemical impedance spectroscopy (EIS) 44, 77, 300
Electrochemical Impedimetric Spectroscopy (EIS) 39
electrochemically detectable label 40–1
electrochemically reduced graphene oxide (ERGO) 460
electrochemical microbiosensor 111
for bacterial cells detection 79–80
electrochemical oxygen biosensor 125–6
electrochemical transducers 74
electrochemiluminescence (ECL) detection 427
electrochemistry capacitance 307
electrode 342
electrode designs, effect of 332–4
electrode functionalization, sample preparation and 324–6
electrodeposited polymer films 28
electrode surface, capacitive detection of biomolecular binding on 319–20
Electrogram (EGM) 380
electrolyte-electrode system 320–1
electro membrane extraction (EME) 430
electron chemical capacitance 303, 307
electron transfer 6–7, 48, 144, 293–5, 460
electroosmotic pumping 432
electrophoresis 55
electrostatic capacitance 302
electrostatic/geometrical capacitance 302
electrostatic immobilization 448, 452
encapsulated enzymatic microreactor (EMR) 27
endogenous small noncoding RNAs: *see* microRNAs (miRNAs)
Enlite (Medtronic) 22
entrapment 347, 449–50
entrapment immobilization 347
environmental monitoring, biosensors for 50
genotoxicants 51
heavy metals 51
pesticides 50
toxic gases 51
enzymatic biosensors 461–5
enzymatic blood glucose biosensors mediators 22
enzyme-based electrochemical biosensors 42, 112
direct detection of analytes 42–3
indirect detection of analytes via inhibition of enzyme activity 43
enzyme field-effect transistors (ENFETs) 39
enzyme immobilisation methods 129
enzyme-linked immunosorbent assay (ELISA) 73, 182–3, 217, 297, 317, 431, 473, 586–7
enzymes 184, 261
as an aid to the electrochemical detection 41–2
ephedrine 426, 432
Epic BenchTop optical biosensor 167–9
epidermal growth factor receptor (EGFR) 454
epitaxial graphene (EG) 467
epithelial cell adhesion molecule (EpCAM) 363, 367
epoxypolyurethane membrane 123–4
epoxy rubber 514
equilibrium swelling, of hydrogel 444–6
error prone PCR 221–3
Escherichia coli 181

detection of 53
detection system 83
determination of 148
O157:H7 181
O157:H7 eaeA gene 10
ethyl-(dimethylaminopropyl) carbodiimide 506
ethyleneglycol dimethacrylate 124
evanescent field 167, 344–5
exfoliated graphite nanoplatelets (xGnP) 462
extraordinary optical transmission (EOT) 476

fabrication of microchip 67
Fano-resonance 478–9
faradaic electron transfer 294
Faraday constant 23, 294
'far field' effects 380
Fe_3O_4 magnetic nanoparticles 153
ferric reducing ability of plasma (FRAP) assay 523–4
ferricyanide 114
ferrocene 9, 114
Fibre Bragg's grating 199
fibre optical biosensors (FOBS) 342, 354
fibre optical technology 341–5
 advantageous and disadvantageous 350–1
 bioreceptors 345–6
 cancer applications, biosensors for 354
  biosensors in cancer disease 355
  cancer biomarkers 354–5
 cardiovascular diseases applications, biosensors for 353
  biosensors in cardiovascular disease 353–4
  cardiovascular disease biomarkers 353
 clinical and diagnostic applications 351
 diabetes applications, biosensors for 352
  biosensors for glucose measuring 352–3
  glucose as diabetes biomarker 352
 immobilization 346
  adsorption 346
  covalent bonding 347
  cross-linking 347
  entrapment 347
  microencapsulation 346–7
 sensing schemes 347
  absorbance 348–9
  fluorescent 349–50
 surface plasmon resonance (SPR) 350
fibre-optic biosensors 199
fibre tapering 344
fibrous encapsulation 109
Fickian diffusion 446
Fick's law 446
field amplified sample injection (FASI) 63
field amplified sample stacking (FASS) 63, 318
field-effect transistor (FET) 148
 -based biosensors 570
 electrochemical-based methods 298
filopodia 365
first-generation biosensors 112, 116, 118, 129
flavin adenine dinucleotide (FAD) cofactors 468
flexible carbon fiber (FCF) 25
flow cytometer, smartphone-based 240
flow-over sensing mode 476
flow-through nanohole array sensor 476, 478
flow-through sensing mode 476
fluorescence 188, 202
 auto-fluorescent protein (AFP) 189
 bioluminescence resonance energy transfer (BRET) 189
 quantum dots (QDs) 189–95
fluorescence lifetime using fluorescence lifetime imaging (FLIM) 190

fluorescence polarization immunoassay (FPIA) 432
fluorescence quenching 349, 354
  metal-induced 547–8
fluorescence resonance energy transfer (FRET) 77–8, 284
fluorescent detection 243
fluorescent measurement 349–50
fluorescent microscope, smartphone (SP)-based 242
fluorescent resonant energy transfer (FRET) 29, 189
fluorophore/reporter, metal NPs and 546
  metal-enhanced fluorescence (MEF) 548–9
  metal-induced fluorescence quenching 547–8
  surface-enhanced Raman scattering (SERS) 549
focused ion beam milling (FIB) 478
folded-cascode OTA, circuit implementation of 393
food borne pathogens, detection of: *see* optical biosensors for detection of food borne pathogens
food industry, biosensors in 51–2
Förster resonance energy transfer (FRET) 547
Fourier-Transform Infrared (FTIR) attenuated total reflection (ATR) spectroscopy 438
free-solution conjugate electrophoresis (FSCE) 66
Freestyle enzymatic electrode 22
Freestyle Navigator CGM system, biosensor of 24
FreeStyle Navigator II (Abbott) 22
fullerene into poly (methylmethacrylate) 155

G4AP 129
G4 Platinum (DexCom) 22–3, 122, 129
genosensors 346
genotoxicants 39, 51
  detection of 40
geometrical capacitance 302, 306
Giardia lamblia cysts 242, 246
Gibbs free energy of redox reaction 299
glassy carbon (GC) 460, 464, 468
glassy carbon electrode (GCE) 63, 77, 531
glucose, monitoring of 24
glucose as diabetes biomarker 352
glucose-binding proteins (GBPs) 29
glucose biosensors 22, 27, 112–15, 124, 126–7
glucose level, monitoring
  in blood 49
glucose measuring, biosensors for 352–3
glucose oxidase 22, 25–7, 112, 145, 352, 428, 446, 450, 461–2, 567
GlucoTrack 49
glutamate 25–6, 28, 116
glutamate oxidase (GmOx) biosensor 25
glutaraldehyde (GA) 324, 326, 449
  -treated collagen scaffolds 124
glutathione (GSH)
  detection of, using biosensor 530–1
  levels, in RBCs 66
glutathione reductase (GR) 531
GlySens device 129
gold colloids, self-assembled monolayer of 96
gold nanoparticles (AuNPs) 1–3, 48–9, 144, 152, 197, 513, 531, 571
  based assay, for biomarker of oxidative stress 530
  chemical synthesis of 4
  coated QCM electrode 152
  coated SPR gold chip 152
  electrodeposition of 3–4
  functions of, in electrochemical biosensors 4
    immobilization of biological recognition element 7
    improvement of electron transfer efficiency 5–7
    signal generation and amplification 8–14

and two-component oligonucleotide modified MBs 152
gold nanoslits 478, 487, 491
-based Fano resonance biosensors 490
gold nanostructures arrays 476
GO modified light addressable potentiometric sensor (GO-LAPS) 468
Gonorrhoea 53
Gouy-Chapman model 304
graphene 25, 48, 148, 568
enzyme-based graphene nanobiosensors 468
N-doped graphene 462
stacked graphene nanofibers (SGNFs) 468
graphene-based bioplatforms 465
graphene-based biosensors 467, 567
for in vitro detection 571–4
graphene microelectrodes' applications in clinical analysis 459
electrochemical biosensors fabrication, graphene nanomaterials used in 460–1
miniaturized graphene electrochemical biosensors for health monitoring 461
DNA sensors 467–8
enzymatic biosensors 461–5
immunosensors 465–7
nanostructured materials, biosensors based on 459–60
graphene nanomaterials used in electrochemical biosensors fabrication 460–1
graphene oxide (GO) 81, 368, 460
graphene oxide-thionine-Au@SiO_2 functional nanocomposite 9
graphene quantum dots (GQDs) 547
graphite 148
graphite microparticle-based electrodes (GMPs) 468
graphite nanosheets (GNSs) 462
graphite oxide (GO) 460, 568
graphitized carbon chromatography (GCC) 66
green fluorescent protein (GFP) 60, 189
guanine oxidation 40
Guillian-Barre Syndrome (GBS) 52

H1N1 influenza virus, clinical diagnosis of 150
half-power beamwidth (HPBW) 406
Haptoglobin phenotyping (Hp) 66
Hartman interferometer 199–200
heart beat sensing techniques 415–16
heavy metals 51
Helmholtz capacitance 294, 304
Helmholtz Inner Plane (IHP) 294
hemin/G-quadruplex complex 9
hepatitis C virus (HCV) NS3 protein detection 145
HER2 protein and HER2-overexpresing SK-BR-3 breast cancer cells 14
1,6-hexanedithiol 6
high-throughput laboratory machines 73
horseradish peroxidase (HRP) 7, 9, 41, 58, 451
horseradish peroxidase-labeled *Staphylococcus aureus* enterotoxin B antibodies 148
human chorionic gonadotropin hormone (HCG) 309
human epidermal growth factor receptor 2 (HER2) 52
human serum albumin (HSA) 543, 553
-stabilized AuNCs 550
humoral immunity 211–12
hybridisation, detection of 40–2
hybrid nanoarchitectures 466
hybridoma cell production 215–16
hydrazine-AuNP-aptamer bioconjugate 13–14
hydrogel-based biosensors 443
general properties of hydrogel 444
equilibrium swelling 444–6
pore size/porosity of the gels 447–8
swelling kinetics 446–7

immobilization of biomolecules and applications as biosensors 448
affinity-based immobilization 453
covalent immobilization 450–2
electrostatic immobilization 452
entrapment 449–50
physical deposition and cross-linking 449
multi-analyte detecting system 453–5
hydrogel-based microchips 454
hydrogel-based molecularly imprinted polymers (HydroMIPs) 450
hydrogel-entrapped *Escherichia coli* sensor 450
hydrogel microlenses 453
hydrogel patterning and transferring (HPT) method 450
hydrogels 124–7, 368, 371
8-hydroxy-2'-deoxyguanosine, detection of
using immunosensor 533
hydroxyethyl methacrylate 124
hypoxanthine-guanine-phosphoribosyl transferase (HGPRT) 215–16
hypoxia 25–6

iHealth Lab 238
IL-1β 279–81
illicit drugs analysis
analysis of drugs in blood 437
analysis of drugs in saliva and other subtracts 438
analysis of drugs in urine 430–2
imidazole-intermediate 451
immobilization 346
adsorption 346
affinity-based 453
of biological recognition element 7
biomolecule 262–3
of biomolecules and applications as biosensors 448–53
covalent 450–2
covalent bonding 347
cross-linking 347
electrostatic 452
entrapment 347
microencapsulation 346–7
immunoassay-capillary electrophoresis (IA-CE) 432
ImmunoChip 433
immunoglobulin new antigen receptors (IgNAR) 210
immunoglobulins (Igs) 209–10
immunohistochemistry 73
immunological field-effect transistors (IMFETs) 39
immunomagnetic separation 186–7
immunosensor 43, 465–7
detection of 8-hydroxy-2' -deoxyguanosine using 533
direct 44
indirect 43–4
impedimetric biosensors 300–1
implantable biosensors 27–8, 123, 125–7, 129, 444, 469
implantable cardioverter defibrillator (ICD) 381, 384–5
components of 385–7
implantable microbiosensors 109
analyte-specific biosensors 115–22
future prospects 129–30
improving the *in vivo* stability of 122–8
microbiosensor technologies 111–15
infrared spectroscopy 426
infrared surface SPR-based technique 489
InN QDs 146, 153
iNPx system 480
in situ hybridization (ISH) 282–3, 286
Integrity Applications 49
interdigitated microelectrodes (IDMEs) 318, 324–5, 333–4
interfacial capacitance, direct detection of 320–1
interferometry 199
interleukin-2 309
internal amplification control (IC) line 144
'interparticle crosslinking' 540

interparticle-distance dependent color change 540–3
interstitial glucose 120
Intracardiac Electrogram 379
intrinsic luminescent properties of metal NCs, sensing based on 549
  formation process of luminescent metal NCs 553
  NC luminescence turn-off 550–2
  NC luminescence turn-on 552–3
in-vivo microbiosensors 21
  enzymatic biosensors 22
    continuous glucose monitoring systems (CGMS) 22–4
    in development 24–9
  non-enzymatic in-vivo biosensors, development of 29–30
in vivo microdialysis 116–17
ion affinity chromatography (IMAC) 221
ionic liquid (IL) 60
ionic liquid-functionalized graphene (IL-graphene) 464
ion-sensitive field-effect transistors (ISFETs) 38–9
iOS-enabled Wireless Smart Gluco-Monitoring System 238
isotachophoresis (ITP) 427
isothermal amplification methods 266

Kaposi's sarcoma associated herpes virus (KSHV) 241
kinetic mass action law (KMAL) 173
Krebs'–Ringer phosphate buffer (KRP) 524
Kretschmann's geometry 503

labeled detection methods 317
label-free biosensing strategies 317
label-free conductivity measurement 489
label-free detection methods 317, 426
label-free optical biosensors, in cell adhesion research 165–8
lab-on-a-chip (LOC) 56, 83–4, 158, 266, 421, 423, 438
lab-on-chip system, for point-of-collection testing (POCT) 423
  blood, analysis of drugs in 432
    illicit drugs analysis 437
    therapeutical drugs analysis 432–7
  detection 425
    electrochemical detection 427–8
    mass spectrometry 428
    optical detection 425–7
  future directions 438
  materials and fabrication 423–5
  saliva and other subtracts, analysis of drugs in 437
    illicit drugs analysis in saliva 438
    therapeutic drugs analysis 437–8
  urine, analysis of drugs in 428
    illicit drugs analysis 430–2
    therapeutical drugs analysis 429–30
lactate 24–5, 115–16
lactate oxidase 26, 129, 450
LactatePro analyser 116
lamellipodia 365
l-ascorbic acid 62
laser induced fluorescence (LIF) 56, 59
lateral flow assays (LFAs) 82, 555–6
lateral flow immunoassay (LFIA) 236, 253
  applications of 264–5
  components 255
    antibodies 257–8
    membrane 258–9
    pads 261–2
    tracers 260–1
  future perspectives 266–7
  important parameters for 262
    biomolecule coverage on the tracer 264
    biomolecule immobilization 262–3
    buffer and pH 264

major hurdles facing 265–6
mechanism of 253–5
types of 255–6
competitive immunoassay 255
noncompetitive immunoassay 255
Lateral Flow Immunochromatographic Assay (LFIA) 82
latex beads 260
ligand 97
ligase detection reaction (LDR) 66
light-addressable potentiometric sensing (LAPS) 584
light emitting diodes (LEDs) 232
light scattering of metal NPs, sensing based on 543
NP-enabled dynamic light scattering (DLS) 545–6
scattered light intensity or wavelength change 544–5
limit of detection (LOD) 79, 97, 329, 334, 348
linear sweep voltammetry (LSV) 531
lipid-based cationic liposomes 285–6
lipid peroxidation, method for monitoring 524
liposomes 261
liquid crystalline lipid-based nanoparticles (LCNPs) 60
liquid–liquid extraction (LLE) 430, 438
lithium 433
Lithium Perchlorate (LP) 47
localized surface plasmon resonance (LSPR) 96, 247, 474–6, 500, 504–5, 537, 540, 543
locked nucleic acid (LNA) 285
long-term grating 199
lower critical solution temperature (LCST) 368
LPR receptor-targeted nanocomplexes (RTNs) 285
luminescent detection 232, 244

Mach-Zehnder interferometer 199–200
magnetic beads (MBs) 144
magnetic bead with multi-layers quantum dots labeling 153
magnetic fluorescence detection nanoparticles (MFAS) 284
magnetic nanoparticles (MGNPs) 146–8, 487, 491
magnetic particles 260
malonaldehyde (MDA) 521, 524
mass-produced SPR-sensors 509
mass sensitive transducers 74
mass spectrometry 67, 428
mean absolute relative difference (MARD) 24, 122
membrane biodegradation 109
membrane biofouling 109
mercapto-carboxylic acid (MCA)-modified Au-NPs 451
mesoporous silica nanoparticles (mSi NPs) 585
metal-enhanced fluorescence (MEF) 538, 548–9
metal-induced fluorescence quenching 546–8
metallic nanobiosensors 537
commercialization potentials 558
future challenges 558
paper-based POC diagnostic devices, development of 554
dipstick assays 555
lateral flow assays (LFAs) 555–6
microfluidic paper analytical devices 556–7
sensing based on absorption of metal NPs 540
interparticle-distance dependent color change 540–3
refractive index change 543
sensing based on interaction between metal NPs and fluorophore/reporter 546
metal-enhanced fluorescence (MEF) 548–9
metal-induced fluorescence quenching 547–8
surface-enhanced Raman scattering (SERS) 549

sensing based on intrinsic luminescent properties of metal NCs 549
formation process of luminescent metal NCs 553
NC luminescence turn-off 550–2
NC luminescence turn-on 552–3
sensing based on light scattering of metal NPs 543
NP-enabled dynamic light scattering (DLS) 545–6
scattered light intensity or wavelength change 544–5
metalloproteinase-13 (MMP-13) 279–80
metal nanoparticles (MNPs) 48, 144–5
sensing based on absorption of 540
interparticle-distance dependent color change 540–3
refractive index change 543
metastasis 363
methacrylic acid (MAA) 532
N,N′-methylenebisacrylamide 61, 449–50
methylene blue (MB) 40, 149
methyltrimethoxysilane (MTMOS) 62
micellar electrokinetic chromatography (MEKC) 426, 430
microarray 282–3, 286
microchip 56
microchip-based separation and detection methods 55
challenges and future outlook 67
DNA, separation and extraction of 57–8
miscellaneous separation 64–7
proteins, separation of 58–62
small biological analytes, separation of 62–4
microchip capillary gel electrophoretic (MCGE) separation step 57
microchip-CE (MCE) platform 58, 67
microchip electrophoresis (MCE) 58–60, 63, 427, 429
microencapsulation 346–7
microfabrication 28, 122
microfluidic chip 27, 236, 474, 476, 487
integration of SPR sensors with 480
microfluidic device 65, 423–7, 430–2, 437–8, 480, 491
microfluidic diffusion immunoassay (DIA) 433
Microfluidic Electrochemical Aptamer-based Sensor (MECAS) chip 437
microfluidic paper analytical devices 556–7
microfluidics 194, 202, 421, 480
for bacterial cells detection 81
microfluidic SPRi platform 514
micro-ribonucleic acids (miRNA) 485
microRNAs (miRNAs) 277
biomarker detection technologies 282–4
as early diagnostic biomarkers for OA 278
miR-140 280
miR-146 279–80
miR-22 280–1
miR-27b 281–2
nano-biomaterials for molecular beacon-based miRNA detection 284–6
microscopy 141, 236
microsensor arrays 533
micro total analysis systems (μTASs) 56, 266, 421, 423
microwave-induced plasma optical emission spectrometry (MIP-OES) 63
Milenia® QuickLine kits 265
milli-Q water (MQW) 570
miniature mass spectrometer (MS) 432
miniaturisation of biosensors 109
miniaturized graphene electrochemical biosensors for health monitoring 461
DNA sensors 467–8
enzymatic biosensors 461–5
immunosensors 465–7
modified Cottrel's equation 23
molecular beacon (MB) technology 282–3, 286

molecular beacon-based miRNA detection, nano-biomaterials for 284–6
molecular imprinting technology (MIT) 532
molecularly imprinted polymer (MIP) 532
molecular recognition elements (MREs) 73, 187, 532
monoclonal antibodies 257
monoclonal antibody generation 215
  DiCAST 218–19
  hybridoma cell production 215–16
  purification of monoclonal antibodies 216
  recombinant antibody
    expression of 220–1
    generation 216–17
    purification of 221
    selection through phage display 217–18
    selection using Biacore 4000 219–20
monomode fibres 343
morphine 431
multi-analyte detecting system 453–5
multimode fibres 343
multiple biomarkers 15, 77, 453, 480
multiplexing, SPR sensors for 480–2
multiwalled carbon nanotubes (MWCNTs) 148–9, 468
  onto SiO_2 grown Si wafer 155
mycobacterium tuberculosis 9, 151
myoglobin 353–4

Nafion 28–9, 118, 462
N-alkylthiols 506
nanoaggregate-embedded beads (NAEBs) 197, 199
nanocarrier for signal amplification 8–10
nanocatalyst for signal amplification 10–14
nanocomposite hydrogels 127
nanoelectrospray ionization mass spectrometry (nESI-MS) 437
nanohole array based sensors 476
nanoimprinting lithography 478–9, 548
nanomaterials 2, 78–9, 81
nanomaterials based biosensors 139
  challenges and future prospects 158
  clinical diagnosis, conventional techniques for 141
  clinical diagnosis, nanomaterials for 141
    carbon nanostructures 148–9, 150
    magnetic nanoparticles (MGNPs) 146–8
    metal nanoparticles (MNPs) 144–5
    nanostructured conducting polymers (NCPs) 149, 151
    nanostructured metal oxide (NMO) 151–7
    quantum dots (QDs) 145–6
nanoparticle-based sensing 583
  of oligonucleotides 584–6
  of protein 586–90
nanostructure array SPR 476–9
nanostructured conducting polymers (NCPs) 149, 151
nanostructured materials, biosensors based on 459–60
nanostructured metal oxide (NMO) 151–7
nanosurface energy transfer (NSET) 539
nanotechnology 2
NanoZrO_2-CNT/ITO electrode 157
Narcotics 431
nasopharyngeal carcinoma (NPC) 285
Navigator 122
'near field' effects 380, 539
needle-like biosensors 22
needle-type biosensor 24, 28–9
needle-type enzymatic electrode 23
Nernst potential 299
Neutral Red (NR) electrochemical mediators 25
N-hydroxy succinimide (NHS) 451, 506

nicotinamide adenine dinucleotide coenzyme in its reduced form (NADH) 62
Ni-histidine 453
nitration of tyrosine by peroxynitrite 532
nitric oxide 22, 118
nitrocellulose 259
3-nitro-L-tyrosine (3NT), detection of
  using solid phase extraction (SPE) sorbent material 531–2
2-nitrophenyl octyl ether (NPOE) 430
noncompetitive immunoassay 255–6
non-contact-based ECG sensor 381
Non-Contact Vital Signs (NCVS) Monitoring 380
non-contact vital signs (NCVS) sensor, Doppler-based: *see* Doppler-based non-contact vital signs (NCVS) sensor
non-covalent binding 507
non-crosslinking aggregation 540
non-enzymatic implantable microbiosensors 21
non-enzymatic in-vivo biosensors, development of 29–30
non-faradaic capacitive transducer signal 301
non-faradaic current 294
non-faradaic electron transfer 294
Non-Fickian diffusion 446
non-fouling on biacore sensing surfaces 101–2
non-laboratory diagnostics, SPR-sensors for 509
  commercial portable SPR-sensors 509–13
  recent works in portable SPR-sensors development 513–15
nordihydroguaiareticacid (NDGA)-treated collagen scaffolds 124
normoglycemia 21
Norovirus 182
northern blotting 282–3
NovioSense 49
nuclear factor kappa B (NF-kB) 279
nucleic acid (NA) biosensors 39
  detection of genotoxicants/pesticide 40
  detection of hybridisation 40
    electrochemically detectable label 40–1
    electrochemical molecular beacons 42
    enzymes as an aid to the electrochemical detection 41–2
    monitoring guanine oxidation 40
    redox mediators 40
nucleic acid amplification techniques 141
nucleic acids 184–5, 346
  detection of 266
  SPR-based biosensors for detection of 483
    detection of DNA 483
    detection of RNA 483–8
nucleic acids lateral flow (NALF) 265
numerical aperture (NA) 343
N-vinyl-2-pyrrolidinone 124
nylon 259
Nyquist plot 39, 296, 329

o-dopaquinone 118
Ohm's law 302
oligonucleotides, sensing of 584–6
operational transconductance amplifier (OTA) 393, 395
o-phenylenediamine (o-PD) 26
optical (fluorescence) receptor-based biosensors 29
optical-affinity biosensors 145
optical biosensing system 348
optical biosensors 499
optical biosensors for detection of food borne pathogens 181
  biosensors 183
    antibodies 184
    biorecognition techniques 184
    enzymes 184
    nucleic acids 184–5

carbon nanotubes (CNT) 200–2
enzyme-linked immunosorbent assay (ELISA) 182–3
fluorescence 188
auto-fluorescent protein (AFP) 189
bioluminescence resonance energy transfer (BRET) 189
quantum dots (QDs) 189–95
future prospects 202–4
interferometry 199
optical fibre 199–200
polymerase chain reaction (PCR) 183
sample preparation 185–6
Surface Enhanced Raman Spectroscopy (SERS) 195–8
surface plasmon resonance (SPR) 186–8
transduction techniques 185
electrochemical biosensors 185
piezoelectric biosensors 185
optical detection 425–7
optical fibre 199–200
optical fibre biosensors
advantageous and disadvantageous of 350–1
optical fibre sensors (OFS) 341
optical nanobiosensors for bacterial cells detection 79–80
optical transducers 74, 81
optical waveguide-based biosensor 165
cell adhesion kinetics
dependence of, on surface density of integrin ligands 170–4
cell adhesion on tailored surfaces 169–70
cell adhesion research, label-free optical biosensors in 165–8
Epic BenchTop optical biosensor 167–9
optical waveguide lightmode spectroscopy (OWLS) 166
Optrode 342
organophosphate (OP) 43, 450
organophosphate hydrolase (OPH) enzyme 450
osmium-based redox polymers 122
osmotic fragility (OF) experiments 529
osteoarthritis (OA), applications of microRNAs in 277
biomarker detection technologies 282–4
miR-22 280–1
miR-27b 281–2
miR-140 280
miR-146 279–80
nano-biomaterials for molecular beacon-based miRNA detection 284–6
Otto–Kretschmann method 499
Overoxidized Polyaniline (OPANi) 28
over-oxidized polypyrrole (OPPy) 28
over-the-counter HIV lateral flow test 267
oxidants 521
endogenous 522
exogenous 522
oxidative stress (OS) 50, 118
oxidative stress (OS), monitoring 521
advanced nanodiagnostic methods 529
detection of 3-nitro-L-tyrosine (3NT) using solid phase extraction (SPE) sorbent material 531–2
detection of 8-hydroxy-2'-deoxyguanosine (8OHdG) using immunosensor 533
detection of glutathione using biosensor 530–1
gold nanoparticle based assay for biomarker of oxidative stress 530
microsensor arrays 533
antioxidants 522–3
conventional methods 523
method for monitoring lipid peroxidation 524
reduced glutathione (GSH)/oxidized glutathione (GSSG) ratio 524–5

total antioxidant activity, determination of 523
measurement of oxidative status using various oxidative stress biomarkers 525
acetylcholinesterase activity, determination of 525–6
protein carbonyl content, determination of 527–8
red blood cell osmotic fragility, determination of 529
sulfhydryl (–SH) group, determination of 526–7
oxidants 521
endogenous 522
exogenous 522
oxidoreductases 22, 25
oxygen deficit 113

paclitaxel (PTX) 575
pads 261–2
p-aminophenol 62
paper-based microfluidic devices 424–5
paper-based nanobiosensors 82
paper-based POC diagnostic devices, development of 554
dipstick assays 555
lateral flow assays (LFAs) 555–6
microfluidic paper analytical devices 556–7
pathogens, biosensors for 52–3
PEGylated ligand 99
peptide-based hydrogels 449
peptide-templated luminescent AuNCs 550
permselective membranes 23, 28
peroxidase 114, 295
peroxynitrite, nitration of tyrosine by 532
pesticides 50
detection of 40
phosphate-buffered saline (PBS) 217, 264, 324
photoinduced electron transfer (PET) 539
photonic band gap (PBG) structure 366
photonic crystal (PC) biosensors 166
piezoelectric biosensors 185
plasma 432
plasma frequency (PF) 500
plasmonics 473
platinum-ceria nanoparticles 26
PLL-*g*-PEG-RGD 170
point-of-care (POC) diagnostics 253
point-of-care testing 1, 73, 84, 355
point-of-collection testing (POCT) drugs analysis
in blood 432
illicit drugs analysis 437
therapeutical drugs analysis 432–7
in saliva and other subtracts 437
illicit drugs analysis in saliva 438
therapeutic drugs analysis 437–8
in urine 428
illicit drugs analysis 430–2
therapeutical drugs analysis 429–30
poly(3,4-ethylendioxythiophene) (PEDOT) 47
poly(acrylamidophenylboronic acid) (polyAAPBA) 370
poly (amidoamine) (PAMAM) dendrimer 149
polyaniline (PANI) 27, 47, 149, 156
PANI electrochemically deposited onto a Pt disk electrode 156
PANI/ITO 156
PANI-MWCNT nanocomposite onto ITO electrode 157
polyaniline (PANi) nanohairs 367
polyaniline-iron oxide-carbon nanotubes nanobiocomposite 157
polyaniline-iron oxide nanocomposite 157
polycarbonate (PC) 424
polyclonal antibodies 257
polyclonal antibody generation 209, 211
adaptive immune response, process of 211–12

hosts for 212–14
purification of polyclonal antibodies 214
chicken IgY purification 215
receptor-ligand-based affinity chromatographic purification 214
using antigen-antibody binding-based affinity chromatographic strategies 215
polydimethylsiloxane (PDMS) 27, 424
microchip 58, 60, 62, 66, 156
microfluidic device 480
template 450
polyelectrolyte hydrogels 445
polyester-toner (PeT) microfluidic device 57–8
polyethylene glycol (PEG) 102, 215, 285, 575
-based hydrogel 450
-coated PMMA plastic microchip 58
hydrogel microspheres 29
poly(ethylene glycol) diacrylate (PEGDA) 450
poly (ethylene glycol) epoly (lactic acid) (PEGePLA) polymeric vesicles 466
poly(ethylene oxide) (PEO) 57
polyethylenimine (PEI) 83, 285
poly(lactic-co-glycolic)acid (PLGA) 125
polymerase chain reaction (PCR) 183, 221, 266, 473
polymeric ionic liquid (PIL) 462
polymer microchips 67
polymethylmethacrylate (PMMA) 57, 59–60, 424
polymethylsiloxane (PDMS) 514
poly-N-isopropylacrylamide (PNIPAAM) 126–7, 368, 450
polyphenol oxidase 111
poly(phenylenylenediamine) (PPD) 28
polypyrrole 46–7
Polypyrrole-poly(2-naphthol) 28
polystyrene (PS) microspheres 367
poly(styrenesulfonate) (PSS) 47
polyunsaturated fatty acids (PUFA) 524
poly(vinyl alcohol) (PVA) hydrogels 125
poly(vinylpyrrolidone) (PVP) 57
pore size/porosity of the gels 447–8
porogens 447
porous graphitized carbon (PGC) 66
portable SPR-sensors development, recent works in 513–15
positron emission tomography (PET) 574
post translational modification (PTM) enzymes 550
potentiometric biosensor 38, 111
QDs based 147
potentiometric D-dimer experiments 466
potentiometric transducer principle 299
power-supply rejection ratio (PSRR) specification of amplifier 391
PPAR (peroxisome proliferator activated receptor) 281
p-polarized wave 502
pre-miRNA 277, 284
printed circuit board (PCB) 58
prismatic coupling devices, SPR-sensors with 502–4
prostate specific antigen (PSA) 466
protein binding and detachment
capacitance changes due to 327–8
protein carbonyl content, determination of 527–8
proteins
sensing of 586–90
separation of 58–62
protein transduction domains (PTDs) 286
Prussian Blue (mediator), 27
pseudoephedrine 432
psychotropic drugs 437
Pt-nanoparticles (PtNPs)-polyaniline (PANI) hydrogel coated electrode 449

pulmonary embolism (PE) 328
pyrophosphate 552

quadrature receiver and arc-tangent demodulation for NCVS sensors 401–2
quantitative detection of biomarker protein 328–9
quantitative PCR (qPCR) 487
quantum dots (QDs) 145–6, 189–95, 202–3
quartz crystal microbalance (QCM) 144, 185–6, 531
quencher-free fluorescent method 282–3, 286
quinines, thionine 114

radio-frequency (RF) Doppler sensor 380
radiolabelling 575
RAID 8 and RAID TOX kits 265
Raman spectroscopy 195
range-correlation effect 403
range correlation in NCVS sensors 403–5
reactive ion etching (RIE) 366
reactive nitrogen species (RNS) 521, 527
reactive oxygen species (ROS) 50, 118, 521, 527
receptor–ligand-based affinity chromatographic purification 214
receptor–ligand interaction 173
receptor–ligand reaction 173
recombinant antibodies 209, 257
  advantages of 216
  expression of 220–1
  generation 216–17
  purification of 221
  selection of
    through phage display 217–18
    using Biacore 4000 219–20
recombinant bovine somatotropin (rBST) 242
red blood cell osmotic fragility, determination of 529
redox mediators 39–40, 113–14, 122
reduced glutathione (GSH)/oxidized glutathione (GSSG) ratio 524–5, 530
reduced graphene oxide 155
refractive-index-based sensors 476
refractive index change 543
resonance units (RU) 220
resonant waveguide grating (RWG) 166
resonant wavelength 169
reticuloendothelial system (RES) 575
reverse transcription quantitative polymerase chain reaction (RT-qPCR) 282–3, 286
RGD motifs 169–70
rheumatoid arthritis (RA) 279
RISC (RNA induced silencing complex) 278
RNA
  RNA polymerase II 277
  RNA–protein interactions 104
  SPR-based biosensors for detection of 483–8

saline sodium citrate (SSC) 264
saliva and other subtracts, analysis of drugs in 437
  illicit drugs analysis in saliva 438
  therapeutic drugs analysis 437–8
Salmonella 81
  detection of 52, 181, 194
Salmonella typhimurium, detection of 202
Salmonella typhimurium DNA 242
sandwich assay: *see* noncompetitive immunoassay
scattered light intensity or wavelength change 544–5
second-generation biosensors 113
SELEX (systematic evolution of ligands by exponential enrichment) 76, 257

self-assembly monolayer (SAM) 306, 309
sensing based on absorption of metal NPs 540
sensing schemes 347
absorbance 348–9
fluorescent 349–50
sensor chip L1 99
sensor chip NTA 99
sensor sensitivity 505
sensor surface functionalization 506
covalent binding 506–7
non-covalent binding 507
serodiagnostics 512
serology 141
serum 432
sexually transmitted diseases (STDs) 53
sialylated human milk oligosaccharides (SHMOs) 66
side-lobe level (SLL) 406
silicon nanowire (SiNW) array 370
silk fibroin 450
silver nanoparticle (AgNPs) 197
silver/silver chloride electrodes 381
single nucleotide polymorphisms (SNPs) 483
single-stranded DNA (ssDNA) 467–8, 540
single-walled carbon nanotubes 66, 83, 112, 155, 567–71, 577
based biosensor for in vitro detection 570
SWNT-PTX conjugate 575
synthesis 569
siRNA 285–6
slip chip methods 58
small biological analytes, separation of 62–4
smartphone (SP)-based in vitro diagnostic technologies 231
applications of 241
bio-analytical applications 246
detection of biomolecules, metabolites and biomarkers 241–2
detection of microorganisms 240–6
detection of other analytes 246
challenges and future trends 246–7
signal detection in 232
colorimetric, fluorescent and luminescent detection 232–3
cytometry 239–40
electrochemical detection 236–9
lateral flow IA (LFIA) 236
microscopy 236
SPR detection 233–5
smart phones 515
'smart tattoo' biosensor 29
Snell's law 343
sodium dodecyl benzene sulfonate (SDBS) 463
sodium dodecyl sulfate-protein complexes (SDS-PC) 60
sol–gel derived nano ZrO_2 157
solid-phase extraction (SPE) 429
sorbent 532
sorbent material
detection of 3-nitro-L-tyrosine (3NT) using 531–2
SP-based colorimetric reader (SPCR) 241
SPIRIT^{TM} system 512
s-polarized wave 502
Spreeta 474, 512
stacked graphene nanofibers (SGNFs) 468
state-of-the-art optical cell-based biosensors 165
strept(avidin)-biotin 453
streptavidin coated magnetic particles 153
streptavidin-functionalised QDs (SAv-QDs) 194
streptavidin-modified magnetic beads 542
streptavidin oligonucleotide (SON) complexes 483
subcutaneous-ICD systems (S-ICD®) 386–7

sudden cardiac death (SCD) 384
sulfhydryl (–SH) group, determination of 526–7
superoxide anion 119
superoxide dismutases (SODs) 118
superparamagnetic Fe_3O_4 nanoparticles 146
superparamagnetic microspheres 153
supported liquid membrane (SLM) 430
surface charge using field-effect transistors 38–9
Surface Enhanced Raman Spectroscopy (SERS) 81, 195–8, 202, 438, 549
surface plasma waves (SPWs) 474
surface plasmon coupler and disperser (SPRCD) 485–6
surface plasmon resonance (SPR) 95, 166, 186–8, 317, 348, 350, 473, 499
  -based Autolab Esprit 96
  -based biosensors 482
    for detection of cancer cells 488–91
    for detection of DNA 483
    for detection of RNA 483–8
  -based waveguide sensor 96
  conventional SPR 474
  detection 233–5, 244
  localized surface plasmon resonance (LSPR) 474–6
  microfluidic chip, integration of SPR sensors with 480
  nanostructure array SPR 476–9
  set-up for biacore-based 98
  SPR imaging (SPRi) 480, 509, 514
  SPRmicro analyzer 512
  SPR-sensor resolution 505
  SPR sensors for multiplexing 480–2
surface-plasmon resonance (SPR) biosensors 145
surface plasmon resonance (SPR) sensors 499
  analytical parameters of 505
  localized SPR (LSPR) 504–5
  mass-produced SPR-sensors 509
  for non-laboratory diagnostics 509
    commercial portable SPR-sensors 509–13
    recent works in portable SPR-sensors development 513–15
  principle of 500–2
  sensor surface functionalization 506
    covalent binding 506–7
    non-covalent binding 507
  SPR-analysis formats 507–9
  SPR-analysis formats 508
  with diffraction gratings 504
  with prismatic coupling devices (couplers) 502–4
  with waveguide coupling devices 504
surface plasmon Resonance imaging (SPRI) 483, 487
surface quality control
  capacitive sensing for rapid analysis of 326
surface-sensitive label-free optical biosensors 166
swelling kinetics, of hydrogel 446–7
synthetic antibodies 257
Systematic Evolution of Ligands by Exponential Enrichment (SELEX) 45
System-on-Chip (SoC) technologies 383–4

Taq polymerase 144
TAT-1 286
t-butyl hydroperoxide (t-BHP) 531
T-cross microchip 56
Telomerase 52
template stripping 480
TET (ten-eleven-translocation) 280
tetracyanoquinodimethane (TCNQ)
tetrahedron-structured DNA probes 7
tetramethoxy silane (TMOS) 452
tetramethylbenzidine/hydrogen peroxide 238
tetrathialfulvalene (TTF), 114
Texas Instruments company 509

theophylline 432
therapeutical drugs analysis
  analysis of drugs in blood 432–7
  analysis of drugs in saliva and other subtracts 437–8
  analysis of drugs in urine 429–30
therapeutic drug monitoring (TDM) 422
thermally reduced graphene (TRGO) 460
thermodynamics 103
thiol-modified DNA recognizers 7
thiophene based polymers 47
third-generation biosensors 114
TIRFM 172
TLS11a 77
toll-like receptor (TLR) 279
toner based microfluidic devices 425
total internal reflection (TIR) 343
total peroxyl radical-trapping potential (TRAP) assay 524
toxic gases 51
tracers 260–1
  biomolecule coverage on 264
transducers 74
transduction techniques 185
  electrochemical biosensors 185
  piezoelectric biosensors 185
transmission plasmon biosensing (TPB) 481
2,4,6-tri[2-pyridyl]-s-triazine 523
N-(trimethoxysilylpropyl) ethylenediamine triacetic-acid (TETT) 62
Tris-buffered saline (TBS) 264
trivalent antibodies 224
T-sensor 433
  diffusion immunoassay in 435
TTF-TCNQ 114
tumour detection, CNMs-based biosensor for 574–5
Turkevich method, for gold nanoparticle synthesis 4
Tydall, John 342
Tydall's water experiment 343
tyrosine, nitration of
  by peroxynitrite 532

ultra-violet (UV) LEDs 232
urea, determination of 50
urea biosensor 465
urine, analysis of drugs in 428
  illicit drugs analysis 430–2
  therapeutical drugs analysis 429–30
urine sample-based lateral flow biosensor 267

valproate 427, 432
variable gain amplifier (VGA) 392
vascular endothelial growth factor (VEGF) 447
ventricular fibrillation 384
visualization 166
V-number of a fibre 345
voltage-controlled oscillator (VCO) 404
voltammetry 37

waveguide coupling devices, SPR-sensors with 504
waveguide sensor device 96
wearable cardiac biosensors 381
wearable electrocardiogram (ECG) sensors 379
  components of 381–4
Western Blot 586
whole cells based sensors 44
  based on cellular activity of the cell 45
  based on cellular barrier behaviour 45
Wireless Smart Gluco-Monitoring System 242

xanthine oxidase enzyme (XOD) 27
X-ray photon spectroscopy (XPS) 531

Yagi antenna 406, 410, 413
Young's interferometer 199

zone electrophoresis (ZE) 427